P9-BZZ-676

The Doctors Book®
of
Food
Remedies

The Doctors Book®
of
Food Remedies

FULLY REVISED AND UPDATED

The Newest Discoveries in the Power of Food to
**Treat and Prevent Health Problems—
From Aging and Diabetes to
Ulcers and Yeast Infections**

Selene Yeager and the Editors of **Prevention**®

RODALE®

Notice

This book is intended as a reference volume only, not as a medical manual. The information given here is designed to help you make informed decisions about your health. It is not intended as a substitute for any treatment that may have been prescribed by your doctor. If you suspect that you have a medical problem, we urge you to seek competent medical help.
Mention of specific companies, organizations, or authorities in this book does not imply endorsement by the publisher, nor does mention of specific companies, organizations, or authorities imply that they endorse this book.

© 2007 by Rodale Inc.

All rights reserved. No part of this publication may be reproduced or transmitted in any form or by any means, electronic or mechanical, including photocopying, recording, or any other information storage and retrieval system, without the written permission of the publisher.

The Doctors Book® and *Prevention*® are registered trademarks of Rodale Inc.

Printed in the United States of America
Rodale Inc. makes every effort to use acid-free ♾, recycled paper ♲.

Book design by Christina Gaugler

Library of Congress Cataloging-in-Publication Data

Yeager, Selene.
    The doctors book of food remedies : the newest discoveries in the power of food to treat and prevent health problems—from aging and diabetes to ulcers and yeast infections / Selene Yeager and the Editors of Prevention.—Fully rev. and updated.
        p.   cm.
    Includes index.
    ISBN-13 978–1–59486–753–8 direct hardcover
    ISBN-10 1–59486–753–4 direct hardcover
    1. Diet therapy—Popular works.   I. Prevention (Firm : Emmaus, Pa.)   II. Title.
RM216.Y38   2007
615.8'54—dc22   2007024804

2   4   6   8   10   9   7   5   3   1   hardcover

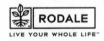

LIVE YOUR WHOLE LIFE™

We inspire and enable people to improve their lives and the world around them

For more of our products visit **rodalestore.com** or call 800-848-4735

Contents

Introduction

Nearly every day, researchers announce more exciting discoveries that show how the foods we eat help fight disease. There is now no doubt that Mother Nature's most delicious foods—from apples and broccoli to yogurt and zucchini—can be your best medicine for cutting cholesterol, losing weight, preventing cancer, beating allergies, reversing heart disease, and managing scores of other conditions.

That's why the editors of *Prevention* are so pleased to bring you this revised and updated version of our best-selling *Doctors Book of Food Remedies,* which features the latest science-based, doctor-approved information on the healing power of foods.

Thanks to the constant deluge of new studies, we now know that it's the remarkable microscopic substances in plants called *phytonutrients* that act in any number of ways to help us prevent illness and achieve optimal health. Quercetin, lycopene, resveratrol, ellagic acid, sulforaphane, alpha- and beta-carotene . . . these are just a few of the powerful phytonutrients you'll read about in this book. Some stimulate your body's immune cells and infection-fighting enzymes, preventing colds and flu, and combating environmental toxins. Others help to balance hormone levels, thus reducing the risk of hormone-related conditions, such as symptoms of menopause, and breast and prostate cancer. And still other phytonutrients function as antioxidants, neutralizing the harmful free radicals (unstable oxygen molecules) that are believed to play a role in the onset of so many degenerative diseases.

Today more than 9,000 phytonutrients have been documented, and this is just the tip of the iceberg. These discoveries have changed everything we thought we knew about foods! Oats, for example, have long been known to lower cholesterol because of the dietary fiber they contain. But that's not the only reason they protect the heart. Scientists now know that oats contain natural chemicals called tocotrienols that are 50 percent more powerful than even vitamin E in reducing the risk of heart disease.

Apples are another food that will surprise you. They've always been thought to be healthy, mostly because they are so chock-full of vitamins and fiber. But it turns out that it's the phytonutrients in apples (found mainly in the skin) that are the powerhouses. In fact, they're so strong that one study of 40,000 women associated the quercetin and other phytonutrients in apples with a 13 to 22 percent lower risk of cardiovascular disease. In addition, the quercetin in apples (and pears) has been found to help improve lung function, reducing the risk of asthma and obstructive pulmonary disease.

Or take red wine. We all know a glass with dinner can be a great relaxer, but who could have predicted that the resveratrol present in red wine could help make bad low-density lipoprotein (LDL) cholesterol less likely to stick to artery walls. Or that wine might even play a role in preventing diabetes.

One of the most exciting discoveries is that some foods can literally stop the chemical changes that can lead to cancer. Watercress, for example, has been found to block some of the harmful effects of cigarette smoke. And strawberries, and other berries that contain ellagic acid, have been shown to block the harmful effects of cancer-causing chemicals in the body.

And as if all this isn't enough to make you head for the produce aisle . . . scientists have also discovered ways to make the foods that we eat even more powerful. You may know, for instance, that beta-carotene (found in carrots, broccoli, mangoes, and other dark orange and dark green vegetables and fruits) is good for your heart. But scientists have learned that your body can't readily absorb beta-carotene unless you eat it with a little fat. That's why a drizzle of olive oil on cooked carrots or broccoli or a dab of yogurt on fresh fruit can vastly increase their healing powers.

Garlic also benefits from a little help. Chop whole cloves fine and suddenly the protective compound allicin is released. It quickly breaks down into a cascade of other healthful compounds, which can help lower triglycerides and cholesterol, reduce the risk of stomach and colon cancers, and much more.

And the list of foods and their seemingly magical healing powers goes on and on.

At *Prevention*, we've always believed that good health comes first from the farm, then the pharmacy. That's why we've spent so much time reviewing the latest scientific journals and talking with hundreds of the country's top doctors and food experts to bring you this important reference. We want to be sure you are armed with the best and most recent advice and information on how to take advantage of something we all love to do (eat) and avoid something we all fear (disease). The new science we've tapped into amazes us—and surely it will amaze you, too.

So grab an apple, or a glass of wine if you like, and start reading—and eating—to your health's content!

—The Editors of *Prevention*

Acerola

A BERRY WITH A HEALTHY PUNCH

HEALING POWER

Can Help:

Strengthen the immune system

Speed wound healing

Prevent heart disease

Protect against cancer

Never heard of acerola? That's no surprise. In America, this small, red, cherrylike fruit and the foods made from it are hard to find. It's far more commonly available in the Caribbean and South America.

Although the acerola is a small fruit, it packs a huge disease-fighting punch. One little acerola fruit, measuring an inch or less across, contains a whopping 81 milligrams of vitamin C! That's well above the Daily Value for C, which is a mere 60 milligrams. A single acerola contains more vitamin C than you'll find in an orange or a cup of broccoli, cantaloupe, or pineapple. The high vitamin C content means that acerola can help your body in a variety of ways, from fortifying your immune system to helping prevent age-related conditions, such as heart disease and cancer.

Decades ago, you could find about 100 acres of acerola plants in Florida, which were grown as a source of vitamin C (the plants, also called Barbados cherry, look like a shrub or a small tree). Nowadays, Brazil is the main commercial grower of acerola, although homeowners in Florida still grow them as ornamentals, says Carlos Balerdi, PhD, an extension agent with the University of Florida/Miami-Dade County Extension Service who specializes in tropical fruits.

When Dr. Balerdi was a boy growing up in Cuba, his mother would make a sweet syrup from the fruit, and "we'd finish the glass or whatever container she stored it in in no time!" he says. The fruit is also used in jellies, jams, and preserves, and people also eat acerola raw.

A Wealth of C

Many of us step up our consumption of orange juice or grapefruit halves at the first sign of the sniffles. It makes sense because vitamin C, found in abundance in citrus fruits, has been shown to help relieve cold symptoms. A major meta-analysis—a type of study that evaluates the results of many previous studies—found that getting at least 200 milligrams daily (less than the amount in three acerola fruits) is linked to shorter and less severe bouts of the common cold.

Doctor's Top Tip

The natural acidity in acerola can give them a sharp taste, says Carlos Balerdi, PhD, an extension agent with the University of Florida/Miami-Dade County Extension Service. Eat them with a little sugar to help reduce the tartness. Acerola is delicious in sherbet and pies (just be sure to add some sugar to these recipes, too).

The benefits of vitamin C go beyond relieving cold symptoms, however. It also helps the body make collagen, a tough, fibrous protein that helps build connective tissue, skin, bones, and teeth, and that also plays a role in wound healing. In addition, vitamin C helps protect the body from free radicals, the cell-damaging oxygen molecules thought to contribute to the development of cancer, heart disease, and many other conditions.

GETTING THE MOST

Grow vitamin C on trees. If you're living in an area that supports acerola growth, like South Florida, grow some plants in your yard. Look for types called "Florida Sweet" and "B-17," recommends the University of Florida Institute of Food and Agricultural Sciences in Gainesville. The plants should start producing fruit in the second year after planting, and *really* produce an abundance of the vitamin C–laden fruit in the following years.

Pick 'em and eat 'em. Acerola plants will grow fruit from April to November. Pick ripe fruits carefully so you don't bruise them, and eat them right away or freeze them. If they're not quite ripe when you pick them, you can keep them for a few days in the refrigerator.

Treat the berries gently. Dried and crushed acerola berries can be used to make tea. Unfortunately, boiling or steeping the berries in hot water can reduce the amount of vitamin C by about half. So to get the most vitamin C per cup, you may want to add extra berries.

Buy acerola products. If you're a resident of the Caribbean or South America, or headed there on vacation, look in specialty markets for acerola jams, jellies, and juices. Although these products contain somewhat less vitamin C than the fresh berries, they're still very good sources.

Aging

LENGTHENING YOUR LIFE, ONE BITE AT A TIME

Every year, more and more Americans are joining a special group: those who've lived to age 100. In the year 2000, only about 72,000 Americans were 100 or older. But by the middle of this century, that number could skyrocket to 834,000!

While most of us probably won't join this group—on average, we can expect to live to our mid- to late-seventies—we certainly have a much longer life expectancy than people did in the early 1900s, when the average person didn't live to be 50.

People are living longer partly because of our success in preventing childhood diseases like polio, as well as finding new treatments and prevention strategies for adult conditions such as heart disease. But it's also because scientists are unlocking the secrets of aging itself. We're finding out why our bodies break down and how to put the brakes on our own destruction. In the process, we're expanding not only our life spans but also what scientists call our health spans—the number of years that we can expect to live in robust good health.

The Power of Antioxidants

Researchers now know that one of the most important contributors to heart disease, wrinkles, cancer, arthritis, and many of the other problems of aging is the same process that causes a variety of objects around us to deteriorate. It's called *oxidation*. The same air that gives us life is what causes iron to rust, fruit to turn brown, and your body's cells to break down and age. Through a series of chemical changes, oxygen molecules in our bodies lose electrons, making them unstable. These unstable molecules are called free radicals.

In frantic attempts to stabilize themselves, free radicals pillage electrons from healthy cells throughout your body. Every time they steal an electron, two things happen: A healthy molecule is damaged, and more free radicals are created. Free radicals can damage vital genetic information within your cells, proteins in tissues throughout your body, and other components that keep you running properly. Unless this process is stopped, more and more cells are damaged every day, and your health pays the price.

To keep this destructive process under control, nature provides an enormous arsenal of antioxidants, which are compounds in foods that can stop free radicals from doing harm. Antioxidants come between free radicals and your body's healthy cells, offering up their own electrons and preventing yours from being pillaged.

Even though your body naturally maintains its own antioxidant system, the antioxidants in foods give you a powerful boost of additional protection against free radicals. Three of the best known antioxidants are beta-carotene and vitamins C and E. Each of these nutrients has been shown to help protect you from age-related illnesses like cancer and heart disease. Although you can get some protection by taking antioxidant supplements, most doctors agree that the antioxidants in foods are a better choice and should be your first line of defense. That's because fruits, vegetables, and other plant foods are brimming with antioxidants and other components that may work together as teams to protect you from disease. Some studies have found that vitamin E may help protect you from heart disease, and beta-carotene and selenium (a mineral that's an ingredient in some of your body's antioxidant enzymes) may help lower your risk of some cancers, but a lot of questions remain about the best ways to get these nutrients. As you'll see in the antioxidants section (page 18), supplements of vitamins C and E are a good idea, but they shouldn't take the place of a diet rich in fruits and vegetables. As far as beta-carotene is concerned, you should just get it from plant foods and skip the supplements.

The quickest way to get vitamin C is to have a glass of grapefruit juice, an orange, or a half-cup of red bell pepper slices—each provides more than 100 percent of the Daily Value (DV). For beta-carotene, deep green or bright orange fruits and vegetables are best. One sweet potato or a large carrot delivers between 12 and 15 milligrams, more than the 6 to 10 milligrams that some experts recommend we get.

Unlike vitamin C and beta-carotene, vitamin E is a bit trickier to get from foods because it's found mainly in high-fat foods, such as vegetable oils, which we'd rather avoid. Still, you can get quite a bit of vitamin E from dry roasted almonds, with 1 ounce providing 7 milligrams, or 40 percent of the DV. Other nuts and seeds are also good sources of vitamin E. And some breakfast cereals offer nearly 100 percent of the vitamin E that you need each day in each serving.

Even though vitamins C and E and beta-carotene are important antioxidants, they're hardly the only ones. Fruits and vegetables are loaded with plant compounds called phytochemicals, which can also have antioxidant abilities.

More than 9,000 phytochemicals have been identified to date, and many more are still unknown, experts say. Research has found that phytochemical extracts taken from fruits demonstrate anticancer power, and the combination of these chemicals in fruits and vegetables adds to their antioxidant and cancer-fighting ability.

Future Youth

While it's important to eat well to prevent aging, you also need to adjust your eating habits *as* you age. As the years pass, your nutritional needs can change dramatically.

"As we age, we produce less saliva, and our swallowing reflexes slow down, so food may not be as easy to digest and swallow," says Susan A. Nitzke, PhD, RD, professor in the nutritional sciences department at the University of Wisconsin in Madison. "Many of us experience changes in taste and appetite as we get older, so we may eat less. We also have less stomach acid, which means that we don't digest foods or absorb some nutrients as well as we used to."

An Israeli study that looked at 414 elderly patients in hospitals found that less than 20 percent were well nourished. The study also found that those with poor dietary habits had less successful outcomes from their visit to the hospital. But even with information from this and other studies available, doctors don't always think to check for nutritional deficiencies in older adults. This is unfortunate because a simple lack of nutrients can easily be mistaken for a more serious illness. Nutritional deficiencies in older people can even be misdiagnosed as dementia.

Vitamin B_{12} is essential for maintaining healthy blood and nerve function. It's also one of the nutrients that requires adequate amounts of stomach secretions in order to be absorbed. When acid levels decline, getting enough vitamin B_{12} can be a problem, says Dr. Nitzke. This is of particular concern for people who use antacids, she adds. You can get plenty of vitamin B_{12} in meats and other animal foods. Clams are the top performers: One small steamed clam provides an astonishing 9 micrograms of vitamin B_{12}, more than 100 percent of the DV.

In addition to a B_{12} deficiency, many people in their late fifties and older may be deficient in vitamin B_6. Chickpeas and potatoes are great bets for bringing in the B_6. A cup of chickpeas contains 1.1 milligrams, or slightly more than half of the DV. A baked potato provides 0.6 milligrams, or about one-third of the DV.

Another B vitamin that's important for protecting the cardiovascular and nervous systems is folate, which is found in green vegetables, beans, and whole grains. A cup of canned pinto beans, for example, provides 144 micrograms of folate, or more than 33 percent of the DV. Asparagus is another good source of folate, with 1 cup of cooked fresh asparagus containing 263 micrograms of folate.

As bones get older, it's essential to get extra calcium and vitamin D to prevent them from becoming brittle, says Dr. Nitzke. "Many older people believe that they can't eat dairy foods because they're 'lactose intolerant,' but in fact, most people can eat moderate amounts of dairy without trouble," she says. Low-fat and fat-free (skim) milk, cheese, and yogurt are your best sources of calcium. One cup of fat-free yogurt contains 415 milligrams of this bone-building nutrient, or 41 percent of the DV. One

Doctor's Top Tip

As you get older, make extra sure that the foods you eat are as nutrient-dense as possible, advises Susan A. Nitzke, PhD, RD, of the University of Wisconsin in Madison, and make empty-calorie foods like candy and sodas an even smaller part of your diet. Nutrient-dense foods are those that are loaded with vitamins, minerals, and phyto-chemicals, and relatively low on calories. As people get older, they tend to lose muscle mass, and consequently, they burn off fewer calories each day. Thus, if you eat the same amount of calories as you did when you were younger, you'll gain weight! So, it's more important to make sure that the foods you eat carry plenty of nutrients into your body, without extra calories.

glass of fat-free milk provides 302 milligrams, or 30 percent of the DV.

Iron is one of several minerals that can be tough to get in the correct amounts. Some people don't get enough, while others get too much, says Dr. Nitzke. In fact, women's need for iron declines in their later years after they stop menstruating.

To ensure that you're getting the right amount of nutrients for your particular needs, Dr. Nitzke recommends talking to your doctor to find out whether or not you need to take supplements of certain nutrients, such as iron, calcium, vitamin D, and vitamin B_{12}.

Eat Less, Live Longer

Even though we may need to eat more of certain foods in order to live longer, researchers are finding that the opposite can also be true: People who eat less may live more years.

Researchers have long known that a concept called "calorie restriction"—essentially, taking in fewer calories—extends the lives and helps slow down age-related diseases in a variety of creatures, including worms, flies, and mice. It's also been shown to improve some markers of aging in monkeys, such as their body-fat percentage and levels of free-radical damage.

Now scientists are working to learn more about how calorie restriction may help humans age better, says George Roth, PhD, a gerontology researcher and CEO of the Maryland-based company GeroScience.

Human research is taking two approaches, he says: observations of people who voluntarily restrict their calories for many years for the potential life-lengthening results, and controlled experiments in which subjects are instructed to restrict their calories for a shorter period.

A Louisiana State University study followed 48 people for 6 months as they either followed a normal diet or different types of calorie-restricted diets. It found that prolonged calorie restriction can lower people's fasting insulin levels and their body temperature, which are both markers of longevity.

Experts think that calorie restriction "resets" your metabolism so it works more efficiently, and your body shifts its focus from growth and reproduction to long-term survival, says Dr. Roth. And when you take in fewer calories, your body naturally produces fewer free radicals as it turns food into energy. Thus, you have less oxidative damage.

However, it's hard for humans to reap the benefits from calorie reduction that lab animals have shown. Tests on rodents have cut back their calories by more than 30 percent, and tests on monkeys lower their calorie intake by about 30 percent, says Dr. Roth. "For those of us who like to eat, that's probably not going to be a viable strategy." In addition, drastically reducing your calories without medical supervision can leave you malnourished.

For now, a good way to potentially get some benefit from calorie reduction is to make sure that you eat a "prudent" diet that provides the nutrients you need without excessive calories, he says. If you do decide to restrict your calories, talk to your doctor to make sure your diet meets your nutritional needs.

GO FOR LOW-AGE FOODS

A 2004 study in the *Journal of the American Dietetic Association* listed common foods and the amount of advanced glycation endproducts (AGEs) they contained. Here's a quick look at some foods high and low in AGEs to give you some sense of how to steer your diet to cut down on the amount you consume. They're measured by AGE kilounits per serving.

High Foods	AGE per Serving
Frankfurter, broiled for 5 minutes	10,143
Chicken breast with skin, breaded and oven-fried for 25 minutes	8,965
Whiting fish, breaded and oven-fried for 25 minutes	7,897
Pizza, thin crust	6,825
Pork sausage, microwaved for 1 minute	5,349

Low Foods	AGE per Serving
Canned red kidney beans	191
Raw onion	36
Canned corn	20
Bran flakes	10
Banana	9

Age Better with Fewer AGEs

Researchers are discovering that substances called advanced glycation endproducts—or AGEs—may be linked to a variety of age-related problems including wrinkles, cataracts, and atherosclerosis (fatty deposits blocking your arteries). AGEs result from sugar attaching to proteins, which causes proteins in your tissues to develop unwanted linkages between them, altering their ability to function normally. They also contribute to extra inflammation and oxidative damage in your body.

AGEs can develop within your body, particularly when you have high blood sugar, and you can also take them in through the foods you eat. Research has shown that foods that are particularly high in AGEs include meats that have been cooked at high temperatures by methods such as frying or broiling.

To cut down on AGE-related damage in your body, it's a wise idea to keep your blood sugar in a normal range. If you have diabetes, be sure to keep your blood sugar well controlled. If you have prediabetes, talk to your doctor about using diet and exercise to lower your risk of developing full-blown diabetes.

And be sure that your diet relies heavily on foods that are low in AGEs, such as fruits, vegetables, whole grains, fish, and low-fat dairy. Be careful with foods high in AGEs, such as meats cooked at high temperatures, processed foods, and full-fat cheeses, and eat them more sparingly.

Alzheimer's Disease

FOODS FOR LIFELONG THOUGHT

Roughly 4.5 million Americans now have Alzheimer's disease—the most common form of dementia, which causes a decline in mental abilities. That number has more than doubled since 1980, according to the Alzheimer's Association. And by 2050, that number could skyrocket as high as 16 million.

Doctors aren't sure what causes Alzheimer's disease. What is known is that in people who have this condition, portions of the brain shrivel and shrink, twisted tangles of protein develop within brain cells, and other deposits of protein develop between brain cells.

Since no cure for Alzheimer's has been found yet, some researchers have focused their attention on nutrition. "I think it's worthwhile to consider diet as a potential factor in Alzheimer's," says James G. Penland, PhD, a research psychologist at the USDA Human Nutrition Research Center in Grand Forks, North Dakota.

A Role for Antioxidants

Research has uncovered evidence that free radicals, which are harmful oxygen molecules that damage tissues throughout the body, including in the brain, may play a role in Alzheimer's disease.

Even though the body produces protective substances called antioxidants that help control free radicals, there aren't always enough of them to stop the onslaught. But you can get more antioxidants into your body simply by eating foods, such as fruits and vegetables, that contain antioxidant substances.

Researchers from Vanderbilt University in Nashville and the University of South Florida in Tampa did a study involving more than 1,800 men and women and found that those who drank fruit and vegetable juices at least three times a week had a 76 percent lower chance of developing suspected Alzheimer's disease than people who drank juice less than once a week. The researchers concluded that "fruit and vegetable juices may play an important role in delaying the onset of Alzheimer's disease."

Bs for the Brain

Researchers are also investigating B vitamins as a way of treating Alzheimer's disease. The body uses B vitamins to help maintain the protective covering on nerves and to

Doctor's Top Tip

According to the National Institute on Aging, two of the most important steps you can take to possibly lower your risk of Alzheimer's disease are to lower your cholesterol and homocysteine levels. A diet rich in folate and vitamins B_6 and B_{12} can lower your blood levels of homocysteine. Eating a diet low in saturated fat (found in meat and full-fat dairy foods), dietary cholesterol (found in animal foods), and trans fat (processed foods are a significant source) can improve your cholesterol.

manufacture chemicals that nerves use to communicate. When levels of B vitamins decline, mental performance may suffer, says Dr. Penland. In addition, an increased level of homocysteine—an amino acid—may raise your risk of Alzheimer's disease. B vitamins help lower your homocysteine level by breaking it down.

An Australian study gave 299 older men either a placebo (dummy pill) or supplemental folate (a B vitamin), B_6, and B_{12} for 2 years. The men who took the B vitamins had smaller increases of a substance that's found within the damaging deposits in the brains of people with Alzheimer's. Thus, B vitamins may play a role in preventing Alzheimer's disease, according to the researchers.

Good sources of thiamin, a B vitamin, include pork, sunflower seeds, and enriched grain products. For vitamin B_{12}, meats such as turkey, chicken livers, and lamb, and seafood such as steamed clams, bluefin tuna, and sardines, are all good sources. For folate, good sources include enriched cereals and enriched flour. For B_6, toss some chickpeas, potatoes, chicken, and bananas into your shopping cart.

One to Watch

Among some Alzheimer's researchers, interest is brewing in a natural substance called acetyl-L-carnitine, which resembles amino acids found in dairy foods, kidney beans, eggs, and red meats. Research suggests that carnitine, which helps carry fats into brain cells, may help slow the progression of the disease.

British researchers compiled the results of multiple studies on acetyl-L-carnitine that looked at the substance's effect on mild cognitive impairment and early Alzheimer's disease. They found that the substance had a "beneficial effect" after just 3 months, and the improvement got even better over time.

Eat Like the Mediterraneans Do

The so-called Mediterranean diet, which is rich in fruits and vegetables, fish, whole grains, and unsaturated fats such as olive oil and canola oil, may help protect you from Alzheimer's, as well as heart disease and cancer. Researchers from Columbia University in New York City tracked the eating habits and cognitive health of 2,258 New Yorkers for 4 years and found that those who most closely followed the Mediterranean eating style were 40 percent less likely to develop Alzheimer's than the people whose eating habits least resembled the Mediterranean diet.

Heavy Metal

According to the Alzheimer's Association, researchers in the 1960s suspected that aluminum may play a role in the disease. Since then, however, research has uncovered so much conflicting information about whether or not the metal is connected with the disease that it's hard to say with any certainty that it plays a role. Nowadays, most scientists conclude that if aluminum plays any role in Alzheimer's, it's a small one, the association says.

According to the National Institutes of Health, it's hard to avoid aluminum, since it's one of the most abundant elements found in the environment. However, if you do want to reduce your exposure, just to be on the safe side, the following steps will help:

- Avoid storing or cooking foods in aluminum foil.
- Avoid processed cheese, which contains a significant amount of aluminum.
- Avoid cooking highly acidic foods, such as tomato products, in aluminum pans.
- Although aluminum beverage cans usually have a coating to minimize the metal that leaches into the drink, buying beverages in bottles will eliminate this exposure.

Dijon Pork Chops with Cabbage

4 center-cut pork chops (4 ounces each), trimmed

4 teaspoons Dijon mustard

½ head red cabbage (about 1 pound), cored and thinly sliced

2 Granny Smith apples, peeled and grated

¼ teaspoon salt

1 teaspoon plus 1 tablespoon canola oil

1 tablespoon grated fresh ginger

½ teaspoon ground cinnamon

¼ teaspoon ground cloves

1 tablespoon pure maple syrup

2 teaspoons cider vinegar

Brush both sides of the pork chops with the mustard and set aside. In a large bowl, combine the cabbage, apples, and salt; toss well.

In a large covered skillet, heat 1 teaspoon of the oil over medium-low heat. Add the ginger, cinnamon, and cloves. Cook, stirring, until fragrant, 10 to 15 seconds. Stir in the cabbage mixture and the maple syrup. Reduce the heat to low, cover, and cook until the ingredients are softened and cooked through, about 30 minutes.

Meanwhile, in a large heavy skillet, heat the remaining 1 tablespoon of oil over medium heat. Add the pork in a single layer. Cook, turning halfway through, until the pork is no longer pink in the center, about 9 minutes.

Uncover the cabbage, stir in the vinegar, and increase the heat to medium. Cook until the liquid is nearly evaporated, about 5 minutes. Serve each chop with a mound of cabbage.

Makes 4 servings

PER SERVING

Calories: 280	Cholesterol: 70 mg
Total fat: 11 g	Sodium: 316 mg
Saturated fat: 2.5 g	Dietary fiber: 4 g

Anemia

IRONING OUT FATIGUE

In Greek, the word *anemia* means "no blood." But that's an exaggeration. People with anemia have plenty of blood. It's just that they don't have the usual number of red blood cells, or these cells aren't carrying their usual payload of energy-giving oxygen.

There are many forms of anemia, but the most common is iron-deficiency anemia. When you're not getting enough iron in your diet or you are losing blood—as a result of menstruation, for example—the oxygen-carrying capacity of your blood can drop precipitously. Deprived of oxygen, you wilt. Anemia can make you feel sluggish and weak. Your brain feels fuzzy. You're always cold.

It is estimated that about 20 percent of US women and 3 percent of men have low iron stores and are at risk for anemia. Luckily, it's generally an easy condition to correct. And the cure is our favorite thing—food.

Ironing Out the Problem

The Daily Value (DV) for iron is 18 milligrams. Pregnant women need a much higher amount—30 milligrams a day. It can be difficult to get that much iron in the diet, so obstetricians may prescribe supplements for pregnant women.

For the rest of us, how hard is it to get enough iron in food? It's not too tricky if you eat meat, fish, and poultry. These foods contain substantial amounts of iron. For example, 3 ounces of steamed blue mussels has 6 milligrams of iron. A 3-ounce serving of lean, broiled top round steak has 3 milligrams, and the same amount of roasted white turkey meat has 1 milligram.

If you eat little or no meat, though, you'll need to pay more attention to your diet. It's not that vegetables don't have iron. A cup of canned pumpkin, for example, has 3.4 milligrams of iron. Kidney beans and lentils have about 3 milligrams in a half-cup serving. As

Doctor's Top Tip

If you notice the signs of anemia—such as shortness of breath, dizziness, and coldness in the extremities—visit your doctor for a checkup, urges the National Institutes of Health. Sometimes anemia may be caused by bleeding in the digestive tract, and treating the underlying problem can solve the anemia, plus limit other complications caused by the bleeding.

you can see, the total amount of iron isn't the problem with these foods. Something called *bioavailability* is.

Increasing Absorption

Bioavailability refers to how well our bodies absorb the nutrients we eat. There are two forms of iron with vastly different levels of bioavailability. The iron found in meat, fish, and shellfish, called heme iron, is readily absorbable. The iron found in plant foods, called nonheme iron, is less so.

Here's an example. Of the 6 milligrams of iron in 3 ounces of mussels, roughly 15 percent will be absorbed by your body. Only 3 percent of the 3 milligrams of iron in a half-cup of lentils, however, will be absorbed.

It's possible to boost the bioavailability of iron with savvy eating. For example, pairing a food that contains vitamin C with a food that contains iron guarantees that you'll get substantially more of the iron into your bloodstream. "Iron is best absorbed in an acidic environment, particularly ascorbic acid—vitamin C," says Carol Fleischman, MD, clinical assistant professor of medicine with the University of Pennsylvania Health System near Philadelphia.

Similarly, combining meats and vegetables in the same meal makes it easier to get more iron. The heme iron in meats "potentiates" the iron in vegetables, making it easier to absorb. Mixing heme iron from meats with nonheme iron from beans and vegetables will increase absorption of the nonheme iron 10 to 15 percent, "an appreciable amount," says Henry C. Lukaski, PhD, assistant director of the USDA Human Nutrition Research Center in Grand Forks, North Dakota.

Dr. Fleischman adds, "Coordinating it all does give the most benefits, but if a woman is iron-deficient, her absorption of iron will be much more avid. So the more iron she eats, the more she absorbs."

Boosting Your Iron Stores

If you suspect that you have anemia, your doctor will probably want to do a complete checkup to make sure that nothing serious is wrong. When the problem is not getting enough iron in the diet, however, it's almost always easy to correct.

If you like clams, you're in business. A bowl of 10 small steamed clams contains an astonishing 26 milligrams of iron. There are also many ways to include vitamin C with your meals to boost your absorption of iron. For example, a large tomato has 23 milligrams of vitamin C, or 38 percent of the DV. You can also get vitamin C by drinking orange juice, or other citrus juices.

Another way to mix vitamin C with iron is to eat more potatoes. One baked potato with the skin contains 17 milligrams of vitamin C, or 28 percent of the DV,

THE BEST SOURCES

The table below offers the best iron sources you can find, both for absorbable heme iron (found in meat and fish) and less absorbable nonheme iron (found in plants), and another list for great sources of vitamin B_{12}.

FOODS CONTAINING HEME IRON

Food	Portion	Iron (mg)
Clams, steamed	Approx. 3 oz	23.8
Chicken livers, simmered	3 oz	7.2
Mussels, steamed	3 oz	5.7
Oysters, steamed	6 medium (1½ oz)	5.0
Quail, whole	1	4.2
Beef, bottom round roast, lean only, braised	3 oz	2.9
Tuna, light meat, water-packed	3 oz	2.7
Shrimp, steamed	3 oz	2.6
Turkey, dark meat, roasted	3 oz	2.0
Chicken leg, roasted	3 oz	1.2

FOODS CONTAINING NONHEME IRON

Food	Portion	Iron (mg)
Cream of Wheat cereal, quick-cooking	¾ cup	7.7
Tofu, regular	¼ block (approx. 4 oz)	6.2
Pumpkin seeds, hulled, dried	1 oz	4.3
Lentils, boiled	½ cup	3.3
Potato, baked	7 oz	2.8
Kidney beans, boiled	1½ cups	2.6
Pinto beans, boiled	½ cup	2.2
Black beans, boiled	½ cup	1.8
Pumpkin, canned	½ cup	1.7
Split peas, boiled	½ cup	1.3

FOODS CONTAINING VITAMIN B_{12}

Food	Portion	Vitamin B_{12} (mcg)
Clams, canned	3 oz	84
Beef liver, pan-fried	3 oz	71
Alaska king crab, steamed	3 oz	9.8
Rainbow trout	3 oz	4.2
Soy milk	1 cup	3
Corn flakes	1 cup	2.7

as well as 1.9 milligrams of iron. Eating the potato with the skin will more than triple the amount of iron it provides.

One nutrient that you don't want to combine with iron is calcium. Especially when you're taking iron supplements, having calcium-rich foods in the same meal may set you back. "They compete for the same receptor sites on your cells," explains Fergus Clydesdale, PhD, distinguished professor and head of the department of food science at the University of Massachusetts in Amherst. The calcium and iron in foods also compete, but not as much as when you're taking supplements. Dr. Clydesdale recommends spacing your calcium and iron 3 hours apart. For example, put milk on your cereal in the morning, but wait until later to take your iron supplement.

The same goes for coffee and tea. Both beverages contain tannins, chemicals that have a mild blocking effect on iron supplements, says Dr. Clydesdale. So don't take your pills with your morning coffee, he advises.

One easy way to get more iron in your diet is simply to cook your meals in cast-iron pots, says Dr. Lukaski. "As a rule of thumb, it increases iron by 2 to 5 percent," he says. And at breakfast, don't hesitate to have an old-fashioned meal. Because it's fortified with iron, a half-cup of cooked Cream of Wheat is loaded with 6 milligrams of iron. Instant oatmeal also contains iron, though not as much: about 3 milligrams in a half-cup.

Vegetarian Dangers

Anemia is much more common in vegetarians than meat eaters. In this case, the problem is due not only to a lack of iron but also to a lack of vitamin B_{12}. This nutrient, which is needed for cells to divide and mature properly, comes mostly from animal foods. Consequently, strict vegetarians may get little or no B_{12} in their diets.

The resulting condition, called pernicious anemia, isn't an immediate problem, if only because the body uses vitamin B_{12} sparingly. Most of us have enough in storage to last 6 years or so—"a grace period," says Dr. Fleischman. Because of this, strict vegetarians may not notice symptoms of B_{12} deficiency, which include fatigue and tingling in the hands and feet, for a very long time.

As with iron-deficiency anemia, being low in B_{12} is easily reversed. "Vegans— strict vegetarians who eat no meats, dairy foods, or eggs—will probably have to take B_{12} supplements or brewers' yeast," says Dr. Fleischman. "Check with your doctor to see which is best for you."

New England Clam Chowder

1 slice bacon

2 teaspoons vegetable oil

½ cup chopped onion

½ cup chopped celery

1 clove garlic, minced

1 bay leaf

½ teaspoon dried thyme

2 cups bottled clam juice

1½ cups diced Yukon Gold potatoes (½-inch size)

1½ cups 2% milk

1½ tablespoons all-purpose flour

3 cans (6.5 ounces each) minced clams, drained

¼ cup chopped parsley

Cook the bacon in a microwave, according to package directions, until crisp. Crumble the bacon into small pieces and set aside.

In a large saucepan, heat the oil over medium-low heat. Add the onion, celery, and garlic, and cook for 5 minutes. Add the bay leaf and thyme, and continue to cook, stirring occasionally, until the onion is softened but not browned, about 3 minutes. Add the clam juice and potatoes. The liquid should just cover the potatoes. Bring the chowder to a simmer, and cook the potatoes for about 10 minutes (they should be tender but not mushy).

In a small bowl, whisk ¼ cup of the milk with the flour until smooth. Add to the chowder with the remaining 1¼ cups milk. Increase the heat to high, and bring to a boil, stirring constantly, until the soup has thickened slightly, about 3 minutes. Remove the pan from the heat, and stir in the clams. Remove the bay leaf. Divide the chowder among 4 bowls, and sprinkle each serving with the parsley and crumbled bacon.

Makes 4 servings

PER SERVING

Calories: 200
Total fat: 7 g
Saturated fat: 2 g

Cholesterol: 25 mg
Sodium: 810 mg
Dietary fiber: 1 g

Antioxidants

BODYGUARDS FOR YOUR CELLS

HEALING POWER

Can Help:

Reduce the risk of heart disease

Prevent certain cancers

Protect your vision

Protect your brain

Prevent muscle soreness

Slow the aging process

If you want to know how antioxidants work, picture yourself as the president, a king or queen, a movie star, or another well-known figure.

A threat to your safety could pop up at any time—and that's why you have a team of bodyguards surrounding you. If a source of danger comes your way, your bodyguards are trained to swoop in and get between you and this threat. Your protectors are willing to suffer the consequences themselves, just to keep you from getting hurt.

Every day, the DNA in *each cell* in your body faces about 10,000 attacks from cell-damaging forces known as free radicals, which are unstable oxygen molecules that have lost an electron. Free radicals are naturally produced as your body turns fuel to energy, but you can also get them in your body from pollution, smoking, and other sources. These volatile molecules cruise around your body trying to stabilize themselves by stealing electrons from other molecules. When they succeed, they create still more free radicals, causing a sort of snowballing procession of damage.

Free radicals don't just occasionally pop up here and there. Up to 5 percent of the oxygen that each cell uses is converted into free radicals.

Free-radical damage is thought to play a role in the accumulation of low-density lipoprotein (LDL) cholesterol in the lining of your artery walls. This can lead to a narrowing of the arteries called atherosclerosis, which contributes to heart disease. And when free-radicals damage DNA inside the cells, the result can be cell mutations that lead to cancer. Free radical assaults on your eyes may lead to cataracts and macular degeneration, which are common causes of vision loss in people over age 50. Researchers think that free-radical damage—also called "oxidative stress"—plays an important role in Alzheimer's disease. And many scientists believe that free radicals are the primary force behind aging itself.

Free radicals can develop and quickly attack your cells faster than the blink of an eye. And unless something is immediately available to "step in," this free-radical free-for-all can cause irreparable damage. That's where antioxidants come in.

Remember that analogy, in which you were a famous person preyed upon by harmful threats? Those bodyguards forming a human shield around you are the antioxidants in your system. Every time you eat fruits, vegetables, or other antioxidant-rich foods, a flood of these protective compounds enters your bloodstream. They travel throughout your body, stepping between your body's healthy cells and the pillaging free radicals, offering up their own electrons to neutralize the free radicals and keep your cells out of harm's way.

The Big Antioxidant Nutrients

Just as your body produces free radicals, it also produces antioxidants. Some of these are enzymes created solely to squelch free radicals. But these defenders can be overwhelmed if you're under serious attack—from car exhaust or cigarette smoke, for example—and they may be insufficient to handle rising levels of free-radical attacks as you get older. Every day, a small percentage of free radicals slip past your natural antioxidant defenses, allowing them to do their damage.

That's why you regularly need to call in the reserves to supplement your own forces: antioxidant compounds from your diet. There are literally hundreds of natural food compounds that act as antioxidants in the body. And the nice thing about them is that you never have to run out, because you can just eat more.

Though researchers are investigating new antioxidant compounds every day, most scientific study has focused on three types in particular—vitamins C and E and carotenoids.

"There is no doubt that antioxidants play a crucial role in reducing the risk for all kinds of diseases," says Roc Ordman, PhD, professor of chemistry and biochemistry at Beloit College in Beloit, Wisconsin. "The published scientific evidence is simply overwhelming."

Vitamin C

Like Navy SEALs, molecules of vitamin C (also called ascorbic acid) patrol the waters of your body, including the fluids in your blood, lungs, and eyes. Vitamin C is quick to give up its electrons, yet it easily picks up more electrons to become "reactivated," making it an efficient protector against free radicals. Getting lots of vitamin C in your diet can help protect against damage in many of your organs and tissues, including your heart, arteries, and eyes.

An important attribute of vitamin C, which is found in foods like tropical and citrus fruits, red bell peppers, and broccoli, is that it works so quickly. Vitamin C has been shown to block free radicals before other antioxidant compounds even arrive on the scene.

When the National Cancer Institute (NCI) explains where to find antioxidants, it sounds like they're describing a rainbow: You'll find beta-carotene in orange pumpkins, sweet potatoes, and carrots, and green spinach and kale; lycopene in red tomatoes and watermelon; lutein in collard greens and other leafy greens; and vitamin C in all sorts of colorful fruits and vegetables, from oranges to red peppers. Be sure to constantly rotate a variety of antioxidant-rich fruits and vegetables across your plate—at least five servings a day, recommends the NCI—to ensure that you provide your body with a wide variety of antioxidants that attack cell-damaging free radicals in different ways. Once you get to five a day, set your sights on nine. And don't forget plant foods that *aren't* colorful fruits and vegetables, such as nuts, whole-wheat bread, beans, and vegetable oils, for their antioxidant nutrients, including vitamin E and selenium.

Vitamin C may possibly reduce your risk of heart disease by helping prevent your LDL (or bad) cholesterol from becoming damaged by free radicals. Experts think that oxidized LDL plays an important role in the plaque buildup that can develop in artery walls and reduce the blood supply to your heart.

In a major study, researchers analyzed a national survey of vitamin C intake and death rate in 11,348 people ages 25 to 74 during a 10-year span. They found that men and women with high intakes of vitamin C—about 300 milligrams a day—from both food and supplements had much lower death rates from heart disease than those with low intakes. Specifically, men had a 42 percent lower death rate from heart disease, and women had a 25 percent lower death rate. Even when vitamin C intakes were less than 50 milligrams a day, women had a 10 percent reduction in death rates from heart disease, while men had a 6 percent reduction from the disease.

Vitamin C may also help protect against certain forms of cancer. Research has found that a diet high in vitamin C is related to a lower risk of stomach cancer. Vitamin C–rich foods may also help protect you from cancer of the mouth, larynx, and esophagus. However, since fruits and vegetables are the main source of vitamin C, these results may be due to *other* disease-fighting components found in produce. As a result, it's a good idea to eat a wide variety of fruits and vegetables daily to ensure that you get plenty of vitamin C. Eating five servings a day—the minimum amount that the federal government recommends—will provide you with up to 300 milligrams of vitamin C.

Maintaining your vitamin C stores is especially important if you're a smoker or you live with one. It takes about 20 milligrams of vitamin C to squelch the free-radical effects of one cigarette.

Good sources of vitamin C include bell peppers, broccoli, oranges, papaya, strawberries, grapefruit, kiwifruit, cabbage, and potatoes.

In addition, Dr. Ordman recommends taking 500 milligrams of vitamin C in supplement form twice a day, once in the morning and once at night, a practice confirmed by a major study at the National Institutes of Health. But remember—this isn't a substitute for eating a variety of foods that are naturally rich in vitamin C, since you want to get the other disease-fighting components they offer, too.

Vitamin E

While vitamin C is hard at work patrolling the waters of your body, vitamin E (also known as alpha-tocopherol) is delving into denser territories, protecting your fat tissues from free-radical invasion.

It's precisely this fat-protecting prowess that makes vitamin E particularly effective in the fight against heart disease. Researchers have found that vitamin E, which dissolves in fat, plays a powerful role in keeping your bad LDL cholesterol from oxidizing and contributing to atherosclerosis.

A number of large population studies involving tens of thousands of people have linked high vitamin E intake with a significant decrease in risk for heart disease. In a study of 80,000 nurses, researchers found that women with the highest vitamin E intake—about 200 IU a day—were one-third less likely to suffer from heart disease than their counterparts who were only getting about 3 IU a day.

A more recent study followed nearly 30,000 middle-aged and older male Finnish smokers for 19 years, and measured the association between their vitamin E levels at the beginning of the study and their risk of death. Men with higher amounts of vitamin E in their systems were about 20 percent less likely to die during the 19 years than the men at the low end of the scale.

In addition, the men whose vitamin E levels put them at the top of the scale were less likely to die of lung cancer, prostate cancer, stroke, heart disease, and lung disease than the men at the bottom of the scale.

Many cardiologists must think the vitamin is important: Research has found that roughly half of these physicians take vitamin E supplements.

One of the most promising findings for female health emerged from a study at the State University of New York at Buffalo in which researchers examined vitamin E levels in women with a high family risk for breast cancer. They found that women who maintained high levels of vitamin E had significantly lower risks for the disease than women who had low levels. The benefits were most pronounced among younger women, although those past menopause were also protected.

Getting enough vitamin E in the diet—it's found in vegetable cooking oils, wheat germ, kale, sweet potato, and sunflower seeds, to name a few sources—is important for men as well. More than 50 percent of men with diabetes, for example, have difficulty achieving erections, often because of free-radical damage to the arteries supplying blood to the penis. Research suggests that getting enough vitamin E in the diet can help keep blood flowing smoothly through those arteries.

While vitamin E is effective in its own right, it works more efficiently when combined with vitamin C, says Dr. Ordman. "It's like vitamin C helps vitamin E get back on its feet again. After vitamin E becomes oxidized by free radicals, vitamin C comes along and regenerates it so that it's ready to work again," he explains. In the summer of 2006, Dr. Ordman published a clinical study showing that 400 IU of vitamin E and 500 milligrams of vitamin C twice a day protect people from free radicals better than other combinations.

The Daily Value for vitamin E is 30 IU, but based on published studies of its benefits to our immune systems, Dr. Ordman recommends 200 to 400 IU in supplement form daily in order to get the maximum protection. Experts agree that this is well within the safe limits for the vitamin. It's difficult to get more than 15 to 30 IU each day just from a balanced diet, since one of the main sources of vitamin E is plant oils, and many people are trying to follow a reduced-fat diet.

Beta-Carotene and Friends

Beta-carotene, a red-yellow food pigment that turns to vitamin A in the body, has been on quite a roller-coaster ride during the past few decades. It enjoyed enormous popularity when scientists linked it with lower rates of heart disease and cancer. The mood changed, however, when researchers discovered that taking beta-carotene supplements seemed to increase the risk for some of these diseases.

"We know that beta-carotene has established benefits, but the amounts that people need are well within the range they can get from eating five or more servings of fruits and vegetables a day," explains Dr. Ordman. "So you don't need extraordinary amounts. There are definite risks with supplementation. It has recently been reported that nearly half of Americans are being harmed by consuming too much vitamin A and beta-carotene."

Why are food sources of beta-carotene so much better than supplements? Scientists still aren't sure, but they suspect that it may be because beta-carotene has more than 600 siblings, collectively known as carotenoids. It's possible, they say, that it's not just the beta-carotene that's causing the benefits, but the combination of beta-carotene plus its less-recognized kin.

Interestingly, researchers have backed off further investigating connections between beta-carotene and cardiovascular disease in recent years, due to previously disappointing results. Some have shifted their focus to other carotenoids found in fruits and vegetables, such as lycopene, lutein, and zeaxanthin, which show promise in reducing the risk of cardiovascular disease and other conditions.

THE BEST SOURCES

All fruits and vegetables are great sources of antioxidant compounds. But which are the best? Researchers at Tufts University in Boston compiled a list of foods that are extremely high in vitamin C and beta-carotene. (It's difficult to get enough vitamin E in foods alone, although cooking oils, nuts, seeds, and wheat germ are all good sources.) Here are some of their favorites.

Food	Portion	Vitamin C (mg)	Beta-Carotene (mg)
Broccoli, cooked	½ cup	37	1.0
Brussels sprouts, cooked	4	36	0.3
Butternut squash, baked and cubed	½ cup	15	4.3
Cantaloupe	¼	56	2.6
Kiwifruit	1	89	0.1
Navel orange	1	80	0.2
Papaya	½	94	0.3
Strawberries	½ cup	42	—
Sweet potato, baked	1	28	15.0
Sweet red pepper, chopped	½ cup	95	1.7
Watermelon, cubed	½ cup	8	0.2

In the American diet, the food that most commonly provides bioavailable lycopene (in other words, the kind your body can use) is tomato sauce. A meta-analysis that grouped the findings of 21 previous studies on tomatoes and prostate cancer found that a diet high in tomatoes may provide up to a 20 percent decreased risk of the disease. Cooked tomatoes seem to be more helpful than raw tomatoes.

In a study that shows that carrots really are good for your eyes, researchers found that people with the highest levels of carotenoids had one-third to one-half the risk of macular degeneration than those with lower levels. Another study, from the National Eye Institute, found that taking high doses of vitamins C and E, beta-carotene, and zinc may cut the risk of advanced macular degeneration by about 25 percent. A diet that's high in lutein and zeaxanthin may help reduce your risk of the condition, too.

While antioxidants have shown their mettle against major health threats like heart disease and cancer, they are also useful in preventing lesser ailments. An example is muscle soreness. One study found that folks who are sedentary most of the time and then suddenly exercise intensely may find relief from aching muscles with vitamin E. It appears that vitamin E may reduce free-radical damage that can lead to muscle soreness.

So the next time you're in the produce aisle, be sure to fill your cart with plenty of carotenoid-rich foods like spinach and other dark green leafy vegetables, and deep orange fruits and vegetables like pumpkins, sweet potatoes, carrots, and cantaloupe. Don't bother with beta-carotene supplements, Dr. Ordman advises. When you eat plant foods rich in beta-carotene, you'll get the countless other antioxidant chemicals they contain as well.

The Rest of the Troops

Despite the importance of vitamins C and E and beta-carotene, they're only a small part of a massive army of protective compounds found in foods. For example, the mineral selenium is needed for its role in supporting your natural antioxidant enzymes. Flavonoids and other types of phenolics in green tea, chocolate, and red wine also act as potent antioxidants. "We all agree that everyone should eat at least five servings of fruits and vegetables a day to ensure that they get healthy amounts of all of these antioxidants, and the latest guidelines ask us to get nine or more servings," explains Dr. Ordman. "But as far as taking extra antioxidant supplements, you should stick with those that have been studied extensively and proven safe in long-term clinical trials. Those are vitamins C and E. Everything else should come solely from food."

Appendicitis
THE FORCE OF FIBER

The next time you want to impress your friends with a bit of appendix-related trivia, toss out this fact: The most commonly performed emergency surgery in the world is the appendectomy, a procedure for treating appendicitis, or an inflammation of the appendix.

But not everyone in the world is equally likely to need this operation. Researchers have wondered for years why appendicitis is relatively rare in places like Africa and Asia, while in the United States it's extremely common, affecting about 7 percent of people during their lives. What are we doing wrong?

"There's always been speculation that high-fiber diets protect against appendicitis," says David G. Addiss, MD, MPH, senior project officer for the private Fetzer Institute in Kalamazoo, Michigan, and a former medical epidemiologist for the division of parasitic diseases at the Centers for Disease Control and Prevention in Atlanta. People in Africa and Asia eat tremendous quantities of fruits, vegetables, whole grains, and other fiber-rich foods. In this country, however, most of us get only 11 to 12 grams of fiber a day. This is less than half of the Daily Value (DV) of 25 grams.

But for a brief time in the 1940s, a curious thing happened. Due to wartime rationing, people started eating less meat and more high-fiber foods, and appendicitis rates started dropping. A coincidence? Some researchers don't think so.

Digestion Made Easy

Experts don't know why we have an appendix. Whatever useful role it plays—if any—is a mystery. But it can certainly cause trouble. Your appendix is a little hollow tube that hangs like a tail off the first part of your colon, also known as your large intestine. Appendicitis most often occurs when a firm piece of stool blocks the pea-size opening of the appendix, allowing bacteria to flourish inside.

Appendicitis is most common in kids and young adults between the ages of 10 and 30. Acute appendicitis is typically treated with surgery to remove the problematic appendix. Appendicitis is a serious problem; if the appendix ruptures, it can trigger a life-threatening infection in the abdomen.

Experts don't know much about preventing appendicitis, but the one step they do recommend is an easy one: Eat more fiber.

Doctor's Top Tip

When you increase the amount of fiber in your diet, make sure to drink plenty of water and other fluids, too, urges the American Dietetic Association. Be sure to get 8 cups daily. Fiber fights constipation by soaking up fluid, making stool soft and bulky. Ironically, though, if you're getting extra fiber but not enough fluid, the fiber can *cause* constipation. When you're making the effort to keep your appendix happy, you don't want that happening.

Since the fiber found in foods absorbs water, a high-fiber diet causes the stool to become larger, softer, and less likely to break apart. This can help prevent stray pieces from blocking the appendix.

Getting more fiber in your diet also causes stool to move more quickly through the digestive tract. "Anything that will decrease the resident time of all the waste products in your large intestine can only help," says Frank G. Moody, MD, professor of surgery at the University of Texas Medical School in Houston. Even though doctors aren't positive that getting more fiber will prevent appendicitis, it clearly provides some protection.

A Greek study relating fiber to a decreased risk of appendicitis looked at 203 kids who'd had appendectomies (appendix-removing surgery) to treat their appendicitis, and compared their diets with that of 1,922 who hadn't had appendix problems. The researchers found that the kids who'd had appendix surgeries got significantly less daily fiber in their diets.

One of the easiest ways to get more fiber into your diet is to start the day with cereal. Most breakfast cereals, both hot and cold, are wonderful sources of fiber, says Pat Harper, RD, a dietitian based in Pittsburgh. Some cereals, in fact, contain 10 or more grams of fiber per serving. That's roughly half of the DV, all in one bowl. So the next time you're at the supermarket, be sure to put a few boxes of cereal in your cart. And take a few minutes to read the labels, Harper adds. A cereal should have at least 5 grams of fiber per serving. If it doesn't, you may want to pick another brand. Or if your favorite cereal is fairly low in fiber, you can mix it with a higher-fiber kind to get the extra protection.

Another way to get more fiber is to eat whole-grain foods. Foods like white bread, white rice, and white flour, which are made from processed grains, have been stripped of much of their protective fiber. In fact, you'd have to eat 20 slices of white bread to get just 10 grams of fiber. Foods made from whole grains, however, are loaded with fiber. A slice of whole-wheat bread, for example, has 2 grams of fiber, more than four times the amount in its processed counterpart. A half-cup serving of cooked barley has 3 grams of fiber, while a half-cup of cooked oatmeal has 3 grams. All whole grains are super fiber choices, says Harper.

Legumes are even better sources. A half-cup of cooked split peas, for example,

GIVE PRODUCE A SHOWER BEFORE YOU EAT IT

Since the peel of fruits and vegetables is rich in fiber, it makes sense to eat this part of the produce, rather than peeling it off and throwing it away. However, the peel may also harbor unhealthy dirt, bacteria, and other contaminants.

So before you sink your teeth into any fruit or veggie (even if you *are* going to peel it), you should clean it first. If the vegetable has outer leaves, such as lettuce, discard them. Wash firm fruits and vegetables under warm, clean running water. Rinse veggies that will go into salads with cool water, to preserve crispness. Don't bother with soap, detergent, or washes commercially marketed for produce, says the FDA. If the piece of produce is hardy enough to handle a little scrubbing, clean it with a clean produce brush as well.

If you're eating more delicate fruits, like berries, pour them into a colander and hose them off with a kitchen sink sprayer. Jostle the colander from time to time to turn the berries so you can wash them all over.

has 8 grams of fiber, nearly a third of the recommended daily amount. The same amount of cooked kidney beans has nearly 6 grams of fiber, and a half-cup of boiled black beans has almost 8 grams.

While fruits and vegetables can't compete with legumes for sheer fiber force, they're still significant sources. A half-cup of broccoli, for example, has 2 grams of fiber. Apples and oranges have about 3 grams of fiber each. And don't forget dried fruits. A half-cup of raisins has 4 grams of fiber, while 10 dried apricot halves have 3 grams.

Even though the juicy flesh of fruits contains some fiber, most of the fiber is found in the peel. So whenever possible, eat fruits (and vegetables, including potatoes) with the skin intact.

Citrus fruits, of course, are an exception to this rule, since you don't eat the skin. Fortunately, though, much of the fiber in oranges, grapefruit, and other citrus fruits is found in the white pith just beneath the skin. To get the most fiber, don't slice citrus fruits. Instead, peel and eat them whole to get the most fiber in each bite.

White Bean and Chicken Chili

1 tablespoon olive oil

2 scallions, thinly sliced, white and green parts separated

1 clove garlic

¾ teaspoons chili powder

½ teaspoon ground cumin

1 can (15 ounces) white beans, rinsed and drained

1 can (14.5 ounces) salt-free diced tomatoes (with juice)

¾ cup chicken broth

4 ounces leftover cooked chicken breast meat, shredded (about ¾ cup)

Hot pepper sauce to taste (optional)

In a medium saucepan, heat the oil over medium-high heat. Add the scallions (saving some greens for a garnish) and the garlic, and cook, stirring, until golden. Add the chili powder and cumin, and continue to cook, stirring, for 1 minute longer. Add the white beans, tomatoes and their juice, and broth. Simmer until the liquid is slightly reduced, about 15 minutes. Stir in the chicken, and simmer 5 minutes longer.

Divide the chili among 4 bowls, and garnish with scallion greens. Serve with hot pepper sauce, if desired.

Makes 4 servings

PER SERVING

Calories: 382
Total fat: 9 g
Saturated fat: 1.5 g

Cholesterol: 45 mg
Sodium: 273 mg
Dietary fiber: 10 g

Apples
THEIR BENEFITS ARE SKIN DEEP

HEALING POWER
Can Help:

Lower the risk of heart disease

Prevent constipation

Improve lung function

Lower the risk of lung cancer

John Chapman, a Massachusetts resident who liked to travel, isn't remembered for his groundbreaking efforts to prevent heart disease and cancer and improve Americans' overall health. But he certainly did his part. As he wandered around the eastern states and the Midwest for the first half of the 1800s, he planted apple seeds, transplanted seedlings, and established apple orchards to help supply pioneers with the tasty fruit.

He's now remembered as Johnny Appleseed, and nowadays, chemists, doctors, and other researchers are expanding his legacy as they discover new reasons why apples are so good to have around.

Apples are more than just a wholesome snack. Studies suggest that eating apples can help reduce the risk of heart disease, and they may also help protect you from lung cancer. In addition, they may lower your risk of asthma and improve your over-all lung function. Indeed, it appears that having an apple or two a day really can help keep the doctor away.

Filled with Antioxidants

Some of the most powerful disease-fighting components in apples are phenolics, and they've been getting a lot of research attention lately. Phenolics are a type of phytochemical that can act as powerful antioxidants, neutralizing free radicals before they have the chance to harm your DNA and other important components within your body.

Research conducted by scientists at Cornell University in Ithaca, New York, and Seoul University in South Korea found that these phenolics, rather than the vitamin C in the fruit, may provide the bulk of apples' antioxidant power.

Other research from Cornell set out to rank the total phenolic content in many popular fruits. Apples came in second place, behind the cranberry, and beat out other favorites such as the red grape, strawberry, pineapple, banana, peach, lemon, orange, pear, and grapefruit.

This study also found that apples had the second highest total antioxidant activity

Doctor's Top Tip

Put away the peeler, and eat your apples with the peel intact. "The peel contains three-quarters of the fiber and most of the antioxidants in the apple," says Wendy Davis, RD, director of communications and consumer health for the US Apple Association. Cornell University food scientists who tested four varieties of apples found that the peels better inhibited the growth of cancer cells than the rest of the apple. As a result, apple peels "may impart health benefits when consumed and should be regarded as a valuable source of antioxidants," the researchers wrote.

of these fruits (again, the cranberry beat it). Finally, the study also measured the ability of extracts of these fruits to inhibit liver-cancer cells in the lab. Apples came in third place, behind cranberries and lemons.

If you factor in their tastiness, easy preparation time, and versatility, apples are hard to beat as an easy way to get a quick dose of antioxidants—after all, have you ever grabbed a handful of cranberries or a lemon and eaten them?

Getting to the Heart of the Matter

The phytochemicals lurking in apples may make them useful tools in warding off heart disease. A study that followed almost 40,000 women for about 7 years associated apples with a 13 to 22 percent lower risk of cardiovascular disease.

Research from Finland has found that intake of flavonoids—a type of phenolic found in apples—was inversely associated with death from heart disease in women. Data gathered from the same group of people also found that those who ate the most apples had a lower risk of a type of stroke than the people who ate the fewest apples.

Another study, involving more than 30,000 older Iowa women, found that consuming catechin and epicatechin—both flavonoids found in apples—was associated with a lower risk of death from coronary heart disease.

Even though many people favor the flesh, much of an apple's healing power resides in the skin, which contains large amounts—about 4 milligrams—of an antioxidant compound called quercetin. Like vitamin C and beta-carotene, quercetin can help prevent harmful oxygen molecules from damaging individual cells.

Even in the healing world of antioxidants, quercetin is thought to be exceptional. Another Finnish study, this one following more than 10,000 men and women, found that the people who ate the most quercetin had a 20 percent lower risk of dying from coronary heart disease than those who ate the least.

"So eating an apple a day is not a bad idea," says Lawrence H. Kushi, ScD, associate director for etiology and prevention research at Kaiser Permanente's division of research in Oakland, California.

Keeping Cancer Away

Apples may also be helpful in warding off the dreaded disease of lung cancer. A study involving more than 120,000 men and women found that women who ate at least one serving of apples or pears daily had a lower risk of this form of cancer.

A Hawaiian study looking at the diet history of 582 people who had lung cancer and 582 without the disease found that the people who ate the most apples, onions, and white grapefruit had roughly half the risk of lung cancer than those who ate the least amounts of these foods. Apples and onions are both high in quercetin. In another study, Finnish researchers found that men who consumed more quercetin were 60 percent less likely to have lung cancer than men with lower quercetin intakes.

"When you subject cells to a carcinogen and then put in the quercetin, you prevent mutation from occurring—you prevent the carcinogen from acting," says Dr. Kushi.

Apples' Effect on Lung Problems

Apples may also help reduce your risk of asthma and improve your lung health. An Australian study involving 1,600 adults associated apple and pear consumption with a lower risk of asthma. Finnish researchers—who seem to be pretty busy when it comes to studying apples—found fewer cases of asthma among people with high levels of quercetin in their diets.

And a study of more than 13,000 adults in the Netherlands found that those who ate more apples and pears had better lung function and less chronic obstructive pulmonary disease.

Maintaining Digestive Health with Apple Fiber

Recent discoveries aside, apples are also excellent sources of fiber. They contain both soluble and insoluble fiber, including pectin. A 5-ounce apple with the skin has about 3 grams of fiber. "They're a good source," says Chang Lee, PhD, professor of food science and technology at the Cornell University–New York State Agricultural Experimental Station in Geneva.

Insoluble fiber, found mostly in the skin, is the kind that we used to call roughage, which has long been recommended for relieving constipation. More is at stake, though, than just comfort. Studies show that a smoothly operating digestive tract can help prevent diverticulosis, a condition in which small pouches form in the large intestine, and also cancer of the colon. Plus, insoluble fiber is filling, which is why apples are such an excellent weight-control food for people who want to lose weight without feeling hungry.

The soluble fiber in apples, which is the same kind that is found in oat bran, acts differently from the insoluble kind. Rather than passing through the digestive tract more or less unchanged, soluble fiber forms a gel-like material in the digestive tract that helps lower cholesterol and, with it, the risk of heart disease and stroke.

It's not just the soluble fiber that's so helpful, but a particular type of soluble fiber called pectin. The same ingredient used to thicken jellies and jams, pectin appears to reduce the amount of cholesterol produced in the liver. An average-size apple contains 0.7 gram of pectin, more than the amount in strawberries and bananas.

GETTING THE MOST

Store them cold. If you're buying more apples than you can eat quickly, store them in a plastic bag or a produce drawer in your refrigerator.

In the Kitchen

There are 2,500 kinds of apples in the United States alone. Even if you can't sample all of the world's apples, you can try some of the more notable varieties. Here are a few types to look for.

Braeburn. Ranging in color from greenish gold to almost solid red, Braeburn apples combine sweetness and tartness. A great eating apple.

Fuji. Available year-round, Fuji apples are crisp and sweet, with just a hint of spice. They are wonderful eating apples. The Fuji actually becomes more flavorful while you store it.

Gala. These apples have distinctive red stripes running down yellow-orange skin. Both crisp and sweet, they are used for munching and also for making applesauce.

Golden Delicious. The most commonly grown apple in many countries, it's firm, sweet, and crisp. It's a good choice for recipes that require baking or cooking, since it retains its shape.

Granny Smith. Probably best known for its bright green color, even when ripe, this apple is crisp and tart, and good for baking and sautéing.

Jonagold. Tangy and sweet, Jonagold apples are used both for eating and baking.

Liberty. A favorite of organic growers, Liberty apples are resistant to many diseases and don't require large amounts of pesticides. They're excellent for eating and cooking.

Northern Spy. Greenish yellow with red stripes, these apples have a tart taste that's wonderful for cooking and baking.

Rome. These apples are firm and crisp, and they're great for baking.

Winesap. Spicy and tart, these are often used for ciders and also for baking and adding to salads.

Protect their color. If you're serving apple slices, dip them in a citrus juice—such as lemon or grapefruit juice—after you cut them to help preserve their bright color.

Don't count on processed apples. Although apple juice contains a little iron and potassium, it's no great shakes compared with the whole fruit. By the time apples wind up as juice, they've given up most of their fiber and quercetin. In addition, the antioxidant-rich peel is discarded when producers make applesauce and canned apples. If you have a choice, eat a whole fresh apple rather than the processed versions.

Of course, if you're choosing between sugary soda and apple juice, by all means choose the juice. But don't use juice as a substitute for the real thing.

Apple Crumble with Toasted-Oat Topping

- 6 **medium Jonagold apples**
- ½ **cup unsweetened applesauce**
- ¾ **cup old-fashioned or quick-cooking rolled oats**
- 3 **tablespoons toasted wheat germ**
- 3 **tablespoons packed light brown sugar**
- 1 **teaspoon ground cinnamon**
- 1 **tablespoon canola oil**
- 1 **tablespoon unsalted butter, cut into small pieces**

Preheat the oven to 350°F. Coat a 12- × 8-inch baking dish with cooking spray.

Cut the apples in half lengthwise. Remove the cores and stems and discard. Cut the apples into thin slices.

Place the apples and the applesauce in the prepared baking dish. Toss to coat the apples evenly with the applesauce, and spread the apples out evenly in the baking dish.

In a small bowl, mix the oats, wheat germ, brown sugar, and cinnamon. Drizzle with the oil. Add the butter. Mix with your fingers to work the oil and butter into the dry ingredients.

Sprinkle the oat mixture evenly over the apples. Bake for 30 to 35 minutes, or until the topping is golden and the apples are bubbling. Serve warm.

Makes 6 servings

PER SERVING

Calories: 197
Total fat: 5.7 g
Saturated fat: 1.6 g

Cholesterol: 5 mg
Sodium: 3 mg
Dietary fiber: 4.7 g

Apricots

A BOUNTY OF BETA-CAROTENE

HEALING POWER

Can Help:

Protect the eyes

Prevent heart disease

Prevent cancer

When you think of Chinese food, apricots might not be the first item that comes to mind. But food historians think that apricots were first cultivated in China more than 4,000 years ago! The tasty fruit spread through the Middle East and the Mediterranean in ancient times, and now it's grown in Europe, Africa, Australia, and America, too.

Not only is this sweet, velvety fruit a delicious treat, but it's also loaded with a variety of compounds that research shows can fight infections, blindness, and heart disease.

Most of apricots' health benefits are due to their copious and exceptionally diverse carotenoid content. Carotenoids are the pigments in plants that paint many of our favorite fruits and vegetables red, orange, and yellow. In humans, they have a wide range of health-protecting properties. Researchers have identified more than 600 different carotenoids, with some of the most powerful, including beta-carotene, being found in apricots.

"Apricots are one of the best foods to look to for carotenoids," says Ritva Butrum, PhD, senior science advisor at the American Institute for Cancer Research in Washington, D.C.

Fruit for the Heart

The apricot's unique mix of healing compounds makes this food a powerful ally in fighting heart disease. Along with beta-carotene, apricots contain another carotenoid called lycopene, and both compounds have been shown in studies to fight the process by which the dangerous low-density lipoprotein (LDL) form of cholesterol becomes oxidized, or altered by free radicals. This is important because experts consider oxidized LDL to be a major player in atherosclerosis, which stiffens and narrows arteries, such as the ones supplying your heart.

A Japanese study that followed more than 3,000 men and women for nearly 12 years found that those with high levels of carotenoids, such as beta-carotene and lycopene, were less likely to die of cardiovascular disease.

Another study, which followed more than 73,000 American women for 12 years, found that those whose diets provided the most beta- and alpha-carotene had significantly less risk of coronary artery disease. Yet another study, this time following nearly 5,000 Dutch men and women for 4 years, found that those with the most beta-carotene in their diets had a significantly lower risk of heart attack.

Potential Cancer Fighter

Although tomatoes (more specifically, processed tomato products) seem to provide more than 85 percent of the lycopene in Americans' diets, apricots are another source of this carotenoid. Lycopene is one of the most potent antioxidants that experts know about. It could help prevent cancer by protecting your cells' DNA from free-radical attacks. (Its antioxidant properties explain why it might also be helpful in preventing the atherosclerosis involved in cardiovascular disease.)

Research looking at the possible role of lycopene in cancer prevention has focused on tomatoes and prostate cancer. A meta-analysis—which synthesizes research results from a number of studies—found that men who ate a lot of cooked tomato products had 19 percent less risk of prostate cancer than men who seldom ate tomato products. So what does this have to do with apricots?

Researchers point out that the protective effects from tomatoes could come from other components in them. If you enjoy the taste of apricots anyway, the knowledge

In the Kitchen

Although most of us eat apricots straight from the fruit bin, there are many other ways to prepare—and enjoy—these little golden gems.

Grill them. Grilled apricots take on a smoky, slightly sweet flavor as the sugars caramelize. Simply thread whole or halved fresh apricots on skewers, brush with honey, and cook for 7 to 10 minutes, turning frequently.

Broil them. To cook apricots indoors, cut the fruit in half, brush with honey, and broil in the oven, cut side up.

Poach them. Poached apricots are a great way to warm up a cool evening. Put fruit juice and whole cloves or a cinnamon stick in a small saucepan, and bring to a simmer. Add whole or halved apricots, and cook for 6 to 8 minutes. Remove the apricots, and continue cooking the sauce until it thickens. Then use it as topping for the apricots.

Slip them into a recipe. Health-savvy cooks know that they can use applesauce in some baked goods in place of some of the oil called for in the recipe. The next time you reach for the applesauce in one of these instances, use apricot purée instead. Just run some canned apricots through a food processor or blender until they're smooth.

Doctor's Top Tip

You don't have to seek out fresh apricots to enjoy their benefits—dried or canned versions are quite nutritious, too, says Adel Kader, PhD, professor of post-harvest physiology in the department of plant science at University of California, Davis. According to the USDA, five raw apricots contain 3,370 IU of vitamin A and 1,915 micrograms of beta-carotene. A half-cup of canned apricots contains 2,063 IU of vitamin A, and 1,232 micrograms of beta-carotene. And 10 dried apricot halves contain 1,261 IU of vitamin A and 757 micrograms of beta-carotene.

that the lycopene within them might be helpful for fighting cancer makes them even sweeter.

Good for the Eyes

You can also get lots of vitamin A by eating apricots. (The beta-carotene in apricots is converted to vitamin A in the body.) This nutrient helps protect the eyes, and as it turns out, the eyes need all the help they can get.

Every time light passes through the eyes, it triggers the release of tissue-damaging free radicals. Left unchecked, these destructive oxygen molecules attack and damage the lenses of the eyes, possibly setting the stage for cataracts. Free radicals can also attack blood vessels supplying the central portions of the retinas, called the maculas. If the blood supply gets cut off, the result can be macular degeneration, the leading cause of vision loss in older adults.

Vitamin A has been shown in studies to be a powerful antioxidant—that is, it helps block the effects of free radicals. A study of more than 50,000 nurses, for example, found that women who got the most vitamin A in their diets reduced their risk of getting cataracts by more than one-third. Three apricots provide 2,769 IU of vitamin A, 55 percent of the Daily Value (DV) for this vitamin.

Help from Fiber

It's almost impossible to exaggerate the benefits of getting enough fiber in your diet. High-fiber foods can help you lose weight, control high blood sugar, and lower cholesterol levels. They're also essential for keeping digestion regular.

So here's another reason to add apricots to your fruit bowl. Three fruits contain 3 grams of fiber, 12 percent of the DV. Better yet, that's at a minimal calorie cost—just 51 calories for all three. When you're eating apricots for fiber, however, be sure to eat the skin, which contains a substantial amount of the fruit's fiber.

GETTING THE MOST

Eat them firm. Even if you enjoy your fruit nice and soft, it's best to eat apricots while they're still slightly firm. Apricots contain the most nutrients when they're

Dangerous Claims

The idea that apricot pits could be used as medicine dates back to the 1920s, when Dr. Ernst T. Krebs put forth a theory that amygdalin, a compound found in apricot pits that is converted to cyanide in the body, could destroy cancer cells.

Some 30 years later, his son reformulated the extract and named it Laetrile. By the 1970s, people with cancer who felt that they couldn't be helped by modern medicine were traveling to obscure clinics and paying exorbitant prices for this new "miracle" cure. So popular was Laetrile that at one time, it was available in health food stores in 27 states.

Today, Laetrile is not approved by the FDA, although it's readily available in Mexico and other countries. Actor Steve McQueen was treated with the drug in a Mexican clinic shortly before he died of cancer. Does Laetrile work? According to most experts, the answer is an emphatic no.

"Laetrile is not only useless but also potentially fatal," says Maurie Markman, MD, vice president of clinical research at the M. D. Anderson Cancer Center in Houston. Indeed, a study at the Mayo Clinic in Rochester, Minnesota, found that Laetrile frequently caused nausea, vomiting, headache, and other symptoms of cyanide poisoning.

Laetrile is dangerous for another reason, Dr. Markman adds. Some people depend on it instead of turning to a safer and more effective cancer therapy.

at their peak of ripeness; once they start getting soft, these compounds quickly begin to break down.

Shop for color. Unlike most fruits, apricots can be yellow or orange and still be ripe. Both colors are acceptable when you're trying to get the most healing benefits. However, apricots that have green in them were picked early and may never ripen, which means that you lose out on much of their healing goodness.

Store them carefully. It's important to keep apricots cool to prevent them from getting overripe. Unless you're going to eat them within a day or two, it's best to store them in the fruit bin in the refrigerator, where they'll keep for about a week.

Here's another storage tip. Because apricots are such a soft, delicate fruit, they readily pick up flavors—from other fruits they're stored with, for example, or even from refrigerator smells. It's a good idea to store them in a paper or plastic bag.

Apricot-Mango Smoothie

6 apricots, peeled, pitted, and chopped (about 2 cups)

2 ripe mangoes, 10 to 12 ounces each, peeled and chopped (about 2 cups)

1 cup reduced-fat milk or plain low-fat yogurt

4 teaspoons fresh lemon juice

¼ teaspoon vanilla extract

6–8 ice cubes

Lemon peel twists (garnish)

Place the apricots, mangoes, milk or yogurt, lemon juice, and vanilla extract in a blender. Process for 8 seconds. Add the ice cubes, and process 6 to 8 seconds longer, or until smooth.

Pour into tall glasses, garnish with lemon twists, if desired, and serve immediately.

Makes 2 servings (12 ounces each)

PER SERVING

Calories: 213
Total fat: 1.7 g
Saturated fat: 0.9 g

Cholesterol: 6 mg
Sodium: 84 mg
Dietary fiber: 5.5 g

Arthritis

FOODS TO EAT (AND AVOID) FOR JOINT PAIN

Although there isn't a specific food that will help relieve arthritis in all people, doctors today recognize that what you eat—or, in some cases, don't eat—can help ease discomfort and even slow the progression of the disease.

Joints Out of Joint

Arthritis, which causes pain, stiffness, and swelling in and around the joints, isn't just one disease, but many. The most common form of arthritis is osteoarthritis, which is caused by wear and tear on cartilage, the shock-absorbing material between the joints. When cartilage wears away, bone grinds against bone, causing pain and stiffness in the fingers, knees, feet, hips, and back.

A more serious form of the disease is rheumatoid arthritis. It occurs when the immune system, instead of protecting the body, begins attacking it. These attacks cause swelling of the membrane that lines the joints, which eventually eats away at the joints' cartilage. It is the form of arthritis most affected by diet.

The Fat Connection

These days, it's difficult to think of an illness that isn't made worse by a diet high in saturated fats. Arthritis, it appears, is no exception.

A diet low in saturated fats reduces the body's production of prostaglandins, hormonelike substances that contribute to inflammation. In addition, a low-fat diet may hinder communications sent by the immune system, thereby interrupting the body's inflammatory response and helping the joints heal.

Some doctors recommend limiting dietary fat to no more than 25 percent of total calories, with no more than 7 percent of these calories coming from saturated fats. "There's a very simple way to reduce your intake of saturated fats—just don't add them to food," says David Pisetsky, MD, PhD, director of the Duke University Arthritis Center in Durham, North Carolina. "When you have a sandwich, for example, use low-fat mayonnaise instead of the real thing."

Replacing butter, sour cream, and cheese with their lower-fat or fat-free counterparts can also lower your intake of saturated fats. Even if you don't cut them out of your diet completely, just cutting back can make a difference.

Eating a diet that's largely vegetarian can also help reduce the amount of saturated fat that you eat, plus provide other arthritis-relieving benefits, as you'll see later in this chapter.

Fish for Relief

Even though it's generally a good idea to cut back on fats, there is one type of fat that you should consider including in an antiarthritis diet. The omega-3 fatty acids, found primarily in cold-water fish like Spanish mackerel, trout, and salmon, reduce the body's production of prostaglandins and leukotrienes, both substances that contribute to inflammation.

A number of studies have found that fish oil offers benefits to people with rheumatoid arthritis, including less morning stiffness, fewer painful joints, more strength in the hands, and less need for anti-inflammatory drugs.

Scientific studies often require the use of fish oil supplements in order to provide high enough doses of omega-3s. Some experts recommend getting a daily dose of 3 grams of EPA and DHA, which are types of omega-3s, in supplement form. (You'd likely need a very large serving of fish to get an equivalent amount.)

However, you can still get healing benefits from fish oil by eating fish two or three times a week. In addition to the fish mentioned above, bluefin tuna, rainbow trout, halibut, and pollack are also good sources of omega-3 fatty acids. Canned fish such as salmon, herring, sardines, and chunk light tuna are also high in omega-3s.

Nutritional Triggers

Since there's evidence that rheumatoid arthritis is triggered by a faulty immune system, and the immune system is affected by what we eat, it makes sense that, for some people, diet can make a difference in how they feel.

"Diet is critical in the treatment of this form of arthritis," says Joel Fuhrman, MD, a specialist in nutritional medicine at Hunterdon Medical Center in Flemington, New Jersey, and author of *Eat to Live*. "In populations that consume natural diets of mostly unprocessed fruits, vegetables, and grains, autoimmune diseases are almost nonexistent."

For people with rheumatoid arthritis, Dr. Fuhrman recommends a vegan diet—which means no meat or other animal products—that also minimizes the use of wheat, salt, and oils. Instead, you'd eat lots of leafy green vegetables in salads, vegetable-rich soups, and vegetable juice. Dr. Fuhrman also suggests making room for plenty of cruciferous vegetables, such as broccoli and cabbage.

In a study at Norway's University of Oslo, 27 people with rheumatoid arthritis followed a vegetarian diet for 1 year. (After the first 3 to 5 months, they could eat dairy products if they wished.) They also avoided gluten (a protein found in wheat), refined sugar, salt, alcohol, and caffeine. After a month, their joints were less swollen and tender, and they had less morning stiffness and a stronger grip than people who followed their usual diets.

But more may be involved in an arthritis-treating diet than just getting more fruits and vegetables. Some people are sensitive to certain foods—like wheat, dairy foods, corn, citrus fruits, tomatoes, and eggs—which can switch on the body's inflammatory response. For the most part, food sensitivities are rarely involved in arthritis flare-ups, says Dr. Pisetsky. Since there are so many things that can exacerbate the pain of rheumatoid arthritis, knowing which foods, if any, to avoid can be difficult. He recommends starting a food diary so that you can keep track of what you were eating around the time a flare-up occurred. If you discover a pattern—for example, you remember eating tomatoes shortly before an attack—you'll have an idea of what to avoid in the future. Once you've identified a possible culprit, stop eating that food (or foods) for at least 5 days, says Dr. Pisetsky. Then try the food again and see if your symptoms return.

> ## Doctor's Top Tip
>
> If you have rheumatoid arthritis, cut animal protein from your diet, recommends Joel Fuhrman, MD, a specialist in nutritional medicine. A vegetable-based diet can make significant improvements in many cases of arthritis. When you eat meat and other animal foods, the proteins they contain can slip through the walls of your digestive tract and get into your blood circulation, he says. Your body's reaction to these proteins can contribute to autoimmune diseases like rheumatoid arthritis. A diet free of animal protein won't help everyone, but it's a standard part of his approach to treating his patients with this type of arthritis.

Help for Wear and Tear

For years, doctors didn't suspect that there could be a link between diet and osteoarthritis. After all, they reasoned, this condition is a "natural" result of wear and tear on the joints. What could diet possibly do?

According to a preliminary study, however, what you eat can make a difference. Researchers at Boston University School of Medicine studied the eating habits of people with osteoarthritis of the knee. They found that those getting the most vitamin C—more than 200 milligrams a day—were three times less likely to have the disease get worse than those who got the least vitamin C (less than 120 milligrams a day).

Since vitamin C is an antioxidant, it may protect the joints from the damaging effects of free radicals, unstable oxygen molecules that can cause joint inflammation.

"Vitamin C may also help generate collagen, which enhances the body's ability to repair damage to the cartilage," says study leader Timothy McAlindon, MD, MPH, who's now an associate professor of medicine at Tufts University School of Medicine in Boston.

Dr. McAlindon recommends that people get at least 120 milligrams of vitamin C a day in their diets, twice the Daily Value. "That's the amount in a couple of oranges," he says. Other fruits and vegetables rich in vitamin C include cantaloupe, broccoli, strawberries, peppers, and cranberry juice.

But it's not only what you eat that can affect osteoarthritis. It's also how much you weigh.

"There's good evidence that people who are overweight are at increased risk for developing osteoarthritis in weight-bearing joints like the knee," says Dr. Pisetsky. Research also suggests that overweight people are at higher risk for developing osteo-arthritis in non-weight-bearing joints, such as those in the hands. "Losing weight leads to less pain and improved mobility," he says.

Artichokes

HEARTS FOR GOOD HEALTH

HEALING POWER
Can Help:
Provide antioxidants
Protect the heart
Prevent birth defects

When you walk through the produce section of your supermarket, you may view the artichoke as a bit of an oddity. It's actually a member of the thistle family, and the portion you purchase and eat is actually the bud of a flower head!

The artichoke is covered in layers of pointy, green, petal-like leaves called "bracts," which guard a central area called the "choke," which in turn contains the delectable artichoke heart. The fleshy base of the bracts is edible and so, of course, is the heart.

If you've passed by these tasty treats because they look like too much work to enjoy—or just too much like a decorative plant—you've been missing out on a wholesome addition to your diet. Plucking the leaves and plunging them into a dip or sauce is a hands-on, interactive experience—or you can take a shortcut and buy frozen artichoke hearts.

Big Antioxidant Power

As researchers have explored the health benefits of antioxidants in recent years, some have been compiling lists of the antioxidant value of commonly eaten foods.

A survey of more than 1,000 popular foods conducted by Norwegian and American researchers found that artichokes ranked in the top 50 for highest antioxidant content per 100 grams of food. Most of the foods that ranked higher were spices, which you eat in much smaller amounts.

Another survey, headed up by a research unit of the USDA, measured the antioxidant capacity of more than 100 foods. In this study, artichokes again scored high. When its total antioxidant capacity per serving size is taken into account, it beats peppers, apples, blackberries, cherries, plums, and strawberries—and these fruits and veggies aren't slouches when it comes to their antioxidant power.

As the authors note in the study, oxidative stress—or free-radical attacks—has been linked to cancer, heart disease, Alzheimer's disease, and general aging. And studies looking at the use of antioxidants to prevent diseases have found more success in using whole fruits and vegetables than supplements of antioxidants like vitamins C and E and carotenoids.

So as you're assembling an array of fruits and vegetables to improve your anti-oxidant consumption, remember: The artichoke may not be the prettiest on the produce stand, but it's one of the hardest-working, healthwise.

Hearts for Your Heart

As Americans continue to enjoy the convenience of drive-thru, fast-food living, they often come up short on many significant food components, particularly the fiber that only comes from plant foods.

Even though dietary fiber does not have nutritional value, it's of tremendous importance. By adding bulk to the stool, it causes wastes to be excreted from the body more quickly. This is essential for sweeping toxins and cholesterol from the intestinal tract before they cause problems. In addition, getting enough fiber in your diet (the Daily Value, or DV, is 25 grams) can help prevent high cholesterol, heart disease, high blood pressure, high blood sugar (a precursor of diabetes), and certain kinds of cancer, particularly colon cancer.

In the Kitchen

At first glance, the artichoke is kind of like the *New York Times* crossword puzzle—it looks inviting and intriguing, but you may not be sure that you're up to the challenge.

Appearances can be deceptive. If you follow a few easy tips, preparing and eating artichokes is simple.

- When shopping for artichokes, look for those that are bright green—not brown—to ensure freshness and lots of nutrients.
- Dirt readily gets lodged beneath their scaly leaves, so it's important to rinse artichokes thoroughly before cooking them.
- Pull off the tough, outer, lower petals. With a sharp knife, slice off the stems so that they're level with the bottoms of the

artichokes. You can also trim off the spiny tips of the leaves using scissors if you like.

- Stand the artichokes in a large saucepan. Cover them halfway with water and simmer, covered, for 30 to 40 minutes. Or place them on a steaming rack, and steam for the same amount of time.
- To test for doneness, pull on a center petal. If it comes out easily, the artichoke is done.
- To eat the leaves, hold them by the tip, curved side down, and draw them between your teeth to remove the tender flesh.
- When the leaves are gone, use a fork or spoon to scoop out the hairy layer, called the choke. Discard the hairy choke, then dig into the best part—the tender heart.

Artichokes are an excellent fiber source. One medium cooked artichoke contains more than 6 grams of fiber, providing about a quarter of your daily requirement. Even if you don't eat the leaves, you can get plenty of fiber from the hearts alone. Frozen or fresh, a half-cup serving of artichoke hearts delivers about 5 grams of fiber, or 20 percent of the DV.

Artichokes are also a good source of magnesium, a mineral that has been found to be helpful in controlling high blood pressure. Magnesium helps keep muscles running smoothly and lessens the risk of arrhythmia, which is a potentially dangerous variation in the heart's normal rhythm. Studies have shown that 20 to 35 percent of people who have heart failure also have low levels of magnesium.

One medium artichoke delivers 72 milligrams of magnesium, or 18 percent of the DV. A half-cup serving of artichoke hearts alone provides 50 milligrams, nearly 13 percent of the DV.

> ## Doctor's Top Tip
>
> Artichoke hearts are very versatile—so be creative with them, urges Reed Mangels, PhD, RD, a dietitian in Amherst, Massachusetts, and an editor of the *Vegetarian Journal*, a publication of the Vegetarian Resource Group. Try them on salads, in sandwiches, or as a topping for pizza. Or use them to make a spinach artichoke dip.

Filled with Folate

Pregnant women would be especially wise to sink their teeth into the sweet layers of artichokes because, as researchers have discovered, artichokes are loaded with folate, a B vitamin known for its importance in fetal development. Folate is called folic acid when it's included in supplements or added to fortified foods.

According to the Centers for Disease Control and Prevention, up to 70 percent of cases of a birth defect known as neural tube defect may be prevented by women getting enough folic acid before and during pregnancy. Spina bifida, a condition in which the baby's spine doesn't properly form, is an example.

Even if you're not pregnant, folate is an essential nutrient. It helps the nerves function properly, and studies show that it may be important in protecting against heart disease.

Folate and other B vitamins help break down homocysteine, an amino acid in your blood. According to the American Heart Association, homocysteine is related to a higher risk of coronary heart disease and stroke. A diet rich in folate and vitamins B_6 and B_{12} can help lower your levels.

Unfortunately, folate deficiency is one of the most common vitamin deficiencies in this country. We simply don't eat enough okra, spinach, and other folate-rich foods to get the 400 micrograms we need each day.

One medium artichoke contains 61 micrograms of folate, or 15 percent of the DV. A half-cup of artichoke hearts contains about 43 micrograms, which is 11 percent of the DV.

A Burst of C

As with most fruits and vegetables grown in the sun-drenched California soils, artichokes are a good source of vitamin C.

Vitamin C is a potent antioxidant, so it squelches free radicals before they do damage. Studies also show that eating plenty of vitamin C helps maintain healthy skin and strong immunity against bacteria and viruses. One medium artichoke contains about 12 milligrams of vitamin C, or 20 percent of the DV.

GETTING THE MOST

Enjoy the convenience. The one problem that many people have with artichokes is that they're too much work to prepare and eat. Fresh is best, but if you just don't have the time, an easy alternative is to buy a bag of frozen hearts. They're a snap to prepare, and although they lose some nutrients during processing, they actually have more folate than their fresh counterparts.

For vitamin C, eat it fresh. Vitamin C is easily destroyed during processing. So when you're trying to boost your intake of this important vitamin, fresh artichokes are the way to go.

Go easy on the dip. In their natural state, artichokes are a low-fat food—a benefit that's quickly lost when you dip the leaves in butter. To maintain their low-fat profile while still adding a bit of zest, replace the butter with a dip of low-fat yogurt seasoned with garlic or lemon juice. Or dip the leaves into healthy extra-virgin olive oil.

Artichoke Gratin

2 packages (9 ounces each) frozen artichoke hearts

1 tablespoon fresh lemon juice

3 tablespoons plain bread crumbs

1 tablespoon grated Parmesan cheese

1 teaspoon dried Italian herb seasoning

1 clove garlic, minced

1 teaspoon olive oil

Preheat the oven to 375°F. Coat a 9-inch glass pie plate with cooking spray.

Place the artichokes in a colander and rinse well with cold water to separate. Drain well, then pat dry with paper towels. Place in the prepared pie plate, and sprinkle lightly with the lemon juice. Toss to coat.

In a small bowl, combine the bread crumbs, cheese, herb seasoning, garlic, and oil. Toss with a fork to mix. Sprinkle the mixture evenly over the artichokes.

Bake until the topping is golden, 15 to 20 minutes. Serve warm.

Makes 4 servings

Cook's Notes: *Use the artichokes straight from the freezer—there's no need to thaw them. Also, if Italian herb seasoning is unavailable, substitute ½ teaspoon dried oregano, ½ teaspoon dried basil, and a pinch of crushed dried rosemary.*

PER SERVING

Calories: 95	Cholesterol: 1 mg
Total fat: 2.5 g	Sodium: 137 mg
Saturated fat: 0.7 g	Dietary fiber: 7 g

Artificial Sweeteners

SWEETS WITHOUT SIN

Humans have long been looking for ways to satisfy our urge for sweetness. Ancient civilizations used honey, and mankind later learned to glean sugar from sugar cane and other crops. Long ago, when people's daily labors were physically demanding and food wasn't always available, the calories in sugar were more appreciated.

Nowadays, many of us have sedentary jobs and leisure activities. We can generally get food from the nearest refrigerator, vending machine, convenience store, supermarket, or restaurant whenever we want it. Thus, nowadays, we often prefer a calorie-free sweetener to satisfy our sweet tooth.

For decades, people have consumed saccharin (found in Sweet'N Low) and aspartame (found in NutraSweet and Equal) in sodas and as sweeteners for tea, coffee, and other beverages and foods. More recently, other artificial sweeteners have become available: acesulfame potassium (Sweet One and Sunette), sucralose (Splenda), and neotame. In addition to processed foods and drinks, some of these are available as a tabletop sweetener.

Even though such sweeteners tickle the sweet buds on your tongue, they contribute hardly any calories (between 0 and 4, depending on the brand) to your diet. They're much sweeter than sugar—aspartame and acesulfame potassium are 200 times sweeter, sucralose is 600 times sweeter, saccharin is 200 to 700 times sweeter, and neotame is up to 13,000 times sweeter, according to the FDA. So you don't need to use as much of them as you would sugar to get the same sweetness in your foods or drinks.

Because artificial sweeteners are chemically

Doctor's Top Tip

According to the American Dietetic Association, artificial sweeteners will only affect your overall energy balance—or the amount of calories coming into your body versus the ones you burn off with physical activity—if you substitute foods and drinks containing these sweeteners for higher-calorie foods and drinks. In other words, if you consume foods and drinks with calorie-free sweeteners *in addition* to regular ones, you're going to have a harder time losing or maintaining your weight.

One mistake people sometimes make is rewarding themselves for "saving" calories. If you have a diet cola, for example, you'll save over 100 calories and about 30 grams of sugar over the regular kind. But that won't do you any good if you splurge on a high-calorie drink later on, or accompany your diet soda with a candy bar.

---

different from sugar, they don't cause the same problems. When you eat sugary foods, for example, bacteria in your mouth quickly multiply, creating acids that can damage the soft enamel on your teeth. Artificial sweeteners, however, don't encourage these bacteria to grow. So if you substitute artificially sweetened foods for those with "natural" sugar, you'll have a much lower risk of tooth decay.

In addition, artificial sweeteners are a real boon for people with diabetes. Unlike sugar, which can cause dangerous swings in blood sugar, artificial sweeteners don't affect it at all.

Different Sweeteners, Many Concerns

If you enter the names of any of these sweeteners into an Internet search engine, you'll quickly discover many Web pages detailing their alleged dangers. And while a thorough look at these controversial claims might fill a book all by itself, there is some precedent for why people may be wary about sugar substitutes.

In 1969, the FDA banned the use of a sweetener called cyclamate due to concerns that it could raise the risk of bladder cancer. Subsequent research found those concerns to be unfounded, and as of 2007, the FDA was reviewing a petition to reapprove the substance. In the 1970s, the FDA considered banning saccharin over concerns that it was linked to bladder cancer in lab rats. Foods with saccharin had to carry a warning label for many years, though they no longer must do so. However, according to the National Cancer Institute, the effects seen in rats don't apply to humans, and studies on groups of people "have shown no consistent evidence that saccharin is associated with bladder cancer incidence."

According to the FDA, these sweeteners "must be approved as safe before they can be marketed," and "for each of the approved sweeteners, the typical amount used by US consumers is well within designated 'acceptable daily intake levels,' or levels that can be consumed safely every day over a lifetime."

The Artificial Sweetener Blues

Despite their benefit for those with diabetes, artificial sweeteners have actually failed in their main mission—to help people enjoy sweets without gaining weight. If anything, people have been getting heavier since the sugar substitutes were first introduced, says Christina M. Stark, MS, RD, an extension associate at Cornell University in Ithaca, New York.

In a landmark study of more than 80,000 nurses, Harvard researchers found that the single best dietary predictor of weight gain was how much saccharin the women ate. A later study revealed that people who used artificial sweeteners were, on average, 2 pounds heavier than people who did not.

Artificial Sweeteners and Phenylketonuria

Children and adults with a rare condition called phenylketonuria—which prevents them from breaking down an amino acid called phenylalanine—must avoid NutraSweet, which contains phenylalanine.

Eating foods containing this amino acid causes it to build up in the body, where it can cause brain damage and retardation.

A newer sweetener, neotame, is safe for people with this condition, experts say, even though it's similar to aspartame. It doesn't break down into phenylalanine in the body, and foods containing it won't require a warning label for people with phenylketonuria.

Even though artificial sweeteners add little or no calories, they'll only help you lose weight if you use them *instead* of sugar. "Since artificial sweeteners came out, consumption of both regular sugar and artificial sweeteners have gone up," explains Stark. "We just added them to our sugar consumption, so we're getting more total calories."

Artificial sweeteners can help you lose weight if you're smart about using them. You can't assume, for example, that "sugar-free" means "calorie-free." A cake made with artificial sweeteners may not contain sugar calories, but it could have a lot of calories from fats or other carbohydrates besides sugar.

Asian Diet

EAST EATS BETTER

HEALING POWER
Can Help:

Ease menopausal discomfort

Lower cholesterol

Reduce the risk of cancer and heart disease

Improve longevity

Americans spent nearly $2 trillion in 2004 to stay healthier, prevent and treat diseases, and live longer. But if we *really* wanted to improve our health, perhaps we should take some of that money and get on the next boat to China or Japan. Studies show that many people living in Asian countries are slimmer and have lower cholesterol and lower rates of heart disease and cancer than people in America.

The general good health of elderly Okinawans has attracted particular interest in recent years. This island in southwest Japan is home to a much higher percentage of centenarians (people who are at least 100 years old) than you'll find in America. Okinawans also reach an older average age than Americans, and they have lower rates of heart disease and cancer.

Why are Asians traditionally healthier? Although exercise and close family relationships certainly play a role, the main reason appears to be the traditional Asian diet, which has been called the healthiest in the world.

"I saw people eating a diet similar to the Asian diet when I was a young doctor on a plantation in Hawaii, taking care of Filipinos of all generations," recalls John A. McDougall, MD, medical director of the McDougall Program, a residential medical program in Santa Rosa, California, and author of *The McDougall Plan* and other books. "The older, first-generation people never got sick. But their children who adopted American eating habits eventually got fat and got all the diseases we see today."

Nowadays, research is finding that the risk of problems like obesity and breast cancer goes up in Asians who move to America and also in their offspring. And as American-style eating patterns spread around the world, other cultures are starting to see higher numbers of the kinds of health problems that plague the United States.

The traditional Asian diet is surprisingly simple and satisfying. Rice, noodles, breads, and other grains make the foundation, which is topped with generous portions of bok choy, mushrooms, and other fruits and vegetables. The diet also includes beans, seeds, nuts, fish, eggs, and poultry, a few sweets, and occasionally some meat.

Although the term *Asian diet* was taken to mean the foods that the Chinese and Japanese typically eat, in more recent years Americans have become more acquainted with cuisines from Thailand, Korea, and Vietnam. In all of these countries, people enjoy a rich array of foods, but the fundamentals of the Asian diet remain the same.

It's easy to incorporate more foods found in the Asian diet into your own meal plans. At the very least, you can bring the healthy *philosophy* of Asian eating into your usual diet without having to explore unfamiliar dishes.

Where's the Beef?

While the Asian diet has many important components, perhaps the most healthful element is what it doesn't have—specifically, lots of meat and the accompanying saturated fats and cholesterol.

In China, for instance, people eat an average of 4 pounds of beef a year. In Japan, they eat more, about 23 pounds of beef and veal a year. The average American, in contrast, eats more than 60 pounds of beef, plus chicken, pork, and other meats. Americans get approximately 33 percent of their calories from fat, while in Japan, it's only about 11 percent.

As you would expect, cholesterol levels tend to be much lower in Asian countries, at least among people who eat traditional diets. The benefits can be profound, since lower cholesterol levels reduce not only the risk of heart disease but also the risk of cancer.

If you look at typical meals in these countries, you'll tend to see meat used as a condiment or side item, says Lola O'Rourke, RD, a spokesperson for the American Dietetic Association and a nutrition consultant in Seattle. That's in stark contrast with America, where meat is often the centerpiece of the meal, from summer barbecues to holiday dinners.

The Benefits of Soy

It's not only the absence of meat and highly processed foods that makes the Asian diet so healthful. People in Asian countries also eat a lot of soy foods—3 to 4 ounces a day of tempeh, tofu, defatted soy flour, and more.

There are several reasons that soy foods are so healthful, says Christopher Gardner, PhD, assistant professor of medicine at the Stanford Prevention Research Center in Stanford, California. They're rich in a group of natural compounds called phytoestrogens, which the body converts into hormonelike substances that act like a weak form of estrogen. These faux estrogens block the body's estrogen receptors, lowering the amount of estrogen in the body. This may help lower the risk of breast cancer in premenopausal women, particularly if they've been eating soy foods since an early age, but studies are inconclusive.

Later in life, the phytoestrogens in soy may ease menopausal symptoms such as hot flashes but not vaginal dryness by replacing the estrogen lost during this time. In fact, Asian women rarely experience hot flashes. (However, research looking into a connection between phytoestrogens and hot flashes hasn't demonstrated much effectiveness.) Asian women are also less likely than American women to have heart disease, which may be due to the low-fat, high-fiber nature of soy, not the phytoestrogens.

Natural Goodness

The National Cancer Institute has been preaching "five or more fruits and vegetables a day," and nutritionists have been begging us to get the Daily Value of 25 grams of fiber instead of the paltry 11 to 12 grams most of us get each day.

The Asian diet, which is packed with fresh fruits, vegetables, and other fiber-rich foods, is on the cutting edge and sets an enviable standard. In China, for example, many people get 33 grams of fiber every day. That's serious heart protection, according to researchers at the Harvard School of Public Health, who in a 6-year study of almost 41,000 men found that those who increased their daily fiber intake by just 10 grams were able to decrease their risk of heart disease by almost 30 percent.

Each day, the average Okinawan eats seven servings of vegetables, two to four servings of fruit, and seven servings of grains, says O'Rourke.

These fruits and vegetables are also rich sources of vitamin C, carotenoids (including beta-carotene), and other antioxidant compounds that help protect the body from disease. "We see again and again that people who eat lots of plant-based foods tend to have lower rates of chronic diseases, like heart disease and cancer," she says.

Doctor's Top Tip

Although the traditional Asian diet includes many of the foods that you probably eat every day, there is one notable exception: You won't find a lot of milk, cheese, or other dairy foods. This is one reason that Asian diets are so low in fat. It also may explain why Asians' bones aren't as strong as they could be.

Even though you can get a lot of calcium from plant foods like bok choy and broccoli, most scientists agree that dairy foods play a critical role in keeping bones strong. In fact, when researchers compared calcium intake and bone density, they found that women who got their calcium largely from dairy foods had bone densities 20 percent higher than those who got their calcium mainly from plant foods.

"Bone density is a concern in countries like China," explains Robert M. Russell, MD, director and senior scientist at the Jean Mayer USDA Human Nutrition Research Center on Aging at Tufts University in Boston. So even if you find yourself following a traditional Asian diet, be sure to supplement it with low-fat milk and cheese, and other reduced-fat dairy foods, he says.

A Cup of Health

The next time you walk into an Asian restaurant, order a pot of tea. But don't stop with one cup. At home, make some tea to accompany your meal. Research suggests that having 4 small cups of tea a day can substantially lower your risk of heart disease and stroke. Asians drink tea by the potful, which may explain their robust good health.

Tea contains potent antioxidant compounds called phenols, which protect the body from disease. In a study of 552 men, researchers in the Netherlands found that those who drank about 5 cups of black tea a day had about one-third the risk of stroke of those drinking fewer than 2½ cups. Green tea, the kind preferred in Eastern countries, has even more antioxidant power than black tea.

A meta-analysis (or a type of study that evaluates the results of many previous studies) of studies on green tea conducted at the University of Minnesota found that those who drank the most green tea had a 22 percent lower risk of breast cancer. Several studies from Japan and China have shown an association between greater green tea consumption and lower risk of stomach cancer. And laboratory studies have found evidence that suggests that green tea can help lower the risk of prostate cancer.

In the world of antioxidants, the phenols in tea are "absolutely exquisite," says Gary Stoner, PhD, professor and cancer researcher at Ohio State University in Columbus.

Fishy Business

Japan and Okinawa are islands, which means that people there eat a lot of fish. Numerous studies show that even small amounts of fish, as little as 3 ounces a week, provide powerful protection. "Fish contains fats that thin the blood and help prevent heart disease," says Dr. McDougall.

According to the *Journal of the American Medical Association*, the omega-3 fatty acids in fish—especially oily fish like salmon, tuna, and herring—can help lower your blood pressure and heart rate. Omega-3s also reduce your risk of heart disease, may lower your risk of stroke, and may help protect you from cognitive decline in your later years. Another way fish can help protect your heart is by providing a good source of protein without the saturated fat that you'd get from red meat.

The American Heart Association recommends that people eat fish—especially the fish high in omega-3s—at least twice a week. (See page 256 for some mercury cautions, however.)

Eat Just the Right Amount

The Okinawans use the phrase *hara hachi bu,* which means only eating until one is 80 percent full. Using this philosophy helps you avoid overeating and taking in unnecessary calories at a meal, says O'Rourke. Thus it's a useful tool for keeping yourself at a normal weight and avoiding the added risks for cancer and heart disease that obesity causes.

It takes your brain about 20 to 30 minutes to know that you've had enough to eat, says O'Rourke. So as you enjoy your meal, take a moment to think, "Am I almost full yet?" If so, stop eating. In just a few minutes, you'll probably feel completely satisfied—and happy that you didn't keep eating until you were uncomfortably stuffed.

GETTING THE MOST

Make the meat hard to find. Whenever you prepare a meal, use large amounts of plant foods and small amounts of meat, O'Rourke suggests. If you're making a stir-fry, fill the skillet 80 percent full of vegetables, with just a little chicken or pork thrown in. Serve the stir-fry over brown, not white, rice.

Even non-Asian meals will benefit from this treatment. Instead of adding a pound or more of ground beef to your spaghetti sauce, stir in chopped-up mushrooms, onions, peppers, and tomatoes instead, and serve the sauce over whole-wheat pasta or noodles.

Investigate the world of soy. A wide variety of soy foods are now available at supermarkets, ranging from soy milk to edamame (fun-to-eat soybeans that come in the pod or frozen and shelled) to soy "crumbles" that look like browned ground beef. It's easy to reap the benefits of this Asian staple by incorporating these foods into your familiar meals.

Make the switch. Start replacing your usual cans of soda or cups of coffee with green tea until you're up to a couple of cups of green tea each day.

Asian Noodles with Vegetables

1 egg, lightly beaten

9 ounces dry eggless chow mein noodles or baked ramen noodles

1 tablespoon canola oil

1 tablespoon minced garlic

4 cups thinly sliced bok choy stems and leaves

1 medium carrot, shredded

1 tablespoon reduced-sodium soy sauce

1 teaspoon sugar

1 teaspoon dark sesame oil

Coat a small nonstick skillet with cooking spray. Warm over medium heat. Add the egg, and swirl the pan so the egg coats the bottom. Cook for about 1 minute, or until almost set. Carefully turn and cook a few seconds until the egg is set on the bottom. Remove from the pan, and place on a cutting board to cool slightly. Roll up tightly, and cut into strips. Set aside.

Cook the noodles (discard the seasoning packet or reserve for another use) in a pot of boiling water for 3 minutes, or according to the package directions. Drain, rinse with cold water, and drain again. Set aside.

In a large nonstick skillet or wok heat the canola oil over medium heat. Add the garlic and cook for 30 seconds, or until fragrant. Add the bok choy and carrot. Stir-fry until the bok choy starts to wilt, 1 to 2 minutes. Add the noodles, soy sauce, sugar, and sesame oil. Cook, tossing until the noodles are heated through, 1 to 2 minutes. Add the reserved egg strips, and toss to combine.

Makes 4 servings

PER SERVING

Calories: 338	Cholesterol: 53 mg
Total fat: 7.2 g	Sodium: 197 mg
Saturated fat: 1 g	Dietary fiber: 3.9 g

Asparagus
SPEARS OF PROTECTION

HEALING POWER
Can Help:

Prevent birth defects

Reduce the risk of heart disease and cancer

Keep skin and other tissues healthy

Support healthy eyes

Maintain a healthy immune system

People have called this vegetable a lot of things over the centuries: Ancient Greeks and Romans called it asparagus, and its name in English evolved from "sperage" to "sparrow grass," and then back to its original name. Now many people call it a delicious treat that's perfectly shaped for dipping.

The slim green rods with the "braided" tips give a great health boost, too, since asparagus contains compounds that can help fight birth defects, heart disease, and cancer and can help strengthen your immune system and help your skin and other tissues.

Filled with Folate

One of the most critical medical breakthroughs of the 20th century was the discovery that the incidence of brain and spinal cord birth defects (called neural tube defects) could be cut in half if women who are of childbearing age got 400 micrograms of folate a day.

Asparagus is richly endowed with folate, a B vitamin that is essential for helping cells regenerate. Five asparagus spears contain 110 micrograms of folate, about 28 percent of the Daily Value (DV).

If you're pregnant, you may want to enjoy a double serving of the green spears. Although the government recommends that adults get 400 micrograms of folate daily, pregnant women need 600 micrograms daily, and women who are breastfeeding need 500, according to the National Institutes of Health.

Not only is folate good for women who are in their childbearing years, this vitamin also appears to fight heart disease in everyone. Folate may act as a floodgate, controlling the amount of homocysteine (an amino acid that appears to damage the lining of arteries) that's in the bloodstream. When your folate levels drop, your homocysteine levels rise, which can cause damage to the arteries supplying blood to your heart and brain.

The American Heart Association isn't yet calling high homocysteine in the blood a major risk factor for heart disease like high cholesterol or blood pressure, but it does recommend that you get plenty of folate in your diet.

And research is beginning to show possible connections between folate intake, homocysteine, and risk of cognitive problems, particularly Alzheimer's disease. One review of data on a large group of people found that their risk of Alzheimer's was doubled if they had elevated homocysteine levels.

Getting sufficient folate in your diet is also associated with a lower risk of some cancers, particularly colorectal, cervical, and breast cancer. Studies have shown that people with the most folate in their blood are the ones least likely to develop colon cancer.

Protection against Cancer

As you've come to expect from green vegetables, asparagus offers powerful protection against cancer. It contains a number of compounds that essentially double-team cancer-causing substances before they do harm.

In addition to folate, another protective compound in asparagus is glutathione, a powerful antioxidant. This means that it helps mop up free radicals, which are altered oxygen molecules that, when left unchecked, ricochet wildly through the body, scarring and punching holes in cells, and doing the types of damage that can lead to cancer, atherosclerosis, and many other conditions. In an analysis of 38 vegetables, freshly cooked asparagus ranked first for its glutathione content.

FOOD ALERT
Strange Smells

It's not something that will send you running to the emergency room, but you may have noticed a curious fact about asparagus. After you eat even a small amount, your urine seems to have an unpleasant odor.

It's not your imagination. Asparagus contains an amino acid called aspartic acid. Many people lack the enzyme needed to break aspartic acid down. As a result, it stays in the body and gets converted to a related compound—one with that distinctive sulfurous smell.

While there isn't a "cure" for this telltale aroma, neither is it anything worth worrying about. So have an extra helping of asparagus, enjoy all those health-preserving nutrients it contains, and ignore the temporary odor.

In the Kitchen

Asparagus is among the easiest vegetables to prepare and cook. What's more, its natural freshness means that you don't need butter or sauces to bring out its flavors. To enjoy great taste with little effort, here's what cooks advise.

Check the tips. When buying asparagus, take a close look at the tips. Fresh asparagus tips are compact and tightly furled. If the tips look loose and frayed, the asparagus is getting old, and you should pass it by.

Remove the stalk. Although you can eat asparagus from top to bottom, the tough, woody stalk is usually discarded. The easiest way to do this is simply to bend the stalk; asparagus naturally snaps off at the point where the tough end stops and the tender part begins.

When the spears are thick, however, the snap method can waste perfectly good flesh. To preserve more of the stalk, use a vegetable peeler to peel the bottom area of each spear. Use a knife to find the point where the flesh turns woody (it will be tough to slice) and cut the bottom off there.

A Dose of Vitamin C

A cup of raw asparagus (just the tender tips—not the tougher base ends) contains 7.5 milligrams of vitamin C, which is roughly 13 percent of the DV for this vitamin. This is more vitamin C than you'll find in a cup of canned peaches, a cup of plums, a cup of carrots, or a pear.

Vitamin C is a valuable antioxidant, neutralizing free radicals throughout your body. It also plays an important role in maintaining the integrity of collagen, which is found in your bones, the walls of your arteries, and elsewhere in your body.

Load Up on Vitamin A

A cup of raw asparagus also contains 1,013 IU of vitamin A, which is a sizeable 21 percent of your DV for this vitamin. Not only does vitamin A help maintain the health of your eyes, it actually plays a role in the transmission of images from your eyes to your brain.

Vitamin A also helps maintain the integrity of epithelial tissues that line surfaces inside and outside of your body, such as your skin, the lining of your digestive system, and the lining of your lungs. This helps them maintain their status as a barrier against germs that are always trying to enter your body.

Doctor's Top Tip

Since most of asparagus's nutrients are in the tip, if you're going to cook it on the stovetop, it's better to cook it upright in a tall container than piling it at the bottom of a baking dish, says Gertrude Armbruster, PhD, RD, of Cornell University. Add a few inches of water to the pot, cover with a lid, and bring to a simmer. Keeping the tips out of the water will not only preserve nutrients but will also help the stalks cook evenly and more quickly.

The vitamin also helps keep your immune system working properly, perhaps by helping lymphocytes—a type of white blood cell—do a better job of battling infections, according to the National Institutes of Health.

GETTING THE MOST

Store it carefully. Folate is destroyed by exposure to air, heat, or light, so you need to store asparagus carefully, says Gertrude Armbruster, PhD, RD, professor emeritus of nutritional science at Cornell University in Ithaca, New York. She recommends storing it away from light in the back of the refrigerator or in a produce drawer.

Cook it gently. Asparagus is a tender vegetable, and vigorous boiling isn't necessary. "Microwaving asparagus definitely destroys fewer nutrients than does boiling or even steaming," says Dr. Armbruster. A USDA survey that measured the antioxidants in commonly eaten foods found that boiled asparagus was "significantly lower" in water-soluble antioxidants than raw asparagus. Its total antioxidant capacity dropped from 2,021 units per serving when raw down to 1,480 when boiled.

Asparagus, Spring Onion, and Mushroom Pasta

1 **pound thin asparagus**

¾ **pound mushrooms (morel, cremini, oyster, or a mixture)**

2 **tablespoons extra-virgin olive oil**

¼ **pound spring onions (or scallions or baby leeks), trimmed and sliced**

¼ **cup dry white wine**

½ **cup vegetable broth**

4 **tablespoons unsalted butter**

Sea salt and freshly ground black pepper

8 **ounces dry pappardelle or fettuccine**

1 **tablespoon chopped flat-leaf parsley**

Cut off the tough ends of the asparagus and slice crosswise into 2-inch pieces. Trim the tough stems from the mushrooms. If the mushrooms are dirty, quickly rinse in cold water and pat dry before slicing into bite-size pieces.

In a large skillet, heat the oil over medium-high heat. Add the mushrooms and cook, stirring, until lightly browned, about 5 minutes.

Add the onions and cook until softened, 1 to 2 minutes. Add the asparagus and cook, stirring, for 2 minutes. Add the wine and simmer until the liquid has evaporated, 1 to 2 minutes. Add the vegetable broth and bring to a boil. Add the butter and toss until melted into the vegetables. Season to taste with salt and pepper.

Meanwhile, in a large pot of boiling, salted water, cook the pasta according to package direcctions until al dente. Drain and transfer to a large bowl. Mix in the sauce and the parsley. Season to taste with additional salt and pepper.

Makes 4 servings

PER SERVING

Calories: 436	Cholesterol: 30 mg
Total fat: 20 g	Sodium: 104 mg
Saturated fat: 8 g	Dietary fiber: 4.5 g

Asthma

FOODS FOR EASY BREATHING

If you have asthma, it doesn't take much: A fast walk, a sudden shot of cold air, or even a whiff of pollen can cause airways inside your lungs to narrow suddenly, making each breath seem unbelievably precious.

But asthma can be controlled. A vital part of the strategy is what you eat. "Diet is the key," says Richard N. Firshein, DO, medical director of the Firshein Center for Comprehensive Medicine in New York City and author of *Reversing Asthma*.

Fighting Inflammation

Much of the battle against asthma is a battle against inflammation. When pollen, pollution, or other airborne irritants enter the lungs, the immune system releases chemicals to confront the invaders. Unfortunately, the chemicals that are meant to defend you can actually do a lot of harm. They cause the airways to become inflamed and swollen, which makes breathing difficult. At the same time, the body releases clouds of free radicals, the harmful oxygen molecules that make the inflammation even worse. This is why, in people with asthma, the airways tend to stay inflamed long after the attack is over.

One way to stop asthma is to reduce the inflammation. There's some evidence that foods high in vitamin C and other antioxidants, which block the effects of free radicals, can help the airways return to normal. "We know an asthma attack is inflammatory, and we know it produces a lot of oxygen radicals," says Gary E. Hatch, PhD, a research pharmacologist and branch chief of the pulmonary toxicology branch of the Environmental Protection Agency. "So antioxidants should help."

Three antioxidants that are thought to have special protective power against asthma are vitamins C and E and the trace mineral selenium. In addition, there are a number of foods, such as cold-water, fatty fish, that have been shown to reduce inflammation throughout your body, including in the lungs.

Giving Asthma the Juice

Studies on large groups of people have found a relationship between a diet rich in fruits and improved lung function. As a result, some experts think it's a good idea for people with asthma to eat a diet that supplies an ample amount of the antioxidant nutrient vitamin C.

Two large studies, the National Health and Nutrition Examination Surveys, found that people who got the most vitamin C in their diets were much less likely to have respiratory diseases, including asthma, than those who got the least.

In a British study, researchers compared the diets of 515 adults with asthma to 515 adults without the condition. Compared with people who ate no citrus fruits, those who ate just a small amount each day had roughly 40 percent less risk of diagnosed asthma. Also, the more vitamin C the diet contained, the less risk that subjects would have symptomatic asthma.

It doesn't take a lot of vitamin C to get the benefits, says Dr. Hatch. Research suggests that getting 200 milligrams a day—less than four times the Daily Value (DV) of 60 milligrams—will go a long way toward keeping your lungs strong. A 6-ounce glass of freshly squeezed orange juice, for example, delivers 93 milligrams of vitamin C, a third more than the DV. Other super sources include other citrus fruits and juices, red and green bell peppers, broccoli, Brussels sprouts, and strawberries.

Doctor's Top Tip

Remember that airborne allergens and irritants aren't the only asthma triggers—foods can set off an attack, too, according to experts at the American Academy of Allergy, Asthma and Immunology. If you've ever suspected that a food such as peanuts, tree nuts, soy, wheat, milk, eggs, or seafood was to blame for an attack, approach it with caution in the future.

Breathe Deep with E

Research suggests that vitamin E can dramatically lower your risk of asthma. In a large study of 75,000 nurses, for example, Harvard University researchers found that those getting the most vitamin E in their diets were 47 percent less likely to have asthma than those getting the least.

The advantage of vitamin E is that it appears to target free radicals that are caused by air pollution, a common asthma trigger. In addition, vitamin E stimulates the release of chemicals that help relax muscles that make up the airways in the lungs. As with vitamin C, it doesn't take a lot of vitamin E to get the benefits. In the nurses' study, for example, women in the low-asthma group were getting no more than the DV of 30 IU.

Since vitamin E is found mainly in cooking oils, however, it's not always easy to get the necessary amounts. Perhaps the best way to get more of this nutrient in your diet is to put wheat germ on the menu by adding it to other foods, like muffins or meat loaf. One serving of wheat germ has 5 IU of vitamin E, nearly 17 percent of the DV. Vitamin E is also in almonds, sunflower seeds, whole-grain cereals, spinach, and kale.

A Nutty Solution

Selenium is one of the trace minerals, which means that you don't need a lot of it. Research suggests, however, that a little selenium goes a long way, especially for people with asthma. Selenium is an ingredient in a natural antioxidant enzyme, glutathione peroxidase, which keeps free radicals from forming.

In a study of 115 people, researchers in New Zealand found that those getting the most selenium in their diets were five times less likely to have asthma than those getting the least. In a British study comparing the diets of people with asthma to the diets of people without the disease, researchers found that those who got the most selenium had about 44 percent less risk of the disease.

The DV for selenium is 70 micrograms. Meats, chicken, and seafood are good selenium selections. Even better, one Brazil nut contains 120 micrograms.

Cut Out the Salt

Some research has indicated that if you have asthma, consuming a diet high in sodium may worsen your condition. Conversely, a low-sodium diet may reduce the severity of a problem common in people with asthma called exercise-induced bronchorestriction, in which symptoms are triggered by exercise.

Although more studies are needed to further test the relationship between sodium and asthma, a low-sodium diet is known to bring other health benefits, such as a reduced risk of high blood pressure. If you have asthma, consider trying a low-sodium diet—such as the DASH diet discussed in the blood pressure chapter of this book—in addition to your normal treatment regimen. Eating a diet rich in fruits and vegetables and low in processed foods is a good way to eat less sodium.

Catching Your Breath

Finally, you might try fishing for asthma relief at your local fish market. Studies show that the omega-3 fatty acids found in oily fish such as salmon and sardines can help reduce inflammation in the lungs. What's more, these oils appear to reduce the tissue damage that often follows asthma attacks, says Dr. Firshein. In one large survey, Australian researchers found that in families where people ate very little oily fish, almost 16 percent of the children had asthma. In families where these fish were frequently on the menu, however, only 9 percent of the children had asthma. And in families where no fish was served, the rate of asthma in children was 23 percent.

Interestingly, Americans eat roughly 20 times more omega-6 fatty acids—which are found in soy, corn, safflower, and sunflower oils—than omega-3s. In general, omega-6s *promote* inflammation in the body, and omega-3s dampen it. Thus, the usual American diet may actually play a contributing role in some cases of asthma.

Avocados

NO LONGER A FORBIDDEN FRUIT

HEALING POWER

Can Help:

Control cholesterol

Lower blood pressure

Prevent birth defects

Maintain bone and immune health

The usual image you apply to fruit—light, low-calorie, and virtually fat-free—doesn't apply to the avocado. Within the dense, dark green mass of an avocado lurk a lot of calories—360 or more. And it also has the dubious distinction of being one of the few fruits with a measurable fat content, with around 30 grams each. That's nearly half the daily recommended amount for an average adult.

You wouldn't think that a food that's so fattening could be good for you. But that's the word from dietitians, who say that adding a little avocado to your diet could actually improve your health.

Avocados are great sources of folate and potassium. They also contain high amounts of fiber and monounsaturated fat, both of which are good news for people who are concerned about diabetes or heart health.

Part of a Diabetes Diet

People with diabetes have traditionally been told to eat more carbohydrates and cut back on fat. Overall that's good advice, but it's not necessarily the best advice for everyone.

Doctors have discovered that when some people who have diabetes eat a lot of carbohydrates, they tend to develop high levels of triglycerides, a type of blood fat that may contribute to heart disease. Surprisingly, when people replace some of those carbohydrates with fat, particularly the kind of fat found in avocados, the dangerous fats in the bloodstream tend to decline.

Avocados are a rich source of monounsaturated fats, particularly a kind called oleic acid. "We've found that these monounsaturated fats improve fat levels in the body and help control diabetes," says Abhimanyu Garg, MD, professor in the Center for Human Nutrition at the University of Texas Southwestern Medical Center at Dallas.

A study from the Oregon Health and Science University put 11 people with type 2 diabetes on a low-fat, high-carb diet and on a diet high in monounsaturated fat, each for 6 weeks. Subjects' total cholesterol and LDL (bad) cholesterol tended to

FOOD ALERT

Easy on the Avocados if You're Taking this Drug

People who are taking warfarin (Coumadin), a heart medication designed to keep blood from clotting, should go easy on the avocados. Though scientists aren't sure why, the natural oil in avocado seems to prevent the drug from working, at least in some people.

In one small study, researchers in Israel found that eating between one-half and one avocado could make the drug work less efficiently. While the effects didn't last long—when people stopped eating avocado, the drug started working better again—this could be dangerous for some people. So if you're taking warfarin, check with your doctor before adding avocados to your meals.

go down with each diet. Their triglyceride levels, blood sugar control, and insulin sensitivity were about the same with each diet, too.

In an earlier study, scientists in Mexico put 16 women with diabetes on a relatively high-fat diet, with about 40 percent of calories coming from fat. Most of the fat came from avocados. The result was a 20 percent drop in triglycerides. Women on a higher-carbohydrate plan, by contrast, had only a 7 percent drop in triglycerides.

"What's nice about avocados is that they provide a lot of these monounsaturated fats," adds Dr. Garg. Someone on a 2,000-calorie-a-day diet, for example, might be advised to eat 33 grams of monounsaturated fat. "You can get about 20 grams from just one avocado," he points out.

Help for High Cholesterol

People with diabetes aren't the only ones who benefit from eating a little more avocado. The oleic acid in avocados can also help people lower their cholesterol.

In a small study from Mexico, where guacamole is considered almost a food group, researchers compared the effects of two low-fat diets. The diets were the same except that one included avocados. While both lowered levels of dangerous low-density lipoprotein (LDL) cholesterol, the avocado diet raised levels of healthful high-density lipoprotein (HDL) cholesterol while slightly lowering triglycerides.

Another way in which avocados help lower cholesterol is by adding healthful amounts of fiber to the diet, adds Dr. Garg. Fiber adds bulk to the stool, causing it, and the cholesterol it contains, to be excreted from the body more quickly. One avocado packs more fiber than a bran muffin—10 grams, or 40 percent of the Daily Value (DV) for fiber.

More Help for Your Heart

Avocados also pack a big potassium punch. Half an avocado provides 548 milligrams of potassium, 16 percent of the DV for this mineral. That's more than you'd get in a medium banana or a cup of orange juice.

Studies show that people who eat diets high in potassium-rich foods like avocados have a markedly lower risk of high blood pressure and related diseases like heart attack and stroke.

In addition, some research has shown that oleic acid can reduce markers of inflammation in your body. Inflammation plays an important role in the development of artery-clogging atherosclerosis.

A Fortune in Folate

Avocados may be one of the perfect foods when you're eating for two, particularly when it comes to getting enough folate, a B vitamin that helps prevent life-threatening birth defects of the brain and spine. Many women don't get enough folate in their diets, but avocados can go a long way toward fixing that. Half an avocado contains 57 micrograms of folate, 14 percent of the DV, or nearly 10 percent of the 600 micrograms that pregnant women need daily.

Moms-to-be aren't the only ones who should be dipping their chips in guacamole, though. Everyone needs folate. It's an essential nutrient for keeping nerves functioning properly. It may also help fight heart disease by reducing levels of

In the Kitchen

A lot of people have never picked, prepared, or eaten an avocado. But they're very easy to work with. Here are a few hints for getting started:

Help them ripen. Like bananas, avocados ripen better off the tree, so they are picked and sold unripe. Once you get them home, leave them on the counter for several days or until the fruit is slightly soft. Or, if you're in a hurry to use them, place them in a paper bag with an apple or banana to soften. Never place hard avocados in the refrigerator, or they will ripen too slowly.

Make a pit stop. To open an avocado, cut it lengthwise, rotating the knife all the way around the seed. Then twist the halves in opposite directions to separate them. To remove the pit, slip the tip of a spoon underneath, and pry it free. Or poke the tip of a knife into it and twist.

Doctor's Top Tip

Avocado tends to turn brown when it's exposed to air, says Reed Mangels, PhD, RD, a dietitian in Amherst, Massachusetts, and an editor of the *Vegetarian Journal*, a publication of the Vegetarian Resource Group. This discoloration doesn't hurt anything—it just looks unattractive. If you're setting out an avocado dish that you might not eat for a while—like guacamole—mix a little lemon juice with the avocado to preserve its green color.

homocysteine, an amino acid that's harmful to blood vessels if it gets too high.

Minerals for Your Bones

If you're concerned about bone health, think avocado. A cup of mashed avocado contains 120 milligrams of phosphorus, which is 12 percent of the DV. This mineral is a major component of your bones and teeth, and having plenty of phosphorus on hand also helps your body produce energy from the foods you eat.

Think Zinc for Good Nutrition

You'll also find 1.47 milligrams of zinc swimming in the green depths of a cup of mashed avocado. That's just under 10 percent of the DV. Zinc conducts countless activities in your body. The mineral helps keep your immune system working properly, for example, and plays a role in wound healing.

Zinc also aids in your senses of smell and taste, which are necessary if you want to fully enjoy the recipes throughout this book!

GETTING THE MOST

Find fruit from Florida. Even though the monounsaturated fat in avocados is good for your cholesterol, it's not so good for your waistline. To get the nutrients from avocado without all the fat, shop for Florida avocados. They have about two-thirds the calories and half the fat of Hass avocados grown in California.

Know when to buy them. A good way to find avocados with a little less fat is to buy those harvested between November and March. They may have one-third the fat of those picked in September or October.

Avocado-Jícama Salad

- 2 **cups peeled, matchstick-cut jícama**
- ¼ **cup fresh orange juice**
- 2 **tablespoons finely chopped onions**
- 1 **small serrano pepper, sliced (wear plastic gloves when handling)**
- ⅛ **teaspoon chili powder**
- 1 **Florida avocado**
- 1 **tablespoon chopped fresh cilantro**

Place the jícama on a serving plate.

In a small bowl, mix the orange juice, onions, pepper, and chili powder. Pour about half of the dressing over the jícama, and toss to coat. Spread the jícama out evenly on the plate.

Cut through the avocado lengthwise, then twist gently to separate the halves. Remove the pit and discard it. Peel each half of the avocado, then cut it into thin lengthwise slices. Arrange the slices in spoke fashion on the bed of jícama.

Drizzle with the remaining dressing. With the back of the spoon, spread the dressing gently over the avocado slices to cover thoroughly. Cover and refrigerate for 15 to 30 minutes. Sprinkle with the cilantro.

Makes 4 servings

PER SERVING

Calories: 121	Cholesterol: 0 mg
Total fat: 6.9 g	Sodium: 9 mg
Saturated fat: 1.4 g	Dietary fiber: 4 g

Bananas

A BUNCH OF POTASSIUM

HEALING POWER

Can Help:

Decrease risk of heart disease and stroke

Lower high blood pressure

Relieve heartburn

Speed recovery from diarrhea

We seem to take bananas for granted. They're a commonly accepted punch line, guaranteed for a laugh when someone slips on a banana peel. We say we're "going bananas" when we feel out-of-sorts. Harry Belafonte is famous for singing about them.

And bananas make few demands on our attention. They're simple to eat—they don't get your hands messy or dribble juice as you eat them—and they're extremely portable. The average American eats about 30 pounds of the fruit each year. And, according to the American Diabetes Association, they outsell apples, which are as American as, well, apple pie.

It's time to honor the banana instead of laughing at it, or stripping its peel and eating it without a second thought! Studies have shown that the fruit beneath that slippery skin can do wonders for our health.

Bananas for the Heart

If the needle on the blood pressure cuff has been inching up in recent years, it may be time for a tropical vacation. If the sun and surf don't bring your pressure down, the bananas sure will.

Bananas are one of nature's best sources of potassium, with a large banana providing about 487 milligrams, or 14 percent of the Daily Value (DV) for this essential mineral. Study after study shows that people who eat foods rich in potassium have a significantly lower risk of high blood pressure and related diseases like heart attack and stroke.

According to the National Institutes of Health, by adopting its DASH diet—which is rich in fruits and vegetables that provide potassium—you can lower your systolic blood pressure (the top number) by 8 to 14 millimeters of mercury.

Even if you already have high blood pressure, eating plenty of bananas may significantly reduce or even eliminate your need for blood pressure medication, according to scientists at the University of Naples in Italy. Researchers believe that one of the ways that bananas keep blood pressure down is by helping to prevent plaque from sticking to artery walls. They do this by keeping the bad low-density lipoprotein cholesterol from oxidizing, a chemical process that makes it more likely to accumulate. That's why bananas may be a good defense against atherosclerosis, or hardening of the arteries, another contributor to high blood pressure, heart attack, and stroke.

And the best part is that you don't have to eat a boatload of bananas to get these benefits, says David B. Young, PhD, professor emeritus of physiology and biophysics at the University of Mississippi Medical Center in Jackson.

"Studies show that you can get a significant impact from relatively small changes," says Dr. Young. "My advice would be to think of potassium-rich foods like love and money: You can never get too much."

Stomach Relief

According to the National Library of Medicine, bananas can help relieve heartburn and upset stomach. They do this by encouraging your stomach to produce more of the mucus that naturally protects it from the acidic digestive fluid it contains. And as you'll see below, bananas can soothe and encourage the normal function of other digestive organs, too!

Doctor's Top Tip

Morning is a great time to get the benefits of an easy-to-eat banana, according to the National Heart, Lung, and Blood Institute. Some statistics say that more than 35 percent of Americans don't eat breakfast, most likely because they're in a rush. The NHLBI offers meal plans to show people how to eat a low-sodium diet to maintain good blood pressure. By combining a medium banana with a bowl of bran flakes, low-fat milk, a slice of whole-wheat bread with trans-fat-free margarine, and a cup of orange juice, you get a quick breakfast that's high in fiber and potassium and low in sodium.

Restoring Balance

When you've been run ragged by a case of the runs, it's important that you replenish all the vital fluids and nutrients that diarrhea depletes. And a banana is just the food to do it, says William Ruderman, MD, a gastroenterologist in Orlando, Florida.

"Bananas are a very good source of electrolytes, like potassium, which you lose when you become dehydrated," he explains. Electrolytes are minerals that turn into electrically charged particles in the body, helping to control almost everything that happens inside, from muscle contractions and fluid balance to the beating of the heart.

Bananas are also the bland type of food that the National Institute of Diabetes and Digestive and Kidney Diseases recommends as you're recuperating from a bout of diarrhea. Along with bananas, they suggest centering your recovery meals around rice, toast, crackers, baked skinless chicken, and cooked carrots.

Bananas also contain some pectin, a soluble fiber that acts like a sponge in the digestive tract, absorbing fluids and helping to keep diarrhea in check.

Promote Digestive Health

Though bananas may not "feel" like a food that's high in fiber as you're eating them, the yellow fruit is actually a decent source of fiber. One large banana contains 3.5 grams of fiber, or 14 percent of the DV for fiber.

A diet rich in fiber may help protect you from a variety of diseases ranging from potentially fatal conditions like heart disease and cancer to problems in the digestive organs, like appendicitis, diverticulosis, and hemorrhoids.

GETTING THE MOST

Buy a bunch. One reason that some people may avoid bananas is that they tend to get soft and mushy if you don't eat them quickly enough. Here's a trick for keeping them fresh. When bananas are getting soft too quickly, put them in the refrigerator. This will quickly stop the ripening process. (Don't be alarmed when the cold turns the skin black—the fruit inside will still be fresh and tasty.) On the other hand, when you're waiting for that bunch of green bananas to ripen, it's easy to speed up the process. Put them in a brown paper bag at room temperature. The ethylene gas that bananas produce naturally will speed up the ripening.

Frozen Chocolate-Banana Pops

4 **wooden sticks for making pops**

2 **bananas, peeled and cut in half crosswise**

½ **cup chocolate sauce (the kind that forms a shell)**

4 **tablespoons finely chopped unsalted peanuts**

Insert a wooden stick into the cut end of each banana piece. Pour the chocolate sauce over the bananas until they're completely coated, then roll the chocolate-coated bananas in the peanuts. Place pops in the freezer for at least 2 hours, or until frozen.

Makes 4 servings

PER SERVING

Calories: 318
Total fat: 22 g
Saturated fat: 9 g

Cholesterol: 0 mg
Sodium: 21 mg
Dietary fiber: 3 g

Barley

A GREAT GRAIN FOR THE HEART

HEALING POWER

Can Help:

Lower cholesterol

Reduce the formation of blood clots

Improve digestion

Reduce the risk of cancer and heart disease

If you're a vitamin E enthusiast, you've probably heard about tocotrienols. Like vitamin E, tocotrienols are antioxidants, meaning that they help reduce damage to the body from dangerous oxygen molecules called free radicals. And barley is one of the richest sources of these compounds.

"Tocotrienols are potentially more powerful antioxidants than other chemical versions of vitamin E," says David J. A. Jenkins, MD, DSc, PhD, professor of nutritional sciences at the University of Toronto. "They have at least 50 percent more free-radical-fighting power than other forms." That translates into a lot of disease-fighting might.

Tocotrienols fight heart disease in two ways. One, they help stop free-radical oxidation, a process that makes low-density lipoprotein (LDL) cholesterol, the dangerous type, more likely to stick to artery walls. And two, they act on the liver to reduce the body's production of cholesterol.

Tocotrienols may also help lower your risk of cancer. A number of studies have shown that these antioxidants can help protect lab rodents from liver and breast cancer. More recently, research has shown that tocotrienols can encourage breast cancer cells to die.

Barley also contains lignans, compounds that have antioxidant ability and thus provide still more protection. According to Lilian Thompson, PhD, professor of nutritional sciences at the University of Toronto, lignans can help prevent tiny blood clots from forming, further reducing the risk of heart disease.

Lignans may also play a role in cancer prevention. After you eat them, your body turns them into phytoestrogens, which can block the cancer-supporting effect of women's own estrogen. A study of more than 3,000 women compared the diet history of women who'd had breast cancer and women who hadn't. Premenopausal women with the highest amount of lignans in their diets had 34 percent less risk of breast cancer.

Finally, barley is exceptionally high in both the trace mineral selenium and vitamin E. Although research results are mixed, there's evidence that both help protect

Unless you're extremely fond of cooked barley, it's unlikely that you're ever going to eat 1 cup a day, the amount that's recommended for maximum health benefits by David J. A. Jenkins, MD, DSc, PhD, of the University of Toronto. Here's another way to get more barley into your diet. Add it to baked goods. You can substitute about 1½ cups of barley flour for every 3 cups of regular flour. Or add barley flakes to cookies, muffins, or bread. They will add a distinctly nutty taste while delivering more fiber and nutrients than you'll get from white flour alone.

against cancer. Indeed, some researchers believe that selenium may work best as an anticancer agent when combined with other antioxidants, which, as we've seen, barley has in abundance.

One cup of cooked pearl barley contains 36 micrograms of selenium, more than half the Daily Value (DV) for this mineral, and 5 IU of vitamin E, 17 percent of the DV for this vitamin.

Fiber Protection

Besides helping to reduce damage from dangerous LDL cholesterol, there's another way in which barley helps keep blood vessels healthy. It's loaded with beta-glucan, a type of soluble fiber that forms a gel in the small intestine. Cholesterol in your body binds to this gel, which is then excreted from the body.

Soluble fiber does more than lower cholesterol, however. It also binds to potential cancer-causing agents in the intestine, keeping them from being absorbed. And because soluble fiber soaks up lots of water in the colon, it helps digestion work more efficiently, thereby preventing constipation.

A 5-week USDA study involving 25 people with elevated cholesterol required them to eat a heart-healthy diet containing varying amounts of beta-glucan from barley, such as barley flakes, barley flour, and pearl barley. The people eating a diet containing 3 or 6 grams of beta-glucan daily saw their total cholesterol drop significantly, compared with people whose diets didn't have the soluble fiber.

You'd need about a half-cup of barley to get 3 grams of soluble fiber.

GETTING THE MOST

Buy it whole. Although pearl barley is the most common form found in American grocery stores, it may be refined no less than five times to scrub off the healthful outer husk and bran layer.

A more nutritious choice is hulled barley. Stripped only of the outer, inedible hull, it's the best source of fiber, minerals, and thiamin. It also has a more distinctive, nuttier flavor than its highly processed counterparts. You can generally find hulled barley at health food stores.

In the Kitchen

Unlike rice and wheat, which are quite mild, barley has a robust, slightly pungent taste that complements highly flavored dishes like lamb stew or mushroom soup. But you prepare it in much the same way as other grains by mixing it with water and letting it simmer, covered, until the kernels are tender. Here are a few additional tips.

Plan for expansion. One cup of dried barley will expand to about four times that amount during cooking, so be sure to use a pan that is slightly oversized.

Give it time to tenderize. Hulled barley can be extremely tough and slow to cook, so it should be soaked overnight before cooking. Pearl barley, on the other hand, has had the tough outer husk removed and doesn't require soaking.

Use it as an add-in. Even properly prepared barley is somewhat chewy, so it's rarely served as a side dish. Most cooks prefer to make barley ahead of time, then add it to soups or stews.

Barley Salad with Squash and Black Beans

1 cup pearled barley

3 tablespoons olive oil

2 leeks, white and light green parts only, thinly sliced

2 cups chopped butternut squash (about ½ medium squash)

¼ cup water

3 tablespoons chopped parsley

1 can (15 ounces) black beans, rinsed and drained

2 tablespoons fresh lemon juice

½ teaspoon salt

¼ teaspoon freshly ground black pepper

Grated lemon zest for garnish (optional)

Cook the barley according to package directions. Rinse and set aside.

Meanwhile, in large nonstick skillet, heat 2 tablespoons of the oil over medium-high heat. Add the leeks and squash, and cook, stirring, until slightly softened and lightly browned, about 10 minutes. Add the water and 1½ tablespoons of the parsley, and cook 2 to 3 minutes more. Transfer the vegetables to a large bowl.

Add the barley, black beans, lemon juice, salt, pepper, and the remaining 1 tablespoon olive oil and 1½ tablespoons parsley. Stir to combine. Garnish with lemon zest, if desired.

Makes 6 servings

PER SERVING

Calories: 233	Cholesterol: 0 mg
Total fat: 7 g	Sodium: 207 mg
Saturated fat: 1 g	Dietary fiber: 8 g

Basil

LEAVES FOR GIVING EASE

HEALING POWER
Can Help:
Ease digestion
Lower the risk of cancer

Pizza lovers from Boise to Brooklyn dust their slices with dried basil. Foodies with a taste for simple pleasures live for the first tomato of the season, drizzled with olive oil and garnished with freshly snipped basil. Gardeners bask in the aroma of a just-plucked basil leaf rubbed between the fingers.

Whether it's used dried or fresh, basil's sharp aroma and spicy flavor pleasure the nose as well as the palate. When you treat yourself to foods flavored with basil, you may also be treating yourself to a serving of health benefits. Substances in this herb can help calm your stomach and even, researchers believe, play a role in preventing cancer.

Keeping Cells Healthy

Laboratory studies have suggested that compounds found in basil may help disrupt the dangerous chain of events that can lead to the development of cancer.

In one study, researchers in India spiked the food of a group of laboratory animals with basil extract, while animals in a second group were given only their usual diet. After 15 days, animals given the extract had higher levels of enzymes that are known to deactivate cancer-causing substances in the body.

Basil's ability to prevent cancerous changes was linked not to one particular compound in the herb but instead to several compounds working together, the researchers speculated.

A survey by Norwegian and American researchers found that basil is a rich source of antioxidants, which neutralize dangerous oxygen molecules called free radicals in your body before they can contribute to a variety of conditions, including heart disease, cancer, and Alzheimer's disease. Per 100 grams, basil has more antioxidant content than dark chocolate, blackberries, strawberries, and blueberries, according to the researchers.

Of course, a serving size of basil is tiny compared with the amount of berries (or chocolate!) that you'd eat in one sitting. But if you love the taste of the herb on your food, at least you know that you're helping yourself to an extra dose of antioxidants.

Doctor's Top Tip

When shopping for dried basil, look for a brand that's organically grown. Some basil is irradiated, which can significantly reduce the antioxidant content of the herb, says Mildred Mattfeldt-Beman, PhD, RD, LD, of St. Louis University. Buying organic is the best bet for ensuring that your basil wasn't irradiated.

Or just raise your own, and enjoy it fresh! The professor says basil plants are quite easy to grow, and you can grow them outdoors during the warm months, and bring them inside before the fall frost.

Keeping Your Stomach Happy

The next time your stomach sends out a postmeal SOS, try sipping a cup of basil tea. This herb has a reputation for easing a variety of digestive disorders, especially gas. One possible explanation is a compound found in basil called eugenol, which has been shown to help ease muscle spasms. This could explain why basil appears to help ease gas and stomach cramps.

To make a soothing basil tea, pour ½ cup of boiling water over 1 to 2 teaspoons of dried basil. Let the brew steep for 15 minutes, then strain and serve. People who frequently have gas may benefit by drinking 2 to 3 cups a day between meals.

Basil may also prove to be a useful tool against ulcers. In one lab study, Indian researchers tested the effects of eugenol on *H. pylori*, the bacteria that's to blame in most ulcers. They found that eugenol inhibited the growth of 30 different strains of the bacteria. Although much more research needs to be done to find out if basil will have this effect in humans, it's nice to know that an herb so tasty to the palate may also be good for the stomach.

Another way basil may help keep your digestive system happy is through its antimicrobial properties. Since outbreaks of illness from contaminated lettuce and spinach have made the news in recent years, it may be helpful to add fresh basil to dishes containing fresh spinach or lettuce, says Mildred Mattfeldt-Beman, PhD, RD, LD, the department chairperson of nutrition and dietetics at St. Louis University in Missouri, who has taught courses about culinary and medicinal herbs. The herb might offer a bit of protection against germs contaminating your food.

GETTING THE MOST

Mix it up. While many fresh foods are more nutritious than their dried counterparts, basil is good both ways. One teaspoon of crumbled dried basil contains more essential minerals, like calcium, iron, magnesium, and potassium, than 1 tablespoon of fresh-snipped leaves.

On the other hand, crumbled basil has a larger surface area exposed to the environment, which can accelerate the natural breakdown of its beneficial compounds. "Dried basil loses its punch pretty quickly," says Dr. Mattfeldt-Beman. Keep it in a

In the Kitchen

Your friend with the green thumb hands you a bouquet of fresh basil, still warm from the sun. It smells heavenly—but how do you use it? Here are a few suggestions:

Treat it gently. Basil is delicate. Rough handling will cause the leaves to blacken around the edges, says Mildred Mattfeldt-Beman, PhD, RD, LD, of St. Louis University. She recommends handling it gently—and as little as possible—before you put it into your recipe.

Keep it happy in the fridge. To store fresh basil for the short term, wrap the lower stems with a damp paper towel, place it in an unsealed plastic bag, and store in your vegetable drawer.

Freeze it for later. For long-term storage, fill an ice cube tray with basil leaves, top off the little compartments with water, and put the tray in a sealed freezer container. When you need basil, you'll have premeasured chunks that you can drop into a soup or sauce, says Dr. Mattfeldt-Beman.

tightly sealed container in a cool, dark, dry place, then pitch it after about 6 months. After that, "you'll just be adding grass to your dish," she says.

Put it in last. Since most of the flavor from basil comes from its volatile oils, which break down in hot temperatures, add basil to recipes in the last 10 minutes of cooking, Dr. Mattfeldt-Beman suggests.

Pasta with Pesto and Tomatoes

¼ **cup blanched almonds**

2 **cups loosely packed fresh basil leaves**

2 **cloves garlic**

3–4 **tablespoons defatted reduced-sodium chicken broth**

2 **tablespoons extra-virgin olive oil**

2 **tablespoons grated Parmesan cheese**

¼ **teaspoon salt**

¼ **teaspoon freshly ground black pepper**

   Pinch of ground nutmeg

8 **ounces penne or rotini**

2 **medium tomatoes, cut into thin wedges**

Place the almonds in a food processor, and process with on/off turns until finely chopped. Pour into a small bowl.

Add the basil and garlic to the food processor. Process until coarsely chopped. Add 3 tablespoons of broth, the oil, cheese, salt, pepper, and nutmeg. Process until the garlic is finely minced. Add the reserved almonds, and process until combined. If the mixture is very dry, add another 1 tablespoon broth, and process to mix.

Cook the pasta in a large pot of boiling water according to the package directions. Drain and place in a large serving bowl. Pour the pesto over the pasta, add the tomatoes, and toss.

Makes 4 servings

PER SERVING

Calories: 398
Total fat: 12 g
Saturated fat: 2 g

Cholesterol: 3 mg
Sodium: 211 mg
Dietary fiber: 10 g

Beans

SMALL BUT MIGHTY

HEALING POWER

Can Help:

Lower cholesterol

Stabilize blood sugar levels

Reduce the risk of cancer

Prevent heart disease in people with diabetes

In the annals of the International Federation of Competitive Eating—where men and women stuff their bellies with shocking amounts of food at one sitting—several bean-related records have been set. One man ate 6 pounds of baked beans in less than 2 minutes. Another eater scarfed down more than 5 pounds of pork and beans in less than 2 minutes.

Although gulping this many beans at one time might not be the wisest activity, at least these competitors had *sort* of the right idea: Beans are a superb addition to a healthy diet.

Despite their small size, beans pack a surprisingly rich and varied array of substances that are vital for good health. Take fiber, for example. "What's so good about beans, I think, is the high fiber in particular. They're one of the better sources of dietary fiber there is," says Joe Hughes, PhD, assistant professor in the nutrition and food sciences program at California State University in San Bernardino, whose research is centered on beans.

What's especially nice is that they're high in soluble and insoluble fiber, which have different effects in the body. Oats are one of the few other foods high in both types of fiber, but beans can be used in many more types of dishes than oats, and it's easier to eat a hearty portion of beans, he points out.

Beans are also a good source of minerals, protein, and, you may be surprised to learn, antioxidants.

Sending Cholesterol South

While beans aren't the only food that can help lower cholesterol, they're certainly one of the best. The soluble fiber in beans is the same gummy stuff found in apples, barley, and oat bran. In the digestive tract, soluble fiber traps cholesterol-containing bile, removing it from the body before it's absorbed.

"Eating a cup of cooked beans a day can lower total cholesterol about 10 percent in 6 weeks," says Patti Bazel Geil, MS, RD, a diabetes educator and nutrition author in Lexington, Kentucky, who's written about the benefits of beans. While 10 percent may not seem like much, keep in mind that every 1 percent reduction in total

Doctor's Top Tip

Even though he sings the praises of beans, Joe Hughes, PhD, of California State University, acknowledges that it takes time to work your way up to being a regular bean aficionado. If you suddenly start eating them daily, you're likely to develop gas and bloating. Start out having beans with a meal once a week. After a month, go to twice a week. Keep building gradually. Your digestive tract, and the gas-producing bacteria it contains, will adapt better to this routine.

cholesterol means a 2 percent decrease in your risk for heart disease.

Beans can lower cholesterol in just about anyone, but the higher your cholesterol, the better they work. In a study at the University of Kentucky, 20 men with high cholesterol (over 260 milligrams per deciliter of blood) were given about ¾ cup of pinto and navy beans a day. The men's total cholesterol dropped an average of 19 percent in 3 weeks, possibly reducing their heart attack risk by almost 40 percent. Even more remarkable, the dangerous low-density lipoprotein (LDL) cholesterol—that's the artery-plugging stuff—plunged by 24 percent.

It appears that all beans can help lower cholesterol, even canned baked beans. In another University of Kentucky study, 24 men with high cholesterol ate 1 cup of canned beans in tomato sauce every day for 3 weeks. Their total cholesterol dropped 10.4 percent, and their triglycerides (another blood fat that contributes to heart disease) fell 10.8 percent.

In further research into the cholesterol-lowering effects of beans and other legumes, authors of a report in the *British Journal of Nutrition* compiled the findings of 11 studies that looked at the relationship between cholesterol and different types of legumes, such as pinto beans, chickpeas, white beans, and mixed beans (but not soybeans). They found that the beans in these studies lowered total cholesterol by 7.2 percent, LDL (bad) cholesterol by 6.2 percent, and triglycerides by 16.6 percent. The soluble fiber in these foods appeared to be the most important factor responsible for their cholesterol-lowering effect.

Beans play another, less direct role in keeping cholesterol levels down. They're extremely filling, so when you eat beans, you'll have less appetite for other, fattier foods. And eating less fat is critical for keeping cholesterol levels low.

Keeping Blood Sugar Steady

Keeping blood sugar levels steady is the key to keeping diabetes under control. "Many people don't realize how good beans are for people with diabetes," says Geil. In fact, eating between ½ and ¾ cup of beans a day has been shown to significantly improve blood sugar control. And beans provide yet another benefit for people with diabetes, she says. "People with diabetes are four to six times more likely to develop heart

In the Kitchen

If you roll right by the dried beans at the supermarket because you don't have time for all the soaking and boiling and waiting around, put on the brakes. Cooking beans from scratch doesn't have to be a daylong project, says Patti Bazel Geil, MS, RD. With the quick-soaking method, you can shave hours off the cooking time. Here's how to do it:

Rinse the beans in a colander, put them in a large pot, and cover with 2 inches of water. Bring to a boil, reduce the heat to medium, and simmer for 10 minutes. Drain the beans, and cover with 2 inches of fresh water. ("Discarding the water that the beans were cooked in gets rid of most of their gas-producing sugars," Geil explains.) Soak for 30 minutes. Then rinse, drain, and cover with fresh water again. Simmer for 2 hours or until the beans are tender.

---

disease," she says. "Eating more beans will help keep their cholesterol low, thereby reducing their risk."

Beans are rich in complex carbohydrates. Unlike sugary foods, which dump sugar (glucose) into the bloodstream all at once, complex carbohydrates are digested more slowly. This means that glucose enters your bloodstream a little at a time, helping to keep blood sugar levels steady, says Geil.

Foods' effect on blood sugar is commonly measured on a scale called the glycemic index, or GI, and beans are a "very good low-GI food" because of their soluble fiber, says Dr. Hughes. This should be good news for the approximately 21 million Americans with diabetes, and the 54 million with "prediabetes," a condition that causes a rise in blood sugar and usually occurs in people before they develop diabetes.

Unfortunately, Americans on average only eat 17 grams of fiber daily—and people with diabetes only eat 16 grams—according to a survey from the federal government. The American Dietetic Association recommends 25 grams daily.

In a small study from the University of Texas, researchers had 13 people with diabetes follow two diets for 6 weeks each. One diet had 24 grams of daily fiber (8 grams were soluble fiber), and the other diet provided a whopping 50 grams of fiber, half of which was soluble. Compared with when they ate the regular-fiber diet, the people eating the high-fiber diet had better control over their blood sugar and lower insulin. Perhaps the best news is that the subjects were eating regular foods—not taking fiber supplements or eating foods specially fortified with fiber. (Experts had previously declared that it's difficult to consume a lot of soluble fiber each day without the use of supplements or fiber-fortified foods.)

A nice quality about beans is that they're available in so many varieties—and you can prepare them in so many ways—that it's easy to eat beans even several times a day in relatively large quantities to reap their fiber-giving benefits, says Dr. Hughes.

Cancer-Licking Legumes

Fruits and vegetables tend to get the spotlight during discussions of foods rich in antioxidants. Indeed, when USDA researchers compiled the antioxidant capacities of hundreds of foods in the American diet, many of these foods stood out. The Granny Smith apple, for example, scored a 5,381 on the measurement of total antioxidant capacity per serving. The artichoke scored 7,904. And the lowbush blueberry got a whopping 13,427.

But several beans more than held their own, too. The pinto bean scored 11,864. And the red kidney bean scored 13,259!

Beans are rich sources of phytochemicals, which are plant components that have antioxidant and other disease-fighting properties, says Dr. Hughes. Beans may contain hundreds of types of antioxidant chemicals. Remember that antioxidants help protect you from cancer by limiting damaging attacks on your cells from free radicals. Plus, unlike some antioxidant-rich plant foods like blueberries, you can put lots of different beans on your plate meal after meal without getting bored or overwhelmed by the flavor.

Some other compounds in beans—like lignans, isoflavones, saponins, phytic acid, and protease inhibitors—have been shown to inhibit cancer-cell growth. These compounds appear to keep normal cells from turning cancerous and prevent cancer cells from growing.

The Healthy Alternative to Meat

Beans used to be called the "poor man's meat." But a more accurate name would be the healthy man's meat. Like red meat, beans are loaded with protein. Unlike meat, they're light in fat, particularly dangerous, artery-clogging saturated fat.

For example, a cup of black beans contains less than 1 gram of fat. Less than 1 percent of that comes from saturated fat. Three ounces of lean, broiled ground beef, on the other hand, has 15 grams of fat, 22 percent of which is the saturated kind.

Beans are also a great source of essential vitamins and minerals. A half-cup of black beans contains 128 micrograms, or 32 percent of the Daily Value (DV) for folate, a B vitamin that may lower risk of heart disease and fight birth defects. That same cup has 2 milligrams of iron, 11 percent of the DV, and 305 milligrams of potassium, or 9 percent of the DV. Potassium is a mineral that has been shown to help control blood pressure.

GETTING THE MOST

Go for the fiber. While virtually all dried beans are good sources of fiber, some varieties stand out from the pack. Black beans, for example, contain 6 grams of fiber in a half-cup serving. Chickpeas, kidney beans, and lima beans all weigh in at about 7 grams of fiber, and black-eyed peas are among the best, with about 8 grams of fiber.

Enjoy them canned. In general, the dry beans that you cook for yourself have a slight edge over canned beans in terms of retaining nutrients, says Dr. Hughes. However, the average American these days just doesn't have the time needed to cook dry beans (even with the expedited method featured in the sidebar). If you only have time for canned beans, then by all means eat canned beans, he says. However, canned beans may be higher in sodium, so if that's a concern, drain and rinse canned beans before using them.

Use gas-deflating spices. Has the fear of uncomfortable and embarrassing gas kept you from reaping beans' nutritional benefits? Try spicing them with a pinch of summer savory or a teaspoon of ground ginger. According to some university studies, these spices may help reduce beans' gas-producing effects.

Read the label. Some canned refried beans contain a lot of fat, and some contain little to none, says Dr. Hughes. Be sure to pick a kind that's low in fat—they still taste great.

Go dark. Buy darker beans for more disease protection. In general, the darker the beans, the more powerful the antioxidants they contain, says Dr. Hughes.

Cannellini Seafood Pouches

- 2 cans (15 ounces each) cannellini beans, rinsed and drained
- 12 ounces sea scallops (halved if very large)
- 8 ounces large shrimp, peeled and deveined
- 1 cup diced plum tomatoes (¾-inch dice)
- 1 jar (6 ounces) marinated artichoke hearts, drained
- 1 tablespoon extra-virgin olive oil
- 2 teaspoons chopped fresh rosemary
- 1 teaspoon finely chopped garlic
- ½ teaspoon salt (optional)
- ¼ teaspoon crushed red pepper flakes

Preheat the oven to 425°F. Tear off 4 pieces of parchment paper, each about 15 inches long. Fold each sheet in half lengthwise, and then open it up so you can see the crease.

In a large bowl, combine all of the ingredients; toss well.

To make each pouch: Mound 1½ cups of the bean mixture on 1 side of the crease. Lift the other side of the parchment over the filling, and fold the edges together around the filling to seal. Repeat with remaining ingredients to make 3 more pouches, then place them on a baking sheet.

Bake until the scallops and shrimp are slightly opaque in the centers, 10 to 12 minutes. To serve, cut an "X" in each pouch, and tear the paper back to reveal the filling.

Makes 4 servings

Cook's Note: *You can use any canned white beans you prefer in this recipe.*

PER SERVING

Calories: 430	Cholesterol: 140 mg
Total fat: 12 g	Sodium: 655 mg
Saturated fat: 2 g	Dietary fiber: 9 g

Edamame and Escarole Salad

1 cup shelled frozen edamame

1 tablespoon fresh lemon juice

1 tablespoon minced shallot

2 tablespoons extra-virgin olive oil

   Sea salt and freshly ground black pepper

1 head escarole (5 pounds), torn into bite-size pieces

2 teaspoons chopped fresh mint

2 teaspoons chopped flat-leaf parsley

¼ pound Pecorino Romano cheese

Bring a large pot of salted water to a boil. Add the edamame, and cook for 2 minutes. Drain well.

In a small bowl, whisk together the lemon juice and shallot; slowly whisk in the olive oil. Season to taste with salt and pepper.

In a large serving bowl, combine the edamame, escarole, mint, parsley, and the dressing; season to taste with salt and pepper. Shave the cheese over the salad.

Makes 4 servings

Cook's Notes: *If you like, use arugula or mixed greens instead of escarole. You can also shell and steam fresh edamame for this recipe if you have time.*

PER SERVING

Calories: 318	Cholesterol: 28 mg
Total fat: 18 g	Sodium: 583 mg
Saturated fat: 7 g	Dietary fiber: 13 g

Gingered Lentils

1¼ cups lentils

2 teaspoons canola oil

2 tablespoons grated fresh ginger

2 cloves garlic, minced

1¼ teaspoons curry powder

¼ teaspoon salt

1 lemon, halved

Place the lentils in a colander and rinse with cold water, then drain. Transfer the lentils to a large saucepan, and add 4 cups water. Bring to a boil over high heat. Reduce the heat to low. Partially cover, and cook until the lentils are tender but not mushy, about 30 to 35 minutes.

Drain the lentils, and set aside. Wipe the pan dry. Add the oil and heat over medium heat. Add the ginger, garlic, curry powder, and salt. Stir for a few seconds, until fragrant. Add the lentils, and stir well to reheat. Remove from the heat.

Squeeze the juice from one half of the lemon, and stir it into the lentils. Cut the remaining half into 4 wedges. Serve the lentils with the lemon wedges.

Makes 4 servings

Cook's Note: *This makes a great meatless meal. Serve it with bread or rice and a steamed vegetable.*

PER SERVING ———————————————

Calories: 208

Total fat: 3 g

Saturated fat: 0.3 g

Cholesterol: 0 mg

Sodium: 137 mg

Dietary fiber: 7.4 g

Beets

BETTER LIVING THROUGH BORSCHT

HEALING POWER
Can Help:

Protect against cancer
Prevent birth defects

If you travel through Eastern Europe, you're likely to encounter borscht, an eye-catching red soup that's especially common in Ukraine, where many consider it to be the national soup.

Served hot or cold, this sweet crimson soup is made from fresh beets, and that means that it's brimming with nutrients that may help stave off heart disease and cancer and fight birth defects.

Giving Heart Disease and Cancer the Red Flag

Beets get their bright color from a combination of two compounds: betacyanins, which lend a ruby color, and betaxanthins, which provide a yellow hue. A substance called betanin in beets is a particularly generous donor of electrons. If you're familiar with free radicals, you know this is a beneficial quality. Free radicals are rogue molecules that are missing one or more electrons, and they zip around in your body attempting to steal electrons from other cells. The ensuing damage can contribute to a spectrum of diseases like cancer and heart disease, and many experts think it's the underlying mechanism of aging itself.

But back to the beets. Substances beets contain make very good antioxidants—or tools your body uses to neutralize free radicals. Researchers conducting laboratory studies on beets (the things they did to those beets make the world's hardest recipe look like a simple task) found that components within them have "strong antioxidant effects." The researchers concluded that ". . . beet products used regularly in the diet may provide protection against certain oxidative stress-related disorders in humans."

In one study, researchers did lab tests to see how betanin and other plant pigments may work to protect your health. Not only did betanin prove to be effective in inhibiting free-radical damage, it also inhibited the growth of breast, stomach, colon, lung, and nervous-system tumor cells!

It can be a long route from the science lab to your dinner table, but it looks like beets are a helpful ally in your ongoing confrontation with free radicals and the problems they cause. As you're loading your grocery cart with a spectrum of colorful vegetables, make sure you include the familiar purplish red of beets.

Doctor's Top Tip

Most people choose the canned version when they're hungry for beets, says Reed Mangels, PhD, RD, a dietitian in Amherst, Massachusetts, and an editor of the *Vegetarian Journal*, a publication of the Vegetarian Resource Group. However, if you're choosing beets from the produce section, give them a little squeeze. Pass up the soft and squishy beets, since they've been sitting out too long, and take home the firm ones.

A Font of Folate

Meeting your daily requirement for the B vitamin folate is essential for normal tissue growth. It also may lower your risk of heart disease, and according to the National Institutes of Health, it helps protect your DNA from damaging changes that can lead to cancer. Plus, doctors have found that folate is a pregnant woman's best friend because it helps protect against birth defects. The Daily Value (DV) for folate is 400 micrograms, but pregnant women need 600 micrograms daily.

A half-cup of boiled, sliced beets contains 68 micrograms of folate, which is 17 percent of the DV.

Increasing Iron Stores

For providing iron, beets can't match such mineral powerhouses as lean beef. But if you're among the millions of Americans who are cutting back on meat or giving it up entirely, then boning up on beets is one way to go. That half-cup of sliced beets also contains 0.7 milligrams of iron, or about 4 percent of the DV for this mineral.

GETTING THE MOST

Eat them raw or cook them lightly. Studies have shown that the antitumor power of beets is diminished by heat. So peel and grate beets, and toss them into salads, or cook them lightly to get the most nutrients.

Try the canned kind. One of the neat things about beets is that they're nearly as nutritious out of a can as they are fresh from the ground. So you can enjoy their health benefits in and out of season.

Beet and Goat Cheese Salad

SALAD

- 1 cup walnut halves (optional)
- 6 ounces (about 3 generous handfuls) baby greens, such as arugula, spinach, or mesclun mix
- 8 medium canned beets (about 8 ounces), drained and sliced
- 4 ounces aged goat cheese, sliced or crumbled

DRESSING

- 2 tablespoons extra-virgin olive oil
- 1 tablespoon walnut oil
- 3 tablespoons tarragon white wine vinegar

  Salt and freshly ground black pepper

Preheat the oven to 350°F.

To prepare the salad: Toast the walnuts (if using) in a single layer on an ungreased baking sheet until golden brown and fragrant, about 6 minutes, stirring occasionally. Allow to cool.

In a large serving bowl, combine the walnuts, greens, and beets; toss gently.

To make the dressing: In a small bowl, whisk the oils together, then gradually whisk in the vinegar. Add salt and pepper to taste.

Gently drizzle the dressing over the salad and toss. Sprinkle with the cheese.

Makes 6 servings

PER SERVING

Calories: 170	Cholesterol: 20 mg
Total fat: 14 g	Sodium: 150 mg
Saturated fat: 5.5 g	Dietary fiber: 1 g

Easy Chilled Beet Soup

- **2 cans (15 ounces each) reduced-sodium beets**
- **2 tablespoons red wine vinegar**
- **1 teaspoon packed light brown sugar**
- **½ cup chopped cucumbers**
- **4 tablespoons fat-free sour cream**
- **1 tablespoon chopped fresh dill**

Drain the beets, reserving 1½ cups of the liquid. Chop the beets, and set aside ½ cup.

Place the remaining beets in a blender or food processor. Add the vinegar, sugar, and the reserved beet liquid. Process for 1 to 2 minutes, or until the mixture is a chunky purée. Chill for up to 12 hours.

Serve sprinkled with the cucumbers and the reserved chopped beets. Top each serving with 1 tablespoon of the sour cream and a sprinkle of dill.

Makes 4 servings

Cook's Notes: *If you use regular canned beets, the sodium will increase 305 milligrams per serving. Also, for variety, you could replace 1 cup of the beet liquid with apple juice.*

PER SERVING

Calories: 89	Cholesterol: 0 mg
Total fat: 0.3 g	Sodium: 116 mg
Saturated fat: 0.1 g	Dietary fiber: 3.9 g

Berries

MORE THAN JUST DESSERT

The Romans believed that strawberries could cure everything from loose teeth to gastritis. Raspberries, according to folklore, had the ability to soothe inflamed tonsils.

While long-ago folk healers may have somewhat exaggerated the curative powers of berries, these small colorful fruits do still have a reputation for their beneficial effects in the body. Researchers around the world are analyzing a wide variety of substances in berries that show promise for preventing such serious problems as cataracts and cancer.

HEALING POWER

Can Help:

Prevent cataracts

Ward off cancer

Prevent constipation

Reduce the risk of infection

Protect brainpower

Filled With Healing Components

More than 9,000 phytochemicals have been identified in plant foods, with many more still to be named, scientists say. These are chemicals in the plants that have a variety of beneficial health effects. And berries, despite their diminutive size, can be powerful sources of phytochemicals.

One such phytochemical is a compound called ellagic acid, which is believed to help prevent cellular changes that can lead to cancer. All berries contain some ellagic acid, with raspberries and strawberries ranking among the top providers. "Ellagic acid is a good friend to us, helping fight the cancer process," says Hasan Mukhtar, PhD, vice chairman for research in the department of dermatology and professor of cancer research at the University of Wisconsin in Madison.

In fact, berries—and the ellagic acid they contain—may help fight cancer on several fronts, says Gary Stoner, PhD, professor and cancer researcher at Ohio State University in Columbus, who has worked on a number of studies involving blackberries. Ellagic acid is a powerful antioxidant, meaning that it can reduce damage caused by free radicals, harmful oxygen molecules that can literally punch holes in healthy cells and kick off the cancerous process. "It also detoxifies carcinogens," says Dr. Stoner.

But ellagic acid is just one of a host of cancer fighters in berries. They also contain flavonoids, tannins, phenolic acid, and lignans, which may help keep you cancer-free through a variety of mechanisms, including their antioxidant power.

A Cornell University study found that extracts from eight different types of

FOOD ALERT

Dangerous Pickings

Even though elderberries are a treasure trove of nutrients, you don't want to pick them in the wild. Before they get ripe, they may contain compounds called cyanogenic glycosides, which can be poisonous, says Ara DerMarderosian, PhD, professor of pharmacognosy and director of the Complementary and Alternative Medicine Institute at the University of the Sciences in Philadelphia.

It's not only the berries that are dangerous, he adds. The leaves and bark of the tree also contain the poisonous compounds. In fact, there have been a number of cases of poisoning in children who carved elderberry branches, used them as peashooters, and didn't even eat the berries.

You don't have to avoid elderberries to be safe, however. Just treat them as you would wild mushrooms—a tasty food that's best picked at your favorite fruit stand instead of in the woods. It's also a good idea to cook the berries, because heat destroys the dangerous compounds, Dr. DerMarderosian notes.

strawberries significantly inhibited liver-cancer cell growth in a lab study.

A University of Georgia lab study found that phenolic compounds extracted from blueberries could limit colon cancer cells' ability to multiply and also trigger these renegade cells to die. Cancer cells can develop into tumors when they multiply too fast and stubbornly refuse to die—and even a little pressure to keep these cells in line can decrease the chance that a cancer will progress, the study authors write. Thus, their findings "suggest that blueberry intake may reduce colon cancer risk."

Need more tantalizing clues that a bowl of berries may help keep you cancer free? Okay, here's some more data. Some berries may have an ingredient that can help "starve" cancer. Louisiana State University researchers found that an extract from black raspberry can inhibit the growth of new blood vessels. Tumors coax your body to grow new blood vessels to feed them nutrients, and they can't grow beyond a few millimeters in size without this food supply. The researchers found that a compound called gallic acid in the black raspberries was partially responsible for this potentially cancer-starving activity.

Help for the Eyes and More

Berries are also very high in vitamin C, which is a powerful antioxidant. Getting a lot of vitamin C in your diet may help reduce your risk of heart disease, cancer, and infections. Vitamin C seems particularly important in preventing cataracts, which are thought to be caused by the oxidation of the protein that forms the lenses of the eyes.

All berries contain large amounts of vitamin C. A half-cup of strawberries, for example, has 42 milligrams, or 70 percent of the Daily Value (DV) for this vitamin. (That's more vitamin C than you'll get in a similar amount of grapefruit.) A half-cup of elderberries has 26 milligrams of vitamin C, or 43 percent of the DV, and a half-cup of blackberries has 15 milligrams, or 25 percent of the DV.

Berry Full of Fiber

One of the pleasant things about berries is that they're a sweet solution to a distinctly unpleasant problem: constipation. Berries contain large amounts of insoluble fiber, which is incredibly absorbent. It draws rivers of water into the intestine, which makes stools heavier. Heavy stools travel through the intestine faster, which means that you're less likely to become constipated.

The fiber in berries is helpful in yet another way. It helps prevent bile acid (a chemical that the body uses for digestion) from being transformed into a more dangerous, potentially cancer-causing form.

Elderberries are an incredible source of fiber, with a half-cup containing 5 grams. A half-cup of blackberries has more than 3 grams of fiber, while a half-cup of raspberries has 4 grams.

Ward Off Urinary Tract Infections

Native Americans used cranberries to treat bladder problems, and people were still using them in modern times to treat urinary tract infections (UTIs) before the advent of antibiotics. Even now, the tart red berry plays a valuable role in preventing UTIs,

---

FOOD ALERT

Cranberry Juice and Warfarin

The medical literature contains several reports about possible interactions between warfarin—an anticlotting drug also known as Coumadin—and cranberry juice. Drinking cranberry juice if you're taking warfarin could possibly lead to bleeding or excessively "thin" blood. Until more is known about their possible interactions, it's prudent to limit your consumption of cranberry juice if you're taking warfarin, a team of researchers advised in the *British Medical Journal*.

Doctor's Top Tip

If you'd like to preserve some berries to ensure that you'll always have a backup supply when you get a craving, stick them into the freezer—berries freeze very well, according to the Mayo Clinic. Spread them out on a cookie sheet, and pop them into the freezer. Once they're frozen, put them into resealable freezer bags, and tuck them away for later.

which may strike as many as half of women in the United States before they reach the age of 30.

One study following 150 women found that drinking a combination cranberry-lingonberry drink daily reduced the risk of infection by 20 percent, compared with women who didn't drink the juice. Another study, which also involved 150 women, found that cranberry juice or tablets of cranberry extract significantly cut down on the number of women who had a UTI over the course of a year.

Experts aren't sure how cranberry juice works to prevent UTIs, but it appears to keep bacteria from gaining a foothold on the surface of the urinary tract—thus they can't trigger an infection. Drinking at least two 8-ounce glasses of pure, unsweetened cranberry juice daily should help protect you from the infections.

Keep a Youthful Brain

According to researchers from the USDA, your brain is particularly vulnerable to free-radical damage as you go through life. It uses 20 percent of the oxygen you breathe (cells produce free radicals from oxygen). Its natural antioxidant system to protect it from free radicals is not particularly robust, and long-living neurons in your brain tend to be exposed to lots of damage from free radicals during your lifetime. Oxidative stress—a term for free-radical damage—probably plays a role in some of the cognitive (a fancy word for thinking) declines that occur with age, researchers say.

However, antioxidant polyphenols, such as those found in blueberries, cranberries, and strawberries, may help preserve brain function. One of the researchers' studies in rats found that a long-term diet that included strawberry extracts helped prevent age-related cognitive declines. Another found that feeding older rats strawberry or blueberry extracts reversed age-related effects on neurons and cognitive function—and the blueberry extracts helped improve the rats' balance and coordination.

These studies are still a long way from proving that berries will offer specific protections to humans, but since berries taste so good and offer so many other health benefits, it's nice to know that brain health is yet one more potential benefit you may enjoy years down the road.

In the Kitchen

Fresh berries are highly perishable and need special handling to maintain peak freshness.

Look for leakage. Berries that are leaking from the bottom of the package are either old or have been crushed and are giving up their juice. Look for a fresher, drier batch.

Give them room. When storing berries at home, don't crowd them together, which will cause them to deteriorate rapidly. It's best to store them, unwashed and uncovered, in a large bowl in the refrigerator or spread out on a platter.

GETTING THE MOST

Shop by color. To get the most nutrients in each bite, it's important to buy (or pick) berries that are at their peak of freshness. Perhaps the easiest way to tell is by checking the color. Blackberries should be jet black; raspberries should be black, golden, or red; blueberries, a powdery blue; and strawberries, a bold red.

Eat them fresh. Cooking destroys large amounts of vitamin C in berries. In fact, even slicing strawberries, for example, can cause vitamin C levels to decline because it causes the release of an enzyme that quickly destroys the vitamin. So to get the most vitamin C from strawberries, it's best to buy those that are still wearing their little green caps and slice them just before serving.

Double-Berry Sundaes

- ½ pint raspberries
- 12 ounces blueberries
- 2 tablespoons fresh orange juice
- 1 tablespoon honey
- 1 teaspoon vanilla extract
- ¼ teaspoon almond extract
- 1 pint fat-free vanilla frozen yogurt

Place half of the raspberries in a medium glass bowl. Mash lightly with a fork. Add the blueberries, orange juice, honey, vanilla and almond extracts, and the remaining raspberries. Stir well to mix. Cover and let stand for at least 30 minutes to allow the flavors to blend.

Scoop the frozen yogurt into 4 dessert dishes. Stir the berry mixture and spoon over the yogurt.

Makes 4 servings

PER SERVING

Calories: 170	Cholesterol: 0 mg
Total fat: 0.6 g	Sodium: 45 mg
Saturated fat: 0 g	Dietary fiber: 4 g

Strawberry Tart with Oat-Cinnamon Crust

CRUST

- ⅔ cup old-fashioned or quick-cooking rolled oats
- ½ cup all-purpose flour
- 1 tablespoon sugar
- 1 teaspoon ground cinnamon
- ¼ teaspoon baking soda
- 2 tablespoons canola oil
- 2–3 tablespoons fat-free plain yogurt

STRAWBERRY FILLING

- 1½ pints strawberries
- ¼ cup all-fruit strawberry spread
- ½ teaspoon vanilla extract

To make the crust: Preheat the oven to 375°F. Coat a baking sheet with cooking spray.

In a medium bowl, combine the oats, flour, sugar, cinnamon, and baking soda. Mix with a fork until blended. Stir in the oil and 2 tablespoons of the yogurt to make a soft, slightly sticky dough. If the dough is too stiff, add the remaining 1 tablespoon yogurt.

Place the dough on the prepared baking sheet, and pat evenly into a 10-inch circle. If the dough sticks to your hands, coat them lightly with cooking spray. Place a 9-inch cake pan on the dough, and trace around it with a sharp knife. With your fingers, push up and pinch the dough around the outside of the circle to make a 9-inch circle with a rim ¼ inch high.

Bake for 15 minutes, or until firm and golden. Remove from the oven, and set aside to cool. With a pancake turner, gently ease the crust onto a large, flat serving plate.

To make the strawberry filling: Wash the strawberries, and pat dry with paper towels. Slice off the stem ends and discard.

In a small microwaveable bowl, combine the strawberry spread and vanilla. Microwave on high for 10 to 15 seconds, or until melted.

Brush or dab a generous tablespoon evenly over the crust. Arrange the strawberries, cut side down, evenly over the crust. Brush or dab the remaining spread evenly over the strawberries, making sure that you get some of the spread between the strawberries to secure them.

Refrigerate for at least 30 minutes, or until the spread has jelled. Cut into wedges.

Makes 6 servings

Cook's Note: *You can serve the tart with a scoop of fat-free vanilla frozen yogurt on the side.*

PER SERVING

Calories: 161	Cholesterol: 0 mg
Total fat: 5.5 g	Sodium: 73 mg
Saturated fat: 0.5 g	Dietary fiber: 2.6 g

Birth Defects
FOCUS ON FOLATE

Women who are preparing to have a baby have long known the importance of eating a healthful diet, with lots of fruits, vegetables, legumes, and whole grains. Especially important, researchers say, is getting more foods high in folate, a B vitamin that has been shown to reduce the risk of certain birth defects.

For a long time, folate didn't get a lot of awareness from the public. Doctors knew that we needed it, but it wasn't considered to be all that important. Then, in the early 1990s, studies proved just how important it is. A study of more than 3,600 mothers found that those who got the Daily Value (DV) of 400 micrograms of folic acid (the form of folate that's in supplements and added to fortified foods) each day were 60 percent less likely to have children with neural tube defects, in which the skull or spinal cord doesn't fuse properly, than those who got less.

Now the federal government and other organizations concerned with preventing birth defects have made it a priority to make sure that women get enough folic acid. Getting enough of this nutrient every day before and during pregnancy can reduce the risk of brain and spinal birth defects by 50 to 70 percent.

Still, most women in the United States aren't getting enough folic acid to help prevent birth defects, according to the Centers for Disease Control and Prevention (CDC). Women who are pregnant need 600 micrograms of folate daily.

But it's not only women who are *planning* to have babies who should be getting more folate, adds J. David Erickson, DDS, PhD, an epidemiologist with the National Center on Birth Defects and Developmental Disabilities at the CDC. Since many birth defects occur very early in pregnancy—often before a woman knows she's pregnant—getting enough folate is important for *all* women of childbearing age, he says. Brain and spinal defects in babies develop in the first few weeks of pregnancy, according to the CDC, so you want to make sure you have enough folate in your circulation already.

To get more folate into your diet, some of the dark green leafy vegetables are good choices, says Patricia A. Baird, MD, professor emerita at the University of British Columbia in Vancouver. One cup of canned spinach, for example, has 210 micrograms of folate, more than half of the DV for nonpregnant women. Lima beans are also a good source, with a cup providing 120 micrograms, or 30 percent of the DV for

Doctor's Top Tip

If you're a woman of childbearing years and choose not to get your folic acid in supplement form, fortified breakfast cereals are a great source of the nutrient. In fact, the CDC recommends that all women who may become pregnant make sure that they get their 400 micrograms daily by eating a daily bowl of cereal containing 100 percent of the DV for this nutrient, as an alternative to taking a folic acid supplement.

folate. In addition, packaged foods such as flour, pasta, and rice are fortified with this essential nutrient.

Incidentally, to get the most folate from the foods you eat, it's important not to overcook them. Boiling or overcooking foods can destroy up to 90 percent of the folate. To maximize this nutrient, either munch foods raw, or cook them gently, using a microwave or a steamer.

Off the A-list

Taking a multivitamin may help prevent other kinds of birth defects, too. A team of CDC researchers, including Dr. Erickson, reviewed the previous literature on multivitamins and birth defects for a report in 2004. They pointed out that an earlier Hungarian study found that using a multivitamin around the time of conception (from a short period beforehand to the first portion of the pregnancy) was associated with roughly *half* as many birth defects. A large American study associated multivitamin use with a 20 percent lower risk of birth defects.

The authors estimate that women worldwide could prevent up to 5,200 birth defects *each day* by using multivitamins. These defects include brain and spinal defects, heart defects, urinary tract defects, and limb malformations. They determined that "for the time being, women should consider the daily use of a folic acid–containing multivitamin supplement."

Of course, if you're pregnant or thinking about getting pregnant, discuss with your doctor whether a multivitamin is appropriate for your needs.

Dangerous Spirits

The ancient Greeks didn't have microscopes or maternal-care units, but they knew that pregnancy and alcohol don't mix. In fact, they had laws prohibiting newly married couples from drinking.

The Greeks were ahead of their time. Studies have shown that drinking alcohol—not just hard liquor but also beer and wine—during pregnancy can cause problems. Children with a condition called fetal alcohol syndrome are small in size, have abnormal facial features, and brain abnormalities, according to the US Surgeon General. Since alcohol-related birth defects are totally preventable, the surgeon general recommends that women should completely avoid alcohol during pregnancy, and even abstain from alcohol if they're *thinking* about becoming pregnant.

Diabetes Control

If a pregnant woman has diabetes—either type 1 or type 2—that is not kept under good control, the condition can cause a variety of problems in the developing fetus. According to the CDC, high blood sugar during the first 2 months of pregnancy (when women may not even know they're pregnant) can cause serious defects in the baby's spine, heart, brain, and other organs.

In addition, high blood sugar later in the pregnancy can cause the baby to grow excessively large in the womb. This can cause a greater risk of nerve injuries to the child during the birthing process. The child may also have a greater risk of obesity and type 2 diabetes later in life.

Finally, according to the CDC, diabetes-related problems that lead to a premature birth can cause a host of complications in the child related to prematurity.

If you're a woman of childbearing age with diabetes, make sure to keep your blood sugar well controlled before and during your pregnancy. Discuss your condition with your doctor and a dietitian before you get pregnant, and follow their recommendations on any steps you need to take to control your condition, such as exercise, diet, checking your blood sugar, and possibly taking medications.

Blood Pressure Control

GETTING THE NUMBERS DOWN

High blood pressure quietly sneaks around your body, causing damage here and wreaking havoc there. It can cause so much strain on your heart that the organ fails from working so hard. It can make arteries in your brain rupture or develop blockages, potentially leaving you disabled. It can hurt your kidneys so badly that you need to use a dialysis machine, and your eyes so much that you become blind.

If you think that's bad, here's the *really* scary part: Since high blood pressure usually causes no symptoms, you might not even know you have it until you develop a serious health problem.

But while high blood pressure works quietly, it's frequently deadly (for this reason, high blood pressure is often called the silent killer). "High blood pressure is just a reflection of a cardiovascular system that's about to burst internally," says John A. McDougall, MD, medical director of the McDougall Program in Santa Rosa, California, and author of *The McDougall Program for a Healthy Heart*. "But if you eat a good diet—lots of fruits and vegetables and whole grains versus rich foods—you can help change all that," he says.

According to the National Institutes of Health, nearly one in three adults has high blood pressure. By eating a healthy diet, you can help ensure that you won't be one of them.

The How of Hypertension

Everyone has blood pressure, and it can go up or down frequently during the course of a day, and even from minute to minute. Your heart pumps blood throughout your body through a system of arteries. Each time your heart beats, it sends out a new wave of blood, and your blood pressure goes up. This is your systolic blood pressure. Between beats, your heart briefly relaxes and the pressure subsides. This is your diastolic blood pressure. When you have your blood pressure tested, you're given two numbers, one over the other (your systolic over your diastolic), measured in millimeters of mercury, or mm Hg. A sample blood pressure might be 135/86 mm Hg.

Your heart, brain, kidneys, eyes, and other organs depend on a reliable flow of blood that courses through your delicate "plumbing." When you develop chronic high blood pressure, or hypertension, trouble follows.

High-pressure blood whooshes through the arteries with damaging force. Your heart has to struggle harder to push out the blood, and it may grow enlarged and unable to bear the extra strain. Your arteries, which should be elastic and flexible, may more rapidly grow stiff and narrow. They may deliver less blood to your organs, and a blood clot can more readily get "stuck" and totally block the flow, causing a heart attack.

In most cases, doctors don't know the exact cause of high blood pressure. But they do know the preventable lifestyle factors that increase your risk of the problem: being overweight or obese, excessive alcohol use, a diet that provides too much salt or too little potassium, smoking, a sedentary lifestyle, chronic stress, and taking certain medications. Other risk factors can't be changed: your age (high blood pressure is more common in middle age and after), your race (it's more common in African Americans than Caucasians), and family history of high blood pressure.

The National Institutes of Health (NIH) and the American Heart Association use the following classifications to identify normal and high blood pressure:

Blood Pressure Classification	Systolic Blood Pressure (in mm Hg)		Diastolic Blood Pressure (in mm Hg)
Normal	Less than 120	and	Less than 80
Prehypertension	120 to 139	or	80 to 89
Stage 1 hypertension	140 to 159	or	90 to 99
Stage 2 hypertension	More than 160	or	More than 100

Even if your blood pressure falls into the normal or "prehypertension" categories, it's not time to breathe a sigh of relief. Your risk of death from heart disease or stroke rises progressively as your blood pressure goes up, and according to the NIH, the risk starts going up in these early stages. In other words—you need to start getting concerned well before you have a diagnosis of hypertension.

Research from the major, long-running Framingham Heart Study shows that having systolic blood pressure between 130 and 139 or diastolic blood pressure between 85 and 89 may more than double your risk of cardiovascular disease versus having blood pressure in the "normal" range.

According to the NIH, people in the prehypertension category should be "firmly and unambiguously advised to practice lifestyle modifications in order to reduce their risk of developing hypertension in the future."

Mild high blood pressure responds well to nondrug therapies. If you feed and exercise your body well, you may be able to avoid blood pressure drugs (and their often troublesome side effects) and calm your rushing blood. Don't be misled by the "mild"

Doctor's Top Tip

In a scientific statement from the American Heart Association on dietary approaches to prevent and treat high blood pressure, the first suggestion from the expert panel was to maintain a healthy weight. Almost all studies have documented that "weight loss lowers blood pressure," they wrote. You don't have to get down to a perfect weight before your blood pressure starts dropping, either. Just a few pounds will make a difference. But the more weight you lose as you pursue your goal of a healthy target weight, the more your blood pressure will drop. Ideally your body mass index, or BMI (a way to classify your weight's effect on your health), should be no higher than 25. That translates to a person who's 5 feet 4 inches weighing no more than 145 pounds, or someone who's 6 feet tall weighing 184 pounds max.

As an added bonus, losing weight may improve your blood pressure enough that you can stop taking hypertension medications (although you shouldn't change your medication regimen without your doctor's guidance).

label, though. "Most heart attacks and strokes that occur do so in people with stage 1 high blood pressure," says Norman Kaplan, MD, professor of internal medicine and hypertension specialist at the University of Texas Southwestern Medical Center at Dallas.

A major study published in the *Journal of the American Medical Association* measured the effects of lifestyle changes on 810 adults with "above optimal" blood pressure. They were divided into three groups. One received many counseling sessions on how to reduce blood pressure with lifestyle measures such as weight loss, physical activity, and a low-sodium diet. Another got counseling, plus lots of information on the DASH diet for lowering blood pressure, which is rich in fruits and vegetables (more on that later). The third group received a single 30-minute counseling session covering these basics on lowering blood pressure.

After 6 months, the first group reduced their systolic blood pressure by an average of 3.7 mm Hg, and the DASH diet group reduced theirs by 4.3 mm Hg. The third group had less impressive changes in their blood pressure. At the beginning of the experiment, 38 percent of the subjects had hypertension, but after 6 months, only 17 percent in the first group had it, and only 12 percent in the DASH group. This contrasted with a considerably higher 26 percent in the advice-only group.

Giving Your Heart a Break

Losing weight—even just 10 pounds—can reduce your blood pressure or prevent you from developing hypertension.

What's the connection between excess weight and hypertension? The more tissue you have in your body, the harder your heart has to pump to feed it. And that work exerts more pressure on artery walls.

Everybody knows that losing weight is no piece of cake. But exercise makes it easier. And the best weight-loss diet is the same as the best diet for controlling blood pressure: low-fat foods and lots of fruits and vegetables.

"We really emphasize following a low-fat, high-fruit-and-vegetable diet. It's almost certain to lower your blood pressure because it lowers sodium and increases all the good stuff that's hypothesized to lower blood pressure—fiber, calcium, and potassium—and it's an effective avenue to weight loss," says Pao-Hwa Lin, PhD, assistant research professor of medicine at Duke University in Durham, North Carolina, and coauthor of *The DASH Diet for Hypertension*.

A diet low in fat won't include large amounts of red meat, which is packed with saturated fat. Nor will it include many processed foods, because they're high-fat minefields. Processed foods also tend to be high in salt and low in potassium, so when you get rid of them, you wipe out three bad birds with one dietary stone.

The Story of Salt

Experts believe that many people with high blood pressure are salt "responders," meaning that their blood pressure levels depend on the amount of salt they eat. "But there is some controversy about the issue," says Lawrence Appel, MD, professor of medicine and epidemiology at Johns Hopkins University School of Medicine in Baltimore. "Some people have a greater response than others. Older people tend to be more sensitive to salt, as are African Americans." Some research shows that roughly 26 percent of Americans with normal blood pressure—and about 58 percent of those with hypertension—are salt sensitive.

Here's what happens. When you eat the typical American's ration of sodium— 3,000 to 6,000 milligrams or more a day, compared with the recommended 2,400-milligram limit—your blood pressure rises. If you're sensitive to salt, the sodium it contains makes your body attract water like a sponge. You soak it up, and your blood vessels expand with it, producing higher pressure.

Some experts feel that you shouldn't worry much about whether you're salt sensitive or not. It's hard to determine an individual's sensitivity to salt—you're better off just reducing your salt intake to the recommended limits to be safe.

"If you have high blood pressure, your sodium needs to be reduced by half," says Dr. Kaplan. "Don't put salt on the table or in the food you cook. Avoid most processed foods, which is where 80 percent of the sodium in American diets comes from. If that doesn't bring your blood pressure down, then sodium isn't the culprit," he says.

According to the NIH, reducing sodium in your diet to no more than 2,400 milligrams daily (equal to about a teaspoon of table salt) will lower your systolic blood pressure by 2 to 8 mm Hg. An even better goal is to reduce daily sodium to 1,500 milligrams, or ⅔ teaspoon of table salt, to lower your blood pressure even further.

Mining for Minerals

Potassium and calcium are two minerals that act like a massage on a tense body. They help the blood vessels relax. When arteries relax, they dilate, or open up, and give blood the room it needs to move calmly.

"You can think of potassium as the opposite of sodium," says Harvey B. Simon, MD, associate professor of medicine at Harvard Medical School. Potassium helps the body excrete sodium, so the more potassium you get in your diet, the more sodium you get rid of. In fact, the landmark INTERSALT study looked at more than 10,000 people from 32 countries and found that people with the highest amounts of potassium in their blood had the lowest blood pressures, and those with the lowest amounts had the highest.

"Fruits and vegetables are naturally low in sodium and high in potassium," says Dr. Lin. "A diet high in vegetables and fruits almost mimics a vegetarian diet, which is known to be linked to lower blood pressure," she says. Foods that are especially rich in potassium include beans, potatoes, avocados, steamed clams, lima beans, bananas, and apricots.

Calcium has shown similar ties to blood pressure in studies. Some have found that low intake is actually a risk factor for developing high blood pressure. The landmark Framingham Heart Study looked at the calcium intakes of 432 men. Those who ate the most (between 322 and 1,118 milligrams a day) had a 20 percent lower risk of developing high blood pressure than those who ate the least (8 to 109 milligrams a day).

A study in the journal *Hypertension* that analyzed the diet habits of nearly 5,000 people found that as they consumed more dairy, they became less likely to have hypertension. In fact, the people who consumed the most dairy were nearly 40 percent less likely to have hypertension as the people who consumed the least. However, this association was mainly seen in people whose diets were relatively low in saturated fat. Since regular dairy foods contain saturated fat, it's wise to make sure that you get your calcium from low-fat or fat-free dairy products.

A cup of fat-free yogurt contains about 415 milligrams of calcium and a glass of fat-free milk has about 352. Besides low-fat and fat-free dairy products, your best sources of calcium include tofu, calcium-fortified orange juice, kale, broccoli, and collard greens.

The government-promoted DASH diet—for Dietary Approaches to Stop Hypertension—is heavy on whole grains (six to eight daily servings) and fruits and vegetables (eight to 10 servings). It calls for two or three servings of low-fat dairy; moderate amounts of lean meat, nuts, and seeds; and limited amounts of fats and oils and sweets. It urges you to eat processed foods sparingly, since these are the main source of sodium in the American diet.

Adopting the DASH plan can lower your systolic blood pressure by 8 to 14 mm Hg. As you can see, by cutting out the salt and sodium and boosting fruits, vegetables, and other plant foods, the blood pressure reductions really add up.

Eating Right

For starters, you should practice what Dr. Appel calls active shopping. In other words, read the nutrition labels and be sure to glance at the sodium content. One 8-ounce can of stewed tomatoes can contain over 800 milligrams of sodium, while another can might have only 70. "You often have to look hard for low-sodium cereals," he adds. "Shredded wheat is one of the low-salt ones."

Sodium-free is a good phrase to look for on a label. So is *low-sodium*. The word *light*, however, is not as conclusive. Light soy sauce, for instance, can still have 605 milligrams of sodium per tablespoon. *No salt added* doesn't mean a food is sodium-free, either. In the Nutrition Facts box on a food label, also look to see how the sodium in the food relates to the Daily Value (DV). Go for foods containing less than 5 percent of the DV. If the product contains 20 percent or more of the DV, it's high in sodium.

While bread is often a nutritious, wholesome food, it too is occasionally high in salt. If you buy bread fresh at a bakery where it isn't labeled, don't be shy about asking how much salt is in each loaf.

When you're buying canned foods, like the tomatoes mentioned above, salt can be a real problem. In many cases, however, rinsing the food will eliminate a good percentage of the salt. If you don't have a can of beans that states it's low-sodium, for example, you can rinse off at least half the salt the food was packed in, says Neva Cochran, RD, a nutrition consultant in Dallas.

Since produce is the cornerstone of a diet for healthy blood pressure, you should always be looking for ways to eat more fruits and vegetables. Here are a few of Dr. Lin's suggestions:

- Buy prepackaged salads for busy days (best to rinse it before using, however).
- Order a fruit plate as an appetizer before your meal in a restaurant.
- Eat two vegetarian dinners a week.

When you're picking up produce, be sure to grab some apples, pears, and oranges. These three fruits are fiber kings. And heart researchers are starting to find that not only does fiber decrease dangerous cholesterol, it may also lower blood pressure. Fruit fiber made a strong showing in a study at Harvard Medical School, where scientists tracked more than 30,000 men. The men in the study who ate less than 12 grams of fruit fiber a day (about four oranges or three apples or

STAY OUT OF THE SALT MINES

If you're sodium savvy and watching your blood pressure, you already know to say no thanks to foods such as chips and salty pickles. Yet sodium appears in many foods in which you might not expect it. Baking soda and baking powder, for instance, are both sodium bicarbonate. Dried fruit contains sodium sulfite, and ice cream often has sodium caseinate and sodium alginate.

Even a sharp-eyed sodium detective can miss a few salt mines. Here are some to watch out for:

Instant chocolate-flavored pudding. A half-cup contains 470 milligrams of sodium, more than the amount in two slices of bacon.

Ketchup. One tablespoon contains 156 milligrams of sodium.

Pastries. A fruit Danish has 333 milligrams of sodium, while a cheese Danish has 319. Scones and baking-powder biscuits also tend to be high in sodium.

Cheese. Most types are high in sodium. This includes cottage cheese, which has 425 milligrams in a half-cup serving.

pears) were 60 percent more likely to develop high blood pressure. The DASH diet is particularly high in fiber, given the amount of grain foods, fruits, and vegetables it recommends.

Finally, it's essential to reduce the amount of fat in your diet. You don't have to be fanatical, however. Instead of cutting out fat with a cleaver, start by slicing it off with a scalpel, bit by bit. Dr. Lin recommends making small, gradual changes that will cut the total amount of fat you use in half. Buy butter substitutes and trans-fat-free versions of margarine. For sautéing, use olive oil cooking spray instead of liquid oils or butter. Use mustard instead of mayonnaise, and snack on low-salt pretzels instead of potato chips.

Keep Drinks to a Minimum

Research has found that 16 percent of hypertensive disease worldwide is due to alcohol use.

The NIH recommends that men drink no more than two drinks daily, and women (and men of slight physical stature) keep their consumption limited to one drink daily. One drink is the equivalent of a 12-ounce beer, 5 ounces of wine, or 1½ ounces of 80-proof liquor.

By staying moderate with your alcohol use, you can reduce your systolic blood pressure by 2 to 4 mm Hg.

Broccoli

KING OF THE CRUCIFERS

If fruits and vegetables had an annual yearbook, broccoli might not win the Tastiest of the Year honor. But it would definitely be in the running for Most Likely to Prevent Cancer.

Scientists around the world are using high-tech methods to learn which compounds contained within this vegetable might be helpful in confronting cancer. And they're finding plenty of them.

HEALING POWER

Can Help:

Protect against heart disease

Fight off cancer

Boost immunity

Multiple Cancer Fighters

Broccoli's impressive power as a cancer fighter is due in part to its multipronged attack. It contains at least two separate compounds—indole-3-carbinol (or I3C, for short) and sulforaphane—that help sweep up cancer-causing substances before they have a chance to do harm.

The compound I3C, which is also found in cabbage and Brussels sprouts, seems to be able to prevent or interrupt cancer in several ways.

The hormone estrogen causes cells in the breasts to multiply and grow. This is a natural and normal process in women. However, if mutated cells that could become cancerous develop in the breasts, estrogen causes these to multiply, too. That's bad. To cause breast cells to perform certain activities, estrogen must first attach to "receptors" on the cells, kind of like a key fitting into a lock. The I3C compound appears to act on these receptors, perhaps by keeping estrogen from attaching to them, or changing the way they work. Thus, estrogen can't have its tumor-encouraging role on the cells.

In addition, I3C may help shift the balance of different types of estrogen in the body so that you have less of a type that *does* promote breast cancer growth, and more of a type that *doesn't*. I3C may also trigger cancerous cells to die, a process called apoptosis, and may raise your levels of enzymes that protect you from cancer-causing substances.

Beyond its potential effects on breast cancer, I3C has been shown to inhibit the growth of prostate and cervical cancer cells. In addition, numerous studies have shown that a diet high in cruciferous vegetables, such as broccoli, may reduce the risk of colon cancer.

Researchers investigating I3C's potential effect on cervical cancer gave supplements of the substance for 12 weeks to 30 women who had precancerous changes on their cervix. In roughly half of the women who took supplemental I3C, these worrisome lesions regressed. This didn't happen in any of the women who took a placebo (dummy pill).

While I3C is conducting its anticancer activities, another component called sulforaphane is offering protection on another front, by boosting the production of cancer-blocking enzymes, says Thomas Kensler, PhD, professor in the department of environmental health sciences in the Bloomberg School of Public Health at Johns Hopkins University in Baltimore.

In one pioneering study, Dr. Kensler and his colleagues at Johns Hopkins exposed 145 laboratory animals to a powerful cancer-causing agent. Twenty-five of the animals had not received any special treatment, while the rest were fed high doses of sulforaphane. After 50 days, 68 percent of the unprotected animals had breast tumors, compared with only 26 percent of those given the sulforaphane.

Other lab studies have found that sulforaphane may help protect against cancer of the prostate, colon, and pancreas. More recent research has also found clues that sulforaphane may have other cancer-fighting properties in addition to boosting your anticancer enzymes. It may help inhibit germs that contribute to cancer, such as the *H. pylori* bacteria that raise the risk of stomach cancer. It may also interfere with cancer cells' growth cycle and may help encourage the cells to die.

It is no wonder that researchers put broccoli at the top of their lists of nutritional superstars. "We know that those people who eat lots of cruciferous vegetables, including broccoli, are protected from many forms of cancer," says Jon Michnovicz, MD, PhD, president of the Foundation for Preventive Oncology in New York City.

In the Kitchen

One of the problems with cooking broccoli is consistency—or, more specifically, a lack thereof. Broccoli consists of both tough stalks and tender florets, the result being that it often ends up with some parts either overdone or underdone.

To help ensure even cooking, it's helpful to cut broccoli into little spears. First, cut off and discard the thick, woody part of the stalk, generally from the bottom up to where the broccoli florets begin to branch. Then cut any large florets and stems in half lengthwise.

If you find that the stems are still too tough for eating, either trim them farther up from the bottom or peel them with a vegetable peeler before cooking.

A Boost from Beta-Carotene

While much recent research has focused on "exotic" compounds like sulforaphane, broccoli is also chock-full of more commonly known, but still powerful, compounds like beta-carotene. This nutrient, which the body converts to vitamin A, is an antioxidant. That is, it helps prevent disease by sweeping up harmful, cell-damaging oxygen molecules that naturally accumulate in the body. High levels of beta-carotene have been linked to lower rates of heart attack, certain cancers, and cataracts.

Broccoli is an excellent source of beta-carotene, providing about 0.7 milligram in a half-cup cooked serving. This provides 7 to 12 percent of the recommended daily amount.

Doctor's Top Tip

While gently cooking broccoli helps release some of its protective compounds, overheating it can destroy others. "Carotenoids like beta-carotene are preserved by heat, but the indoles, like I3C, don't withstand a lot of heat," explains Jon Michnovicz, MD, PhD, president of the Foundation for Preventive Oncology in New York City. "Light steaming is a great way to cook broccoli. And microwaving is okay, too."

Supporting Players

Broccoli isn't called the king of the crucifers for nothing. Besides beta-carotene, sulforaphane, and I3C, broccoli contains a variety of other nutrients, each of which can help fend off a host of conditions, from heart disease to osteoporosis.

For example, just a half-cup of chopped, cooked broccoli contains 85 percent of the Daily Value (DV) for vitamin C. This antioxidant vitamin has been proven in studies to help boost immunity and fight diseases like heart disease and cancer.

Broccoli also ranks highly for women's health, particularly for women who don't get enough dairy food. It's one of the best vegetable sources of calcium, packing in 72 milligrams per cooked cup—about a quarter of the amount in an 8-ounce glass of fat-free milk. Calcium is well-documented as the single most important nutrient that women need to keep osteoporosis (the breaking down of bones) at bay.

Broccoli is also rich in folate, a nutrient that's essential for normal tissue growth and that studies show may protect against cancer, heart disease, and birth defects. Women, especially those who take birth control pills, are often low in this vital nutrient. A cup of chopped, cooked broccoli contains 84 micrograms, or almost one-quarter of the DV for folate.

Finally, if you're looking to keep your digestive system running smoothly, make broccoli your food of choice, experts advise. A half-cup provides 2 grams of fiber, which is a proven protector against constipation, hemorrhoids, colon cancer, diabetes, high cholesterol, heart disease, and obesity.

Experts aren't yet sure how much broccoli you need to maximize its healing potential. Dr. Kensler advises eating at least five servings of fruits and vegetables a day, while reaching for this crunchy crucifer whenever you can.

GETTING THE MOST

Buy it purple. You'll notice at the supermarket that broccoli is sometimes so dark that it's almost purple. That's good. The dark color means that it has more beta-carotene, experts say. If it's yellowish, on the other hand, skip it. That means that it's old, and its nutritional clock is running down.

Look for the sprouts. Studies at Johns Hopkins University in Baltimore found that 3-day-old broccoli sprouts can contain up to 100 times the amount of protective substances in the mature vegetable. These can provide a great alternative if you don't care for the taste of mature broccoli (and you may get the same cancer-fighting benefit by eating a smaller amount of sprouts than regular broccoli). Broccoli sprouts look like white strings with little green heads. They're perfect for salads or sandwiches, but they quickly spoil in the refrigerator, so only buy an amount that you can eat in a few days. You'll likely find them in plastic containers in the produce section of your supermarket.

Broccoli Pesto Pizzas

1 cup packed small broccoli florets

2 large cloves garlic

½ cup fresh basil leaves

1½ tablespoons extra-virgin olive oil

1½ tablespoons fresh lemon juice

2 tablespoons water

⅓ cup grated Parmesan cheese

2 tablespoons chopped walnuts

¼ teaspoon salt

4 mini whole-wheat pitas (4 inches in diameter)

½ cup chopped roasted red pepper

½ cup shredded low-fat mozzarella cheese

Preheat the oven to 375°F.

Place the broccoli and the garlic in a microwaveable bowl. Cover and microwave on high for 45 seconds. Transfer to a food processor, and add the basil, oil, lemon juice, water, Parmesan, walnuts, and salt. Process 1 minute, or until smooth.

Cut around the edge of the pitas, and split in half. Place the pita halves on a baking sheet, rough side down, and bake for 8 minutes. Turn over, and spread each half with 1½ tablespoons of the pesto. Top evenly with some roasted pepper and mozzarella. Bake for 8 minutes longer, or until heated through.

Cook's Notes: *The broccoli pesto can be made ahead and refrigerated in an airtight container for up to a week. It can also be drizzled on pasta and veggies, added to soup, or used as a spread.*

Makes 4 servings (2 pizzas each)

PER SERVING ————————————

Calories: 230	Cholesterol: 10 mg
Total fat: 12 g	Sodium: 540 mg
Saturated fat: 4 g	Dietary fiber: 3 g

Brussels Sprouts
GOOD THINGS IN SMALL PACKAGES

HEALING POWER

Can Help:

Reduce the risk of many forms of cancer

Lower cholesterol

Prevent constipation

Lower the risk of heart disease

If you've never seen Brussels sprouts growing on a farm, you might wonder how farmers harvest them. Do they walk down the rows, bending down to pluck the tiny vegetables, which look like miniature cabbages, off the ground? Do they drive little harvesters across the fields?

Actually, Brussels sprouts grow in bunches of 20 to 40 up and down the sides of a central stalk that's several feet tall—they don't pop up individually. Surprised? It's possible that you may harbor some other, more common misconceptions about Brussels sprouts, too. When many people hear the words "Brussels sprouts," they remember those piles of bitter, overcooked blobs from childhood dinners.

It's time to reevaluate this vegetable with an undeserved bad reputation. Today's Brussels sprouts taste better than those of bygone days, and researchers have uncovered that they may contain great disease-stopping power.

New Taste in the Marketplace

Brussels sprouts are related to cabbage, cauliflower, and broccoli . . . none of which are famous for their pleasing taste. However, while the Brussels sprouts of yore were often strong and bitter, today their taste has changed.

In recent years, Brussels sprouts growers have shifted to growing varieties that are sweeter and milder than those you may remember from your childhood. Plus, if you take care to store and cook them properly, you can maximize their tastiness. So now you'll be smacking your lips instead of holding your nose when you spoon these health-saving leafy nuggets onto your plate.

Belgium's Can-Do Cancer Beaters

Like other cruciferous vegetables, Brussels sprouts are chock-full of natural plant compounds called phytonutrients, which may help protect against cancer. These compounds may be particularly effective against common cancers, like those of the breast and colon.

One of the key protective compounds in Brussels sprouts is sulforaphane.

Research from test tubes to lab animals to humans shows that this component can interfere with cancer at many stages of its development. It can keep cancer-causing chemicals from becoming activated in your body; it may trigger cancer cells to spontaneously die; it can prevent new blood vessels from growing to a tumor to feed it; and it may help prevent cancer from metastasizing, or spreading to new locations.

In one study looking at the effects of vegetables on cancer, researchers from the Fred Hutchinson Cancer Research Center in Seattle compared the diet history of more than 600 men with newly diagnosed prostate cancer with the diet history of more than 600 men without prostate cancer. Although a diet that is rich in vegetables reduced the risk of cancer, cruciferous vegetables—such as Brussels sprouts—were particularly helpful. Men who ate three or more servings of crucifers a week were 41 percent less likely to have prostate cancer than those who ate less than one serving a week.

Another study, which reviewed 80 studies looking at the relationship between consumption of brassica vegetables (such as Brussels sprouts), found that most showed a link between higher consumption of these vegetables and a lower risk of cancer. The results were most consistent with cancer of the lung, stomach, colon, and rectum.

Brussels sprouts contain another protective phytonutrient called indole-3-carbinol, or I3C. This compound works as an antiestrogen, meaning it helps break down your body's estrogens before they contribute to the growth of cancer cells. It also helps boost the production of certain enzymes that help clear cancer-causing toxins from the body.

Lab tests have shown that I3C inhibits the growth of a variety of types of cancer cells, including breast, prostate, endometrial, colon, and leukemia.

In one small study, researchers in the Netherlands found that people who ate more than 10 ounces of Brussels sprouts (about 14 sprouts) a day for 1 week had levels of protective cancer-fighting enzymes in their colon that were, on average, 23 percent higher than people who did not eat Brussels sprouts.

Doctor's Top Tip

Cook your Brussels sprouts using a method that preserves more of their cancer-fighting power. British researchers investigating the effects of different cooking techniques on Brussels sprouts and related vegetables found that boiling caused them to lose "significant" amounts of glucosinolates into the boiling water. (Glucosinolates turn into isothiocyanates—and one of these is sulforaphane, the cancer-fighting component you learned about on these pages.)

Instead, the researchers suggest, prepare your Brussels sprouts (and broccoli, cabbage, and cauliflower, for that matter) by steaming, microwaving, or stir-frying them. You won't lose much of the glucosinolates that way.

In the Kitchen

For such tiny vegetables, Brussels sprouts sure cause some large culinary conundrums. Not only is it challenging to cook them just so, but it's also likely that you'll smell up the house while you do it.

It doesn't have to be this way. If you follow these tips, you'll get the health benefits of Brussels sprouts without the hassles:

Mark the spot. To allow the tough stems to cook as quickly as the leaves, make an "X" on the bottom of each stem, using a sharp knife. Then steam them for 7 to 14 minutes, until they're just tender enough to poke with a fork.

Quell the smell. The big sulfur smell thrown off by these little cabbages discourages some people from taking advantage of their healing power. Try tossing a stalk of celery in the cooking water. It will help neutralize the smell.

Use them fast. Although Brussels sprouts will keep for a week or more in the refrigerator, they start getting bitter after about 3 days, which may discourage you and your family from eating them and reaping their benefits. Buy only as many as you'll use in the next few days.

Brussels for Your Bowels

Aside from all the "sciency" compounds in Brussels sprouts, there are also plenty of good old-fashioned vitamins, minerals, and other substances that can help fight off cancer, heart disease, high cholesterol, and a host of other health problems.

Topping this list is fiber. Brussels sprouts are a decent source of fiber, with about 3 grams in a half-cup serving. That's more than you'd get in a slice of whole-grain bread.

Eating your daily fill of Brussels sprouts can help you avoid all the conditions that a diet rich in fiber is known to prevent, like constipation, hemorrhoids, and other digestive complaints.

A half-cup of Brussels sprouts also provides 48 milligrams of immunity-building vitamin C, more than 80 percent of the Daily Value (DV) for this vitamin. It also provides 47 micrograms of the B vitamin folate, about 12 percent of the DV. Folate is essential for normal tissue growth, and studies show that it may protect against cancer, heart disease, and birth defects. Women, especially those on birth control pills, often have low levels of this important vitamin.

Glazed Brussels Sprouts

1 **pound small Brussels sprouts**

1 **teaspoon unsalted butter**

2 **tablespoons all-fruit apricot spread**

¼ **teaspoon salt**

¼ **teaspoon dry mustard**

Trim the bottoms of the Brussels sprouts and cut them in half lengthwise. Place in a large saucepan and add 2 tablespoons water. Bring to a boil over high heat, then cover, and reduce the heat to medium-high. Cook, stirring once, for 5 to 7 minutes, or until the sprouts are crisp-tender. If the sprouts start to dry out, add another 1 to 2 tablespoons water.

If any water remains in the pan, drain the sprouts in a colander. Transfer to a medium bowl.

Add the butter to the pan and melt over medium heat. Stir in the apricot spread, salt, and mustard. Cook for 30 seconds, or until bubbly and hot. Add the Brussels sprouts to the pan, and toss to coat with the glaze.

Makes 4 servings

PER SERVING

Calories: 83
Total fat: 1.7 g
Saturated fat: 0.7 g

Cholesterol: 3 mg
Sodium: 164 mg
Dietary fiber: 5.7 g

Buckwheat

HOMEGROWN PROTECTION

HEALING POWER

Can Help:

Prevent cancer and
heart disease

Control diabetes

Provide an antioxidant
boost

Supply protein, minerals,
and B vitamins

Buckwheat has been a somewhat neglected food in America. Historically, if you've had a diet heavy in buckwheat, you would most likely be a farm animal, since until recent years, it was primarily grown as feed for livestock.

However, buckwheat is popular in Japan, says Michael Eskin, PhD, professor of food chemistry at the University of Manitoba in Winnipeg, and some researchers suspect that this may partially explain that country's remarkably low cancer rates. If you're familiar with Japanese cuisine, you might recognize soba noodles, which contain buckwheat. It's also commonly available stateside in pancake mixes.

Despite its name, buckwheat is not a grain—it's a seed from a plant related to rhubarb. Want to know more about this underappreciated food? Read on.

Two-Pronged Protection

Buckwheat contains a variety of compounds called flavonoids that have been shown in studies to help block the spread of cancer. Two compounds in particular, quercetin and rutin, are especially promising because they appear to thwart cancer in two ways.

These substances make it difficult for cancer-promoting hormones to attach to healthy cells. They can literally stop cancers before they start. Should cancer-causing substances get into cells, these compounds may be able to reduce damage to DNA, the body's chemical blueprint for normal cell division.

Japanese researchers have found that buckwheat extract can help interfere with colon and breast cancer in rats.

A study from South Carolina researchers looked at the possible relationship of quercetin and rutin and a lower risk of colon cancer in rats. They found that a diet containing quercetin for several weeks decreased the number of lesions that serve as a warning of early colon cancer fourfold. A diet containing rutin decreased these lesions by 20 percent.

FOOD ALERT

A Surprising Allergy

Although buckwheat allergy is rare in America, it's relatively common in Asian cultures that eat more of it. Eating products containing buckwheat can cause red eyes, runny nose, hives, asthma, and even dangerous anaphylactic shock. If you think that you may be allergic to buckwheat, talk to your doctor about whether you should avoid it in foods.

If you are allergic to buckwheat, also avoid pillows filled with buckwheat hulls. These trendy pillows have been implicated in at least one case of a bothersome allergic reaction.

Keeping Blood Flowing

The rutin in buckwheat plays yet another protective role. Working in concert with other compounds, it helps prevent platelets—the components in blood that assist in clotting—from clumping together. By helping to keep blood fluid, buckwheat can play an important part in any heart-protection plan. Rutin has also been reported to stabilize blood vessels and help lower blood pressure, thus helping to protect against heart disease. And it acts as an antioxidant, protecting your cells from damaging attacks from free radicals.

Research suggests that when flavonoids are combined with vitamin E, which is also found in buckwheat, the benefits are even more pronounced. Fat-soluble vitamin E can neutralize dangerous free radicals, harmful oxygen molecules that can damage cells, in the fatty portions of cells. Flavonoids, on the other hand, are water soluble; they attack free radicals in the watery parts of cells. "That puts an antioxidant in both the watery and fatty portions of cells," says Timothy Johns, PhD, professor in the School of Dietetics and Human Nutrition at McGill University in Montreal.

An Italian study tested the antioxidant capacity of a number of spices, fruits, cereal products, and other foods. It found that among the 18 cereal products tested, whole-meal buckwheat and wheat bran had the highest total antioxidant capacity.

Protein Power

Here's great news for vegetarians and others trying to cut back on meat. Buckwheat is the best known grain source of high-quality protein. We need protein for everything from healing wounds to producing brainpower. Yet buckwheat protein does more. It helps lower cholesterol as well.

In laboratory experiments, animals that were fed extracts of buckwheat protein had significantly lower cholesterol levels than their non-buckwheat-eating companions. Levels in the buckwheat-fed animals, in fact, were even lower than in animals given soy protein extract, one of the most powerful cholesterol-busting foods.

In addition, buckwheat is an excellent source of essential nutrients. "It's rich in several minerals, most especially magnesium and manganese but also zinc and copper," says Dr. Eskin.

One cup of buckwheat flour made from whole groats (the grain with the hull removed) contains 301 milligrams of magnesium, or 75 percent of the Daily Value (DV) for this mineral. It also contains 25 percent of the DV for zinc, 40 percent of the DV for phosphorus, 27 percent of the DV for iron, and 20 percent of the DV for potassium.

Help for Digestion

One of the most valuable aspects of buckwheat is its ability to help control blood sugar levels in people with adult-onset, or type 2, diabetes, the most common form of the disease.

In the Kitchen

Unlike rice and wheat, buckwheat has no gluten, a protein with a gluelike consistency. Without gluten to hold the grain together, "it will turn to mush unless you precook it," says Clifford Orr, director of the Buckwheat Institute in Penn Yan, New York. Here's what he advises:

- Put the buckwheat in a hot skillet, and toss gently for 3 to 5 minutes. This expands and strengthens the outer skin, which will help it stay intact during the simmering process.
- If you're using kasha (the roasted form of buckwheat) that's been cracked, toss it

with an egg white before adding it to the pan. The albumen in the egg will help keep it firm. Uncracked kasha, however, can be cooked without the egg.

- Transfer the buckwheat to a saucepan, and add 2 cups of water for each cup of buckwheat. Always begin with boiling water, which will seal the outer surface and help the buckwheat hold its shape during cooking.
- Simmer the buckwheat, covered, until all the water is absorbed and the kernels are tender. Cracked kasha will take 8 to 10 minutes, and whole will require 10 to 12 minutes.

The carbohydrates in buckwheat, amylose and amylopectin, are digested more slowly than other types of carbohydrates. This causes blood sugar levels to rise more evenly. While this is good for everyone, it's especially important for those with diabetes, whose blood sugar levels tend to rise steeply and stay high too long. Keeping blood sugar under control has been shown to reduce or prevent many of the serious complications of diabetes, including kidney damage.

Even if you don't have diabetes, buckwheat can help. Because it's absorbed more slowly than other grains, it leaves you feeling full longer. This makes it easier to eat less and thus control your weight.

British researchers investigating the "filling" effects of meals found that using buckwheat flour in pasta made it more satiating, or filling. One easy way to get buckwheat into your diet is in pancake mixes that contain buckwheat flour; these are commonly available in supermarkets. You may find that buckwheat pancakes "stick with you" better than versions made with regular pancake flour.

And don't forget buckwheat if you or someone you know has celiac disease. This is a potentially serious intestinal problem that occurs in people sensitive to gluten, a protein found in wheat and other grains. Because buckwheat is free of gluten, people with this ailment can eat as much as they want.

> ## Doctor's Top Tip
>
> You know that getting whole grains in your diet provides many health benefits—but it can be hard to tell which grain foods actually contain whole grains. The National Institutes of Health recommends that when looking at labels, you keep in mind that the words "buckwheat" or "kasha" mean that the food contains whole grain.

Think "B" for Buckwheat

Buckwheat is also a good source of several B vitamins. One cup of buckwheat flour provides 37 percent of the DV for niacin, 35 percent of the DV for vitamin B_6, and 33 percent of the DV for thiamin.

Niacin helps your body turn the food it uses for fuel into energy. Your body needs vitamin B_6 because it helps the hemoglobin in your red blood cells carry oxygen, and it plays a role in maintaining a healthy immune system and a healthy nervous system. Like niacin, thiamin also helps your body turn fuel into energy, and like B_6, it helps your nerves function properly.

A Sweet-Tasting Form of Buckwheat

Some honey producers bottle honey made by bees that harvest nectar from buckwheat fields. Honey contains a number of antioxidants, including phenolic acids and flavonoids. However, the dark honey made from buckwheat seems to be particularly powerful. Research has found that 1 milliliter of buckwheat honey has 20 times more antioxidant activity than the same amount of a very light-colored honey.

By sweetening your foods with honey instead of other sweeteners, you could add a "significant" amount of antioxidants to your diet, according to the study authors. However, buckwheat honey has a strong flavor that some people call "full-bodied," and its taste is not for everyone.

Kasha Pilaf

2 teaspoons canola oil

¾ cup chopped onions

¾ cup kasha (toasted buckwheat groats)

½ cup shredded carrots

1 egg white, lightly beaten

1½ cups defatted reduced-sodium chicken broth

1 teaspoon dried marjoram

¼ teaspoon freshly ground black pepper

⅛ teaspoon salt (optional)

1 tablespoon minced parsley

In a large skillet, heat the oil over medium heat. Add the onions, and cook, stirring occasionally, until softened, about 5 minutes. Transfer the onions to a plate, and set aside.

Add the kasha to the skillet. Reduce the heat to low. Cook, stirring, for 30 seconds. Add the carrots, and stir to combine. Add the egg white, stirring constantly with a fork so that it adheres to the kasha and carrots. Cook, stirring to break up any large clumps, for 1 minute, or until the egg white is set and the kasha looks dry and crumbly.

Gradually stir in the broth, marjoram, and the reserved onions. Partially cover, and cook until the kasha absorbs the liquid, 10 to 12 minutes. Add the pepper and salt (if using). Stir to combine. Sprinkle with the parsley.

Makes 4 servings

PER SERVING

Calories: 175
Total fat: 3.2 g
Saturated fat: 0.4 g

Cholesterol: 0 mg
Sodium: 80 mg
Dietary fiber: 4 g

Bulgur
A WHOLE-GRAIN HEALER

Despite its unfamiliar name, bulgur is simply wheat in its whole form. And as you would expect, this wholesome grain is one of the healthiest foods you can eat.

Research shows that bulgur may play a role in preventing colon and breast cancers as well as heart disease and diabetes. In addition, it's extremely high in fiber, which means it can help prevent and treat a variety of digestive problems, including constipation and diverticular disease.

HEALING POWER

Can Help:

Prevent constipation

Prevent colon and breast cancers

Reduce the risk of diabetes and heart disease

Chemical Repair

No matter how carefully you watch your diet, you're probably being exposed to dangerous chemicals nearly every day. Two of the most common are nitrates and nitrites. Nitrates occur naturally in lots of vegetables, including beets, celery, and lettuce. Nitrites are common ingredients in processed foods such as cured fish, poultry, and meat.

These compounds themselves aren't harmful. But when you get them from food, your body transforms them into related compounds called nitrosamines, which have been linked to cancer.

While it's difficult to avoid nitrates and nitrites, a diet high in bulgur can help reduce the potentially dangerous effects. Bulgur contains a compound called ferulic acid, which helps prevent these compounds from making the troublesome conversion into nitrosamines.

Bulgur protects against cancer in yet another way because it contains lignans. According to Lilian Thompson, PhD, professor of nutritional sciences at the University of Toronto, "Lignans are potent cancer warriors, especially against colon and breast cancer."

Lignans have antioxidant properties, which means that they gobble up dangerous oxygen molecules (free radicals) before they damage individual cells. "Lignans also subdue cancerous changes once they've occurred, rendering them less likely to race out of control," says Dr. Thompson.

In addition, lignans contribute important phytoestrogens to the American diet.

Phytoestrogens are plant estrogens that may help protect you from a variety of cancers by "blocking" the cancer-promoting action of your own estrogen in tissues such as your breasts. However, a lot more research will be needed to determine what role lignans from foods such as bulgur may play in protecting us from cancer.

Help for the Heart

We've seen that free radicals can contribute to cancer. The same vicious molecules can also damage blood vessels, setting the stage for heart disease.

Somewhat paradoxically, the lignans in bulgur can help protect the heart by protecting cholesterol. Why would you want to protect a bad guy? Because when cholesterol is damaged by free-radical molecules, it is more likely to stick to artery walls, contributing to the development of heart disease.

Bulgur can help in yet another way. This grain has a low glycemic index, meaning that the sugars it contains are released relatively slowly into the bloodstream, says David J. A. Jenkins, MD, DSc, PhD, professor of nutritional sciences at the University of Toronto. Not only does this help keep blood sugar levels stable, which is important for people with diabetes, it also may play a role in reducing the risk of heart disease.

Rich in Fiber

Getting more fiber in your diet helps lower cholesterol, reduces cancer and diabetes risk, and helps treat or prevent many digestive complaints, from constipation to

In the Kitchen

Even if you've never cooked bulgur, don't let the exotic name put you off. It's extremely easy to prepare. Here's how:

Choose the right kind. Bulgur comes in three grinds, each of which is recommended for different types of recipes.

- The **coarse grind,** which has a consistency similar to rice, is recommended for making pilaf or when using bulgur in any rice recipe.

- The **medium grind** is used when making breakfast cereal or bulgur filling.
- The **fine grind** is usually used for making tabbouleh.

Start it hot. You don't have to cook—and cook and cook—bulgur the way you do other grains. Just cover it with about 2 cups of boiling water for each cup of bulgur. Then let it stand, covered, for 15 to 20 minutes for "al dente," or longer if you like it softer.

hemorrhoids. Bulgur is a good fiber source, with 1 cup of cooked bulgur providing over 8 grams, almost a third of the Daily Value (DV) for fiber. Compare that to a cup of cooked oatmeal, which has 4 grams of fiber, or a cup of cooked white rice, which has a measly 0.8 gram.

Many of bulgur's benefits come from insoluble fiber. This type of fiber doesn't break down in the body. Instead, it stays in the intestine, soaking up large amounts of water. This makes wastes heavier, so they move through the digestive system faster. Potential cancer-causing substances are ushered out of the body more quickly, giving them less time to create problems.

Doctor's Top Tip

Experts at the USDA say if you're trying to fill your diet with whole grains, it can be difficult sometimes to surmise whether a bread or other grain food actually contains whole grains or just something that *sounds* like whole grains. If you see "bulgur" on a package, rest assured that it contains whole grain.

In a 4-year study at the New York Hospital–Cornell Medical Center in New York City, researchers studied 58 men and women with histories of intestinal polyps. (While polyps themselves aren't dangerous, over time, they may become cancerous.) In the study, those given bran cereal containing 22 grams of insoluble fiber were more likely to have their polyps shrink or disappear entirely than were those who were given a low-fiber look-alike.

Insoluble fiber has also been shown to prevent (and relieve) constipation. This isn't just a matter of comfort. Moving wastes more quickly through the digestive tract reduces the time that harmful substances are in contact with the intestine. In addition, preventing constipation also helps relieve conditions such as hemorrhoids and diverticular disease.

Minerals for Health

Finally, bulgur is a virtual metal warehouse, rich in minerals essential to health. In addition to iron, phosphorus, and zinc, 1 cup of cooked bulgur contains the following minerals:

- 1 milligram of manganese, or half the DV for this mineral. Manganese is needed to ensure healthy bones, nerves, and reproduction.
- 15 micrograms of selenium, or 21 percent of the DV for this mineral. Selenium is needed to help protect the heart and immune system.
- 58 milligrams of magnesium, or 15 percent of the DV for this mineral. Magnesium helps keep your heart beating, nerves functioning, muscles contracting, and bones forming.

GETTING THE MOST

Have it with hot dogs. Since bulgur can help block the process that converts the nitrites in processed foods into cancer-causing substances, it's a good idea to combine it with these foods whenever possible. Tabbouleh, which is made from cooked bulgur mixed with chopped tomatoes, onions, parsley, and mint, and flavored with olive oil and lemon juice, makes a wonderfully fresh salad that goes well with any meal.

Buy it in bulk. Unlike many whole grains, which can be extremely slow-cooking, bulgur is steamed, dried, and crushed before it gets to the store. Essentially, it's precooked, meaning that it's ready to go in about 15 minutes. If you always have it on hand, you'll find out how easy it is to get more of this healthful grain into your diet.

Keep it cold. Since bulgur is cracked open during processing, the fatty portion of the germ is exposed to air and tends to go rancid. To keep bulgur fresh and ready to eat, be sure to keep it refrigerated until you're ready to use it.

Bulgur Salad with Currants

1 cup fine bulgur

3 cups cold water

¼ cup dried currants

¼ cup minced parsley

¼ cup chopped scallions or onions

2 tablespoons fresh lemon juice

1 tablespoon extra-virgin olive oil

⅛ teaspoon salt (optional)

In a medium bowl, combine the bulgur and water; stir to mix. Let stand for 30 minutes, or until the bulgur has absorbed the water. If the bulgur is tender but has not completely absorbed the water, drain through a fine sieve and return to the bowl.

Add the currants, parsley, scallions, lemon juice, oil, and salt (if using). Toss to combine. Serve at room temperature.

Makes 4 servings

PER SERVING

Calories: 180
Total fat: 3.9 g
Saturated fat: 0.5 g

Cholesterol: 0 mg
Sodium: 77 mg
Dietary fiber: 7.4 g

Cabbage Family

A HEAD ABOVE THE REST

HEALING POWER

Can Help:

Prevent breast, lung, and prostate cancers

Lower the risk of cataracts

Prevent heart disease and birth defects

Ancient Roman healers thought that they could cure breast cancer by rubbing on pastes made from cabbage. Not long ago, modern scientists would have dismissed that practice as so much folklore. Now they're not so sure.

"Studies have shown that if you make cabbage into a paste and rub it on the backs of laboratory animals, you can prevent tumors from developing," says Jon Michnovicz, MD, PhD, president of the Foundation for Preventive Oncology in New York City.

Of course, the best way to absorb the healing properties of cabbage is simply to eat it. Cabbage fights a variety of cancers, and it also contains a wealth of nutrients that can ward off heart disease, digestive problems, and other conditions, according to research. In fact, one study found that eating four servings of cruciferous vegetables, such as cabbage, a week slashed the risk of dying from any cause by 26 percent.

Cabbage against Cancer

Like other members of the cruciferous vegetable family, cabbage contains several compounds that studies show can help prevent cancers from occurring. Researchers reviewed almost 100 studies that evaluated the relationship between brassica vegetables, such as cabbage, and cancer. They found that in 70 percent of the studies, cabbage consumption was associated with a lower risk of cancer. Cabbage is particularly effective in preventing cancers of the breast, lung, and prostate gland.

Scientists believe that two compounds in particular help make cabbage a potent cancer-fighting food. The first of these, indole-3-carbinol, or I3C, is especially effective against breast cancer, research shows. The compound acts as an antiestrogen, which means that it sweeps up harmful estrogens that have been linked to breast cancer.

"There was no doubt that if we gave women pure I3C, it would work," says Dr. Michnovicz. But for the average person, eating cabbage or a cabbagelike vegetable, such as broccoli, would have the same effect.

Doctor's Top Tip

"For the most protective dose of this healing food, eat 100 grams (about ½ cup) every other day, raw or cooked for no longer than 5 minutes," says Allan Magaziner, DO, director of the Magaziner Center for Wellness and Anti-Aging Medicine in Cherry Hill, New Jersey.

Another compound in cabbage, called sulforaphane, has been shown to be protective against breast cancer. (It's believed to inhibit carcinogens and aid in DNA repair.) Women in Poland eat three times as much cabbage as women in the United States—30 pounds a year compared with 10 pounds here in the United States. Women in Poland also tend to eat more raw cabbage, sauerkraut, and short-cooked cabbage as a side dish, instead of boiled or slow-cooked cabbage. Scientists think perhaps that's why the breast cancer risk of Polish women who immigrate to the United States triples, to match that of US-born women.

Researchers studied hundreds of Polish women and Polish-born women living in the United States. They asked how often the women had eaten cabbage when they were 12 and 13 years old, and how often they eat it now as adults. The researchers found that the women who ate four or more servings of cabbage a week while preteens were 72 percent less likely to develop breast cancer as adults than the women who ate one serving or less of cabbage a week while preteens. Eating lots of cabbage as adults also provided significant cancer protection.

Compounds in cabbage and other cruciferous vegetables are also protective against lung cancer. A study of Chinese women in Singapore, a city with high levels of air pollution, found that nonsmokers who ate cruciferous vegetables lowered their risk of lung cancer by 30 percent. Smokers who ate cruciferous vegetables reduced their lung cancer risk by 69 percent!

Another type of cancer that cabbage protects against is prostate cancer. A study of men at the Fred Hutchinson Cancer Research Center in Seattle found that men who ate three or more servings of cruciferous vegetables each week had a 44 percent lower risk of prostate cancer than men who ate fewer cruciferous vegetables.

Antioxidant Protection

You've heard a lot about antioxidants such as vitamins C and E and beta-carotene, which help ward off disease by mopping up harmful oxygen molecules called free radicals that naturally accumulate in the body. Free radicals damage healthy tissues throughout the body, causing changes that can lead to heart disease, cancer, and other serious conditions.

Members of the cabbage family are packed with these nutritious compounds. In fact, researchers found that a half-cup of red cabbage contains more antioxidants than

In the Kitchen

As produce goes, cabbage is a cook's best friend. It's versatile, inexpensive, readily available, and easy to prepare. Sure, there's that cabbagy smell, but that's easily remedied.

The next time you're cooking cabbage, add a celery stalk or whole English walnut (in the shell) to the pot. This will help neutralize the powerful odor. Or simply cook the cabbage quicker, stir-frying it in a skillet or wok rather than boiling it for a long time. Long cooking times release more of the strong-smelling sulfur compounds.

---

1 cup of green tea, which has long been considered to be an antioxidant powerhouse!

Two cabbages of note—bok choy and savoy—are also super sources of beta-carotene, a nutrient that other cabbages don't have in abundance. High blood levels of beta-carotene are related to lower incidences of heart attacks, certain types of cancer, and cataracts.

Not only are these cabbages high in beta-carotene, they're also a good source of vitamin C, which has been shown to boost immunity as well as reduce blood pressure and fight heart disease. A half-cup serving of uncooked bok choy provides 16 milligrams of vitamin C, or 27 percent of the Daily Value (DV) for this vitamin, while the same amount of uncooked savoy cabbage supplies 11 milligrams, or 18 percent of the DV.

Both bok choy and savoy cabbage are also decent sources of the B vitamin folate, with a half-cup of either providing about 35 micrograms, or 9 percent of the DV. Your body uses folate for normal tissue growth. Studies show that folate also may protect against certain forms of cancer, including cervical, colorectal, and lung cancers, heart disease, and birth defects. Research shows that women are at high risk for folate deficiency, especially if they take birth control pills.

GETTING THE MOST

Keep a cool head. To preserve cabbage's beneficial compounds at maximum levels, experts recommend eating cabbage raw.

Cook it right. If you must cook your cabbage, steam it lightly (5 minutes or less) to retain the phytonutrients and maximize their availability. Don't microwave cabbage because it decreases the amount of sulforaphane. Don't boil cabbage either. In one study, 90 percent of the glucosinolates were found in the cooking water. (Glucosinolates turn into isothiocyanates—one of which is sulforaphane.)

Buy it whole. Avoid buying halved or shredded cabbage because it loses its vitamin C content quickly once cut. When you get your cabbage home, place the whole head in a plastic bag in the fridge.

Let it sit. To promote the production of the most glucosinolates, slice or chop cabbage and let it sit for 5 to 10 minutes before cooking.

Tangy Red Cabbage and Apples

1½ tablespoons unsalted butter

1 onion, halved and thinly sliced

1 package (10 ounces) shredded red cabbage or 1 small head red cabbage, shredded

2 apples, peeled, cored, and cut into ½-inch cubes

¼ cup packed brown sugar

2 tablespoons red wine vinegar

½ teaspoon salt

¼ teaspoon ground allspice or cinnamon

½ cup water

In a large skillet, melt the butter over medium heat. Cook the onion until wilted, about 6 minutes. Add the cabbage, apples, brown sugar, vinegar, salt, and allspice or cinnamon, and stir to combine.

Add the water and bring to a simmer. Cook, covered, until the cabbage and apples are just tender, about 15 minutes, stirring twice during cooking.

Makes 6 servings

PER SERVING

Calories: 110
Total fat: 3 g
Saturated fat: 2 g

Cholesterol: 10 mg
Sodium: 210 mg
Dietary fiber: 2 g

Cancer

FOODS AS THE ULTIMATE PROTECTOR

According to the American Cancer Society, cancer is the leading killer of Americans under age 85, causing about 25 percent of all deaths. Thankfully, when it comes to cancer prevention, food is powerful medicine. Study after study shows that a healthful diet—eating less fat and getting more fruits, vegetables, whole grains, and legumes—can vastly reduce the risk of cancer. In fact, research indicates that if we all ate more of the right foods and less of the wrong ones, the incidence of all cancers would be reduced by at least 30 percent.

"Food goes beyond being crude fuel, as we once believed," says Keith Block, MD, medical director of the Block Center for Integrative Cancer Care in Evanston, Illinois. "Our experience over the past 2 decades indicates that diet plays an important role when dealing with cancer. We're discovering that there are compounds in foods that can actually both prevent and help fight cancer at the cellular level."

Protection from the Garden

Researchers have known for a long time that people who eat the most fruits, vegetables, and other plant foods are less likely to get cancer than those who fill up on other, less wholesome foods. Recent research suggests that eating five servings of fruits and vegetables each day reduces cancer deaths by 35 percent. One study in particular found that a diet rich in fruits and vegetables slashes the risk of pancreatic cancer—a particularly deadly kind—in half.

But it's only recently that researchers have discovered the reason why plant foods offer such powerful cancer protection. Certain substances found only in plant foods and known collectively as phytonutrients (*phyto* is a Greek word meaning "plant") have the ability to stop cancer.

Research has shown, for example, that eating just one serving of watermelon or pink grapefruit a day can reduce a man's risk of developing prostate cancer by 82 percent! Watermelon and pink grapefruit are high in a phytonutrient called lycopene. In fact, watermelon contains about 40 percent more lycopene than do fresh tomatoes—the produce most people probably think of when they think of lycopene.

When processed into sauce, juice, or ketchup, however, tomatoes do yield more usable lycopene. Interestingly, a recent study found that organic ketchup has up to three times more lycopene than ordinary kinds. Why? Perhaps because organic ketchups are made with riper tomatoes than other types of ketchup. The darker red a ketchup is, the greater its lycopene content.

Another common garden dweller, garlic, has a long tradition as a healing food, and it turns out it is also very rich in phytonutrients. Some of the most impressive are called allyl sulfides, which appear to help destroy cancer-causing substances in the body. In a study of nearly 42,000 women, researchers at the University of Minnesota School of Public Health in Minneapolis found that those who ate more than one serving of garlic—either one fresh clove or a shake of powder—a week were 35 percent less likely to get colon cancer than those who ate none.

The Power of Antioxidants

Every day, your body is attacked, again and again, by a barrage of harmful molecules called free radicals. These are oxygen molecules that have lost an electron, and they careen around your body looking for replacements. In the process of pilfering electrons, they damage healthy cells, possibly kicking off the cancer process.

Nature anticipated this threat by packing fruits, vegetables, and other foods with antioxidants, protective compounds that either stop the formation of free radicals or disable them before they do harm.

There are many compounds in foods that act as antioxidants in the body, but two of the best studied and most powerful are beta-carotene and vitamin C.

Beta-carotene is the pigment that gives many fruits and vegetables their lush, deep orange to red hues. It's more than nature's palette, however. Beta-carotene has been shown to stimulate the release of natural killer cells, which hunt down and destroy cancer cells before they have a chance to cause damage.

Literally dozens of studies have shown that people who get a lot of beta-carotene in their diets can reduce their risks of certain cancers, especially those of the lungs, intestinal tract, mouth, and gums.

It doesn't take a lot of beta-carotene to get the benefits. Evidence suggests that getting 15 to 30 milligrams a day—the amount provided by one or two large carrots—is probably all it takes. Cantaloupes, sweet potatoes, spinach, and bok choy all are excellent sources of beta-carotene.

Another antioxidant is vitamin C, which has been shown to help prevent cancer-causing compounds from forming in the digestive tract. In one large study, Gladys Block, PhD, professor of epidemiology and public health nutrition at the University of California, Berkeley, analyzed dozens of smaller studies that looked at the relationship between vitamin C and cancer. Of the 46 studies she examined, 33 showed that people who consumed the most vitamin C had the lowest risk of cancer.

The DV for vitamin C is 60 milligrams, an amount that's very easy to get in foods. One green bell pepper, for example, contains 66 milligrams of vitamin C, while a half-cup of broccoli has 41 milligrams.

Beans, Beans, They're Good for . . . Fighting Cancer

They may not be glamorous, but beans are showing their stuff as cancer fighters. A University of Minnesota study found that women who ate the most high-magnesium foods, such as beans, reduced their risk of developing colon cancer by 23 percent. Just a half-cup of beans provides 43 milligrams of magnesium, almost 11 percent of the 400-milligram DV. The optimum intake is 310 to 420 milligrams per day.

Another study, this one from the M. D. Anderson Cancer Center in Houston, found that people who ate the most foods containing phytoestrogens, such as beans, were the least likely to get lung cancer. Interestingly, men reduced their risk more than women—by 72 percent compared with 41 percent.

Beans also offer protection from breast cancer. A Harvard School of Public Health study found that women who ate beans twice a week had a 24 percent lower risk of developing breast cancer than women who rarely ate them.

Drink Some Protection

Drinking a 4-ounce glass of red wine a day may cut a man's prostate cancer risk in half, according to a study of more than 1,400 men by the Fred Hutchinson Cancer Research Center in Seattle. Which wine is best? Order a Pinot Noir from California. Researchers at the University of Mississippi tested 11 red wines and found that Pinot Noirs from California have the most resveratrol, an antioxidant that can help ward off cancer and even heart attacks.

Although the Fred Hutchinson researchers didn't find an association between beer and prostate cancer in their study, researchers in Italy found that an antioxidant in hops called xanthohumol inhibits the growth of cancer cells. The results have been shown only in test tubes so far, but studies in humans are planned.

The world's second most popular beverage (next to water) is tea, which has long had a reputation as a cancer fighter. It was known to defeat cancer cells in test tubes, but now it's been shown to fight cancer in people, too. A Swedish study of 61,000 women found that those who drank 2 cups of tea a day decreased their risk of ovarian cancer by 46 percent.

Yet one more beverage, milk, really does do a body good. Researchers reviewed 63 studies and revealed that high levels of vitamin D cut the risk of colon, ovarian, and breast cancer by up to 50 percent. The researchers recommend getting 1,000 IU of vitamin D per day. One cup of milk contains 100 IU. However, the FDA recently

Doctor's Top Tip

Eating just one Brazil nut a day could help ward off colon cancer. Brazil nuts are high in the trace mineral selenium, and doctors at the University of Arizona found that men with high levels of selenium are six times less likely to develop colon cancer than men with low levels.

changed its vitamin D fortification guidelines so that food manufacturers can now add nearly three times more vitamin D to dairy products.

The Fiber Solution

For a long time, no one took dietary fiber seriously. It's not a nutrient. It isn't absorbed by the body. In fact, it doesn't seem to do much of anything.

As it turns out, fiber does more than anyone ever imagined. "Consuming a high-fiber diet is essential for reducing the risk of certain types of cancer, particularly colon cancer," says Daniel W. Nixon, MD, a scientific counselor with the Cancer Treatment Research Foundation in Schaumburg, Illinois.

Fiber works against cancer in several ways, he explains. Since fiber is absorbent, it soaks up water as it moves through the digestive tract. This makes stools larger, which causes the intestine to move them along more quickly. And the more quickly stools move, the less time there is for any harmful substances they contain to damage the cells lining the intestine. In addition, fiber helps trap cancer-causing substances in the colon. And since the fiber itself isn't absorbed, it exits the body in the stool, taking the harmful substances with it.

According to doctors at the National Cancer Institute, you need between 20 and 35 grams of fiber a day to keep your risk of cancer low. That may sound like a lot, and it would be if you ate it all at once. (And truth be told, most people get only 11 grams of fiber per day.) But since many foods contain at least some fiber, it's fairly easy to get enough if you pick the right foods. Simply make it a point to eat more fruits and vegetables—raw, when possible, and with their skins rather than peeled—than you're currently eating. If you do this regularly, you'll soon find that you're getting most of the fiber you need, says Dr. Keith Block.

Beans and certain vegetables are among the best sources of fiber you can find. Eating one of them a few times a day will automatically bring your fiber intake into the comfort zone. A half-cup of kidney beans, for example, contains 7 grams of fiber, while the same amount of chickpeas contains 5 grams. As for vegetables, a half-cup of cooked okra contains 3 grams of fiber, while the same amount of Brussels sprouts has 3 grams.

Whether you're eating whole-wheat toast (2 grams of fiber per slice) for breakfast or a bowl of kasha (about 3 grams per half-cup, cooked), whole grains are also great sources of fiber. If you can, get 6 to 11 servings of whole grains a day.

Cantaloupe

SWEET FRUIT FOR BETTER SIGHT

Cantaloupe—what an odd word! But it makes more sense once you learn that cantaloupes were first cultivated in the Italian village of Cantalupo, around AD 1700. This brightly colored fruit belongs to the same family as the cucumber, squash, pumpkin, and gourd, and it is filled with healing substances that can help protect your sight, control blood pressure, lower cholesterol, keep the blood running smoothly, and protect against cancer.

"Cantaloupe is one of the few fruits or vegetables rich in both vitamin C *and* beta-carotene," says John Erdman, PhD, professor of nutritional sciences at the University of Illinois in Urbana. Both of these antioxidant compounds have been shown to protect against cancer, heart disease, and other age-related health conditions, such as cataracts.

HEALING POWER
Can Help:
Reduce risk of macular degeneration and cataracts
Lower blood pressure and cholesterol
Reduce the risk of heart disease and cancer

Save Your Sight

Cantaloupes are rich in carotenoids, the pigments that give fruits and vegetables their bright colors and offer powerful health protection. A study in the Netherlands found that eating carotenoid-rich fruits was linked to a 35 percent lower risk of developing age-related macular degeneration, the leading cause of irreversible blindness in developed countries.

Cantaloupe also offers protection against another sight stealer: cataracts. A study found that women who got the most vitamin A through diet had a 39 percent reduced risk of developing cataracts. Once beta-carotene is inside the body, it is converted to vitamin A. Another study found that people whose diets included the most vitamin A, including from foods like cantaloupe, had half the risk of cataract surgery.

The Dynamic Duo

As we mentioned earlier, cantaloupe is a rich source of two potent antioxidants, vitamin C and beta-carotene. Antioxidants are compounds that neutralize free radicals—cell-damaging molecules that occur naturally and that are thought to cause cellular changes that can lead to heart disease, cancer, and cataracts.

Doctor's Top Tip

Cut cantaloupe under water to keep it fresher longer. Scientists at the USDA found that slicing cantaloupe under water short-circuits the signals plant cells send to each other when they detect an injury, such as being sliced.

Like potassium, vitamin C helps keep the arteries clear and blood moving smoothly by preventing bad LDL cholesterol from oxidizing and gumming up the artery walls. The body also uses vitamin C for producing collagen, a protein that makes up skin and connective tissue. Cantaloupe is an excellent source of vitamin C, with 1 cup containing 68 milligrams, or 113 percent of the Daily Value (DV) for this vitamin.

Cantaloupe is also a good source of beta-carotene, which fights heart disease and cancer. Half a cantaloupe provides 5 milligrams of beta-carotene—about half of the daily amount recommended by most experts.

GETTING THE MOST

Buy them ripe. The riper the cantaloupe, the more beta-carotene it contains, says Dr. Erdman. The challenge is that melons are often picked while unripe to make it through the shipping process undamaged. To check for ripeness, tap the melon and listen for a hollow sound. Then heft the fruit to make sure that it's heavy for its size. Last, smell the cantaloupe to make sure that it exudes a sweet, musky perfume (the smell shouldn't be too strong; an overly strong smell indicates an overripe fruit). If there's no smell, put it down and try another.

Check the stem. There shouldn't be one. Mature cantaloupes will only have a smooth, symmetrical basin where the stem once was and flesh that yields slightly to pressure.

Set it out. Leave a firm cantaloupe at room temperature for several days to allow it to become softer and juicier. Once it's ripe, move it to the fridge.

Eat it quickly. Vitamin C degrades quickly when exposed to air, so it's important to eat cantaloupe fairly soon after cutting, says Dr. Erdman. This is especially true when the fruit is cut into small pieces, which substantially increases the amount of air to which it's exposed. One study found that after 6 days, cantaloupe cubes lost 25 percent of their vitamin C and 10 to 15 percent of their carotenoids.

Carotenoids

MORE THAN PRETTY COLORS

HEALING POWER

Can Help:

Lower cholesterol

Reduce the risk of heart disease and cancer

Protect eye tissue

All great chefs know that the eyes eat first. That's why they put so much effort into presentation, livening up the plate with vivid vegetables.

For a long time, in fact, nature's colorful bounty—an emerald bed of lettuce, shiny scarlet tomato wedges, or bright orange slivers of carrot—was used mainly as a bit of colorful warmth to fill up the empty spaces between the meat and potatoes.

Now we know that there's a better reason to serve vegetables. The pigments that give fruits and vegetables their cheery hues, called carotenoids, are more than pretty colors. They could save your life.

Researchers have found that people who eat the most carotenoid-rich yellow, orange, and red vegetables—such as pumpkins, sweet potatoes, watermelons, and sweet red bell peppers—have significantly lower risks of dying from heart disease and cancer. The same is true of the dark green leafy vegetables, such as spinach and kale. (The chlorophyll they contain masks the lighter carotenoid hues.)

How can a simple food coloring be so good for you? The reason, as is often true with nutrition, comes down to chemistry. Our bodies are constantly under attack by free radicals—oxygen molecules that have lost an electron and zip through the body trying to steal replacement electrons from healthy cells. In time, this process causes internal damage to tissues throughout the body, possibly causing heart disease, cancer, and many other serious conditions. The carotenoids in vegetables neutralize free radicals by offering up their own electrons. This effectively stops the destructive process, helping prevent your cells from being damaged.

Researchers have pinpointed more than 600 carotenoids, but only 50 to 60 of them are found in common foods. The key carotenoids identified so far are alpha-carotene, beta-carotene, gamma-carotene, beta-cryptoxanthin, lutein, lycopene, and zeaxanthin, and scientists continue to investigate others.

Carotenoids for Your Heart

People have been fighting the cholesterol war since doctors first uttered the words "hardening of the arteries." Along with avoiding high-fat foods, you can make

Doctor's Top Tip

"Enjoy a variety of fruits and vegetables," says Allan Maga-ziner, DO, director of the Maga-ziner Center for Wellness and Anti-Aging Medicine in Cherry Hill, New Jersey. "There are hundreds of carotenoids, and different foods offer different ones. So eat many different fruits and vegetables. And choose deeply pigmented fruits and vegetables over lightly colored ones because they have more carotenoids. For example, spinach contains more carot-enoids than iceberg lettuce."

progress in winning this war by eating carotenoid-rich fruits and vegetables—such as sweet potatoes, spinach, and cantaloupe—every day.

Carotenoids contribute to heart health by helping prevent the dangerous low-density lipoprotein (LDL) cholesterol from oxidizing—the process that causes it to stick to artery walls. Studies show that people with high levels of carotenoids have significantly lower risks for heart disease than those who don't.

Researchers at Johns Hopkins University in Balti-more found that smokers who already had one heart attack were less likely to have a second if they had high blood levels of four important carotenoids—beta-carotene, lutein, lycopene, and zeaxanthin.

Keeping Cancer in Check

The same process by which carotenoids protect against heart disease also seems to protect against cancer. Researchers believe that these compounds, by neu-tralizing free radicals, can prevent damage to DNA, the genetic material that controls how cells behave.

For example, in one study, researchers at the National Cancer Institute found that people with the highest intakes of carotenoids were as much as six times less likely to develop skin cancer than those with the lowest intakes. Researchers think that beta-carotene plants itself in the skin, where its pigments help deflect sunlight.

"There are several other studies now yielding the same results," says Harinder Garewal, MD, PhD, professor of medicine at the University of Arizona College of Medicine in Tucson. "These findings are important because they suggest that you can do something to reverse the onset of cancer."

Another carotenoid that seems to be a crusader against cancer is lycopene—the pigment that gives tomatoes their rosy glow and that is also found in watermelons, guavas, and pink grapefruit. Researchers from the Harvard School of Public Health found that people who ate 10 or more servings per week of tomato-based foods had a 45 percent decrease in their risk for prostate cancer. Those who only ate four to seven servings a week—less than one a day—still came out ahead, with a 20 percent reduction in risk. It wasn't only whole tomatoes that provided the benefits either. Pizza, tomato juice, and other tomato-based foods also were protective.

Although evidence clearly shows that people who get the most carotenoids in

THE 24-CARAT CAROTENOIDS

All rich yellow, orange, and red vegetables contain generous amounts of carotenoids. So do the deep green leafy vegetables, like spinach and kale. To get the greatest amounts of these healing compounds into your diet, here are some of the best food sources.

Cantaloupe	Oranges	Spinach
Carrots	Peaches	Sweet potatoes
Dark leafy greens	Pumpkin	Tomatoes
Kale		

their diets tend to get less cancer, the case for taking supplements of carotenoids isn't quite so clear.

For example, when researchers tested the effectiveness of beta-carotene supplements, they found that this compound wasn't effective in preventing cancer. In fact, some studies have shown that taking beta-carotene supplements may accelerate the disease.

"There is very clear evidence that we know less than we thought we did," says Walter Willett, MD, DrPH, professor of epidemiology and nutrition, and chairman of the department of nutrition at the Harvard School of Public Health. It's possible that beta-carotene supplements cause problems because high doses interfere with the body's absorption of other protective carotenoids.

For now, the best strategy for preventing cancer is to get carotenoids from foods rather than supplements. "Our hope is that with more research, we'll be able to pinpoint which compounds are most beneficial and which fruits and vegetables people should emphasize in their diets," says Dr. Willett.

Good for the Eyes

As his name suggests, Popeye has his share of vision problems. But according to research on his favorite leafy elixir, he won't likely have problems with macular degeneration—the leading cause of severe vision loss in older adults.

People who eat spinach, collard greens, and other dark green leafy vegetables five or six times a week have about a 43 percent lower risk for macular degeneration than those who eat such foods less than once a month, according to a large study in Massachusetts.

The carotenoids that seem to be responsible, lutein and zeaxanthin, are believed to block the effects of free radicals in the outer retina, preventing them from damaging healthy eye tissue.

Butternut Squash, Kale, and Tomato Stew

1 small butternut squash

8 ounces kale

1 tablespoon olive oil

1 tablespoon minced garlic

1 can (16 ounces) whole tomatoes (with juice)

½ cup water

1 tablespoon chopped fresh basil

1 tablespoon chopped fresh sage

With a sharp knife, pierce the squash in 3 or 4 places. Microwave on high, turning once, for 2 to 3 minutes, or just until the squash starts to soften under the skin. To test, press with your thumb. Carefully cut the squash into quarters. Scoop out and discard the seeds. Cut off and discard the peel. Cut the squash into 1-inch chunks. Rinse the kale and strip the leaves from the coarse stems. Coarsely chop the leaves.

In a large saucepan, heat the oil over medium heat, Add the garlic and cook for 20 seconds, or until fragrant. Add the squash, tomatoes and their juice, and water.

Cover, and reduce the heat to medium-low. Cook until the squash is tender but not mushy, 25 to 30 minutes . Test for doneness by inserting the tip of a sharp knife into a piece of squash. Add more water if necessary to keep the squash from sticking. With the back of a large spoon, break the tomatoes into smaller pieces. Add the kale, basil, and sage. Cook until the kale softens, 3 to 4 minutes longer.

Makes 4 servings

Cook's Note: *Serve over hot cooked brown rice or quinoa.*

PER SERVING

Calories: 134	Cholesterol: 0 mg
Total fat: 4.1 g	Sodium: 207 mg
Saturated fat: 0.6 g	Dietary fiber: 6.2 g

Carpal Tunnel Syndrome
MORE FLEX WITH FLAX

Just as highways go through tunnels in order to get around (or under) obstacles, some structures in your body, such as nerves and ligaments, also use tunnels to get where they're going. One of the busiest tunnels is the carpal tunnel, which allows a nerve, blood vessels, and ligaments to pass through the wrist and into the fingers.

There's usually a lot of room inside the carpal tunnel. But when you use your hands and wrists a lot while typing, knitting, or doing other repetitive motions, tissues inside the tunnel may become inflamed and swollen, causing them to press against the nerve. This can cause pain in the wrist as well as tingling or numbness in the fingers, says James L. Napier Jr., MD, assistant clinical professor of neurology at Case Western Reserve University School of Medicine in Cleveland. Doctors call this condition carpal tunnel syndrome. It affects about 3 out of every 100 people in the United States, and it's one of the most common causes of partial disability.

One of the best remedies for carpal tunnel syndrome is simply to give your wrists a rest. It may also help to keep your hands warm. Pain and stiffness are more likely to occur if your hands are cold. In addition, there's some evidence that eating flaxseed may help reduce inflammation in the body, including in the wrists, says Jack Carter, PhD, professor emeritus of plant science at North Dakota State University in Fargo and president of the Flax Institute.

Flaxseed contains a compound called alpha-linolenic acid, which has been shown to reduce levels of prostaglandins, chemicals in the body that contribute to inflammation, says Dr. Carter. It also contains other compounds called lignans, which have antioxidant properties that can block the effects of harmful oxygen molecules called free radicals. This is important because free radicals are produced in large amounts whenever there's inflammation, and unless they're stopped, they make the inflammation even worse.

So far, researchers haven't put flaxseed to the test against carpal tunnel syndrome, so there's no way to know for sure how much you might need to get the benefits, says Dr. Carter. Some evidence suggests, however, that getting 25 to 30 grams (about 3 tablespoons) of ground flaxseed or 1 to 3 tablespoons of flaxseed oil might be enough to help ease the symptoms.

Since the body can't digest whole flaxseed, be sure to buy flaxseed that's ground,

Doctor's Top Tip

Relax your grip, according to doctors at the Mayo Clinic in Rochester, Minnesota. When cooking, use tools with wide grips and hold them softly. Two activities in particular—cutting and slicing with knives—are problematic for people with carpal tunnel syndrome. These actions put strain on your wrist and carpal tunnel. Minimize—or delegate!—these tasks whenever possible.

or grind it yourself. You can add the ground seed to hot cereals or mix it into flour when you bake. Refrigerate any leftover ground seeds in an airtight container. Once the oils in flaxseed are exposed to air, they quickly become rancid.

A Weighty Problem

While you're thinking about ways to get more flaxseed into your diet, you should also be thinking about how to get extra calories out. There's scientific evidence that people who are overweight are more likely to get carpal tunnel syndrome than those who are lean, says Peter A. Nathan, MD, hand surgeon and carpal tunnel researcher at the Portland Hand Surgery and Rehabilitation Center in Oregon. In fact, research by Dr. Nathan suggests that people who are overweight have greater risks of getting carpal tunnel syndrome than typists, cashiers, or other folks who use their hands and wrists a lot on the job.

"Heavy people have a tendency to accumulate more fluid in the soft tissues, including in the wrist," Dr. Nathan explains. As fluids accumulate, they may begin putting pressure on the nerve inside the carpal tunnel, while also reducing the amount of oxygen it receives. Losing weight isn't necessarily a "cure" for carpal tunnel syndrome, Dr. Nathan adds. But if you are overweight and having problems, losing even a few pounds might take some pressure off this vulnerable nerve.

Perhaps the best way to lose weight if you have carpal tunnel syndrome is through exercise. In addition to the weight-loss benefit, a study conducted by Dr. Nathan at the Portland Hand Surgery and Rehabilitation Center found that exercise relieved the carpal tunnel syndrome symptoms of pain, tightness, and clumsiness.

Too Much of a Good Thing

One thing you might want to eliminate from your diet if you have carpal tunnel syndrome is the artificial sweetener aspartame. A study found that heavy users of aspartame have developed symptoms of carpal tunnel syndrome. After eliminating aspartame from their diets, symptoms subsided within 2 weeks, even though no changes were made in work habits.

Carrots

GOOD FOR THE EYES—AND MORE

As kids, we all heard how good carrots are for our eyes. But nowadays, researchers are seeing carrots in a whole new light.

The healing potential of carrots goes far beyond their ability to help our vision. They contain a variety of compounds that may help prevent certain cancers, lower cholesterol, and prevent heart attacks.

HEALING POWER

Can Help:

Reduce the risk of cancer and heart disease

Improve night vision

Reduce risk of macular degeneration

Carotene's Namesake

The same substance that gives carrots their brash orange color is also responsible for providing many of their health benefits. Carrots are rich in beta-carotene, an anti-oxidant compound that fights free radicals, the unstable molecules in the body that contribute to conditions ranging from heart disease and cancer to macular degeneration, the leading cause of severe vision loss in older adults. In fact, carrots are by far one of the richest sources of carotenoids. Just 1 cup of carrots provides more than 250 percent of the daily amount recommended by experts.

A study at Brigham and Women's Hospital in Boston found that women who ate just five servings of four raw carrot sticks a week had a 54 percent decrease in their risk of getting ovarian cancer. The researchers credit the carotene in carrots for their protection.

Another study, this one in Sweden, of 61,000 women found that those who ate four to six servings of antioxidant-rich carrots a week cut their risk of the most common form of kidney cancer by 54 percent.

Other large-population studies have shown that having low levels of beta-carotene leaves people more open to developing certain cancers, especially those of the lungs and stomach.

What's good for your body's cells is also very good for your heart. Evidence shows that eating large amounts of carrots and other fruits and vegetables rich in beta-carotene and related compounds may reduce the risk of heart disease. "A half-cup serving of cooked carrots contains 12 milligrams of beta-carotene, about twice the amount you need to get the benefits," says Paul Lachance, PhD, executive director of the Nutraceuticals Institute at Rutgers University in New Brunswick, New Jersey.

Researchers in Germany found that eating foods rich in beta-carotene can reduce your blood levels of an important marker of cardiovascular disease risk, C-reactive protein (also known as CRP). In the study, men who ate eight servings of fruits and vegetables containing beta-carotene decreased their CRP levels by 42 percent in just 4 weeks.

It's not only beta-carotene that gives carrots their protective edge. They contain another antioxidant, alpha-carotene, which also appears to help fight cancer. In one study, researchers at the National Cancer Institute found that lung cancer occurred more often in men with low intakes of alpha-carotene than in men who got more.

Better Vision

The beta-carotene in carrots does double duty. It converts to vitamin A in the body and helps improve vision. This eye appeal is so well known that researchers in World War II cultivated carrots that were high in beta-carotene to help pilots see better at night.

Vitamin A helps vision by forming a purple pigment that the eye needs in order to be able to see in dim light. This pigment, called rhodopsin, is located in the light-sensitive area of the retina. The more vitamin A you get, the more rhodopsin your body is able to produce. Conversely, people with low levels of vitamin A may suffer

---

FOOD ALERT

The Color of Indulgence

Orange and yellow are attractive colors for autumn leaves, but not at all pleasing when it's your own skin that's making the change.

People who enjoy their carrots a bit too much may experience a colorful condition called carotenosis, in which the skin turns a faint orange hue. Doctors tell stories of frantic parents rushing to the hospital because they think their children are jaundiced, when in fact, they just ate a lot of baby-food carrots.

"Children are particularly prone to it because parents will give them puréed carrots or squash or sweet potatoes, usually in a number of servings," says John Erdman, PhD, of the University of Illinois in Urbana.

Carotenosis is harmless, Dr. Erdman says. It's also easy to remedy. Stop eating carrots, and within a day or two, your skin color should return to normal.

In the Kitchen

Roasting carrots brings out their flavors. Toss 1¼-inch pieces of carrot with salt, pepper, and a little extra-virgin olive oil. Bake, covered, for 20 minutes at 400°F. Uncover and bake for 30 minutes longer.

Adding that olive oil is important. Beta-carotene needs a small amount of fat to make the trip through your intestinal wall and into your body, says John Erdman, PhD, of the University of Illinois in Urbana. So the next time you're serving carrot sticks, you may want to accompany them with a small amount of a dip, such as ranch dressing. (As if you needed an excuse!)

---

from night blindness, which can make it difficult to drive after dark or to find your seat in a dark theater.

In addition to giving you better vision, carrots might also help *protect* your vision. A study in Boston at Brigham and Women's Hospital found that eating carotenoid-rich produce was linked to a 36 percent lower risk of the leading cause of severe vision loss in the elderly—age-related macular degeneration.

GETTING THE MOST

Choose a rainbow. At your farmers' market or supermarket, look for new-colored carrots with more powerful pigments: lycopene-rich red and lutein-laden yellow in addition to the usual orange.

Trim them well. When you buy carrots with the greenery still on them, trim it off before storing them. Otherwise, those pretty, leafy tops will act like nutrient vampires, sucking out the vitamins and moisture before you can eat the carrots.

Eat them cooked. While many foods are more nutritious raw than cooked, carrots can benefit from a little cooking. The reason is that carrots have a lot of dietary fiber—more than 2 grams in one carrot—which traps the beta-carotene, says John Erdman, PhD, professor of nutritional sciences at the University of Illinois in Urbana. Cooking carrots helps free beta-carotene from the fiber cells, making it easier for your body to absorb.

Save the nutrients. One problem with cooking carrots is that some of the nutrients escape into the cooking water, says Carol Boushey, PhD, MPH, RD, associate professor of foods and nutrition at Purdue

> ### Doctor's Top Tip
>
> "For improving your overall health, eat two carrots each day," says Allan Magaziner, DO, director of the Magaziner Center for Wellness and Anti-Aging Medicine in Cherry Hill, New Jersey. "Fresh, organic, raw carrots are best."

University in West Lafayette, Indiana. To get nutrients into your body instead of pouring them down the sink, try reusing the cooking water—in a sauce, for example, or for moistening mashed potatoes.

Enjoy some juice. Another way to release more of the beta-carotene from carrots is to make a carrot cocktail. Processing carrots in a blender breaks apart the fibers, allowing the beta-carotene to get out, says Dr. Erdman.

Carrot-Walnut Salad

⅓ **cup golden raisins**

⅓ **cup chopped walnuts**

2 **tablespoons rice wine vinegar**

1 **tablespoon extra-virgin olive oil**

2 **teaspoons fresh lemon juice**

1 **teaspoon honey**

⅛ **teaspoon salt**

4 **large carrots, shredded**

¼ **cup chopped parsley**

Soak the raisins in hot tap water until plumped, about 20 minutes. Drain. Preheat the oven to 250°F. Place the walnuts on a baking sheet, and toast until lightly browned, about 5 minutes; set aside.

In a small bowl, combine the vinegar, oil, lemon juice, honey, and salt.

Just before serving, in a medium bowl, toss the carrots, walnuts, parsley, and raisins with the dressing.

Makes 4 servings

PER SERVING

Calories: 170	Cholesterol: 0 mg
Total fat: 10 g	Sodium: 125 mg
Saturated fat: 1 g	Dietary fiber: 3 g

Cataracts

SET YOUR SIGHT ON ANTIOXIDANTS

It seems as if, with every year that goes by, we have to hold the newspaper a little farther away to read the headlines. Traffic signs get harder to see, and as for reading the menu in a dim restaurant, well, forget it. It's natural for the eyes to undergo slight changes over time. But for people with cataracts—proteins that accumulate inside the lenses of the eyes—the loss of vision can be profound. Cataracts are the leading cause of blindness in the world, and they affect nearly 20.5 million Americans age 40 and older. By age 80, more than half of all Americans have cataracts. Age-related cataracts are the leading cause of blindness in adults 45 years of age and older, and cataract surgery is the most frequent surgical procedure in the United States.

Wearing sunglasses and not smoking may reduce the risk of cataracts, but an even better strategy is to eat more fruits and vegetables, says Allen Taylor, PhD, director of the Laboratory for Nutrition and Vision Research at the Jean Mayer USDA Human Nutrition Research Center on Aging at Tufts University in Boston. These foods contain a variety of protective compounds that can stop damage to the eyes.

The eyes are constantly being bombarded by free radicals, harmful oxygen molecules that are missing electrons and spend their lives looking for replacements. They grab extra electrons wherever they can, damaging healthy cells every time they strike. One way to help stop this damage is by filling your body with antioxidants, such as beta-carotene and vitamins C and E. Each of these compounds blocks the effects of free radicals, says Dr. Taylor.

Seeing Colors

Popeye used spinach to build strong muscles, but it works just as well for strengthening the eyes. In fact, studies show that spinach might be one of your best defenses against cataracts. In a study of more than 50,000 nurses, Harvard researchers found that those who got the most carotenoids, which are natural plant pigments such as beta-carotene, in their diets were 39 percent less likely to develop serious cataracts than women who got the least. And when the researchers looked at specific foods that contained carotenoids, spinach appeared to be the most protective.

Spinach (along with kale, broccoli, and other dark green leafy vegetables) contains more than just beta-carotene, however. It also contains two other carotenoids,

Doctor's Top Tip

According to doctors at the American Optometric Association, the cataract-protective carotenoids lutein and zeaxanthin, plentiful in spinach, are fat-soluble. This means that it's best to eat spinach cooked with a little fat, such as olive oil, to maximize the absorption of these key nutrients by the body.

lutein and zeaxanthin, which concentrate in the fluids of the eyes. This means that you're getting the most protection right where you need it most. Two studies, the Health Professional's Follow-Up Study and the Beaver Dam Eye Study, showed that people eating foods with the highest amounts of lutein and zeaxanthin have a lower risk of developing cataracts and needing cataract surgery.

Another study from Harvard University of almost 40,000 women, found that those who ate the most fruits and vegetables (3½ servings each day) had a 10 to 15 percent reduced risk of cataracts, compared with the women who ate the least fruits and vegetables (2½ daily servings or less). Fruits and vegetables are, of course, great sources of antioxidants, including vitamin C, which appears to be a key player in keeping the eyes clear.

Even though the Daily Value (DV) for vitamin C is 60 milligrams, Dr. Taylor recommends boosting that amount to 250 milligrams for maximum eye protection. It's easy to get that much vitamin C in your diet, he adds. A half-cup of broccoli, for example, has about 30 milligrams of vitamin C, and a large glass of fresh-squeezed orange juice has about 90 milligrams.

Find a Fishy Solution

Wondering what to have with all that produce? Order the catch of the day. One study found that women who consumed fish containing omega-3 fatty acids at least once a week had a 12 percent lower risk of needing cataract surgery. The fish that offer good amounts of omega-3s include salmon, Spanish mackerel, and tuna.

Making the Most of Milk

You wouldn't think to toast your eyes with a glass of Bessie's best, but milk, along with chicken and yogurt, provides some of the best eye protection you can find. All of these foods contain large amounts of riboflavin, a B vitamin that appears to help prevent cataracts from forming. In a study of more than 1,000 people, researchers at State University of New York at Stony Brook found that those getting the most riboflavin were much less likely to have cataracts than those getting smaller amounts.

The connection, once again, appears to be antioxidants. The body uses riboflavin to manufacture glutathione, a powerful compound that battles free radicals. When you don't get enough riboflavin, glutathione levels fall, and that gives free radicals more time to damage the eyes.

Cauliflower

A WHITE KNIGHT AGAINST CANCER

Mark Twain once called cauliflower "a cabbage with a college education"—a bit more refined, perhaps, but essentially the same plain-Jane vegetable.

What Twain didn't know is just how valuable cauliflower is in our quest for good health. (If he had, Huckleberry Finn and Jim might have spent their days eating raw cauliflower instead of greasy catfish fillets.) Like other members of the cruciferous family, cauliflower is loaded with nutrients that seem to wage war against a host of diseases, including cancer. It's also an excellent source of vitamins and minerals that are essential for keeping the immune system strong. One study found that eating just four servings of cruciferous vegetables, such as cauliflower, a week slashed the risk of dying from *any* cause by 26 percent.

HEALING POWER
Can Help:
Inhibit tumor growth
Boost the immune system

Formidable Florets

Although cauliflower's darker-hued brother, broccoli, has gotten most of the attention for its healing potential, cauliflower is also generously endowed with cancer-preventing powers, says Jon Michnovicz, MD, PhD, president of the Foundation for Preventive Oncology in New York City.

Researchers have found two potent munitions in cauliflower's cancer-fighting arsenal: the phytonutrients sulforaphane and indole-3-carbinol, or I3C. These compounds, found in all cruciferous vegetables, may be the reason that studies consistently show that folks who make a habit of crunching crucifers are less likely to get cancer.

In one study, scientists at Johns Hopkins University in Baltimore exposed 145 laboratory animals to high doses of an extremely powerful cancer-causing agent. Of those, 120 were given high levels of protective sulforaphane. Fifty days later, 68 percent of the unprotected animals had breast tumors, compared with only 26 percent of those that received the sulforaphane.

While previous studies showed that sulforaphane can prevent changes that lead to cancer in human breast cells, newer research at the University of Illinois at Urbana-Champaign showed it can halt the growth of cancerous breast cells. In test tube studies, the sulforaphane interrupted the cancer cells' ability to divide, and so they died.

FOOD ALERT

Getting the Gout

Michelangelo, Leonardo da Vinci, and Henry VIII all had one thing in common. They should have stayed away from cauliflower. If you have gout, like they did, you should, too.

Cauliflower contains amino acids called purines that break down into uric acid in the body. The uric acid crystals can trigger a painful case of gout—a form of arthritis that occurs when the sharp-edged crystals jab into the joints, causing pain and swelling. If you have gout and can't eat cauliflower, you can still get the same cancer-fighting benefits from its cruciferous siblings like broccoli, cabbage, and Brussels sprouts, which contain lower concentrations of purines.

Sulforaphane works by stepping up the production of enzymes in your body that sweep toxins out the door before they can damage your body's cells, making them cancerous, explains Dr. Michnovicz.

Cauliflower's other tumor-squelching compound, I3C, works as an antiestrogen, explains Dr. Michnovicz. In other words, it reduces levels of harmful estrogens that can foster tumor growth in hormone-sensitive cells, like those in the breasts and prostate gland. "That's why, although studies show that people who eat cruciferous vegetables are protected from all kinds of cancers, these foods are probably most useful for fighting cancers of the colon, breast, and prostate," says Dr. Michnovicz.

As an interesting example of the latter, prostate cancer is rare in India, where vegetables such as cauliflower are often enjoyed with the spice turmeric. A study conducted at Rutgers University in New Brunswick, New Jersey, found that both phenethyl isothiocyanates (a phytochemical in cauliflower) and curcumin (a phytonutrient in turmeric) retarded the growth of human prostate cancer cells that had been implanted into mice. (See the delicious rice and cauliflower salad recipe on page 152 that uses turmeric.)

Immune Power

Cauliflower does more than protect against cancer. It's also packed with vitamin C and the B vitamin folate, two nutrients that are well-known for keeping your immune system in peak condition.

Just three uncooked florets of this crucifer supply 67 percent of the Daily Value (DV) for vitamin C—more than the amount in a tangerine or a white grapefruit. By upping your level of vitamin C, along with other anti-oxidants like vitamin E and beta-carotene, you can keep your immune system strong while staving off a host of conditions, among them heart disease, cancer, and cataracts.

GETTING THE MOST

Use your head. Avoid cauliflower if it has brown spots on its ivory (or purple) florets. That means that it's already past its nutritional peak. Choose cauliflower heads that are surrounded by many thick green leaves. They are better protected and will be fresher.

Store with care. Store cauliflower with the stem side down to prevent moisture from developing in the floret clusters.

Enjoy it raw. To keep cauliflower's cancer-fighting indoles intact, keep it out of the heat, advises Dr. Michnovicz. Your best bet is either eating it raw or cooking it quickly in a steamer, wok, or microwave, he says. Boiling is the worst way to cook this crucifer. Submerging cauliflower in the hot, roily water will cause it to lose about half of its valuable indoles, he says.

Steam it right. Steaming cauliflower releases the maximum amount of sulforaphane. But be sure to cut cauliflower into large (not small) pieces before you steam it. Larger pieces equal a smaller surface area exposed. The greater the surface area exposed, the more nutrients can leach out.

Doctor's Top Tip

"Enjoy cauliflower raw, steamed, or lightly cooked and then puréed," says Allan Magaziner, DO, director of the Magaziner Center for Wellness and Anti-Aging Medicine in Cherry Hill, New Jersey. "Puréed in a blender or food processor, cauliflower is like mashed potatoes. Plus it's low in calories and high in fiber."

A CRUCIFER COMBO

Maybe you don't like the cabbagy flavor of cauliflower. Or the way those stringy broccoli florets get stuck between your teeth. Is there a way to combine the benefits of crucifers with a taste and texture you enjoy?

Look for that nitro-green vegetable in the produce section—the one that looks like cauliflower on Saint Patrick's Day: broccoflower.

A California-born hybrid that combines the best of broccoli and cauliflower, broccoflower is sweeter, milder, and easier to chew than either of its parents. Plus it has more nutrients: a half-cup serving has as much as 125 percent of the DV for vitamin C. It's also rich in tumor-squelching phytonutrients like sulforaphane and indoles, experts say.

Basmati Rice Salad with Roasted Cauliflower

1 cup brown basmati rice

2¼ cups water

1 cinnamon stick

½ teaspoon ground turmeric

½ cup frozen peas

1 head cauliflower, cut into bite-size florets

2 tablespoons extra-virgin olive oil

1 teaspoon cumin seeds

1 teaspoon salt

1 tablespoon prepared mango chutney

1 tablespoon cider vinegar

1 tablespoon fresh lime juice

   Pinch of dry mustard

¼ cup chopped cashews

¼ cup raisins

2 tablespoons chopped fresh cilantro

Preheat the oven to 450°F. In a saucepan with a tight-fitting lid, combine the rice with the water, cinnamon stick, and turmeric. Bring to a boil, uncovered, over high heat. Cover, reduce the heat, and simmer until the rice is tender and the liquid is absorbed, 35 to 40 minutes. Fluff the rice, add the peas, and let sit, covered, for 5 minutes.

While the rice cooks, toss the cauliflower with 1 tablespoon of the oil, the cumin, and salt, and arrange on a baking sheet in a single layer. Roast in the oven, stirring occasionally, until the cauliflower is tender and browned at the edges, 15 to 20 minutes. Set aside to cool.

In a small bowl, whisk together the remaining 1 tablespoon oil, chutney, vinegar, lime juice, and mustard.

In a large bowl, combine the rice and peas with the cauliflower, cashews, raisins, and cilantro. Pour the chutney dressing over the rice mixture, and toss to combine.

Makes 4 servings

PER SERVING

Calories: 348
Total fat: 13 g
Saturated fat: 2 g

Cholesterol: 0 mg
Sodium: 678 mg
Dietary fiber: 7 g

Celery

STALKS OF PROTECTION

HEALING POWER

Can Help:

Lower cholesterol levels
and high blood pressure

Lower the risk of cancer

The ancient Romans, notorious party animals that they were, wore wreaths of celery to protect them from hangovers, which may explain the practice of putting celery sticks in Bloody Marys.

While there's no evidence that donning a celery chapeau will save you from the consequences of having one too many, celery does have other healing properties. This member of the parsley family contains compounds that may help lower blood pressure and perhaps help prevent cancer. Celery is also a good source of insoluble fiber as well as a number of essential nutrients, including potassium, vitamin C, and calcium.

Clobber Cholesterol with Celery

The humble, pale celery stalk seems like an unlikely warrior in the battle against high cholesterol. Yet, studies of animals have shown celery's cholesterol-lowering activity. In one study, conducted at the National University of Singapore, researchers fed laboratory animals a high-fat diet, plumping them up for 8 weeks and raising their cholesterol. Then they gave some of the animals celery juice. The animals that drank the celery juice had significantly lower total cholesterol and LDL (bad) cholesterol than the animals that weren't given any celery juice.

In a later study, also conducted at the National University of Singapore, researchers gave celery juice for 8 weeks to animals that were bred to have high cholesterol. The researchers found that the celery juice significantly lowered the animals' total cholesterol. Granted, these studies were on rats, so it's not clear whether eating celery will help lower a human's cholesterol or not, but it's certainly not going to hurt.

Chomp Down on Blood Pressure

Celery has been used for centuries in Asia as a folk remedy for high blood pressure. In the United States, it took one man with high blood pressure and persistence to persuade researchers at the University of Chicago Medical Center to put this remedy to the scientific test.

The story began when a man named Mr. Le was diagnosed with mild high blood

FOOD ALERT

A Skin Stalker

Celery is such a sweet, succulent stalk that it has to produce its own pesticides to protect it from hungry fungi.

These compounds, called psoralens, do, in fact, protect the celery. In the process, however, they may do us some harm. For some people, getting psoralens in the diet (or even through the skin) can make their skin extremely sensitive to sunlight—so much so that they can get sunburns after spending even short periods of time in the sun.

If you begin having skin problems after eating celery, you may have to leave it alone. But first, you may want to try washing celery thoroughly before eating it. Washing removes any fungi that may form on the plant, which sometimes causes the production of psoralens.

pressure. Rather than cutting back on salt as his doctor advised, he began eating a quarter-pound (about four stalks) of celery per day. Within a week, his blood pressure had dropped from 158/96 to 118/82.

William J. Elliott, MD, PhD, who was then assistant professor of medicine and pharmacological and physiological science at the University of Chicago, decided to put celery to the test. Researchers injected test animals with a small amount of 3-n-butyl phthalide, a chemical compound that is found in celery. Within a week, the animals' blood pressures dropped an average of 12 to 14 percent.

"Phthalide was found to relax the muscles of the arteries that regulate blood pressure, allowing the vessels to dilate," says Dr. Elliott, who is now an associate professor of preventive medicine at the Rush University Medical Center in Chicago. In addition, the chemical reduced the amount of "stress hormones," called catecholamines, in the blood. This may be helpful because stress hormones typically raise blood pressure by causing blood vessels to constrict.

If you have high blood pressure and would like to give celery a try, employ this strategy recommended by Asian folk practitioners. Eat four to five stalks every day for a week, then stop for 3 weeks. Then start over, and eat celery for another week.

But don't overdo it and start eating celery by the pound, Dr. Elliott warns. Each stalk of celery contains 35 milligrams of sodium, and for some people, this can cause blood pressure to go up rather than down. "Eating a ton of celery can be dangerous if you have salt-sensitive hypertension," he says.

Blocking Cancer Cells

Who'd have thought that crunching celery might help prevent cancer? Celery contains a number of compounds that researchers believe may help prevent cancer cells from spreading.

For starters, celery contains compounds called acetylenics, which have been shown to stop the growth of tumor cells.

In addition, celery contains compounds called phenolic acids, which block the action of hormonelike substances called prostaglandins. Some prostaglandins are thought to encourage the growth of tumor cells.

Also, celery contains compounds called coumarins, which help prevent free radicals from damaging cells. That gives celery a one-two-*three* punch against cancer.

Doctor's Top Tip

While it's tempting to cut up celery ahead of time to eat later, resist! Best to eat it soon after you cut it. After only 24 hours in the fridge, the flavonoids in cut-up celery are considerably decreased, according to researchers in Buenos Aires, Argentina.

GETTING THE MOST

Snap to it. Choose a bunch of celery that looks crisp and snaps easily when pulled apart. Look for celery that's relatively tight and compact, not splayed out.

Leave on the leaves. Celery leaves should be pale to bright green and free from yellow or brown patches. While celery stalks are certainly a healthful snack, it's the leaves that contain the most potassium, vitamin C, and calcium.

Eat it the way you like it. While many foods lose nutrients during cooking, most of the compounds in celery hold up well during cooking. Eating a cup of celery, raw or cooked, provides about 9 milligrams of vitamin C, or 15 percent of the Daily Value (DV); 426 milligrams of potassium, or 12 percent of the DV; and 60 milligrams of calcium, or 6 percent of the DV.

Celiac Disease

LIVING WITHOUT THE LOAF

It's hard to resist the aroma and taste of fresh-from-the-oven bread. But for people with celiac disease, giving in to temptation means intestinal misery.

Celiac disease, also known as celiac sprue, is a lifelong autoimmune disorder that is caused by an immunologically toxic reaction to eating gluten, a protein found in wheat, barley, oats, and rye. In people with celiac disease, even small amounts of gluten can damage millions of villi, the fingerlike projections lining the small intestine that contain many digestive enzymes and that absorb nutrients and fluids. Once the villi are damaged, they're less able to absorb nutrients from food. That's why doctors say that people with celiac disease are "starving in the midst of plenty."

One out of 133 people in the United States has celiac disease, a surprisingly high number. Although there's no cure for the disease, it can be treated with diet.

According to Rallie McAllister, MD, MPH, a board-certified family physician at Nathaniel Mission Clinic in Lexington, Kentucky, and author of *Healthy Lunchbox: The Working Mom's Guide to Keeping You and Your Kids Trim*, the first step is to follow a gluten-free diet, avoiding all foods that contain wheat, rye, barley, and for some people, oats.

In the Kitchen

Baking with gluten-free flours is tricky because they don't "handle" like regular flours. It takes some trial and error to learn tricks for handling each type of flour. Here are some tips:

- Corn flour can be blended with other gluten-free flours and used to make cornbread.
- Potato flour is usually used as a thickening agent in casseroles and soups, while its relative, potato starch flour, makes a great sponge cake.
- Rice flour, with its rather bland flavor, is often mixed with other gluten-free flours, especially potato starch flour.
- Pea, bean, and lentil flours can be used as direct substitutes for wheat flour, as long as egg whites and cottage cheese are added as softeners. They're also good for thickening gravies, soups, and sauces.

HIDDEN DANGERS

For people with celiac disease, staying away from bread and the gluten it contains is an obvious solution. But there are many sources of gluten that aren't so obvious.

For instance, there may be a wheat-derived thickening agent in ice cream that is a source of gluten, says Frederick F. Paustian, MD, of the University of Nebraska Medical Center in Omaha.

Gluten is found in many other processed foods as well, among them yogurt with fruit, ketchup, lunchmeats, cheese spreads, salad dressings, and canned soups. Some food labels may list gluten as an ingredient. Others refer to it by other names. Here's what you need to watch out for:

- Distilled white vinegar
- Hydrolyzed vegetable protein
- Malt or malt flavoring
- Modified starch or modified food starch
- Monoglycerides and diglycerides
- Products that list "natural" or "artificial" flavorings
- Red or yellow food dyes
- Vegetable gum or vegetable protein

"Maintaining a gluten-free diet sounds simple enough, but it's a lot easier said than done," says Dr. McAllister. "Many of the foods that Americans eat and enjoy are rich in gluten, including most pastas, breads, and cereals."

With vigilance, however, it's possible to eat gluten-free. Look for the new labeling "wheat allergen" and "gluten-free" on foods. Also, you can buy many whole grains and flours, for example, that don't contain gluten. Gluten-free flours include corn flour, potato flour, rice flour, soy flour, tapioca, arrowroot, and milo. You can even find pea, bean, and lentil flours, none of which contain gluten, at health food stores.

The second step in taking control of celiac disease is to work with your doctor to correct any nutritional deficiencies you may already have. For example, because people with active celiac disease have difficulty absorbing fats, they may be deficient in fat-soluble vitamins such as vitamins A, D, E, and K. They may have low levels of iron as well, says Frederick F. Paustian, MD, a gastroenterologist at the University of Nebraska Medical Center and a member of the Celiac Sprue Association medical advisory board, both in Omaha.

Doctor's Top Tip

Dealing with celiac disease is deceptively simple. All you have to do is avoid the thing that's making you sick. "Eliminate gluten from your diet, and you get better," says Frederick F. Paustian, MD, of the University of Nebraska Medical Center in Omaha.

Sounds great. The problem is that what is making you sick—gluten—is found in products in practically every aisle in your supermarket, from ketchup and lunchmeat to salad dressings and canned soups. You'll need to become a food detective, and read labels with care to keep gluten off your plate.

People with celiac disease are often unable to drink milk or eat cheese because they lack the enzyme (lactase) that is needed to digest a sugar (lactose) found in dairy foods. Yogurt, however, is a good alternative. "Yogurt contains a type of bacteria that breaks down the lactose," explains Dr. Paustian. "So people with celiac disease can get the benefit of the milk protein as well as the calcium present in yogurt."

An interesting point is that when people with celiac disease have maintained gluten-free diets, they may find that they're able to digest dairy foods without having problems, due to the regrowth of villi in the small intestine.

People with celiac disease are also often deficient in calcium and magnesium, says Dr. Paustian. So it's important to eat plenty of magnesium-rich foods, such as potatoes, avocados, and beans, along with calcium-rich foods such as yogurt.

Cereal

A HEALTHY WAY TO START THE DAY

The cereal aisle in the supermarket can seem more like a playground than a place to buy real food. Many of the colorful boxes are festooned with cartoon characters, puzzles, and promises of prizes inside. And the cereal inside those boxes is often no more substantial. Many popular cereals are essentially sugary snacks. Eating a serving of these is the equivalent of having a couple of cookies or a slice of chocolate cake for breakfast, says Rallie McAllister, MD, MPH, a board-certified family physician at Nathaniel Mission Clinic in Lexington, Kentucky, and author of *Healthy Lunchbox: The Working Mom's Guide to Keeping You and Your Kids Trim.*

HEALING POWER

Can Help:

Prevent cancer and heart disease

Keep digestion regular

Protect against birth defects

But if you read the labels and push on past the worst offenders, you'll find that breakfast cereals, both hot and cold, can be very healthful foods. Many cereals are extraordinarily high in dietary fiber, and almost all are fortified with nutrients, including the B vitamin folate, which can help protect against birth defects. "Cereals are the ideal breakfast," says Pat Harper, RD, a dietitian based in Pittsburgh. "They're convenient, quick, and wonderfully nutritious."

Besides cereals adding life to your years, as you'll read about in this chapter, cereals might also add years to your life. Researchers from the Georgia Centenarian Study discovered that people who reach triple digits consume breakfast more regularly than people who skip the most important meal of the day.

A Spoonful of Serenity

A study conducted in Wales showed that eating breakfast cereal regularly was associated with reduced stress and improved physical and mental health. People who ate cereal each day had lower levels of cortisol, a hormone that rises with stress. Next, researchers hope to find the reason why. (It probably doesn't have anything to do with the free toy at the bottom of the box.)

Two Scoops for Your Heart

Another reason to start your day with a bowlful of a nutritious cereal is heart health. Researchers in Boston found that men who eat more than one serving of whole-grain cereal a day were 20 percent less likely to die from heart disease or other causes than men who rarely ate whole-grain cereals. The study found that men who ate at least one serving of whole-grain breakfast cereal per day had a 27 percent lower risk of dying from any cause compared with the men who rarely ate whole-grain cereal.

Another study—this one from Rush University in Chicago—found that eating breakfast cereal reduced homocysteine levels by 7 percent. Homocysteine is an amino acid that's known to raise heart attack rates.

One of the best things about cereals is that they are often fortified with a host of essential vitamins and minerals that you might not get enough of any other way. "We'd be in big trouble without fortified and enriched foods like breakfast cereals," says Paul Lachance, PhD, executive director of the Nutraceuticals Institute at Rutgers University in New Brunswick, New Jersey. "That's where we get up to 25 percent of many important nutrients. Their contribution to our health is very real."

Flakes of Fiber

Doctors agree that dietary fiber is the key to a healthful diet, not only because it keeps digestion regular but also because it's been shown to lower cholesterol. In excess amounts, cholesterol can stick to artery walls, narrowing blood vessels and increasing the risk of heart disease.

In the Kitchen

The problem with starting the day with hot cereals like oatmeal, Cream of Wheat, and Cream of Rice is that in their plain, unadulterated state, they can leave your taste buds fast asleep. To get the benefits of hot cereals along with some zing, here are some tips you may want to try:

- Substituting orange or apple juice for the cooking water adds a hint of fruity sweetness to hot cereals, along with a nutritional boost.
- You can also use fat-free milk instead of water when cooking hot cereals. Milk adds a touch of creaminess, along with a

healthful shot of calcium. Cooking a half-cup of oatmeal in 1 cup of fat-free milk will deliver 320 milligrams of this important mineral.

- Adding fruit to hot cereals is an easy way to boost the flavor. With hard fruits like apples or pears, simply grate the fruit directly into the cooked cereal. Bananas, berries, and other soft fruits can also be dropped in after cooking. When using dried fruits like raisins, however, add them at the beginning of the cooking time so that they become plump and juicy.

Eating cereal is a good way to get enough of the rough stuff. A serving of Wheaties or Cheerios, for example, has 3 grams of fiber. A total oat bran cereal is even better. One serving provides 6 grams of fiber, or 24 percent of the Daily Value for this nutrient. Other first-rate fiber contenders include Fiber One, with 13 grams per serving, and Uncle Sam cereal, with 10 grams per serving.

In one study, people who got just 3 grams of soluble fiber from oat bran were able to reduce their cholesterol levels five to six points.

The same cereal that's good for your heart can also lower your risk of colon cancer. This is because the fiber in cereal causes stool to move through the intestine more quickly. The faster stool moves, the less time there is for harmful substances to irritate the colon wall, says Beth Kunkel, PhD, RD, professor of food and nutrition at Clemson University in South Carolina.

"The 25 to 30 grams of fiber that is recommended is always a little tough to get in the diet," Harper adds. "By choosing high-fiber cereals more often, you'll have a better chance of getting the fiber you need."

Need more motivation to increase your fiber intake? How about the number on the scale. A study conducted at the University of Rhode Island put one group of people on a 24-week exercise plan, a second group of people on the exercise plan plus a reduced-calorie diet, and a third group of people on the exercise plan plus a reduced-calorie diet including fiber-rich, whole-grain cereal. Both the second and third groups lost an average of 12 pounds, more than the folks in the exercise-only group. But as an added bonus, the people who ate cereal also improved the quality of their diets, by not only taking in more fiber but also getting more magnesium and vitamin B_6.

The Best Picks

Even though many breakfast cereals are high in fiber, others are only middling, and some contain negligible amounts. Here are a few tips to help you find the most fiber in each serving.

Follow the "rule of five." With so many high-quality cereals to choose from, there's simply no reason to settle for second best, Harper says. Cereals that have at least 5 grams of fiber per serving are good choices, so she recommends setting a 5-gram minimum.

Shop for variety. Different cereals contain different types of dietary fiber. To get the best fiber kick, it is a good idea to mix cereals, Harper says. Wheat and rice cereals, for example, are high in insoluble fiber, which is the best kind for preventing constipation and reducing the risk of colon cancer. Oatmeal, on the other hand, contains mainly soluble fiber, which is the cholesterol-lowering kind. Still other cereals,

Doctor's Top Tip

Eating breakfast cereals is a good way to get a start on your fiber intake. But keep in mind that minus the cardboard boxes they're packaged in, most kids' cereals are virtually fiber free, says Rallie McAllister, MD, MPH, a family physician in Lexington, Kentucky. Pass up the marshmallows and free toys and, instead, choose cereals made of bran and shredded wheat, which are rich in fiber, offering 5 grams or more per serving.

such as those that mix grains and fruit, contain both types of fiber, she adds.

Buy the bran. Hot cereals such as corn, wheat, or oat bran are excellent sources of fiber, Harper says. In fact, any cereal that contains the outer portions of grains will contain more fiber than its "lighter" counterparts. So when buying cereals, look for those that say "bran" or "whole grain" on the label.

Keep your guard up. Don't reach for a box just because it says "oats" or "wheat," advises cardiologist Michael H. Davidson, MD, executive medical director of Radiant Research in Chicago. Manufacturers can put almost anything on (or in) a box of cereal. A cereal labeled "wheat," for instance, could have only a trace of the grain and almost no fiber, Dr. Davidson says. So before putting any cereal in your cart, read the label.

Scrutinize the freeze-dried. Think twice about cereal with freeze-dried fruit. Fruits are usually added to low-fiber refined-grain cereals. It's better to add your own fruit to high-fiber cereals.

Look for this label. Choose cereals with the new "help reduce the risk of heart disease" label. These claims are approved by the FDA because cereals bearing this label contain certain heart-healthy ingredients.

Watch portion sizes. One study found that most people eat two times the portion size on the box of cereal. While you may think this is doubling your fiber, it's also doubling your calories.

Cherries

PICK A LITTLE PREVENTION

HEALING POWER

Can Help:

Prevent a variety of cancers

Relieve gout and other forms of arthritis

Reduce the risk of heart disease and stroke

With their hard little pits and rich, shirt-staining colors, cherries take a bit more work to eat than many fruits. But research suggests that this fruit, which contains a compound called perillyl alcohol, are worth the bother—and then some.

"Perillyl alcohol is about the best thing we've ever seen for curing mammary cancer in laboratory animals," says Michael Gould, PhD, professor of oncology and medical physics at the University of Wisconsin Medical School in Madison. In fact, it shows so much promise that it's being tried in cancer patients at the University of Wisconsin.

Perillyl alcohol belongs to a group of compounds called monoterpenes. Limonene, found in the peel of citrus fruits, is another member of this family. These compounds have been shown in studies to block the formation of a variety of cancers, including those of the breasts, lungs, stomach, liver, and skin. Expectations for perillyl alcohol are high, in part, because it is 5 to 10 times more potent than limonene, which itself has been proven to be very effective.

It's not yet known how much perillyl alcohol there is in cherries, adds Pamela Crowell, PhD, associate professor of biology at Indiana University School of Medicine in Indianapolis. Even in small amounts, however, the compound probably has some beneficial effects. So cherries, when eaten as part of a well-rounded diet, can play a small but important role in helping the body ward off cancer.

Vitamin C and More

There's more to cherries than exotic new compounds. They also contain a variety of antioxidants, which help ward off disease by mopping up harmful oxygen molecules called free radicals that naturally accumulate in the body. Unchecked, these free radicals damage healthy tissues throughout the body, causing changes that can lead to cancer, heart disease, and other serious conditions. Researchers have found that 1 cup of sweet cherries has more than twice as many antioxidants as green tea.

Additionally, a half-cup of sour cherries has 5 milligrams of vitamin C, about 8 percent of the Daily Value (DV) for this vitamin. Sour cherries also provide vitamins

A and E. Sweet cherries contain these nutrients, too, but not as much vitamin A and E as their mouth-puckering kin.

The vitamin E in cherries is of particular interest, since one study of postmenopausal women found that those who consumed the most vitamin E had the least risk of heart disease. And there was an interesting twist. The women who got their vitamin E naturally—solely from food—had less risk than women who were also taking vitamin E supplements.

The problem with vitamin E is that it's difficult to get the DV of 30 IU from food alone. In fact, the only foods with a lot of vitamin E are high-fat cooking oils and nuts, which you don't want a lot of. Cherries are one of the better food sources for vitamin E.

Finally, cherries contain a compound called quercetin. Like vitamin C and other antioxidants, quercetin helps block the damage caused by free radicals.

Relief for Gout and Other Forms of Arthritis

Folklore is full of stories about people who relieved the agonizing pain of gout by eating cherries or drinking cherry juice daily. While the Arthritis Foundation still says that there's no absolute evidence to suggest that cherries really can ease the ache of this form of arthritis or any other, many gout sufferers swear by them.

Several studies have found that natural compounds in cherries may reduce the

In the Kitchen

Fresh cherries are at their ever-loving, mouth-watering best from May through July. To get the sweetest taste from the harvest, here are some tips you may want to try:

Check the stems. When buying cherries, make sure that the stems are green. Dark-colored stems are a tip-off that cherries have been sitting in the bin too long.

Buy in small quantities. Cherries are highly perishable. Even when properly stored in the refrigerator, they'll only keep for a few days. So plan on buying only what you're going to eat right away.

Store them dry. Washing cherries ahead of time can cause them to spoil in the refrigerator. So it's best to store them dry, then wash them as needed. It's important, however, to wash them thoroughly. Cherries are often coated with a mixture of insecticides, anti-fungal oils, and moisture seals that producers use to keep them fresh.

Use up the extras. When you're tired of munching cherries, you may want to try a little juice. Simply wash, stem, pit, and crush the cherries. Heat them in a saucepan, then press the mixture through a strainer. Refrigerate several hours, then pour off the clear juice, and add sugar to taste.

painful inflammation of arthritis. The first study, conducted at the University of California, Davis, instructed 10 healthy women to eat 45 fresh Bing cherries one day for breakfast. The women were asked not to eat other fruits or vegetables or to drink tea or red wine for the 2 days before the cherry breakfast because the researchers were concerned that these other high-antioxidant foods would interfere with the results. The researchers measured the women's plasma urate, a marker for gout, before and after the cherry breakfast. The researchers found that the women's urate levels decreased significantly after eating cherries, which suggests that cherries might play an important role in fighting gout.

Doctor's Top Tip

"Eat fresh cherries, organic if possible," says Allan Magaziner, DO, director of the Magaziner Center for Wellness and Anti-Aging Medicine in Cherry Hill, New Jersey. "They're great as a snack."

A second, follow-up study was also conducted at the University of California, Davis. This study asked 18 women and 2 men to eat 45 fresh Bing cherries throughout the day, every day for a month. After the month, the volunteers' levels of three indicators of inflammation—nitric oxide, C-reactive protein, and a marker for T-cell activation—decreased by 18 to 25 percent.

A survey by *Prevention* magazine found that 67 percent of readers who tried cherries for gout had good results. And Steve Schumacher, a kinesiologist in Louisville, Kentucky, enthusiastically recommends them. He advises people with gout to quit eating red meats and organ meats and also to drink two to three glasses of cherry juice a day. He recommends using pure black-cherry juice diluted with an equal amount of water. "Those who have followed this diet faithfully have all gotten results, some within 48 to 72 hours, and some within a week, depending on the severity," Schumacher says.

GETTING THE MOST

Eat cherries uncooked. Because cooking destroys some of the vitamin C and other nutrients in cherries, it's best to eat them uncooked to reap their full nutritional bounty.

Prepare them for baking. While it's easy to eat sweet cherries uncooked, that's really not an option for the sour kinds. Still, sour cherries are high enough in a variety of nutrients that they'll keep some of their value even after baking.

Bing Cherry Topping

- 1 tablespoon cornstarch
- ¾ cup apple juice
- 2 tablespoons honey
- ½ teaspoon vanilla extract
- 3½ cups Bing cherries, stemmed and pitted
- ¼ teaspoon ground cinnamon
- ⅛ teaspoon ground cardamom (optional)

In a medium saucepan, whisk the cornstarch with the apple juice until the cornstarch dissolves. Whisk in the honey and vanilla extract.

Add the cherries, cinnamon, and cardamom (if using). Cook over medium-low heat, stirring frequently, until the sauce thickens and turns transparent, about 4 to 5 minutes. Remove from the heat. Serve warm.

Makes about 4 cups

Cook's Notes: *The sauce can be refrigerated in a covered container for up to 3 days. Reheat gently in the microwave or in a saucepan before serving. Serve over pancakes, waffles, or fat-free frozen yogurt.*

PER ½ CUP

Calories: 77	Cholesterol: 0 mg
Total fat: 0.7 g	Sodium: 1 mg
Saturated fat: 0.2 g	Dietary fiber: 1.1 g

Chicken Soup

FOOD FOR BODY AND SOUL

HEALING POWER
Can Help:
Relieve nasal congestion
Soothe irritated airways

Put a chicken in a pot with water, onions, carrots, peppercorns, and a little salt. Cook until it falls apart. Strain. Discard the fat. Feed the overdone chicken and vegetables to a hungry pet. Add a whole chile pepper to the broth, half a large garlic clove, and thin slices of lemon. Serve steaming hot. This is the cure for the common cold.

Grandma's traditional favorite? Not quite. This recipe was created by Pauline M. Jackson, MD, a member of the board of directors at Gunderson Lutheran Medical Center in La Crosse, Wisconsin, and a firm believer in the soothing powers of chicken soup. "It's hot, it tastes good, and it reminds you of Mom," she says.

You don't need a panel of experts to tell you that chicken soup is soothing when you're sick. But evidence suggests that it's more than a feel-good food. When you're honking and sniffling with a cold or other upper respiratory infection, says Dr. Jackson, virtually no remedy is more effective than chicken soup.

Breathing Easy

The classic chicken soup study was conducted in 1978 by three lung specialists at Mount Sinai Medical Center in Miami Beach, Florida. Intrigued by the healing mystique surrounding the savory brew, they had 15 people with colds sip either hot chicken soup, hot water, or cold water. Then they measured how quickly and easily mucus and air flowed through the patients' noses. The result was that chicken soup eased nasal congestion better than both hot water and cold water.

Chicken soup may relieve cold symptoms, speculated the researchers, because the heat "increases nasal mucous velocity." In other words, it makes your nose run, possibly reducing the amount of time that cold germs spend in your nose and helping you recover more quickly.

So why didn't the hot water work just as well at relieving colds as the chicken soup did? The soup's healing secret may lie in its savory aroma and taste, which "appear to possess an additional substance for increasing nasal mucous velocity," the researchers reported. What this substance might be, however, remains a mystery.

More recently, Stephen Rennard, MD, professor in the department of internal

In the Kitchen

When a cold hits, so might a yearning for homemade chicken soup. But who wants to get out of a cozy sickbed to make it from scratch? You won't have to if you make and freeze a batch of chicken stock before a flu bug bites.

Making stock isn't difficult. Put some skinless chicken parts in a large pot, cover with cold water, add a carrot, onion, a garlic clove, and a bay leaf, and simmer for a few hours. Strain out the solids and set the stock aside to cool.

To reduce the fat in the stock, first ladle it into shallow containers and let cool for up to 2 hours. Then refrigerate overnight. The fat will solidify into a thin sheet that can be peeled right off.

Frozen stock will keep for up to 6 months. For convenience, freeze it in ice-cube trays rather than large containers; the small, frozen cubes will defrost more quickly than large blocks.

---

medicine at the University of Nebraska Medical Center in Omaha, tested chicken soup that was prepared by his wife from her grandmother's recipe. He found that the soup reduced the action of neutrophils—white blood cells that are attracted to areas of inflammation and that may cause common cold symptoms like irritated airways and mucus production. (See page 170 for the recipe.)

Researchers also suspect that part of the healing power of chicken soup lies in the bird itself. Chicken contains a natural amino acid called cysteine, which is chemically similar to a drug called acetylcysteine, says Irwin Ziment, MD, professor emeritus at the University of California, Los Angeles. Doctors use acetylcysteine to treat people with bronchitis and other respiratory infections. "Acetylcysteine was originally derived from chicken feathers and chicken skin," he notes.

More recently, Dr. Rennard polled a group of American Academy of Family Physicians doctors and found that 87 percent agreed that increasing your fluid intake is critical for cold sufferers. Two out of three of the family physicians agreed that eating chicken soup is an effective way to increase your fluids, second only to water.

Doctor's Top Tip

"Eat it hot. The steam from a piping hot bowl of chicken soup acts as a powerful decongestant," says Rallie McAllister, MD, MPH, a family physician at Nathaniel Mission Clinic in Lexington, Kentucky. As you breathe in the steam, it helps break up secretions in your nose, throat, and chest. Drinking the hot liquid also brings about a temporary elevation in your body temperature, which hinders the ability of cold viruses to multiply. A higher body temperature also speeds the rate of chemical reactions, so injured cells can repair themselves more rapidly.

GETTING THE MOST

Sip it often. The therapeutic effects of chicken soup last about 30 minutes, according to the Miami Beach study. So it's a good idea to make a large batch and keep it handy for reheating so that you can sip a cup when symptoms flare up.

Opt for convenience. If you can coax a sympathetic spouse into whipping up a pot of homemade, aromatic soup, enjoy the pampering. But home-cooked broth really isn't mandatory, says Dr. Ziment. Canned chicken soup can also be helpful in breaking up congestion.

Spice it up. Adding hot spices to chicken soup—a clove of garlic, say, or a chopped chile pepper or some fresh grated ginger—will speed up chicken soup's declogging power, says Dr. Ziment.

Grandma's Chicken Soup

This is the recipe used by Stephen Rennard, MD, professor in the department of internal medicine at the University of Nebraska Medical Center in Omaha, for his famous chicken soup study. He stresses that other chicken soup recipes are also effective, including many store-bought soups. Dr. Rennard credits his wife's grandmother, Celia Fleischer, for developing this recipe.

1   **stewing hen or baking chicken (about 5 to 6 pounds)**

1   **package chicken wings**

3   **large onions**

1   **large sweet potato, peeled and cubed**

3   **parsnips, peeled and cubed**

2   **turnips, peeled and cubed**

11–12   **large carrots, sliced**

5–6   **celery stalks, sliced**

1   **bunch parsley**

     Salt

     Freshly ground black pepper

Clean the whole stewing hen or chicken, put it in a large pot, and cover it with cold water. Bring the water to a boil. Add the chicken wings, onions, sweet potato, parsnips, turnips, and carrots. Boil about 1½ hours. Remove the fat from the surface as it accumulates. Add the celery and parsley. Cook the soup about 45 minutes longer. Remove the chicken. (The chicken is not used further for the soup, but the meat makes excellent Chicken Parmesan.) Using a slotted spoon, transfer the vegetables to a food processor and process until they are puréed, or pass the vegetables through a strainer. Refrigerate the broth and puréed vegetables for 1 to 2 hours. Skim any fat that forms on the broth.

Return the puréed vegetables to the soup, stir, and reheat. Add salt and pepper to taste.

Cook's Note: *This soup freezes well. You can also add matzoh balls, prepared according to the recipe on the back of the box of matzoh meal.*

Makes 8 servings

PER SERVING ─────────────────

Calories: 138
Total fat: 1 g
Saturated fat: 0 g

Cholesterol: 5 mg
Sodium: 559 mg
Dietary fiber: 7 g

Chile Peppers
RED-HOT HEALERS

According to an old saying, "Whatever doesn't kill you makes you stronger." This might be the perfect motto for the chile pepper. Not only can many people withstand the heat, they actually enjoy it. Chile pepper fans savor the heat at every opportunity, not just in traditional favorites like tacos and burritos but also in foods such as omelets, stews, and even salads.

More is involved than just a little culinary spice. These thermogenic morsels are prized around the globe for their healing power as well as their firepower. Hot chiles have long been used as natural remedies for coughs, colds, sinusitis, and bronchitis, says Irwin Ziment, MD, professor emeritus at the University of California, Los Angeles. There's some evidence that they can help lower low-density lipoprotein (LDL) cholesterol, the type associated with stroke, high blood pressure, and heart disease. There's also some evidence that chiles can help prevent—of all things—stomach ulcers. And research suggests that chile peppers might help you win the battle of the bulge and prevent cancer.

HEALING POWER
Can Help:

Reduce weight

Prevent the spread of cancer

Clear sinuses and relieve congestion

Stop ulcers

Reduce the risk of heart disease and stroke

Burn Off Pounds

Historically, chile peppers were used to stimulate appetite. But ironically, they may actually do just the opposite. In fact, chile peppers seem to provide a three-pronged attack against obesity. First, eating chile peppers may help fight off cravings. Some experts believe that eating sharp-tasting foods such as hot peppers, pickles, and tomato juice can overwhelm taste buds, cutting off cravings.

Second, chile peppers may help you eat less. Researchers in the Netherlands gave 12 men 0.9 gram of ground chile pepper, either as a pill or mixed into a tomato juice beverage. Thirty minutes later, they turned the men loose at an all-you-can-eat buffet. Compared with men who were given a placebo, the men who had chile pepper reduced their food intake by 10 to 16 percent.

And third, it actually *requires* energy to eat chile peppers. That's right, it burns calories to eat them! That's because the heat you feel when you eat chile peppers takes energy to produce.

Protect Against Cancer

Compounds in chile peppers show promise against cancer. For example, researchers at the University of Pittsburgh discovered that the capsaicin, the compound that gives chile peppers their heat, caused pancreatic cancer cells that had been implanted in mice to die through a process called apoptosis. Pancreatic cancer, one of the most aggressive cancers, is the fifth-leading cause of cancer death in the United States.

Another study, this one by researchers at the University of California, Los Angeles, School of Medicine, found that capsaicin stops the spread of prostate cancer cells. Researchers found it does that in several ways, including causing cancer cells to commit suicide. Researchers gave animals capsaicin three times a week. After a month, the animals' prostate cancer tumor growth and size had decreased significantly.

Heat Up a Cold

Chile lovers have long asserted that hot peppers, from serranos to jalapeños, are the ultimate decongestant, clearing a stuffy nose in the time it takes to gasp "Yow!" In fact, the fiery bite of hot chiles (or chile-based condiments like Tabasco sauce) can work as well as over-the-counter cold remedies, says Dr. Ziment. "Some of the foods used to fight respiratory diseases for centuries, including hot peppers, are very similar to the drugs we now use."

The stuff that makes hot peppers so nose-clearing good is capsaicin, a plant chemical that gives hot peppers their sting. Chemically, capsaicin is similar to a drug called guaifenesin, which is used in many over-the-counter and prescription cold remedies such as Robitussin, says Dr. Ziment.

Of course, eating a chile pepper has more of an immediate impact than taking a spoonful of medicine. When hot pepper meets the tongue, the brain is slammed with an onslaught of nerve messages. The brain responds to this "Ow!" message by stimulating secretion-producing glands that line the airways. The result is a flood of fluids that makes your eyes water, your nose run, and the mucus in your lungs loosen, says Dr. Ziment. In other words, chile peppers are a natural decongestant and expectorant.

Even beyond that, though, researchers in Korea found that capsaicin actually affects the immune system. In one study, mice were given a daily dose of capsaicin and had nearly three times more antibody-producing cells after 3 weeks than other mice that weren't given any capsaicin. What does this mean for humans? More antibodies equals fewer colds and infections.

It doesn't take a lot of pepper to get the healing benefits. Adding 10 drops of hot pepper sauce to a bowl of chicken soup can be very effective, says Paul Bosland, PhD, professor in the department of horticulture at New Mexico State University in Las Cruces and founder of the Chile Pepper Institute at the university. "Most of us here in New Mexico do this when we're sick," he says. "We all feel better after we've had a little bit of chile pepper."

Dr. Ziment recommends treating a cold with a warm-water gargle to which you've added 10 drops of Tabasco sauce. "This remedy can be quite effective, particularly if you want to clear your sinuses," he says.

Help for Heart and Stomach

"Consuming peppers may lower your risk for heart disease," says Rallie McAllister, MD, MPH, a board-certified family physician at Nathaniel Mission Clinic in Lexington, Kentucky, and author of *Healthy Lunchbox: The Working Mom's Guide to*

In the Kitchen

Cooking with hot peppers is like riding a Harley. You have to do it very carefully.

"Approach hot peppers with respect," says Bill Hufnagle, author of *Biker Billy Cooks with Fire*. "People tell me the most unusual stories about their experiences with hot peppers—where they touched, whom they touched, and what happened," says Hufnagle.

To enjoy the heat of peppers without getting burned, follow these Hufnagle tips:

Protect your hands. When you're cooking with very hot peppers—"anything hotter than a jalapeño," Hufnagle says—put on a pair of disposable plastic gloves. (If you have sensitive hands, you may want to wear gloves even when working with milder peppers.) When you're done, thoroughly rinse the tips of the gloves with soapy water before taking them off to avoid transferring the pepper oil to your fingers. Then immediately wash your hands, says Hufnagle.

Use plenty of soap. Chile oil sticks to the skin, and water alone won't get it off. You need to use plenty of soap as well. "You might want to wash your hands more than once, depending on the kind of pepper you were working with and how much of it you handled," says Hufnagle.

Protect against pepper dust. When grinding or crushing dried hot peppers, wear a dust mask and goggles. "The dust can get in your throat and eyes," says Hufnagle.

Crush them by hand. It may be convenient to grind dried hot peppers in a blender or coffee grinder—but you won't appreciate the aftershocks. "How thoroughly can you wash a coffee grinder or blender, anyway?" says Hufnagle. "If you use them to grind peppers, you're going to have some nice hot coffee—or milk shakes." At the very least, you may want to consider getting a separate grinder to use on dried hot peppers only.

The heat source and beneficial compound in chile peppers is called capsaicin. Capsaicin is produced by the pepper membranes, and then drawn into the seeds, says Rallie McAllister, MD, MPH, a family physician in Lexington, Kentucky. Eating the entire pepper—seeds and all—gives you the highest concentration of this healing compound and the most heat.

Keeping You and Your Kids Trim. Capsaicin not only improves circulation, it also decreases the clotting potential of your blood, preventing blockages in the arteries of the heart and brain that can lead to heart attacks and strokes.

In experiments at the Bristol-Myers Squibb Pharmaceutical Research Institute, capsaicin was found to reduce the occurrence of dangerous heart-rhythm disturbances, lower blood pressure, and improve blood-flow to the heart. It seems to function in these roles as a natural calcium channel blocker, analogous to some prescription heart drugs, says Dr. McAllister.

Interestingly, capsaicin has been shown to lower cholesterol levels in turkeys eating high-cholesterol diets. Like humans, turkeys are known to develop hardening of the arteries that can lead to heart disease.

For years, doctors advised people prone to ulcers to abstain from spicy foods. Research now suggests the opposite—that chile peppers may help prevent ulcers from occurring.

Capsaicin appears to shield the stomach lining from ulcer-causing bacteria by stimulating the flow of protective digestive juices. Researchers at National University Hospital in Singapore found that people who consumed the most chili powder had the fewest ulcers, leading them to speculate that chile, or capsaicin, was the protective factor.

Red-Hot Vitamins

Getting more hot chiles into your diet may strengthen your personal antiaging arsenal. That's because they're a rich source of the antioxidants vitamin C and beta-carotene (which is converted into vitamin A in the body).

These antioxidants help protect the body by "neutralizing" free radicals, harmful oxygen molecules that naturally accumulate in the body and cause cell damage. Upping your intake of antioxidant vitamins, researchers believe, may help prevent damage that can lead to cancer, heart disease, and stroke as well as arthritis and a weakened immune system.

One red chile packs 3 milligrams of beta-carotene, between 30 and 50 percent of the amount recommended by most experts. Studies show that people who consume more beta-carotene-rich foods are not as prone to cancer and heart disease.

GETTING THE MOST

Choose with care. Buy fresh chile peppers that have vivid, deep colors. Their skin should be glossy, firm, and taut, and their stems should be hardy and fresh. Look for dried chile peppers with vivid colors as well. Drab chile peppers offer drab flavor.

Go for paper over plastic. Storing peppers in plastic bags isn't a great idea because the moisture accumulation can cause them to spoil more quickly. Instead, keep them in paper bags, or wrap them in paper towels. They should last for a week in the vegetable drawer of the fridge.

Enjoy them raw. Although raw chiles can be uncomfortably hot for some people, that's the best way to get the most vitamin C; cooking destroys the stores of this vitamin, says Dr. Bosland. On the other hand, capsaicin isn't affected by heating, so if that's what you're after—to help relieve congestion, for example—cook the peppers to your taste.

Preserve the powder. Storing chili powder at room temperature will eventually deplete its beta-carotene. "Keep chili powder in a dark, cool place, like in the freezer," says Dr. Bosland.

Eat for comfort. The hottest chile pepper isn't necessarily the most healing, so don't make yourself suffer. From wild to mild, here are a few chiles you may want to try:

- Habanero pepper and Scotch bonnet are among the most mouth-blistering peppers.
- Jalapeño and Fresno peppers weigh in at 50 percent firepower, compared to the habanero.
- Hungarian cherry and Anaheim peppers emit more of a glow than a flame and are a good choice for tamer palates.

Fiery Chile Pepper Salsa

2 medium tomatoes, coarsely chopped

2 small jalapeño peppers, cut in half lengthwise and very thinly sliced (wear plastic gloves when handling)

¼ cup finely chopped red onion

2 tablespoons chopped fresh cilantro

2 tablespoons fresh lime juice

⅛ teaspoon salt

In a small bowl, combine the tomatoes, peppers, onion, cilantro, lime juice, and salt. Mix well. Let the salsa stand for at least 30 minutes to allow the flavors to blend.

Makes 1⅓ cups

Cook's Notes: *The salsa can be covered and stored in the refrigerator for several days. Also, serve with fat-free corn chips or as a condiment for baked potatoes or grilled poultry or meat.*

PER ⅓ CUP ———————————————————————

Calories: 29	Cholesterol: 0 mg
Total fat: 0.2 g	Sodium: 74 mg
Saturated fat: 0 g	Dietary fiber: 0.8 g

Cholesterol Control
KEEP YOUR ARTERIES CLEAN

When you consider that haggis, a favorite food in Scotland, is made of the innards of various animals mixed with animal fat and that many of the people there never eat vegetables, it's easy to understand why the Scots still have one of the highest mortality rates from cardiovascular disease in the world. Of course, Americans are more likely to eat hamburgers than haggis, but when it comes to cardiovascular health, we're only a few chest-clutching steps behind the Scots.

The reason, to a large extent, is high cholesterol. Having high cholesterol levels is one of the primary risk factors for heart attack, stroke, and other vascular diseases. Almost 100 million American adults have cholesterol levels over 200. Of these, about 34.5 million have cholesterol levels of 240 or above.

If there's any good news in these statistics, it's this: While elevated cholesterol puts you at higher risk for heart disease, it's a risk that you can control every day. Eating foods that are low in saturated fats and cholesterol is an efficient way to reduce the amount of cholesterol in your blood. Moreover, making even small reductions in cholesterol can add up to big health benefits. For each 1 percent that you lower your total cholesterol, you lower your risk of having a heart attack by 2 percent.

Understanding Cholesterol

By itself, cholesterol isn't the toxic sludge that people think it is. Indeed, the body uses cholesterol, which is produced in the liver, to make cell membranes, sex hormones, bile acids, and vitamin D. You couldn't live without it. In large amounts, however, this essential substance, which is found in animal foods such as meats, milk, eggs, and butter, quickly becomes dangerous. This is particularly true of a form of cholesterol called low-density lipoprotein (LDL), the bad cholesterol.

As LDL cholesterol circulates in the bloodstream, it undergoes a process called oxidation. Essentially, this means that it spoils and turns rancid. Your immune system quickly spots the decaying LDL and reacts to it as it would to any other invader. Immune cells gobble up the cholesterol molecules. Once engorged, they stick to the walls of arteries, hardening into a dense, fatty layer called plaque. When enough plaque accumulates, there's less room for blood to flow. Eventually, bloodflow may slow or even stop. When this occurs in arteries supplying the heart, the result is a heart attack. When it occurs in arteries supplying the brain, the result is a stroke.

Your body has a mechanism for dealing with this threat. A second form of cholesterol, called high-density lipoprotein (HDL), transports the dangerous cholesterol out of the blood and to the liver for disposal. Normally, it does a good job. (In fact, one study found that every one-point rise in HDL cholesterol protects the heart at least as much as a one-point drop in LDL cholesterol, reducing risk of a fatal heart attack by 2 percent.) But when cholesterol levels get too high, the HDL cholesterol can't keep up, and LDL gradually rises to dangerous levels.

Ideally, you want to have high levels of HDL and low levels of the dangerous LDL. The National Cholesterol Education Program recommends keeping total cholesterol below 200 milligrams per deciliter of blood. More specifically, LDL should be below 130, and HDL should be above 40. Even better, they say that an HDL above 60 is protective against disease.

One way to help keep your blood cholesterol within healthy limits is to eat no more than 300 milligrams of dietary cholesterol a day (a little more than the amount in 1½ egg yolks). But as mentioned, the body makes cholesterol on its own. That's why limiting the amount of cholesterol in your diet is only part of the solution.

Nuts to You

Not long ago, nuts were generally regarded as "fat pills," and people were urged to eat less of them. But that has changed in recent years. One of the many health benefits of nuts is their cholesterol-fighting ability.

Scientists at the USDA found that nuts contain significant levels of nutrients called plant sterols. These nutrients can lower LDL cholesterol, possibly by keeping your digestive system from absorbing the cholesterol in the foods you eat. Researchers in Canada found that when people with high cholesterol ate 1.8 grams of plant sterols a day, their cholesterol levels dropped by 8 percent.

You can buy sterol-fortified foods, such as margarine and juices, that contain extra sterols. Or you can eat them the way Mother Nature intended—in sesame seeds, sunflower seeds, and pistachios, with 144 milligrams, 104 milligrams, and 83 milligrams respectively in ¼ cup.

One nut that's gotten a particularly bad rap, coconut, may actually be especially helpful for battling high cholesterol. It's true that coconut contains more saturated fat (one of the unhealthiest kinds of fat) than butter does, ounce for ounce. However, more than half of coconut's saturated fat is lauric acid. When researchers analyzed 60 studies, they discovered that even though lauric acid raises LDL (bad) cholesterol, it boosts HDL (good) cholesterol even more. So in the end, this is good for your overall cholesterol profile.

A nut that has gotten more favorable press than the coconut is the almond. And here's one reason why. Researchers at Tufts University in Boston found that almonds' skins are particularly rich in antioxidants that help to remove LDL cholesterol. The scientists found that an extract of almond-skin flavonoids reduced LDL oxidation by 18 percent in hamsters.

Help from Fiber

You know that eating whole grains, beans, and fresh fruits will help keep your digestive system in top shape, but you may want to eat these foods to reduce cholesterol, too. They're filled with soluble fiber, a substance that forms a gummy gel in the digestive tract, which helps lower cholesterol.

A study of people in China, conducted by researchers from Johns Hopkins University in Baltimore, found that cholesterol levels in men who ate about 3 ounces of oats a day were 11 percent lower than those of men who rarely ate oats. In addition, the blood pressures of the men who ate oats were 8 percent lower.

"This study suggests that eating a high-fiber diet can have a beneficial effect on blood cholesterol and blood pressure," says Jiang He, MD, PhD, professor and chairman of the department of epidemiology at the Tulane University School of Public Health and Tropical Medicine in New Orleans. "It further suggests that adopting a high-fiber diet could reduce the death rate from cardiovascular disease in the United States."

In another study, researchers from the USDA put 25 people on heart-healthy diets for 5 weeks. They gave some of the people 3 grams of soluble fiber each day from barley—about the amount in a half-cup. When compared with the other people, who didn't get the barley, their total cholesterol levels dropped by 9 percent.

The Daily Value (DV) for fiber is 25 grams. In practical terms, this means eating 2 to 4 servings of fruit, 3 to 5 servings of vegetables, and 6 to 11 servings of breads, cereals, and grains a day, says Joanne Curran-Celentano, PhD, RD, associate professor of nutritional sciences at the University of New Hampshire in Durham. "Eating oatmeal or oat bran cereal several times a week will add even more soluble fiber to your diet," she adds. Other good sources of soluble fiber include pinto beans, red kidney beans, Brussels sprouts, and sweet potatoes.

Drink Up

Two very different beverages—milk and wine—may help improve cholesterol levels, though obviously we don't recommend drinking them together, and fat-free or low-fat milk is best. One study found that after 4 weeks of consuming 1,060 milligrams of calcium and 490 milligrams of phosphorus (a combination found in dairy products such as milk) in supplement form, the cholesterol levels of healthy people were reduced by 6 percent, compared with people who didn't get the supplements. One 8-ounce glass of milk provides about a third of the amounts taken in the study.

Another study, conducted in Boston, found that averaging five wine drinks a week cut the risk of having dangerously low HDL levels by a whopping 78 percent. It's important to keep in mind that while this amount of wine may improve your HDL cholesterol, drinking more heavily can raise blood pressure (another risk factor for heart disease) and have other damaging effects on your health. So be judicious.

The Asian Superfood

We feed soybeans to chickens. But in Asian countries, people eat soybeans as well as soy foods such as tofu nearly every day. These foods contain compounds that help lower cholesterol, and this may explain, at least in part, why cholesterol levels in Japan are so much lower than they are in the United States.

Studies have shown that replacing protein from animal sources with about 1½ ounces of soy protein a day can lower total cholesterol by 9 percent. It lowers dangerous LDL cholesterol even more, by 13 percent.

Now research shows that soy protein can also *raise* your HDL cholesterol. Researchers at the University of Minnesota found that women who consumed 26 grams of soy protein over 6 weeks increased their HDL by 4.2 percent. You could get that much soy protein in two to four servings of soy milk or soy-added cereal or energy bars.

Tofu and other soy foods contain compounds called phytoestrogens, says James W. Anderson, MD, professor of internal medicine in the department of endocrinology and molecular medicine at the University of Kentucky in Lexington. Researchers believe that these compounds help transport LDL cholesterol from the bloodstream to the liver, where it's broken down and excreted. They also may prevent the LDL from oxidizing, making it less likely to clog the coronary arteries.

To get the cholesterol-lowering benefits of soy, you need to eat two or three servings of soy foods a day, says Dr. Anderson.

Cloves of Protection

Garlic lovers say that you can't eat too much of the "stinking rose," and it certainly can't hurt. When it comes to cholesterol, some research suggests that this pungent bulb can significantly lower cholesterol; other research says it does nothing.

Garlic contains a compound called allicin that may change the way in which the body uses cholesterol. When researchers analyzed data from five of the most reliable scientific studies on garlic and cholesterol, they found that eating one-half to one

THE MONOUNSATURATED EDGE

"The component in food that has the biggest effect on blood cholesterol levels is saturated fat," says Mark Kantor, PhD, of the University of Maryland in College Park. Saturated fats, which are found mostly in animal foods such as red meats, whole and 2% milk, egg yolks, butter, and cheese, can increase the amount of harmful low-density lipoprotein (LDL) cholesterol in the bloodstream as well as the total amount of cholesterol.

Every day, the average American eats the fat equivalent of a full stick of butter. Experts strongly recommend decreasing the amount of fat in your diet.

But while it's a good idea to reduce the total amount of fat in your diet, there's one type of fat that you can feel good about eating. Research suggests that having moderate amounts of monounsaturated fat, the kind found in avocados, olive oil, and canola oil, can lower levels of bad LDL cholesterol, while leaving the beneficial high-density lipoprotein (HDL) untouched.

Researchers have known for a long time that people in Greece, Spain, and other Mediterranean countries where olive oil is used every day have some of the lowest rates of heart disease in the world. Indeed, even when their cholesterol levels are fairly high, they're about half as likely to die of heart disease as an American with the same cholesterol reading. Research suggests that olive oil may somehow improve the liver's ability to remove LDL cholesterol from the bloodstream.

Even so, olive oil can't take credit for all the benefits. People in the Mediterranean region also eat a lot of fresh fruits and vegetables, plus they walk more than Americans and are less likely to be overweight.

If you do decide to add more olive oil to your diet, use it in moderation, adds Dr. Kantor. It may be better than other oils, but it's still 100 percent fat. "Cut back on all fats," he says, "and consume olive oil in moderation. Don't increase the total amount of oil in your diet."

clove of garlic a day lowered blood cholesterol an average of 9 percent. Recent research at Stanford University in California, however, found that eating raw garlic didn't affect cholesterol levels at all.

When using garlic, it's a good idea to mince or crush it, since this releases more of the allicin. Even if you eat a lot of garlic, however, don't count on it to be a magic bullet. "Eating garlic on top of a diet high in saturated fat and cholesterol is unlikely to do you any good," says Mark Kantor, PhD, associate professor of nutrition and food science at the University of Maryland in College Park.

Doctor's Top Tip

"Eat one to two small fistfuls of almonds a day," says Cyril Kendall, PhD, a research scientist in the department of nutritional sciences at the University of Toronto. This amount—1 to 2 ounces—of raw, unblanched almonds each day caused a significant reduction in cholesterol in a University of Toronto study. Even better news? The addition of this amount of almonds to the diet didn't result in any weight gain.

Help from the Deep

In addition to knowing your cholesterol levels, there's another number to watch: your level of blood fats called triglycerides. People with high levels of triglycerides are more likely to have low levels of protective HDL. Conversely, lowering your level of triglycerides can help decrease your risk of heart disease.

Salmon, tuna, and other oily fish contain fats called omega-3 fatty acids, which have been shown to lower triglycerides. In a study at the University of Western Australia in Perth, two groups of men followed a low-fat diet. Those in one group ate a variety of protein foods, while those in the second group ate 3 to 5 ounces of fish a day. After 3 months, men in both groups had drops in cholesterol. But the men who ate fish also experienced a 23 percent reduction in triglycerides.

Omega-3s may do more than lower triglycerides. Research suggests that they may raise levels of beneficial HDL cholesterol as well. Men in the Australian study who ate fish had a 15 percent increase in HDL. It appears that as fish is added to a low-fat diet, triglycerides go down, and HDL levels go up.

In another study, researchers at the University of Guelph in Ontario, Canada, found that women who took 2.8 grams of omega-3 fats for a month had 8 percent higher HDL levels than the women who took a placebo (dummy pill).

Finally, fish is also low in calories and saturated fat, making it a perfect addition to a cholesterol-reducing diet. To get the maximum benefits from omega-3s, plan on eating 3 to 4 ounces of fish two times a week, recommends Dr. Curran-Celentano.

Incidentally, if you're a fan of canned tuna, you're in luck since it also contains omega-3s. However, be sure to buy chunk light tuna packed in water (canned albacore tuna has been linked to high levels of mercury). Three ounces contains approximately 90 calories and less than 1 gram of fat, while the same amount of tuna canned in oil contains 168 calories and nearly 7 grams of fat.

Coffee

THIS BREW'S GOOD FOR YOU

HEALING POWER

Can Help:

Reduce the risk of cancer

Increase mood and alertness

Pop quiz: What's the number one source of antioxidants in Americans' diets? Blueberries? Strawberries? Oranges? No, no, and no. It's coffee.

Researchers at the University of Scranton in Pennsylvania found that no other food or beverage comes close to providing as many antioxidants in our diets as coffee. Truth be told, of all the fruits and beverages studied, dates have more antioxidants per serving than coffee, but because people drink a whole lot more coffee than they eat dates, coffee wins out as the number one source of antioxidants.

And perhaps that's not a bad thing at all.

"A lot of new research suggests that coffee—in moderation—is fine," says Molly Kimball, RD, a sports and lifestyle nutritionist at the Ochner Health System's Elmwood Fitness Center in New Orleans. "One or two cups a day can be helpful, but more than that is counterproductive. Coffee has been linked to a decrease in the risk of Parkinson's disease, for example. It also reduces the risk of gallstones, so it may be helpful if you have a family history of them or are prone to them. And the polyphenols—a type of antioxidant—in coffee are the same as those in fruit and wine."

Brew Up Some Antioxidants

Antioxidants are substances that help ward off disease by mopping up harmful oxygen molecules called free radicals, which naturally accumulate in the body. Free radicals damage healthy tissues throughout the body, causing changes that can lead to heart disease, cancer, and other serious conditions. The antioxidants in coffee may protect against colon cancer, diabetes, and Parkinson's disease, studies show. Both regular and decaf coffee offer the same amount of antioxidants.

One study, for example, found that coffee (decaf in particular in this study) offers protection against lung cancer. Researchers at Roswell Park Cancer Institute in Buffalo, New York, studied 993 former smokers. They found that the people who drank at least 2 cups of decaf each day were 36 percent less likely to develop lung cancer than those who drank caffeinated black tea or coffee.

Another study, in Japan, found that people who drank coffee on a daily or almost daily basis had about half the risk of developing a type of liver cancer compared with people who never drank coffee. Most interesting, the risk of cancer decreased with an increase in the amount of coffee consumed each day.

More Cancer Protection

The antioxidants in coffee offer protection against cancer. But there might be another reason why researchers found that drinking two or more cups of coffee (decaf in this study) may lower the incidence of rectal cancer by a whopping 52 percent. Researchers think that by increasing bowel movements, coffee speeds things through the body, decreasing the risk. (They have no idea why decaf offered more protection than regular coffee, however.)

Get a Java Jolt

It's not likely to come as a surprise to anyone that coffee makes you more alert. But researchers couldn't say for sure if it was the coffee that truly had the effect, or if it was merely a reversal of the negative effects of caffeine withdrawal.

A British study found that it's more likely a positive effect of the coffee. Researchers in Wales gave 60 people, all regular caffeine consumers, a long battery of tests in one evening to tucker them out. They were told to drink their regular amounts of beverages with caffeine. Another evening, they were given two beverages without caffeine and given the tests again. A third evening, they were given two beverages with caffeine and given the tests a third time. The researchers found that after drinking the caffeinated beverages, the people had better moods and did better on the tests as well. So, the researchers concluded, a daily cup or two of coffee boosts mood and alertness. (But of course it does! Any Starbucks devotee could have told them that.)

Know When to Say When

But before you chug that 32-ouncer, know that you can have too much of a good thing. Too much regular coffee can give you that feeling that you've had so much caffeine your molecules are vibrating. But also a study found that people who drank two or more

---

Doctor's Top Tip

"The best way to enjoy your coffee is caffeinated with milk, for extra calcium," says Jennifer Ramos Galluzzi, PhD, of Housatonic Community College in Bridgeport, Connecticut.

Why caffeinated? Most of the studies that found benefits to drinking coffee were done on caffeinated coffee, so it's likely that some of those benefits may have come from the caffeine. "Limit your caffeinated coffee drinking to one or two cups a day, though," Dr. Galluzzi adds.

cups of java a day had higher levels of inflammatory markers linked to heart disease.

"Caffeinated coffee can, of course, interfere with sleep," says Kimball. "And you should talk with your doctor before drinking coffee if you have blood pressure issues, because coffee can increase heart rate."

GETTING THE MOST

Don't be cool. For some reason, conventional wisdom says to store coffee beans in the refrigerator or freezer. Ignore it! Coffee stored in the fridge or deep freeze is exposed to fluctuating temperatures, and therefore condensation. Each time the coffee is exposed to water, it's brewed a tiny bit, which waters down the flavor. Instead, keep coffee in an airtight canister in a cabinet.

Filter it out. "Studies have shown that boiled, unfiltered coffee consumption is related to elevated cholesterol levels because of the cafestol, a compound in the coffee," says Jennifer Ramos Galluzzi, PhD, assistant professor in the science department at Housatonic Community College in Bridgeport, Connecticut.

Detox, fast. If you've had too much coffee, you'll know it by a flush on your face or a twitch in your muscles. (Or by noticing the empty Styrofoam cups littering your desk.) Headaches usually start after drinking 200 to 500 milligrams of caffeine, the amount in 2 to 5 cups of coffee. To flush the caffeine out of your system, drink plenty of water.

Colds and Flu

FOODS THAT FIGHT INFECTION

Since the beginning of time, people have been catching colds, and trying—without success—to come up with a cure for them.

The common cold is one of the most prevalent causes of illness in the world, says Rallie McAllister, MD, MPH, a board-certified family physician at Nathaniel Mission Clinic in Lexington, Kentucky, and author of *Healthy Lunchbox: The Working Mom's Guide to Keeping You and Your Kids Trim*. If you're like most adults, you'll succumb to an average of two to four colds each year. With each infection, you can expect to spend somewhere in the neighborhood of 8 to 10 days coughing, sniffling, sneezing, and feeling miserable in general.

The common cold is caused when one of more than 200 cold-causing viruses invades the cells of your nose and throat. These viruses are tiny, but they're practically indestructible. Antibiotic drugs that stop bacteria in their tracks can't even put a dent in viruses. Medicines strong enough to kill most cold-causing microbes would probably kill you in the process, says Dr. McAllister.

The flu, which is also caused by a virus, affects 5 to 20 percent of the people in the United States each year. About 36,000 people die from flu each year.

Fortunately, there is a flu shot. The Centers for Disease Control and Prevention (CDC) in Atlanta recommends that anyone who doesn't want to get the flu should get a flu shot. Studies show that the vaccine is effective in 70 to 90 percent of healthy people under age 65, as long as the match between the vaccine and circulating virus is close.

According to the CDC, among people over age 65 living outside of nursing homes, the flu shot is 30 to 70 percent effective in preventing hospitalization for the flu, and also for pneumonia. Among people over age 65 living in nursing homes, the flu shot is 50 to 60 percent effective in preventing hospitalization for the flu or pneumonia and 80 percent effective in preventing death from the flu.

The only way to avoid colds and flu entirely would be to become a hermit, living far from the sneezes of co-workers, the runny noses of children, and the coughs of strangers on city streets.

Since secluding yourself on a desert island won't pay the bills, however, one of the best strategies is to eat all the immunity-boosting foods you can find. As it turns out, there are plenty to choose from. Research has found that some of the foods we eat every day contain powerful compounds that can help stop viruses from taking hold. Even when you're already sick, choosing the right foods will ease the discomfort and possibly help you get better more quickly.

Eat for Immunity

Colds and flu get their starts when just a few viruses slip into your system. Once they're inside, they immediately set to work making more viruses. If your immune system doesn't stop them early on, they multiply to enormous numbers, and that's when you start feeling sick.

Doctor's Top Tip

While physicians have been at a loss to offer an effective treatment for cold and flu sufferers, mothers haven't. As long as people have been catching colds and the flu, mothers have been recommending rest, fluids, and chicken soup. And it turns out, Mom has been right all along, says Rallie McAllister, MD, MPH, a family physician in Lexington, Kentucky.

One way to stop this microbial invasion is by eating a food that might surprise you—yogurt. Researchers in Sweden gave 262 people either a supplement containing a healthy bacteria that's added to some yogurts, called *Lactobacillus reuteri*, or a placebo (dummy pill). After taking either the supplement or the placebo once a day for 80 days, the researchers found that the people who took the supplement were 2½ times less likely to have caught a cold than the placebo-popping people.

The researchers think that the bacteria in yogurt stop viruses from binding to tissue. The catch is, not just any brand will do. In the United States, the only yogurt brand currently with *Lactobacillus reuteri* is Stonyfield Farm.

The other, less surprising, way to stop the microbial invasion is to eat more fruits and vegetables. These foods contain a variety of substances that strengthen the immune system, making it better able to destroy viruses before they make you sick. Research has shown, for example, that many fruits and vegetables contain a compound called glutathione, which stimulates the immune system to release large numbers of macrophages, specialized cells that seize viruses and mark them for destruction. Avocados, watermelons, asparagus, winter squash, and grapefruit are all rich in glutathione. Okra, oranges, tomatoes, potatoes, cauliflower, broccoli, cantaloupe, strawberries, and peaches are also good sources.

Another powerful compound in many fruits and vegetables is vitamin C. Doctors have been debating for years whether vitamin C can help prevent colds—and they're still debating. When you're already sick, however, getting extra vitamin C in your diet has been proven to relieve cold symptoms and help you get better more quickly.

Vitamin C lowers levels of histamine, a defensive chemical released by the immune system that is responsible for causing stuffiness and other cold and flu symptoms. At the same time, vitamin C appears to strengthen white blood cells, which are essential for fighting infection.

After reviewing 21 scientific studies published since 1971, researchers at the University of Helsinki in Finland concluded that getting 1,000 milligrams of vitamin C a day can reduce cold symptoms and shorten the duration of the illness by 23 percent.

Of course, you'd have to eat a lot of oranges, broccoli, and other foods rich in vitamin C to get that much of this important nutrient. So drink your C instead. Orange juice, which has 61 milligrams of vitamin C in a 6-ounce serving, is probably your best choice, although cranberry and grapefruit juices also contain a lot of vitamin C.

Raise a Glass

To mount an even stronger defense against the flu, consider filling your glass with red wine instead of juice. One study conducted in Rome found that resveratrol, the polyphenol found in red wine, actually stopped influenza cells from replicating. Wondering which wine is best? Pick up a Pinot Noir from California. When researchers at the University of Mississippi tested 11 red wines, they found that Pinot Noirs from California have the most resveratrol. It's important to keep in mind, however, that alcohol can come with some unwanted effects. For example, drinking heavily can raise blood pressure and have other damaging effects on your health. So, if you do drink, do so in moderation.

Bulbs of Health

Garlic has been used throughout history for treating virtually every type of infection. Now there's increasing evidence that it can help protect against colds and flu as well.

Garlic contains dozens of chemically active compounds. Two of them, allicin and alliin, have been shown to kill germs directly. Plus, garlic appears to stimulate the immune system to release natural killer cells, which destroy even more germs.

To get the benefits of garlic, however, you have to eat a lot of it—as much as an entire bulb a day to combat colds and flu, says Elson Haas, MD, director of the Preventive Medical Center of Marin in San Rafael, California, and author of *Staying Healthy with Nutrition.*

Unless you have developed a taste for it, you probably can't eat that much raw garlic. Microwaving or baking garlic until it's tender, however, will take away some of the burn and sweeten the taste, says Irwin Ziment, MD, professor emeritus at the

University of California, Los Angeles. "The softened garlic still seems to be quite potent," he adds.

Hot and Helpful

Research has shown that two traditional treatments for colds and flu—a cup of hot tea and a steaming bowl of chicken soup—are among the most-potent home remedies there are. Both of these, along with chile peppers and other spicy foods, contain compounds that can relieve congestion and keep the immune system strong.

Tea, for example, contains a compound called theophylline, which helps break up congestion. Tea also contains quercetin, a compound that may help prevent viruses from multiplying.

Instead of black tea, though, you might want to sip chamomile. Researchers in London (where else?!) found that people who drank 5 cups of chamomile tea a day for 2 weeks had increased blood levels of polyphenols. These plant-based chemicals have been associated with antibacterial activity.

Chicken soup is another folk remedy that has been proven to be effective. In fact, having a bowl of chicken soup is one of the best ways to relieve stuffiness and other cold and flu symptoms. In laboratory studies, for example, researchers at the University of Nebraska Medical Center in Omaha found that chicken soup was able to prevent white blood cells from causing inflammation and congestion in the airways.

When a cold has your nose so stuffy that you feel like you're breathing through a thick blanket, you may want to take a bite of hot pepper. Jalapeños, ground red pepper (cayenne), and their fiery kin contain a compound called capsaicin. This compound, which is similar to a drug in cold and flu medications, will help you breathe easy again, says Dr. Ziment.

In addition, several studies have shown that capsaicin can help stop sickness before it starts. In one study, researchers in Korea found that mice given capsaicin had nearly three times more antibody-producing cells after 3 weeks than mice that weren't given any capsaicin.

You can get plenty of capsaicin from fresh hot peppers, of course, but the peppers don't need to be fresh for you to get the benefits, adds Dr. Haas. Mixing ¼ teaspoon of ground red pepper in a glass of water and drinking it can be very effective. "It's heating, but not irritating," he says.

Constipation
THE FIBER EXPRESS

There's not much that people don't talk about these days. Spend a few minutes around the water cooler, and you'll hear about sex, divorce, and the details of a colleague's prostate surgery.

The one thing people don't talk about, even with their doctors, is constipation. If they did, constipation probably would no longer be the most common digestive complaint—affecting more than 4 million Americans chronically—because they'd find out that it's easy to treat. For most people, simply getting more fiber and fluids in their diet can put an end to constipation for good.

Just Passing Through

Unlike vitamins and minerals, fiber isn't absorbed by the digestive tract. Instead, it spends a long time in the intestine, absorbing large amounts of fluid. And that's precisely its constipation-fighting secret.

When fiber absorbs water, stools gradually swell, getting bigger and wetter. Unlike small stools, which can accumulate for days before moving on, large stools are moved out of the intestine much more quickly, says Marie Borum, MD, MPH, professor of medicine at George Washington University Medical Center in Washington, D.C. And because large stools are much softer than small ones, there's less straining when they do move, she adds.

All fruits, vegetables, legumes, and whole-grain foods contain healthful amounts of fiber. Doctors once believed that insoluble fiber, the kind found mainly in whole wheat, was the only choice for beating constipation. As it turns out, however, both insoluble and soluble fiber (the kind found primarily in legumes, oats, and many fruits) can help keep the intestine working smoothly. "Both types of fiber add bulk, soften the stool, and speed transit time," says Dr. Borum. The reason that constipation is so common is that most Americans simply don't get enough fiber. On average, we only get about 11 grams a day, a lot less than the Daily Value (DV) of 25 grams, says Pat Harper, RD, a dietitian based in Pittsburgh. Since virtually all plant foods contain healthy quantities of fiber, you don't have to work very hard to get the necessary amounts. A 1-cup serving of Wheaties has 3 grams of fiber, or 12 percent of the DV, and Kellogg's Raisin Bran has 8 grams in the same size serving, or 32 percent

GOOD MORNING, JOE

Coffee drinkers have always known that a morning cup of their favorite jolt does more than pop their eyes open. It appears to wake up the digestive tract as well.

It's not your imagination. The caffeine in coffee stimulates the large intestine, causing it to contract, says Pat Harper, RD, a dietitian based in Pittsburgh. "A cup or two of coffee in the morning can help you stay regular," she says. In fact, some doctors recommend that anyone who is constipated try drinking a cup of coffee rather than taking an over-the-counter laxative. And that recommendation is supported by research. Scientists in Japan found that the women who drank the most coffee were less likely to be constipated than the women who drank the least.

The problem with coffee, of course, is that when you drink a lot of it each day, it removes more fluids from your body than it puts in. It's fine to use coffee as a morning wake-up call, Harper says. It's a good idea, however, to limit yourself to fewer than five cups a day.

of the DV. A half-cup of cooked kidney beans has 3 grams of fiber, or 12 percent of the DV, and an apple also has about 3 grams.

There is one problem with adding more fiber to your diet. When your body isn't used to it, it can cause cramping and gas, Dr. Borum warns. To get the benefits without the grief, she recommends that you gradually add fiber to your diet over a period of several months. "A lifetime of not getting enough fiber can't be fixed in a week," she says. But if you gradually increase the amount of fiber you get each day, you probably won't have any discomfort at all, she adds.

Want to add fiber to relieve constipation without the adverse effects? A combination of rye bread, which is high in fiber, and yogurt containing the bacteria *Lactobacillus GG* might just be the ticket. (One slice of rye bread has 2 grams of fiber, or 8 percent of the DV for this nutrient.) One study, conducted by researchers in Finland, recruited 59 otherwise healthy women with constipation. The researchers divided the women into four groups: Some women ate both rye bread and yogurt, other women ate only rye bread, still other women ate only yogurt, and the rest ate neither. During the 3-week study, the researchers found that the combination of rye bread and yogurt alleviated the constipation the most comfortably. They think that the rye bread treated the constipation, and the yogurt relieved the adverse gastrointestinal effects of the extra fiber. While the study used yogurt containing *Lactobacillus GG*, this type of yogurt is not presently sold in the United States. You can, however, buy *Lactobacillus GG* in supplement form in this country.

Water Works

We often think of water as being sort of an add-on to a healthful diet, not an essential ingredient in its own right. But not getting enough water is a very common cause of constipation, Dr. Borum says. After all, stools can absorb large amounts of water. When they don't get enough, they get hard, sluggish, and more difficult to pass. This is particularly true when you're eating more fiber, which must be accompanied by fluids in order to keep things moving smoothly.

You can't depend on thirst to tell you when it's time to drink, Dr. Borum adds. The thirst mechanism isn't all that sensitive to begin with, and often it stays silent even when your body needs more fluids. What's more, the urge to drink naturally gets weaker with age, which is one reason that constipation is more common in older folks.

To avoid walking on the dry side, Dr. Borum recommends drinking at least six to eight full glasses of water a day. Or, if you don't want to drink that much water, make up the difference by having soups or juices.

Beverages containing alcohol or caffeine, however, really shouldn't count toward your daily fluid total because they're diuretics, meaning that they actually remove more fluids from your body than they put in, says Dr. Borum.

Several studies have proven the link between not drinking enough water and constipation. Scientists in Germany gave eight men 2,500 milliliters (85 ounces) of water each day for 1 week and then 500 milliliters of water (16 ounces) each day for another week. The researchers found that even this relative short period of fluid deprivation decreased stool frequency and weight.

So, fiber is good, and water is good, but both is better! Researchers in Italy divided 117 people with chronic constipation into two groups. For 2 months, both groups ate a standard diet with about 25 grams of fiber a day. The first group was allowed to drink as much water as they wanted (which turned out to be not too much), but the second group drank 2 liters (about 2 quarts) of mineral water each day. The researchers found that the 25 grams of fiber each day relieved the people's constipation, but their constipation was relieved even more when they drank 1.5 to 2 liters of water a day.

Pruning the Problem

Prunes are probably the oldest home remedy for constipation—and, researchers have discovered, one of the most effective.

Prunes contain three ingredients that help keep digestion on track. For starters, they're very high in fiber, with 3 grams of the rough stuff, or about 12 percent of the DV, in just three prunes. They also contain a compound called dihydroxyphenyl isatin, which stimulates the intestinal contractions that are necessary for regular bowel movements. Finally, prunes contain a natural sugar called sorbitol, which soaks up enormous amounts of water in the digestive tract and helps keep the system active.

If you don't happen to care for prunes, you can get some of the same benefits by eating raisins. In one study, for example, people were given 4½ ounces of raisins a day. At the end of the study, the average time it took for stools to move through the digestive tract was cut in half, from two days to one.

Like prunes, raisins are very high in fiber, with a snack-size box providing about 2 grams, or 8 percent of the DV. In addition, they contain a compound called tartaric acid, which acts as a natural laxative, Dr. Borum explains.

Doctor's Top Tip

"Take 2 tablespoons of black-strap molasses before bed," says Allan Magaziner, DO, director of the Magaziner Center for Wellness and Anti-Aging Medicine in Cherry Hill, New Jersey. "Or eat 1 tablespoon of ground flaxseed each day. Sprinkle it on cereal or into yogurt, stir it into water, or mix it into a salad."

Hold the Cheese

For people prone to constipation, limiting foods that have little or no fiber, such as cheese, ice cream, meat, and processed foods, is also important, according to researchers at the National Digestive Diseases Information Clearinghouse.

As a double whammy, cheese and other dairy products contain an insoluble protein called casein, which slows digestion and worsens constipation.

Corn

KERNELS AGAINST CHOLESTEROL

HEALING POWER

Can Help:

Reduce cancer risk

Lower cholesterol

Boost energy levels

In Mitchell, South Dakota, right in the middle of the corn belt, residents pay homage to the harvest. Their shrine is the Corn Palace, a mansion built in 1892 that's decorated—murals, minarets, towers, and all—with 3,000 bushels of corn.

It isn't necessary to take corn that seriously, but it does deserve a place of honor at your dinner table. Because corn is high in fiber, it can help lower cholesterol. And because it's very high in carbohydrates, it provides quick energy while delivering virtually no fat.

"Corn is really an excellent basic food source," says Mark McLellan, PhD, dean of research for the University of Florida's Institute of Food and Agricultural Sciences and director of the Florida Agricultural Experiment Station, both in Gainesville. "When combined with other vegetables in the diet, it is a good source of protein, carbohydrates, and vitamins."

'Ears to Preventing Cancer

Corn, which is native to America, has been a staple food here since primitive times, with meal made from corn dating back about 7,000 years. Today, the United States is still one of the largest commercial growers of corn. But this humble food's health benefits often get overlooked. It turns out that corn might be a powerful ally in the fight against cancer.

One study, conducted at the University of Southern California Keck School of Medicine in Los Angeles, found that an orange-red carotenoid found in corn, beta-cryptoxanthin, was protective against lung cancer. The scientist found that men who ate the most food containing beta-cryptoxanthin had a 15 to 40 percent reduction in lung cancer risk, compared with the men who ate the least.

Another study, this one conducted at the University of Maryland School of Medicine in Baltimore, found that a component of fiber that's found in abundance in corn, inositol hexaphosphate, prevents the growth of colon cancer cells in test tubes. Researchers say it stops the cancer cells from dividing.

FOOD ALERT

Corn Can Be a Problem

When you think of food allergies, the foods that probably come to mind are shellfish, peanuts, or other common offenders. But many people are sensitive to processed corn as well. In fact, cereals made from corn are among the top five allergy-causing foods.

What's more, corn cereals are known for triggering flare-ups in people with irritable bowel syndrome, a condition that causes abdominal pain and cramping. Several studies have found that corn may cause problems in over 20 percent of people with this problem.

Corn is included in many products, so if you're sensitive to it (or think you might be), be sure to read labels carefully before buying. For example, people who are allergic to corn might have to avoid foods containing corn syrup as well.

Kernels against Cholesterol

Corn contains a type of dietary fiber called soluble fiber. When you eat corn, this fiber binds with bile, a cholesterol-laden digestive fluid produced by the liver. Since soluble fiber isn't readily absorbed by the body, it passes out in the stool, taking the cholesterol with it.

You've heard a lot about how oat and wheat bran can lower cholesterol. Corn bran is in the same league. In a study at Illinois State University in Normal, researchers put 29 men with high cholesterol on a low-fat diet. After 2 weeks on the diet, some of the men were each given 20 grams (almost ½ tablespoon) of corn bran a day, while others received a similar amount of wheat bran. During the 6-week study, those on the corn bran plan had a drop in cholesterol of more than 5 percent and about a 13 percent drop in triglycerides, blood fats that in large amounts can contribute to heart disease. Those who were given wheat bran showed no change beyond the initial drop caused by being on a low-fat diet.

A Bushel of Nutrients

The beauty of corn is that it provides a lot of energy while delivering a small number of calories—about 83 per ear.

Corn is an excellent source of thiamin, a B vitamin that's essential for converting food to energy. An ear of corn provides 0.2 milligram of thiamin, 13 percent of the

Daily Value (DV) for this nutrient. That's more than you'll get in three slices of bacon or 3 ounces of roast beef.

And since fresh sweet corn consists primarily of simple and complex carbohydrates, it's a superb energy source, says Donald V. Schlimme, PhD, professor emeritus of nutrition and food science at the University of Maryland in College Park. "It fulfills our energy needs without providing us with a substantial amount of fat," he says. What little fats there are in corn are the polyunsaturated and monounsaturated kinds, which are far healthier than the saturated fats found in meats and high-fat dairy foods.

GETTING THE MOST

Make sure it's mature. When you buy fresh corn at the supermarket, look for ears that have full, plump kernels. "Purchase corn at the optimum stage of maturity," Dr. Schlimme advises. "Under those conditions, the level of nutrients is higher."

To see if corn is ripe, puncture one of the kernels with your fingernail. If the liquid that comes out isn't milky-colored, the corn is either immature or overripe, and you should pass it by.

Get the whole kernel. No matter how diligent you are when eating corn on the cob, you invariably leave a lot behind. To get the most out of each kernel, you're

In the Kitchen

Corn on the cob is so easy to prepare, it's essentially nature's fast food. Just strip off the husk and corn silk, drop the ears in a steamer, and wait until it's done a few minutes later. To maximize the taste, here are a few tips you may want to try.

Gotta wear shades. Heat rapidly converts the sugar in corn to starch, so buy corn that's refrigerated or at least been kept in the shade.

Cook it right away. When corn sits around, its natural sugar turns into starch, giving up the natural sweet taste. So it's best to cook corn soon after it is picked.

Hold the salt. When cooking corn in boiling water, don't add salt. This will draw moisture from the kernels, making them tough and hard to chew.

Strip the kernels. When you have a craving for fresh corn but don't want to wrestle with the cob, just strip the kernels off. Hold the cob upright in a bowl. Using a sharp knife, slice downward, cutting away a few rows at a time. When all the kernels are removed, scrape the dull side of the blade down the sides of the cob to extract the sweet, milky juice.

better off buying frozen or canned corn. Or you can cut the kernels from the cob with a knife. Unlike eating it right off the cob, "you get more of the corn's benefit by having a mechanical cut that takes the entire kernel off," Dr. McLellan says.

Buy it vacuum-packed. While canned corn can be almost as nutritious as fresh, it loses some of its value when it's packed in brine, a salty liquid that leaches nutrients from food during processing, says Dr. Schlimme. To get the most vitamins, look for vacuum-packed corn, which doesn't contain brine. Corn that's vacuum-packed (it will say so on the label) usually comes in short, squat cans, he says. Or choose frozen corn instead. Studies at the FDA showed that frozen corn is just as nutritious as fresh.

Doctor's Top Tip

"Try raw corn," says Allan Magaziner, DO, director of the Magaziner Center for Wellness and Anti-Aging Medicine in Cherry Hill, New Jersey. "It's tasty and very healthy. And there's almost no preparation needed—just husk and wash. If you boil corn, most of the nutrients end up in the cooking water. But if you must boil your corn, you can use that nutritious cooking water as the base for soup."

Spicy Black Bean and Corn Salad

1 can (15 ounces) black beans, rinsed and drained

2 cups frozen corn kernels, thawed and drained

4 jalapeño peppers, seeded and chopped

2 tomatoes, chopped

1 small red onion, chopped

2 cloves garlic, minced

2 tablespoons fresh lime juice

1 tablespoon extra-virgin olive oil

2 teaspoons chili powder

In a large bowl, combine the beans, corn, peppers, tomatoes, onion, and garlic.

In a cup, stir together the lime juice, oil, and chili powder, and pour over the salad; toss well.

Makes 4 servings

PER SERVING

Calories: 193
Total fat: 4.5 g
Saturated fat: 1 g

Cholesterol: 0 mg
Sodium: 283 mg
Dietary fiber: 8 g

Cranberries

A SAUCE FOR ALL SEASONS

HEALING POWER

Can Help:

Prevent and treat urinary tract infections

Protect cells from cancerous changes

Reduce the risk of heart disease and stroke

Pity the lowly cranberry. Like swallows returning to San Juan Capistrano, this Thanksgiving staple finds its way back into our diet every year—then gets lost after the holiday season is over.

And that's a pity. Cranberries contain a number of compounds that show early promise against cancer and heart disease. What's more, cranberry juice has finally earned the scientific stamp of approval for its traditional role in relieving urinary tract infections.

A Role against Cancer

Along with raspberries, strawberries, and blackberries, cranberries are a good source of ellagic acid, an antioxidant compound that has raised high hopes in cancer researchers.

Cousin to the blueberry, the cranberry is an incredible antioxidant star. Dried cranberries actually have the most antioxidants, then fresh, then bottled cranberry drinks, then cranberry cocktails. One cup of fresh cranberries has *four times* as many antioxidants as 1 cup of green tea!

Studies have found cranberries to be protective against breast, colon, prostate, head, and neck cancers. In laboratory tests, ellagic acid has been shown to help prevent mutations in DNA, the genetic stuff that instructs our cells how to function. In addition, ellagic acid has been shown to disarm cancer-causing agents and also to help prevent tumors from growing.

Indeed, one tantalizing aspect of this compound is its apparent ability to battle carcinogens on both ends—before and after they take hold. "Ellagic acid has what we call anti-initiating activity. It inhibits the genetic damage that starts the cancer process," says Gary Stoner, PhD, professor and cancer researcher at Ohio State University in Columbus. Even after a carcinogen has been introduced into cells, he says, ellagic acid helps prevent the cells from becoming cancerous.

Pure ellagic acid—the form in which it's used in laboratory studies—doesn't get into the bloodstream very well. However, Dr. Stoner's research suggests that this

FOOD ALERT

Cranberry Cautions

If you suffer from kidney or gallbladder problems, you should probably pick another fruit. Cranberries are one of the few foods that contain oxalates. When these naturally occurring substances become too concentrated in your body, they can crystallize and cause health problems. For example, researchers think they might play a role in some types of kidney stones.

Another possible side effect of cranberries it that they might strengthen the effects of the drug warfarin (Coumadin). In Great Britain, at least 12 instances of suspected interactions have been reported. The Cranberry Institute, an organization in the United States that researches the health effects of cranberries, investigated these concerns, however, and didn't find any interaction of cranberries with warfarin, or any other medication for that matter.

"Warfarin is a blood thinner, and cranberry juice can increase its blood-thinning effects," says Molly Kimball, RD, a sports and lifestyle nutritionist at the Ochner Health System's Elmwood Fitness Center in New Orleans. "People taking warfarin should talk with their pharmacists before drinking cranberry juice. It might be that you can still drink it; you might just need to keep your cranberry intake steady from day to day."

compound is better absorbed in its natural state in food—good news for those who enjoy their cranberries year-round. Here's just one example of cranberry's cancer-fighting ability. Researchers at Cornell University in Ithaca, New York, found that after 4 hours of exposure to cranberry extracts, breast cancer cells committed suicide 25 percent more than cells not exposed to the berries.

Power from Flavonoids

Another way in which cranberries will help keep you healthy is by putting more flavonoids into your diet. Flavonoids are plant pigments that put the reds and yellows into fruits and vegetables and that have powerful antioxidant abilities—that is, they help block damage from free radicals, harmful oxygen molecules that can lead to cancer, heart disease, and other serious conditions.

Cranberries contain several powerful flavonoids, including quercetin and myricetin. The darker cranberry varieties, like Stevens, Early Black, and Ben Lear, contain a third compound called kaempferol. Each of these compounds has been shown in scientific studies to help prevent the genetic changes that can sometimes lead to cancer.

Here's a bonus: Flavonoids, in general, and quercetin, in particular, are thought to play a role in preventing artery disease, perhaps because their antioxidant ability helps prevent damage to the linings of blood vessels.

Large studies in Finland, the Netherlands, and the United Kingdom have shown that people with very low intakes of flavonoids have high risks of coronary disease. In one study of middle-age men in the Dutch town of Zutphen, those who ate a lot of fruits and vegetables—and consequently had a high intake of flavonoids—had a 73 percent lower risk of stroke than men who consumed few fruits and vegetables.

Help for Urinary Complaints

In the United States, about half of women will develop at least one urinary tract infection before they reach the age of 30, says Rallie McAllister, MD, MPH, a board-certified family physician at Nathaniel Mission Clinic in Lexington, Kentucky, and author of *Healthy Lunchbox: The Working Mom's Guide to Keeping You and Your Kids Trim*. For ages now, grandmothers and mothers—and a few wise doctors— have recommended cranberry juice to clear up urinary tract infections. Scientists were a little later coming on board, but they now concur. A 1994 Harvard Medical School study of elderly women found that those who drank about 10 ounces of cranberry juice cocktail daily for 6 months had significantly lower amounts of bacteria in their urine and were almost 60 percent less likely to develop infections

In the Kitchen

Buying and preparing cranberries is the ultimate no-brainer. If it were any easier, they'd be called fast food.

Whole cranberries usually come in 1-pound bags. The berries are long keepers; they'll last a month or more when kept in the refrigerator and over a year when stored in the freezer. You don't even have to wash them because washing cranberries prior to storage will cause them to spoil.

When preparing fresh cranberry sauce, here's all you need to do:

- Put a pound of cranberries (4 cups) in a medium saucepan, and cover with 2 cups of boiling water. Return to a boil, cover the pan, and continue cooking for about 4 minutes, or until the skins burst.
- Stir in sugar to taste. Because the berries are so tart, you'll probably use about 2 cups of sugar.
- Return the pan to the heat, and bring to a boil. Immediately remove from the heat. Allow to cool before serving.

than women who drank a noncranberry impostor.

Among women who already had infections, those drinking cranberry juice were nearly 75 percent more likely to have their infections clear up.

One long-held belief was that if you could make urine more acidic, bacteria would have a tougher time growing. This was thought to be why cranberry juice helped prevent urinary tract infections.

Now scientists believe that cranberries contain compounds called proanthocyanidins that are responsible for helping prevent infections of the urinary tract, says Dr. McAllister. These compounds prevent certain types of bacteria from latching onto cells that line the bladder. If the bacteria bind to the cell walls, they can reproduce and multiply. But the proanthocyanidins keep the bacteria from attaching so they are flushed out of the body in urine.

Doctor's Top Tip

Drink 8 ounces of cranberry juice cocktail in the morning and in the evening for 24 hours of protection against urinary tract infections, says Rallie McAllister, MD, MPH, a family physician in Lexington, Kentucky.

In his book, *Doctor, What Should I Eat?*, Isadore Rosenfeld, MD, clinical professor of medicine at Weill Cornell Medical College in New York City, suggests that women who have urinary tract infections drink two glasses (8 ounces each) of cranberry juice a day in addition to taking any antibiotics prescribed by their doctors.

In addition to preventing and treating urinary tract infections, it turns out that cranberries may also help prevent the more serious infections of the bladder. In a very small study conducted at the University of Washington in Seattle, researchers gave three women cranberry juice cocktail. (Yes, just three of them. We said it was a small study!) The scientists collected urine samples before the women drank the juice and 4 to 6 hours afterward. Then the scientists combined the samples with human bladder cells and incubated them with *E. coli*, the pesky bacteria that is the most common cause of bladder infections. The scientists found that the number of bacteria able to adhere to the bladder cells (which is the first thing the bacteria have to do to cause an infection) was significantly reduced in the urine of the women after they drank the cranberry juice cocktail. The most protective dose was 8 ounces.

GETTING THE MOST

Choose your colors. Cranberries with a deep, red color have more highly concentrated anthocyanins, a flavonoid abundant in this fruit.

Eat them with relish. Since uncooked cranberries contain considerably more healing compounds than cooked, you may want to try a cranberry relish. (See the recipe on page 202.)

Have a drink. Because uncooked cranberries have a tart taste and tough texture, you're unlikely to eat them this way. But you can still get the nutritional payload by drinking the juice.

Keep in mind that while commercial cranberry juice cocktail drinks are loaded with vitamin C (with one glass containing a full day's supply), unfortunately most also have a full day's supply of sugar and are never more than 30 percent juice.

An alternative to supermarket juice is the juice found in health food stores. You can buy either pure cranberry juice or concentrated cranberry extract, which is used to make cold drinks or hot teas.

Grab a handful. Recently, researchers at Brigham and Women's Hospital found that dried, sweetened cranberries, sold under the brand name Craisins, may offer the same protection as cranberry juice cocktail, says Dr. McAllister. The recommended serving size is ⅓ cup.

Cranberry Relish

1 **bag (12 ounces) cranberries**

1 **medium apple**

1 **thin-skinned orange**

½ **cup sugar**

⅛ **teaspoon ground ginger**

Place the cranberries in a colander. Rinse well with cold water. Discard any soft cranberries. Place the cranberries in a food processor.

Core the apple and cut into chunks. Add to the food processor. Cut the orange, including the peel, into chunks. Add to the food processor. Process, scraping down the bowl once or twice, until finely chopped.

Transfer to a medium bowl. Add the sugar and ginger and stir well. Let stand for at least 15 minutes. Stir again before serving.

Makes 2½ cups

Cook's Notes: *For a sweeter relish, peel the orange. The relish can be refrigerated in a covered container for up to 2 days.*

PER ¼ CUP

Calories: 70
Total fat: 0.1 g
Saturated fat: 0 g

Cholesterol: 0 mg
Sodium: 0 mg
Dietary fiber: 1.7 g

Currants

A GREAT SOURCE OF C

The British adore currant jams and jellies. The French favor black currant liqueur. And until the turn of the previous century, Americans delighted in fresh currants as well as currant jellies and sauces.

Today, unless you're lucky enough to have a currant shrub in your backyard, fresh currants are as scarce in the United States as icicles in July. (Don't be fooled by the black "currants" sold in supermarkets—they're really zante grapes.)

What ended our craving for currants? In the early 1900s, the USDA banned the cultivation of currants because the shrubs harbored a fungus that was destroying white pines. Even though the ban was lifted in the 1960s, currants never really made a comeback.

This is unfortunate because currants, the forgotten fruit, are a superb source of vitamin C and fiber. What's more, they contain a compound with powerful cancer-fighting potential.

HEALING POWER

Can Help:

Counter Alzheimer's disease

Protect against cancer

Reduce cholesterol

Lower the risk for heart disease

Prevent constipation

Fight Alzheimer's Disease

It's ironic that the forgotten fruit might prove to be helpful in keeping your memory sharp. Researchers in New Zealand found that substances in currants could help prevent Alzheimer's disease. Two compounds in the berries, anthocyanins (which give them their deep red color) and polyphenolics (which are also abundant in red wine and chocolate), were found to protect rats' brain cells against the kind of damage that occurs in people's brains afflicted by Alzheimer's disease.

Both anthocyanins and polyphenolics are powerful antioxidants that protect against free radicals. These highly reactive oxygen molecules can damage the brain and other tissues if left to run amok. Much more research is needed to see if these results would actually translate to people, too.

Currant Cancer Protection

Even though currants are extraordinarily high in vitamins—a half-cup of black currants, for example, has 101 milligrams of vitamin C, which is 168 percent of the

Daily Value (DV) and three times that of oranges—but that's not what gets researchers excited. The big news is that the berries contain a compound called ellagic acid, which shows promise for stopping cancer before it starts.

Ellagic acid is a member of a disease-fighting family of compounds known as polyphenols. (Cranberries, raspberries, strawberries, and grapes also contain polyphenols.) In laboratory studies, ellagic acid has been shown to be a powerful antioxidant, meaning that it helps neutralize free radicals, harmful oxygen molecules that are missing electrons, says Gary Stoner, PhD, professor and cancer researcher at Ohio State University in Columbus. Free radicals try to replace their missing electrons by taking electrons from healthy cells, causing cellular changes that can lead to cancer.

It may come as a surprise, but researchers found that currants are a much higher source of antioxidants than blueberries, long regarded as the antioxidant champ.

Ellagic acid has also been shown to block the effects of cancer-causing chemicals in the body at the same time that it stimulates the activity of enzymes that fight cancer growth. This two-pronged approach makes this compound a powerful ally for blocking cancer.

Another antioxidant that's been found in currants is quercetin. Generally, the most common sources of quercetin are onions, tea, apples, and red wine. That's for most of us anyway. People who live in Finland, however, commonly eat certain types of berries that contain quercetin—currants, lingonberries, and bilberries. Researchers in Finland theorized that these berries might be an important source of quercetin in that country. The scientists divided 40 healthy men into two groups. Half of the men ate their usual diets, but the other half ate 100 grams of black currants, lingonberries, and bilberries every day. After 8 weeks, the researchers found that the men who ate the berries had blood levels of quercetin 32 to 51 percent

In the Kitchen

Currants are mouth-puckeringly tart, which is why they're rarely eaten out of hand. Here are several sweeter uses for these berries:

■ Like cranberries, currants make a perfect sauce for livening up meat dishes. They're slightly sweeter than cranberries, however, so you'll want to add less sugar when making the sauce. You can also add currants to meat loaves and stuffings.

■ Putting currants in fruit salads will add a tangy taste. For an even prettier plate, add a combination of red, white, and black currants.

■ To make a tangy dessert, put currants in a bowl, and top them with sugar and just a bit of light cream.

higher than the men who ate their regular old diets. So, the researchers concluded, these berries are a good source of quercetin.

Like ellagic acid, quercetin has long been considered important in possibly helping to prevent cancer. In test tube studies, it inhibits the growth of cancer cells, including those from breast, colon, prostate, and lung tumors.

Doctor's Top Tip

Eat four to six servings of fruits (including currants) and vegetables a day to substantially lower your risk of developing cancer, says Gary Stoner, PhD, of Ohio State University.

Digestion and Heart Helpers

Like most berries, currants are high in fiber; the black, red, and white types all provide about 2 grams, or 8 percent of the DV. Fiber does more than control digestive problems like constipation and hemorrhoids, however. It also helps head off more serious health problems like high cholesterol and heart disease.

In fact, a study of 21,930 Finnish men found that those who got just 10 extra grams of fiber a day were able to reduce their risk of dying from heart disease by 17 percent. Eating one or two servings of currants a day, along with extra fruits and vegetables, will provide all the fiber you need to help keep your circulation in the swim.

GETTING THE MOST

Check the roadsides. The one problem with fresh currants is that they're so hard to find. Since most supermarkets don't stock them, your best bet is to check out roadside stands or farmers' markets since growers will sometimes sell small amounts of these homegrown favorites.

Store them carefully. When you're lucky enough to get your hands on fresh currants, you'll want to make them last. The berries will stay fresh for 2 to 3 days when stored in an airtight container in the refrigerator. Or you can freeze them for use throughout the year.

Apple-Currant Chutney

2 cups chopped tart apples

2 cups fresh red currants

2 cups chopped green tomatoes

1 cup chopped onions

½ cup honey

½ cup cider vinegar

½ cup water

2 teaspoons minced garlic

2 teaspoons brown or yellow mustard seeds

1 serrano pepper, chopped (wear plastic gloves when handling)

1 teaspoon grated fresh ginger

1 lime

In a large saucepan, combine the apples, currants, tomatoes, onions, honey, vinegar, water, garlic, mustard seeds, pepper, and ginger. Bring to a boil over medium-high heat.

Slice the lime into 4 lengthwise wedges. Cut each wedge into thin crosswise slices. Add to the saucepan. Reduce the heat to medium-low. Simmer the mixture until the apples are tender and the mixture thickens slightly, about 15 to 20 minutes.

Cool, then refrigerate in a covered container for several days to allow the flavors to develop.

Makes 4 cups

Cook's Notes: *The chutney can be refrigerated for several weeks or frozen for several months in a covered container. Serve with grilled or broiled turkey breast, chicken drumsticks, or pork tenderloin.*

PER ¼ CUP

Calories: 63

Total fat: 0.3 g

Saturated fat: 0 g

Cholesterol: 0 mg

Sodium: 4 mg

Dietary fiber: 1.6 g

Deficiency Diseases
FOOD OR CONSEQUENCES

S pirit, tell me if Tiny Tim will live," pleads a woeful Ebenezer Scrooge as he gazes at visions of Christmases to come. "I see a vacant seat," replies the Ghost, "in the poor chimney-corner, and a crutch without an owner, carefully preserved. If these shadows remain unaltered by the Future, the child will die."

As we know, the beloved Tiny Tim in Dickens's *A Christmas Carol* doesn't die but lives to romp through the streets of London. But sadly, many real-life children in the 19th century weren't so fortunate, especially those who, like Tiny Tim, may have had rickets, a bone-softening disease that occurs when the body doesn't get enough vitamin D. It was one of the most common crippling diseases of the time.

Perhaps the saddest thing about rickets and other deficiency diseases is that they're entirely preventable. These diseases occur when people don't get even the bare-bones minimum of nutrients that the body needs to thrive.

Severe deficiency diseases are rare in this country, partly because of advances in food technology and distribution that have made it possible for most foods to be available all year long. In addition, manufacturers fortify many foods with vitamins and minerals.

"In today's world, we don't see a lot of full-blown deficiency diseases," says Allan Magaziner, DO, director of the Magaziner Center for Wellness and Anti-Aging Medicine in Cherry Hill, New Jersey. "However, we do see subclinical, or low-level, deficiency diseases. Also, you can have what's called localized tissue deficiencies. That means, you might have enough of a nutrient in your blood, but you might not have enough in specific tissues, such as your lungs or cervix. This puts you at risk for diseases, such as lung cancer and cervical cancer, respectively. And you'd never even know it."

But even though serious deficiency diseases are rare in this country, they still occur, and in fact, they may be becoming increasingly common. People who are ill with digestive disorders or other conditions may not get all the nutrients they need. People who abuse alcohol are particularly prone to deficiency diseases, as are those who live in poverty. In many parts of the developing world, in fact, deficiency diseases regularly occur.

Rickets: Northern Exposure

It's not surprising that Tiny Tim, who lived in London at a time when air pollution got so thick that the sun was barely visible, may have suffered from rickets. The only practical way to get enough vitamin D, with the exception of drinking fortified milk, is by spending time in the sun. In fact, doctors sometimes call vitamin D the sunshine vitamin.

Whenever sunshine touches the skin, the body uses the ultraviolet rays to manufacture vitamin D, which is essential for transporting calcium and phosphorus into the bones. If you don't get enough vitamin D, your bones get soft and weak, sometimes bowing under the body's own weight.

Ever since food manufacturers began fortifying milk with vitamin D, rickets has become much less common. But it's hardly gone, and in fact, it's coming back. Not so long ago, seven children in Minneapolis were discovered to have rickets. Public health officials are becoming increasingly concerned about reports of infants diagnosed with rickets. In 2003, the American Academy of Pediatrics began recommending that all infants 2 months and older, children, and adolescents receive vitamin D supplementation to prevent rickets.

Alarmingly, vitamin D deficiency is now recognized as an epidemic in the United States. In children, in addition to causing rickets, vitamin D deficiency can cause growth retardation. In adults, not getting enough vitamin D causes a painful bone disease called osteomalacia. Vitamin D deficiency also causes muscle weakness, which increases the risk of falling and bone fractures. Scientists think that vitamin D deficiency could play a role in such diverse diseases as type 1 diabetes, multiple sclerosis, rheumatoid arthritis, high blood pressure, heart disease, and many common cancers.

You don't have to bake in the sun to get enough vitamin D. For most people, about 15 minutes of sunshine on the face and hands will provide the Daily Value (DV) of 400 IU of vitamin D. Don't try to do your sunning indoors, though, since window glass absorbs the necessary rays.

Even if you get plenty of sunshine, it's a still a good idea to get a little extra vitamin D in your diet. Having one glass of fortified milk will provide about 100 IU, or 25 percent of the DV.

Beriberi: A Lack of Energy

The word *beriberi*, which originated in the tiny country of Sri Lanka and means "I can't, I can't," became the name of an illness supposedly because a man with the disease was so weak that he couldn't rise to meet the physician who had come to help him.

Beriberi is caused by a deficiency of thiamin, a B vitamin that is essential for helping the body utilize energy. People who don't get enough thiamin become extremely weak and may experience symptoms such as swelling in the legs or a buildup of fluids in the heart.

Although rice and whole grains naturally contain a lot of thiamin, much of this nutrient is lost during processing. Since manufacturers put most of the thiamin back into foods after processing, however, beriberi has become very rare, at least in this country. (People who abuse alcohol, though, may still suffer from severe thiamin deficiencies.) Rice, flours, cereals, and breads are all fortified with thiamin. In addition, pork is naturally high in thiamin, with 3 ounces of pork tenderloin providing 0.8 milligram, or 53 percent of the DV for this nutrient.

Although beriberi is very rare in the United States, bariatric surgery is causing a resurgence of it, and other nutritional deficiencies as well, says Paul Ernsberger, PhD, associate professor of medicine, pharmacology, and neuroscience at Case Western Reserve School of Medicine in Cleveland. The beriberi often shows up about a year after the surgery, once the patient's liver thiamin reserves have been used up. To compound the problem, it doesn't help to treat bariatric surgery patients who develop beriberi with vitamins because the surgery often causes the patients to pass the pills in their stools, completely intact. These patients, says Dr. Ernsberger, "have very nutritious stools."

Pellagra: A Frightening Mystery

In 1914, the year World War I began, there was another threat facing Americans. For a brief time, a terrifying epidemic swept through the South, causing diarrhea, skin inflammation, and in many cases, death. More than 100,000 people were struck down, and worst of all, nobody knew what the cause was.

It wasn't until 1937 that scientists understood that pellagra, as the disease was called—the word means "rough skin"—occurred when people didn't get enough of the B vitamin niacin in their diets. The rural South was particularly hard-hit because people there relied on corn as their main grain, and corn contains a form of niacin that isn't available to the body.

Today, we've all but kissed pellagra goodbye in the United States, thanks to the fortification of flours and cereals, which makes it very easy to get the DV of 20 milligrams of niacin. Meats also contain niacin. A serving of skinless roast chicken breast, for example, contains 12 milligrams of niacin, or 60 percent of the DV. However, pellagra is still common in parts of the world where people have a lot of corn in their diets. And it can develop after gastrointestinal disease or even from alcoholism. It can also be a complication of the eating disorder anorexia.

Doctor's Top Tip

"To prevent deficiency diseases, color your plate," says Allan Magaziner, DO, director of the Magaziner Center for Wellness and Anti-Aging Medicine in Cherry Hill, New Jersey. "Eat plenty of fruits and vegetables of different colors, such as red tomatoes and strawberries, orange oranges and cantaloupe, yellow lemons and onions, green spinach and Brussels sprouts, blue berries, and purple grapes. Up to 80 percent of Americans' meals are made up of 20 foods! But there are so many more healthy foods out there."

Scurvy: The Sailor's Bane

Long before it was understood that certain foods are essential for preventing disease, sailors worldwide often suffered from scurvy, a vitamin C deficiency that causes slow wound healing, bleeding gums, pneumonia, and eventually death. Landlubbers also got scurvy, but because they were more likely to have fresh fruits and vegetables, they didn't get it anywhere near as often as their seafaring friends.

Here's the amazing thing about scurvy: You can reverse it almost instantly by having several servings of foods that are rich in vitamin C. In fact, sailors who were all but depleted of vitamin C were often able to recover in a matter of days after including oranges or lemons in their diets.

Scurvy has been virtually wiped out for centuries, yet today, vitamin C deficiency is cropping up in the most unexpected places. When an Arizona State University researcher tested vitamin C levels in college students, many were just the sunny side of scurvy.

To make sure you get enough vitamin C, just pour some orange juice. One 6-ounce glass contains 73 milligrams of vitamin C, or 121 percent of the DV for this vitamin. Other excellent sources include citrus and tropical fruits, broccoli, and sweet peppers.

Dental Health

A TOOTH-PROTECTION PLAN

Even though teeth are hard and bonelike, they're very much alive. Like your skin, muscles, or any other part of your body, they must be well-nourished to stay healthy. "In fact, selecting nutritious foods is probably as important as staying away from cavity-causing foods," says Dominick DePaola, DDS, PhD, senior consultant to the Education Alliance in Framingham, Massachusetts.

While there's no substitute for regular brushing and flossing, choosing the right foods, particularly those that provide large amounts of calcium and vitamins A, C, and D, will help keep your teeth and gums strong. Here's a case in point: Researchers in Japan analyzed the diets of 57 seventy-four-year-olds and counted their teeth. The scientists found that the people who had eaten the fewest vegetables, fish, and shell-fish also had the fewest teeth.

While you're eating nutritious foods, it's important not to bombard your teeth frequently with sugary, sticky snacks, which make it easy for cavity-causing bacteria to flourish, says Donna Oberg, RD, a nutritionist with the Seattle–King County Department of Public Health in Kent, Washington.

Eating for Strong Teeth

Just as bones need calcium to stay strong, your teeth also depend on this essential mineral, especially during the early years. "Calcium-rich foods are extremely important," says William Kuttler, DDS, a dentist in private practice in Dubuque, Iowa. "Without calcium, teeth won't form," he explains. And in adults, calcium fortifies the bone that supports the teeth so they don't loosen over time.

Getting more dairy foods in your diet is about the best protection teeth can have. A glass of low-fat milk, for example, contains about 300 milligrams of calcium, or about 30 percent of the Daily Value (DV) for this mineral. Eight ounces of low-fat and fat-free plain yogurt contains 448 milligrams and 488 milligrams, respectively. You can get somewhat smaller amounts from reduced-fat cheeses and some leafy green vegetables, including turnip greens, bok choy, and curly endive.

You need more than just calcium for good dental health though. You also need a variety of vitamins, including vitamins D, C, and A. Vitamin D is important for your pearly whites because a shortfall leads to bone loss as well as increased inflammation, which is a symptom of gum disease, according to researchers at the Washington University School of Medicine in St. Louis. The best way to get your D right along with calcium is to drink milk that is fortified with D.

Your body uses vitamin C to make collagen, a tough protein fiber that keeps the gums strong. It's easy to get enough C in your diet. A half-cup serving of cooked broccoli, for example, has 58 milligrams of vitamin C, almost 97 percent of the DV. A half-cup serving of cantaloupe has 34 milligrams, or 57 percent of the DV, and a medium-size navel orange has 80 milligrams, or 133 percent of the DV.

Vitamin A is used to form dentin, a layer of bonelike material just beneath the surface of the teeth. The best way to get vitamin A is by eating foods high in beta-carotene, which is converted to vitamin A in the body. Sweet potatoes are a great source, with a half-cup providing over 21,000 IU of vitamin A, or more than four times the DV. Other good sources of beta-carotene include kale, carrots, and most of the yellow-orange winter squashes. (Despite its hue, acorn squash is a beta-carotene lightweight, with only 0.2 milligram in a half-cup.)

Sticky Problems

As noted above, while some foods help keep the insides of the teeth healthy, others aren't so good for the outside. Because sugary foods make it possible for large amounts of bacteria to flourish in the mouth, over time the bacteria and the acids they produce act almost like little dental drills, wearing away the surface of the teeth and allowing cavities to form, says Dr. Kuttler.

Even fruit juices, which many people drink as a healthful alternative to sodas, can be a problem. "Juice is a very concentrated source of sugar," Dr. Kuttler explains. In fact, researchers in Switzerland found that grapefruit and apple juices did slightly more damage to the teeth than cola did.

While sweet foods can be a problem, sticky foods are even worse, Dr. Kuttler says. The reason for this is that because such foods stick to the teeth, they make it easy for bacteria to remain in the mouth for long periods of time.

Ironically, one food that's known for its stickiness might actually be good for your teeth. Researchers at the University of Chicago discovered in lab studies that oleanolic acid, a compound raisins are high in, prevented plaque-causing bacteria from sticking to surfaces.

The best way to deal with sticky snacks, if you must eat them, is to take a minute to brush your teeth after eating snacks or having a sweet drink. Even if you can't brush, simply rinsing out your mouth with water will help remove sugars before the bacteria have time to do damage.

It's not only what you eat but how you eat that plays a role in keeping teeth strong. Your mouth naturally produces saliva every time you chew, so the more you chew—during a meal, for example, or while chewing gum—the more saliva there is to wash away sugars from the teeth, says Dr. Kuttler. As a bonus, saliva also contains calcium and phosphorus, which help neutralize tooth-damaging acids that form in the mouth after eating.

While you're at the dinner table, you may want to consider having a little cheese. Researchers aren't sure why, but eating cheese appears to play a role in preventing tooth decay. It may be that cheese contains compounds that neutralize acids in the mouth before they do damage, Dr. Kuttler says. In other words, while eating sweets causes the pH level of your saliva to drop, transforming plaque into tooth-dissolving acid, eating cheese helps the pH stay steady. Which cheese to choose? Researchers reviewed a number of studies and found that among 12 cheeses, Cheddar offers the best tooth protection.

Doctor's Top Tip

Rinse your mouth with some black tea. Researchers at the University of Illinois at Chicago College of Dentistry found that people who rinsed their mouths with tea several times a day had less plaque buildup than people who swished with water. Drinking the tea, instead of just swishing it around, can help, too. Experts think it's the polyphenols in tea that do the trick.

Depression

EAT TO BEAT THE BLUES

It's hardly news that many of us, when we're feeling down, seek emotional comfort in foods, particularly such "comfort" foods as potato chips, snack cakes, or macaroni and cheese. But for some people, comfort foods are anything but comforting. The very foods they eat to make themselves feel better may actually make them feel worse—listless, moody, and fatigued.

Researchers have been studying the food-mood link for decades, but the connection is still uncertain. Studies have shown that for some individuals, diet can cause depression, according to Larry Christensen, PhD, chairman of the department of psychology at the University of South Alabama in Mobile and an expert on the effects of sugar and caffeine on mood. What you eat can lift your mood or, if you make the wrong choices, sink it. Moreover, what you don't eat can have as great an impact as what you do.

Food and Mood

Everything you do, from thinking and feeling to taking a walk, is influenced by nerve cells in the brain called neurons. You have billions of neurons—100 billion, in fact. In order to communicate, neurons depend on neurotransmitters, which are brain chemicals with intergalactic-sounding names like serotonin, dopamine, and norepinephrine.

These chemicals do more than just communicate; they can have a powerful effect on mood as well. When serotonin is in short supply, for example, depression—as well as insomnia and food cravings—may result. Conversely, high serotonin levels can impart feelings of calm and well-being, says Elizabeth Somer, RD, author of *Food and Mood* and *Nutrition for Women*. Changing levels of dopamine and norepinephrine in the brain can have similar results.

Fish for a Better Mood

Charlie the Tuna certainly always looks happy. Turns out, it's for good reason. Tuna, and other oily, cold-water fish, are the best sources of omega-3 fatty acids, which studies show are linked to lower rates of depression.

"Omega-3 polyunsaturated fatty acids may be beneficial to good mental health," says Jennifer Ramos Galluzzi, PhD, assistant professor in the science department at Housatonic Community College in Bridgeport, Connecticut.

Experts suggest getting two servings a week of high-omega-3 fish, such as tuna, salmon, herring, and Spanish mackerel. Other sources include canola oil and flax-seed oil.

Interestingly, recent research has found that omega-3s boost mood even in non-depressed people. When scientists at the University of Pittsburgh measured the blood levels of omega-3s in 106 healthy adults and gave them psychological tests, they discovered that the people with the highest omega-3 levels scored 49 to 58 percent better on the tests than the people with the lowest blood levels. (The scientists agree that omega-3 blood levels are a reliable indicator of how much omega-3 fatty acids a person eats.)

Carbohydrates: Nature's Calming Touch

Is life without your morning bagel not worth living? Does your passion for pasta know no bounds? Eat up—your moods will thank you for it.

In research pioneered by husband-and-wife researchers Richard Wurtman, PhD, and Judith Wurtman, PhD, both of the Massachusetts Institute of Technology in Cambridge, diets high in carbohydrate-rich foods have been shown to increase brain concentrations of the amino acid tryptophan. The tryptophan then is converted in the body to mood-boosting serotonin.

This may explain why, for many people, comfort foods that are high in carbohydrates can help ease feelings of depression, anxiety, and fatigue. For others, not eating carbohydrates may leave them grouchy and depressed.

Of course, some people can eat pasta, potatoes, and bread by the bushel without noticing any particular difference. But for others, known to scientists as carbohydrate cravers, the effects can be quite pronounced. It may be that carbohydrate cravings are the body's attempt to counteract low serotonin levels.

"Many people who eat spaghetti with marinara sauce and French bread for lunch get sleepy because that carbohydrate-heavy meal raises the serotonin level," Somer says. "But carbohydrate cravers feel energized by that same meal."

Stopping the Swings

It's hardly news that some people experience mood swings at certain times—during the dark days of winter, for example, or for some women, just before their menstrual periods. And some people, it now appears, can improve their moods during these low times simply by eating more carbohydrates.

In a study conducted by researchers at Harvard University and the Massachusetts

Doctor's Top Tip

"Have a bit of chocolate," says Jennifer Ramos Galluzzi, PhD, of Housatonic Community College in Bridgeport, Connecticut. "In small amounts, it's a mood booster." And who's gonna argue with that?

Institute of Technology, women suffering from premenstrual mood swings were asked to drink about 7½ ounces of a specially formulated high-carbohydrate drink once a month, just before their periods. Within hours of having the drink, they experienced significant reductions in depression, anger, and confusion, the researchers found.

While the women in the study consumed a specially made drink, you can get a similar amount of high carbohydrates by eating a small portion of a carbohydrate-rich food such as a cup of whole-wheat pasta, a baked potato, or a half-cup of raisins.

When Food Brings You Down

You've probably experienced the droopy, let-down feeling that sometimes occurs after sipping a large cappuccino or bingeing on your favorite cookies. It's not your imagination. "Consuming too much sugar or caffeine definitely contributes to feelings of depression for sensitive individuals," says Dr. Christensen. Experts aren't sure why sugar gives some people the blues, but it may be related to the amount you consume, says Dr. Christensen. While indulging in an occasional candy bar or doughnut can trigger a "sugar buzz" that temporarily boosts your spirits, a steady diet of sugar seems to be linked with depression.

In one study led by Dr. Christensen and a colleague, 20 people with serious depression were asked to cut all sugar and caffeine from their diets. After 3 weeks, these folks were significantly less depressed.

While the effects of caffeine on mood haven't been studied extensively, there's evidence that cutting back on coffee (or other high-caffeine drinks) may lift your spirits, especially if you normally drink it by the potful.

Diabetes
THE NEW APPROACH

Most people with diabetes should eat a diet that's higher in carbohydrates, particularly the complex kind, than was formerly believed. While your doctor, dietitian, or nutritionist will determine your personal need for carbohydrates, most people should be getting approximately 50 percent of their total calories from carbohydrates, says Stanley Mirsky, MD, associate clinical professor of metabolic diseases at Mount Sinai School of Medicine in New York City and the author of *Controlling Diabetes the Easy Way.*

It may sound strange, but there's never been a better time to have diabetes. Gone are the days when a doctor handed you a list of what you could and couldn't eat—the same list he gave to everyone else who came in the door. New evidence has significantly altered the one-size-fits-all dietary approach to this condition.

For example, even though it's best to eat sugar in moderation, for most people with diabetes, it's no longer forbidden. Some may be advised to cut back on fat and eat more carbohydrates; others will be told just the opposite. In fact, it's not unusual these days for two people with diabetes, even if they are the same age, same weight, and in the same overall condition, to have totally different diets for controlling it.

Yet one aspect of diabetes has stayed the same. Diet—what you eat, and in some cases, what you don't—is at the heart of any treatment plan. Along with maintaining a healthy weight and getting regular exercise, eating right helps keep blood sugar and fats at steady levels, which is the key to keeping problems under control.

Hunger Amidst Plenty

Before seeing how you can use food to treat or prevent diabetes, here's a quick look at what this condition is. The fuel that keeps our bodies running is sugar. Doctors call it glucose. Soon after we eat, glucose pours into the bloodstream and is carried to individual cells throughout the body. Before it can enter these cells, however, it requires the presence of a hormone called insulin. And therein lies the problem.

People with diabetes either don't produce enough insulin, or the insulin they do produce doesn't work efficiently. In either case, all that glucose in the bloodstream isn't able to get inside the cells. Rather, it hovers in the bloodstream, getting more and more concentrated as time goes by. Not only do individual cells go hungry, which can cause fatigue, dizziness, and many other symptoms, but all that concentrated sugar becomes toxic, eventually damaging the eyes, kidneys, nerves, immune system, heart, and blood vessels.

The most serious form of diabetes—and the least common—is type 1, or insulin-dependent, diabetes. It occurs when the body makes little or no insulin of its own. People with type 1 diabetes must take insulin to replace their own missing supplies.

Far more common is type 2, or non-insulin-dependent, diabetes. People with this condition, which occurs mainly in those over age 40, produce some insulin, but generally not enough. They may take oral medications, but usually don't require insulin injections, at least not in the early stages of the disease.

The Healing Power of Food

Experts have long recognized that what you eat can play a critical role both in preventing and controlling type 2 diabetes. Perhaps the best way to understand the effects of diet on diabetes is to look at two similar groups of people who differ primarily in what they eat.

Consider the Pima Indians. Researchers discovered that Pimas who live in Mexico and eat a lot of corn, beans, and fruits are seldom overweight and rarely develop diabetes. By contrast, the Pima Indians in Arizona eat an Americanized diet that is high in sugar and fat. They commonly develop diabetes by age 50.

Fuel Up with Carbs

Carbohydrates, which are found in most foods except meat, fish, and poultry, are the body's main source of energy. There are two types. Complex carbohydrates, called starches, include foods like rice, beans, potatoes, and pasta. Simple carbohydrates, called sugars, include the natural sugars found in milk, fruits, and vegetables as well as white table sugar and honey. The body turns both complex and simple carbohydrates into glucose, which is either immediately converted into energy or stored until needed.

If you have diabetes, a helpful way to plan your meals is to use a system called the glycemic index (GI). Scientists at the University of Sydney in Australia developed the glycemic index, which ranks carbohydrates according to their effects on your insulin-regulating system. All carbs are not created equal, however. Some carbohydrates are broken down into sugars slowly, and they slowly release those sugars into your bloodstream. Other carbohydrates are broken down lightning fast, and their sugars zip right into your bloodstream.

The index is based on the standard of table sugar, which enters your bloodstream almost instantly, causing a fast spike in your blood sugar levels, which requires a big jolt of insulin to stabilize. The index compares how fast other carbs are broken down into sugars with this table sugar standard. High-GI foods, such as cookies and cakes, affect your body like table sugar does—quickly spiking blood sugar levels. Low-GI foods, such as vegetables and some fruits, release their sugars into the bloodstream more slowly, easing out insulin more slowly.

Look for the glycemic index values of foods on product labels soon. But if you do decide to eat the low-GI way, bear in mind that it's not a perfect system. Because the glycemic index only considers carbs, it can make some healthy foods (like carrots) look bad and other not-so-healthy foods (like peanut M&Ms) look good. That's why researchers have developed an improved system called the glycemic load. The glycemic load (GL) also takes into consideration fiber and fat, both of which affect the digestion of carbohydrates. Like the glycemic index, you can find the GL of foods in books and online.

Toss One Back

Beer is probably the last thing you'd expect to be on a diabetes-friendly diet. But researchers at Boston Medical Center found that mild to moderate alcohol consumption—of beer and wine specifically—was associated with a lower risk of hyperinsulinemia (having too much insulin in the blood, which is often associated with diabetes). The people in the study who drank 20 drinks per month were 66 percent less likely to be diagnosed with an obesity-related condition, such as diabetes, than those who abstained.

Don't look at this as a license to binge, however, and talk with your doctor before adding alcohol to your diabetes diet! Safe upper limits are one drink per day for women and two for men. A drink is defined as 12 ounces of beer, 5 ounces of wine, or 1½ ounces of liquor.

Healing Fiber

A high-fiber diet has been shown to relieve everything from constipation to heart disease. Research suggests that it can also play a powerful role in controlling blood sugar, says James W. Anderson, MD, professor of internal medicine in the department of endocrinology and molecular medicine at the University of Kentucky in Lexington.

There are two types of fiber, soluble and insoluble. Both play a role in stabilizing blood sugar.

Here's how soluble fiber helps: Because it forms a gummy gel in the intestine, soluble fiber helps prevent glucose from being absorbed into the blood too quickly. This in turn helps keep blood sugar levels from rising or dipping too drastically.

In addition, soluble fiber seems to increase cells' sensitivity to insulin, so more sugar can move from the blood into the cells. In studies conducted by Dr. Anderson, people with type 2 diabetes who ate a high-fiber (and high-carbohydrate) diet were able to improve their blood sugar control by an average of 95 percent. People with type 1 diabetes on the same diet showed a 30 percent improvement.

Research now shows that insoluble fiber may play a role in diabetes prevention as well. Insoluble fiber is found in whole-grain products, vegetables such as green beans and dark green leafy vegetables, fruit skins and root vegetable skins, seeds, and nuts. In a study conducted at Harvard University, averaging 10 grams of cereal fiber each day (from foods such as whole-grain breads, rice, and pasta), lowered the risk of type 2 diabetes by 36 percent.

It's really very easy to increase your fiber intake. Try eating at least five servings of fruits and vegetables each day. Eat more whole-grain bread. (The first ingredient should be 100 percent whole-wheat flour or stone ground whole-wheat flour. Another clue is that the bread should provide 1½ to 2 grams of fiber per slice. Don't be fooled by just a brown color, which can simply be molasses!) Use whole-grain cereals and whole-wheat pasta instead of white pasta. And swap out beans for meat in some meals. You don't have to be fanatical about counting fiber grams. You can easily get enough by eating 3 to 5 servings of vegetables, 2 to 4 servings of fruits, and 6 to 11 servings of breads, cereals, pasta, and rice a day.

Two great sources of fiber are Brussels sprouts and beans. A half-cup serving of Brussels sprouts contains 4 grams of fiber, with 2 grams of soluble fiber. (That's more fiber than you'll get in a cup of pasta.) A half-cup of kidney beans contains nearly 7 grams of fiber, almost 3 grams of it soluble.

Increase your fiber intake slowly to avoid some uncomfortable digestive issues, and drink more water to help keep the fiber moving through your system.

Help from Vitamins

Perhaps it's appropriate that vitamin D is helpful for diabetes. Researchers at Tufts University in Boston discovered that getting enough of the "sunshine vitamin" (so-called because your body makes vitamin D from time spent in the sun) may help reduce the risk of type 2 diabetes. The scientists studied 81,700 women for 20 years and found that the women who had the highest intake of vitamin D (which you can get not only from being out in the sun but also from foods) had a 28 percent lower risk of type 2 diabetes than the women who had the lowest intake of vitamin D.

Possibly the easiest way to get vitamin D in your diet is from drinking fortified milk. Having one glass of fortified milk will provide about 100 IU, or 25 percent of the Daily Value (DV) for this vitamin. And another great reason to do that is because you'll also get milk's calcium. One cup of fat-free milk contains more than 300 milligrams of calcium, which is almost a third of the DV for this mineral.

Why is calcium important for people with type 2 diabetes? It turns out that calcium is key in the fight against this disease. When Harvard University scientists studied the diets of more than 41,000 men for 12 years, they found that for every daily serving of low-fat dairy foods the men ate each day, their risk of developing type 2 diabetes dropped by 9 percent. The researchers think that the calcium in low-fat dairy plays a role.

But probably the best strategy is to get both vitamin D and calcium together, and of course you can get that combo in one convenient package—a carton of milk. Researchers at Tufts–New England Medical Center in Boston found that among the 83,779 women studied, those who got the highest levels of both vitamin D and calcium had a 33 percent lower risk of type 2 diabetes than the women who got the least. How high was that highest level? More than 1,200 milligrams of calcium each day and more than 800 IU of vitamin D.

Two other important vitamins for diabetes care are C and E. In fact, if you have diabetes, fruits and vegetables rich in vitamins C and E may be your ticket to healthier eyes, nerves, and blood vessels. These vitamins are known as antioxidants. They help protect your body's cells from free radicals, naturally occurring, cell-damaging molecules that may pose particular risks to people with diabetes.

What's more, vitamin C may provide even more direct benefits. In one study, Italian researchers gave 40 people with diabetes 1 gram of vitamin C every day. After 4 months, the patients' abilities to use insulin had significantly improved, perhaps because vitamin C helps insulin penetrate cells.

The DV for vitamin C is 60 milligrams. Oranges and grapefruit are excellent sources of vitamin C, but they're not the only ones. One cup of chopped, steamed broccoli, for example, contains more than 116 milligrams, or almost twice the DV for vitamin C. Half a cantaloupe has about 113 milligrams of vitamin C, and one red bell pepper has 140 milligrams.

Even though vitamin C is essential for people with diabetes, this nutrient is readily destroyed during cooking. For example, boiled broccoli may retain only 45 percent of its vitamin C. Steaming, which can preserve 70 percent of the C, is better. Best of all is microwaving, which preserves as much as 85 percent.

Another way to increase your intake of vitamin C is to pick the ripest fruits. Scarlet tomatoes, garnet strawberries, and deep chartreuse kiwifruit are much more nutrient-dense than fruits that haven't yet hit their prime.

Vitamin E, which is good for the heart, may be particularly important for people with diabetes, who are two to three times more likely to develop heart disease than people who do not have the disease. And research suggests that, like vitamin C, it may help insulin work better. Finnish scientists studied 944 men and found that those with the lowest levels of vitamin E in their blood were four times more likely to have diabetes than those with the highest levels. Vitamin E may somehow help insulin carry sugar from the blood into cells in muscles and tissues, the researchers speculate.

Vitamin E also helps keep blood platelets, which are elements in blood that help it clot, from becoming too sticky. This is particularly important in people with diabetes, whose platelets tend to clump more readily and lead to heart disease.

To get the most vitamin E, you need to occasionally use oils rich in polyunsaturated fats, like soybean oil, corn oil, and sunflower oil. Of course, these oils don't provide the benefits of the monounsaturated fats found in olive oil and canola oil. Used in moderation, however, they will help boost your vitamin E to healthy levels.

Wheat germ is another excellent source of vitamin E, with ¼ cup containing 6 IU, or 20 percent of the DV. Other good sources of this vitamin include kale, sweet potatoes, almonds, avocados, and blueberries.

Chrome-Plated Protection

It's not just vitamins that can help control diabetes. The trace mineral chromium, found in broccoli, grapefruit, and fortified breakfast cereals, has been shown to help regulate blood sugar, says Richard A. Anderson, PhD, a research chemist with the USDA Human Nutrition Research Center in Beltsville, Maryland.

Tests show that people with diabetes have lower levels of chromium circulating in their blood than people without the disease. In one study, eight people who had difficulty regulating blood sugar were given 20 micrograms of chromium a day. After 5 weeks, their blood sugar levels fell by as much as 50 percent. People without blood sugar problems who were given chromium showed no such changes.

In two more recent studies, scientists found that chromium may help control the health risks of diabetes. In one study, researchers studied 27 people with diabetes for 10 months and found that insulin sensitivity was twice as good in those who took chromium as in people who took a fake supplement. Another study, this one in Slovenia, found that in people with diabetes, taking chromium supplements for 3 months shortened QTc intervals, which is a heart rhythm that may become fatal if the interval lengthens.

It's true that the people in these studies took chromium supplements. But because experts aren't sure that taking chromium supplements is safe, it's best to boost your chromium supplies by eating foods that provide it. One cup of broccoli, for example, contains 22 micrograms, or 18 percent of the DV. A 2½-ounce waffle has almost

7 micrograms, or 6 percent of the DV. And 1 cup of grape juice contains 8 micrograms, or 6 percent of the DV.

When you're trying to get more chromium, barley is a good choice. One animal study done in England found that barley can help keep blood sugar levels under control. This grain makes great soups and breads and is a nice addition to casseroles.

To help your body retain the most chromium, it's helpful to eat lots of complex carbohydrates, like pasta and bagels, says Dr. Richard Anderson. Eating lots of sugary foods, on the other hand, will cause your body to excrete chromium. So even though it's fine to enjoy an occasional sugary snack, the emphasis should really be on the healthier whole foods, he says.

The USDA recommends eating whole grains—such as whole-wheat flour, whole-wheat bread, and brown rice—instead of refined grains—such as white flour, white bread, and white rice—whenever possible. Whole grains provide many health benefits, in addition to helping your body retain chromium.

Doctor's Top Tip

Most people with diabetes should eat a diet that's higher in carbohydrates, particularly the complex kind, than was formerly believed. While your doctor, dietitian, or nutritionist will determine your personal need for carbohydrates, most people should be getting approximately 50 percent of total calories from carbohydrates, says Stanley Mirsky, MD, of Mount Sinai School of Medicine.

Magnesium for Glucose Control

Experts estimate that 25 percent of people with diabetes are low in the mineral magnesium. The problem is even worse in those who have diabetes-related heart disease or a type of eye damage known as retinopathy. Since low levels of magnesium have been linked to damage to the retinas, it's likely that upping your intake of this mineral may help protect your eyes.

Good sources of magnesium include baked halibut, which contains 91 milligrams of magnesium per 3-ounce serving, or 23 percent of the DV. Cooked spinach is also good: 1 cup contains 157 milligrams, or almost 40 percent of the DV. And a half-cup serving of long-grain brown rice has 42 milligrams, or 11 percent of the DV.

Putting It All Together

Treating and preventing diabetes with foods involves more than just eating a few good foods. It's really a whole diet in which all the separate elements—fiber, vitamins, minerals, and so forth—come together in one good plan. Consider working with a dietitian to develop a meal plan that promotes blood sugar control, coordinates with your medications, and is tailored to your preferences and lifestyle.

Diarrhea

FOODS FOR RELIEF

Television commercials often portray a poor guy with diarrhea dashing to the nearest restroom—again and again. When you're the one making the dash, however, it's not so entertaining, particularly when you're doubled over with the cramps and bloating that often accompany this miserable condition.

Diarrhea usually occurs when bacteria or viruses cause inflammation in the intestine. In addition, certain foods, among them honey, sugar substitutes, and dairy foods, aren't completely digested and cause fermentation in the intestine. The body responds by drawing water into the intestine, which is what causes loose stools.

Luckily, diarrhea usually lasts only a day or two and then disappears. When it lasts longer, however, it can remove large amounts of fluids from the body as well as essential minerals that control blood pressure, heart rate, and muscle movement. This is why doctors usually recommend drinking fruit juice, flat cola, or a diluted sports drink whenever you have diarrhea to replace lost sugars and minerals.

Until diarrhea has run its course, it's a good idea to eat only the blandest of foods, such as noodles, white bread, bananas, and applesauce, because they won't irritate an already cranky colon, says Marvin M. Schuster, MD, founder of the Marvin M. Schuster Digestive and Motility Disorders Center at Johns Hopkins Bayview Medical Center in Baltimore. An added advantage is that these foods contain fiber, which acts like a water-absorbing sponge in the intestine and helps to dry things up a bit. "The skin of apples, for example, contains the fiber pectin, which is one of the ingredients in the pill form of Kaopectate," he says.

There's not a lot you can do to avoid all contact with diarrhea-causing viruses or bacteria. But if you're one of the millions of people who are sensitive to certain foods, you can prevent problems simply by watching what you eat.

Doctor's Top Tip

It may seem counterintuitive, but at the first sign of diarrhea, start chugging fluids, says Rallie McAllister, MD, MPH, a board-certified family physician at Nathaniel Mission Clinic in Lexington, Kentucky. "Water and clear broth are okay, but sports drinks may be even better. Because they replace minerals that are lost in your stool, sports drinks help you keep up your strength. But since they're usually loaded with sugar, an ingredient that can cause diarrhea on its own, it's usually a good idea to dilute them with equal parts of water."

Problems with Lactose

For many people, having cheese, a glass of milk, or a milk shake can, well, shake things up. This is because adults often don't have enough of the enzyme (lactase) that's needed to fully digest the sugar (lactose) found in dairy foods. In fact, about half of the world's population has this problem to a certain degree. "Lactose intolerance is a common cause of diarrhea," says Dr. Schuster. "It's a major problem because there are so many products that contain dairy, and people don't make the connection."

If you've been having diarrhea and suspect that dairy foods may be to blame, give yourself this test: Avoid all dairy foods for a week to let your system adjust. Then drink a couple of glasses of milk, says Dr. Schuster. If you're lactose intolerant, your digestive system will let you know within a few hours that it's unhappy.

Even if you have lactose intolerance, however, you probably don't have to forfeit dairy foods completely. Researchers at the University of Minnesota in St. Paul found that people were generally able to drink up to 8 ounces of milk a day without having problems. Small amounts of cheese or other dairy foods may also be safe, especially if you have them as part of a meal rather than by themselves.

In addition, many people with lactose intolerance can eat yogurt without having problems since yogurt is naturally lower in lactose than other dairy foods.

A Honey of a Problem

Hot tea and honey can warm a cold winter's day better than the noontime sun. But too much of the sweet stuff can send some people running for the warm security of

---

A TOAST TO HEALTH

Long before there was Pepto-Bismol, the ancient Greeks sipped wine as a digestive aid. Scientists today are finding that it just might work for traveler's diarrhea as well.

In laboratory studies, researchers from Honolulu doused diarrhea-causing bacteria with either red wine, white wine, or bismuth subsalicylate, the active ingredient in Pepto-Bismol. They found that both types of wine wiped out bacteria just as well as the medication did. In fact, even diluted wine worked better than the diluted pink stuff.

Although the research is promising, it's too early to say for sure whether drinking wine will do the trick against the trots. (And it certainly won't take the place of antibiotics, which are essential for some kinds of infections.) But if you decide to give wine a try, one glass is probably enough. The researchers in the Honolulu study estimate that 6 ounces of wine is all it takes to get the benefits.

GLOBE-TROTTING

After months of planning for an exotic vacation, the last thing you want is to spend it in the bathroom. Unfortunately, that's exactly where a lot of people wind up. Studies show that 30 to 40 percent of people traveling to "exotic" areas, which don't always have the same sanitation standards as the United States, will have encounters with traveler's diarrhea.

It's wise not to drink the water in less-developed countries, since it often harbors large amounts of bacteria. Here are a few additional tips that will help keep you in the loop and out of the loo.

Leave the lasagna. A common cause of traveler's diarrhea is restaurant food that's prepared early in the day, then reheated later on. Foods such as lasagna, quiche, and casseroles are more likely to become contaminated than dishes that go straight from the stove to your plate. To be safe, order foods that are made fresh and served hot.

Be careful in the garden. Salad greens are a common cause of traveler's diarrhea because the leaves may be washed in bacteria-laden water. The same is true of fruits. You can reduce the risk of diarrhea by avoiding raw vegetables and peeling all fruits, even apples, before eating them.

Put dairy out to pasture. When traveling abroad, it's best to leave the dairy to the cows. Local milk, cheese, and other dairy foods may not be pasteurized and can contain large amounts of bacteria.

the bathroom. This is because honey and fruit juices contain a natural sugar called fructose. When you eat a lot of fructose, some of the sugar can slip into the large intestine undigested. Over time it begins to ferment, often causing gas and diarrhea.

Even small amounts of fructose may cause problems. Some of the people in one study had diarrhea after eating 3 tablespoons of honey (nature's greatest source of fructose). Others had problems from just half that amount. The same is true of fruit juices. For some folks, having several glasses of juice a day won't cause problems. For others, the same amount or less may cause diarrhea, says William Ruderman, MD, a gastroenterologist in Orlando, Florida.

If you've been having diarrhea, try cutting down on honey and fruit juices or giving them up entirely, Dr. Ruderman advises. Then gradually start adding them to your diet again. Eventually, you'll find an amount that you can enjoy without having discomfort.

Artificial Problems

Sometimes diarrhea is caused not by what you ate but by what you chewed. Sugarless gums and candies sometimes contain sorbitol, a sweetener that the digestive system has trouble handling, says Dr. Ruderman. As with fructose, sorbitol tends to ferment in the intestine, causing diarrhea.

As little as 5 grams of sorbitol—about the amount you'd get by chewing 2½ sticks of sugarless gum—may cause diarrhea. If you suspect sugarless gum has been causing your problems, you may want to switch to the regular kind. Or simply chew smaller pieces, Dr. Ruderman says.

Other artificial sweeteners can be problematic, too, such as mannitol, xylitol, erythritol, and D-tagatose. Check for these on product ingredients lists. These sweeteners are called sugar alcohols. All sugar alcohols are absorbed slowly and incompletely by the intestine, which is why they have little caloric effect. However, this property can also cause gas and diarrhea if you consume too much. For many people, more than 50 grams per day of sorbitol or 20 grams per day of mannitol can cause these problems.

Diverticulosis

THE FACTS ABOUT FIBER

With the Industrial Revolution came a whole new way of living. We traded sail-boats for steamboats, wagons for freight trains, and whole-wheat bread for white. While the first two innovations made life easier, the last did not. In fact, it was partly responsible for a "new" intestinal disease called diverticulosis.

In the late 1800s, manufacturers developed a process that made it easy to remove the tough fibrous shells from wheat and other grains. Although breads made from these refined grains were softer and smoother, they had considerably less fiber. And this caused a lot of problems.

When there's a lot of fiber in your diet, stools are large, soft, and easy to pass. Take away the fiber, and the stools get small and hard. This makes it harder for the intestines to move them along. When the colon has to strain to do its job, it can stretch out of shape, causing small pouches to form in the muscular wall. Doctors call this condition diverticulosis. While diverticulosis was uncommon before the 1900s, about 10 percent of Americans over age 40 and about half of people over age 60 have it today. Amazingly, though, most of them don't even know they have diverticulosis because it doesn't always cause discomfort or symptoms. Other times, though, it can lead to cramping, infection, and other problems.

To make matters worse, if the pouches become infected or inflamed, it causes a painful, more dangerous condition called diverticulitis. This happens to 10 to 25 percent of people with diverticulosis.

Interestingly, medical textbooks describe diverticulitis as a disease of the more senior set, people over age 50. But sadly, it's becoming more common in obese, younger adults, found researchers at the University of Maryland Medical Center in Baltimore. Obese people are at risk for diverticulitis as early as age 20.

Are men more likely to get diverticulitis than women? Possibly. Researchers in Israel found that young men are more likely to get diverticulitis than women. They found that acute diverticulitis was significantly more common among men younger than age 45 than older—76 percent of the people with diverticulitis in the younger group were men compared with only 33 percent in the older group.

The good news is that these conditions are almost entirely preventable—if you eat the right foods.

The Colon's Best Friend

Our ancestors didn't know it, but the fruits, vegetables, legumes, and whole grains that they ate every day were protecting them from diverticulosis. It's really that simple. High-fiber foods are the secret to keeping the colon healthy, says Marvin M. Schuster, MD, founder of the Marvin M. Schuster Digestive and Motility Disorders Center at Johns Hopkins Bayview Medical Center in Baltimore. Diverticular diseases are common in countries where low-fiber diets are common, such as the United States, England, and Australia. However, these diseases are rare in countries where people eat high-fiber diets, such as Asia and Africa. For example, missionary surgeons in Africa report diverticulosis is rare among Africans eating a native, high-fiber diet. However, descendents of black Africans living in the United States are just as likely to have diverticular diseases as whites.

In a 4-year study of nearly 48,000 men, researchers from Harvard University and Brigham and Women's Hospital in Boston found that those who got the most fiber in their diets were 42 percent less likely to have diverticulosis than those eating the least. And although any fiber is good fiber, the men who got most of their fiber from fruits and vegetables got the best results. The Daily Value (DV) for fiber is 25 grams. Eating several servings a day of fruits, beans, vegetables, and whole-grain cereals and breads will provide all the fiber your insides need to stay healthy.

It's important, however, not to suddenly increase your fiber intake, as that can cause gas and bloating, says William Ruderman, MD, a gastroenterologist in Orlando, Florida. He advises adding fiber slowly to your diet by having an extra piece of fruit

---

IS POPCORN A PROBLEM?

For a long time, doctors advised people with diverticulosis to avoid rough foods like seeds and popcorn. It was believed that hard particles of undigested food would become lodged in pouches in the intestine, possibly causing inflammation.

"That recommendation used to be in all the medical textbooks," says Marvin Schuster, MD, of Johns Hopkins Bayview Medical Center in Baltimore. "But there was never any evidence that these foods ever caused problems for people with diverticulosis. It was all just speculation."

While it's possible, doctors say, for a piece of popcorn or some other particle to lodge where it shouldn't, this really isn't a big concern. What is important, Dr. Schuster says, is getting more fiber, and if eating popcorn helps you get it, then go ahead and munch away. Of course, if you do have discomfort after eating certain foods, you'll know what to avoid in the future, he adds.

Doctor's Top Tip

"To prevent diverticulosis, manmade fiber, such as fiber bars or drinks, are not the answer. We are meant to digest meats, nuts, fruits, and vegetables," says DicQie Fuller, PhD, DSc, scientific advisor for Z-Health Corporation in Chicago. "Instead, eat at least five servings a day of raw fruits and vegetables for their natural fiber."

one day, for example, and a bowl of high-fiber cereal the next, until your body adjusts to the changes.

It's also important to drink at least eight glasses of water a day, which will help the fiber move smoothly through your system rather than getting dry and hard, says Dr. Ruderman.

Give Your Colon a Break

If you're in the middle of a diverticulitis attack (the more serious condition that occurs if your diverticulosis pouches become infected or inflamed), which causes tenderness around the left side of the lower abdomen and might be accompanied by nausea, fever, vomiting, chills, cramping, and constipation, consider trying a clear liquid or low-fiber diet for a few days. This helps your tender colon to heal. After that, ease your fiber intake back up by adding 5 to 15 grams of fiber a day.

The Fat Foes

Although not getting enough fiber is clearly the number one cause of diverticulosis, researchers have found that eating too many red meats or other high-fat foods can also be a problem.

Researchers from the Harvard study mentioned earlier found that people who ate a low-fiber diet and also ate high-fat foods or 4 ounces of red meats a day were significantly more likely to get diverticulosis than those who merely skimped on the fiber.

It's not entirely clear what it is about red meats and high-fat foods that gives us a propensity for intestinal pouches. What is clear is that meats contain no fiber and don't add bulk to stools the way fiber does, says Dr. Ruderman. "And often meats replace healthier fiber foods in people's diets, which adds to the problem," he says.

Fatigue
WHAT TO EAT WHEN YOU'RE FEELING BEAT

Every day is the same. You slap the snooze button five or six times, then crawl out of bed—no time for breakfast. Struggle through the morning, fueled by generous mugs of strong coffee. Drag yourself to lunch. Drag yourself back to your office, and muscle through the afternoon. Then drag yourself back home, where all you want is takeout, TV, your quilt, and the couch.

You're exhausted just thinking about it.

Fatigue in this country is at near-epidemic proportions. Fully half of all adults who seek medical treatment complain of fatigue. But it doesn't have to be this way. Making even small changes in your diet, experts say, can have a substantial effect on your energy levels.

Brain Fuel

There are some foods that make us sleepy and droopy, while others give us energy to burn. It's only in recent years, however, that scientists have begun understanding why. The answer, as it so often does, begins in the brain.

To a large extent our feelings, moods, and energy levels are controlled by neurons—nerve cells in the brain that communicate with the help of chemical messengers called neurotransmitters. Studies have shown that changes in the levels of neurotransmitters such as dopamine and norepinephrine can dramatically affect energy levels, which is why they're sometimes called wake-up chemicals. Studies show that people tend to think more quickly and feel more motivated and energetic when their brains are producing large amounts of these chemicals.

Our diets provide the raw materials needed for the production of these neurotransmitters. What we eat—or don't—can play a large role in how we feel. "We're talking about a whole symphony of brain chemicals that ebb and flow throughout the day," says Elizabeth Somer, RD, author of *Food and Mood* and *Nutrition for Women*.

The building block for dopamine and norepinephrine, for example, is the amino acid tyrosine. Tyrosine levels are elevated when you eat high-protein foods such as fish, chicken, or low-fat yogurt.

"Make sure to eat some protein along with carbohydrates at each meal or snack," says Molly Kimball, RD, a sports and lifestyle nutritionist at the Ochner Health System's Elmwood Fitness Center in New Orleans. "For instance, instead of having whole-wheat toast with jelly or fruit with juice for breakfast, have whole-wheat toast with peanut butter or fruit with cottage cheese. The carbohydrates alone cause a rapid release of blood sugar and a rapid drop in energy, but the protein helps even that out."

You don't have to down huge amounts of protein to get the energizing effects. Eating just 3 to 4 ounces of a protein-rich food, like a broiled chicken breast or a hard-boiled egg, "feeds" your brain enough tyrosine to get the dopamine and nor-epinephrine flowing.

Even though protein-rich foods can help boost energy, the fats that often come with them can drag you down. Digesting fats diverts blood from the brain, which can make you feel sluggish. So don't overload a turkey sandwich with high-fat cheese and mayonnaise; dress it with mustard, lettuce, and tomatoes instead, recommends Somer.

Back to Basics

While much research has focused on the intricacies of brain chemistry, eating for energy can also be as simple as getting more fruits and vegetables and essential minerals like iron.

A study of 411 dentists and their wives found that those who consumed at least 400 milligrams of vitamin C a day reported feeling less fatigue than those consuming less than 100 milligrams. In both cases, of course, the amount of vitamin C was considerably higher than the Daily Value (DV) of 60 milligrams.

It's easy to boost the amounts of vitamin C in your diet. An 8-ounce glass of orange juice, for example, contains 82 milligrams of vitamin C, or about 132 percent of the DV. A half-cup of strawberries has 42 milligrams, or 70 percent of the DV, and a half-cup of cooked chopped broccoli has 58 milligrams, or 97 percent of the DV.

Iron is also essential for energy. This is particularly true among women, who can lose large amounts of iron as a result of menstruation. In fact, 39 percent of premenopausal women may be iron-deficient. What's more, even small iron-deficiencies can leave you weary.

Fortunately, iron is very easy to get in the diet. Eating a half-cup of quick-cooking Cream of Wheat, for example, provides 5 milligrams of iron, 10 percent of the Recommended Dietary Allowance (RDA) for women and 50 percent of the RDA for men. Red meats are another good source of iron. You don't need much. A 3-ounce serving of broiled flank steak, for example, contains 2 milligrams of iron, 13 percent of the RDA for women and 20 percent of the RDA for men.

The Ups and Downs of Carbohydrates

Whereas eating high-protein foods often leaves us feeling energized, eating starchy foods like pasta and potatoes, especially for lunch, often leaves us nodding. The explanation, once again, is found in brain chemistry.

Eating high-carbohydrate foods like potatoes or rice causes an amino acid called tryptophan to be delivered to the brain. This, in turn, jump-starts the production of serotonin, a "calm-down" chemical that regulates mood. And it doesn't take a lot. Eating as little as 1 ounce of rice, for example, can get the serotonin flowing.

In one study, researchers in England gave people a variety of lunches to see how their energy levels fared. One lunch was low-fat, high-carbohydrate; another was medium-fat, medium-carbohydrate; and the third was high-fat, low-carbohydrate. As you might expect, the people eating the high-carbohydrate (and also the high-fat) lunches reported feeling more drowsy and muddled than those getting the lower-carbohydrate fare.

"What you want to do is balance your carbohydrate-protein mix so that the bulk of your diet comes from complex carbohydrates, laced with a bit of protein," Somer says. "That's how most people will improve their energy levels."

Paradoxically, the opposite is true in people known as carbohydrate cravers. Experts aren't sure why, but these people tend to get an energy boost after eating high-carbohydrate meals or snacks. Researchers at the Massachusetts Institute of Technology in Cambridge speculate that carbohydrate cravings are the body's attempt to boost low serotonin levels.

If you're one of those people who seem to get energy after eating starchy foods, don't fight it, advises Somer. Enjoy a baked potato, bread, pasta, or other starchy food at lunch. While you're at it, feel free to eat a starchy snack—like whole-wheat crackers or a banana—to stave off fatigue at midday.

Incidentally, it's generally better to eat several small meals a day instead of two or three large meals. Smaller meals will help keep blood sugar levels stable, which will help stave off fatigue, says Wahida Karmally, DrPH, RD, CDE, a registered dietitian on the Nutrition Advisory Committee at New York–Presbyterian Hospital/Columbia University Medical Center and director of nutrition at the Irving Center for Clinical Research at Columbia University Medical Center.

Snooze Foods

It's 3 p.m. Do you know where your energy is?

Not at the coffee cart. While a cup or two of coffee early in the day has been shown to boost alertness and mental functioning, drinking large amounts day after day tends to lower energy levels. The same thing is true of sweet pick-me-ups like

FOOD FOR THOUGHT

It has been hammered into us since grade school: Start the day with a good breakfast. But while eating breakfast does seem to boost performance in children, it's not so clear whether it's equally important for adults.

While a number of studies have suggested that skipping breakfast can cause fuzzy thinking and fatigue, some experts say that the evidence isn't convincing. "In terms of human evolution, the notion of organized meals is very new," says Arthur Frank, MD, medical director of the Obesity Management Program at George Washington University Hospital in Washington, D.C. Indeed, studies on human performance indicate that people who regularly skip breakfast may actually experience an energy slump on occasions when they do eat it.

While Dr. Frank certainly isn't opposed to the idea of having breakfast, "you shouldn't feel obligated to eat it," he says. "Follow your body's lead."

Of course, if you frequently find yourself feeling tired as the day wears on, skipping breakfast could be making the problem worse, says Wahida Karmally, DrPH, RD, CDE, director of nutrition at the Irving Center for Clinical Research at Columbia University Medical Center. She recommends starting the day with a breakfast that is high in complex carbohydrates blended with protein—whole-grain cereal with low-fat or fat-free milk and fresh fruit, for example, or whole-wheat toast topped with low-fat cheese.

doughnuts. The quick surge of energy, for some people, is often followed by an equally quick—and longer-lasting—crash.

"Sugar can contribute to feelings of fatigue, particularly if you're sensitive to it," says Larry Christensen, PhD, chairman of the department of psychology at the University of South Alabama in Mobile and an expert on the effects of sugar and caffeine on mood.

Unlike starches, which gradually release their energy into the bloodstream, sugars (called glucose) careen in all at once, causing blood sugar to spike. To cope with the sugar surge, the body releases insulin, which quickly removes sugars from the blood and carries them into individual cells. The result, of course, is lower levels of blood sugar. And the lower the level of sugar in your blood, the more fatigued you become.

Sugar can also cause fatigue by indirectly stimulating the production of serotonin, which, as we've seen, is the brain chemical that plays a calming role. That's exactly what you don't need when you're fighting off fatigue.

Experts aren't sure why caffeine tends to sap your energy, says Dr. Christensen.

They do know that the caffeine buzz caused by cup after cup of coffee—or cola, tea, or other caffeine-containing drinks—is often followed by the caffeine crash.

To get reenergized, many people simply drink more coffee. This creates a cycle that can leave you alternately jittery and heavy-lidded.

In one study, people with a history of fatigue, depression, and moodiness were put on a sugar- and caffeine-free diet for 2 weeks. Not surprisingly, many of them quickly improved on this diet. More interesting is what happened later. When they resumed getting caffeine and sugar in their diets, 44 percent got fatigued all over again.

Doctor's Top Tip

"Drink more water," says DicQie Fuller, PhD, DSc, scientific advisor for Z-Health Corporation in Chicago. "It allows the enzymes to work throughout your body, assisting in the proper digestion of food for energy. I personally recommend hydrating with pure water rather than soda, coffee, and juice."

Fat Substitutes
BETTER THAN THE REAL THING

There's nothing quite like the flavor of a tender, juicy burger, the aroma of freshly baked cookies, or the smooth sensation of ice cream on your tongue. The one ingredient that really makes these foods stand out—the one that delivers aroma, flavor, texture, and feelings of satisfaction like nothing else—is fat.

Unfortunately, fat is the "ultimate" in more ways than one. Nothing adds to our waistlines the way fat does. And nothing else puts us more at risk for obesity, high blood pressure, heart disease, stroke, diabetes, and even cancer.

Researchers think that fat is so bad, in fact, that even a taste of fatty foods may cause triglycerides, which are potentially dangerous fats in the bloodstream, to rise. In one study, researchers at Purdue University in West Lafayette, Indiana, gave people crackers topped with either regular or fat-free cream cheese and asked them to chew the food and spit it out. Those who nibbled the full-fat spread ended up with triglyceride levels almost twice as high as those of the people who had the fat-free spread.

It's little wonder, then, that manufacturers are working overtime to create foods using fat substitutes and that we're gobbling them up as quickly as they hit the shelves.

Using these foods is no substitute for a diet that's high in naturally low-fat foods such as fruits, vegetables, and whole grains. The substitutes, however, are a great way to reduce (or even eliminate) the fat in many common foods, like cheese and salad dressings, says Christina M. Stark, MS, RD, an extension associate at Cornell University in Ithaca, New York.

Making the Bad Better

There are many different kinds of fat substitutes. Some are simply made from carbohydrates or proteins that have been processed to mimic the mouth-feel and texture of fat. Others are made from actual fat molecules that have been chemically altered so that they can't get through the intestinal wall and into the bloodstream. These fat fill-ins aren't intended for home use but are used by food manufacturers to whittle calories from snack foods, desserts, and other high-fat favorites.

And the fat savings can be substantial. Using 2 tablespoons of fat-free Italian salad dressing, for example, can save 11 grams of fat and more than 100 calories over the same amount of the regular kind. Similarly, you can slice off 5 grams of fat and 40 calories from a grilled cheese sandwich by using fat-free cheese instead of regular American.

Fat substitutes are good in yet another way. Because they're often made from carbohydrates or proteins, they can provide a few health benefits beyond their ability to cut calories. Here's a quick guide to the most-common faux fats.

Fiber Fillers

The original and possibly the best fat substitutes are those made from carbohydrates, which are listed on food labels as dextrins, maltodextrins, modified food starches, polydextrose, and gums. They contain between zero and 4 calories per gram, instead of the 9 calories provided by fat. Since they can hold up to 24 times their weight in water, they're often used for adding moisture to low-fat baked goods.

The best thing about carbohydrate-based fat substitutes is that they're made from fiber, says Mark Kantor, PhD, associate professor of nutrition and food science at the University of Maryland in College Park. "They not only have fewer fat calories, but because they contain soluble fiber, they can help lower cholesterol levels as well as help control your weight," he says.

In one study, researchers found that when people with mildly high cholesterol ate large amounts of Oatrim, a carbohydrate-based fat substitute, for 5 weeks, their cholesterol went down 15 percent. In addition, their systolic blood pressure readings (which measured how hard their hearts worked to pump blood through their arteries) declined, and their blood sugar levels were steadier.

Although you're not likely to eat as much Oatrim as the people in the study, who essentially had it with every meal, it's good to know that it provides at least a small benefit, says Dr. Kantor.

Ice Cream Clones

There's nothing quite like the smooth, creamy texture of ice cream, which traditionally comes from the high fat content. To duplicate the mouth-feel of full-fat ice cream, manufacturers use fat substitutes made from proteins such as milk or egg whites, which glide across your tongue in the same way that fat does.

Protein-based fat substitutes, such as Simplesse and Trailblazer, are listed on the label as microparticulated protein products. Providing 1 to 4 calories per gram, they're used mainly in ice cream, butter, sour cream, yogurt, mayonnaise, and other creamy foods.

Like their carbohydrate-based kin, protein fat substitutes have health benefits

In the Kitchen

Most fat fill-ins aren't intended for home use. Instead, food manufacturers use them to cut calories from snack foods, desserts, and other high-fat favorites.

You'll find one new product, however, in your grocery store that you can cook with at home. It's a new brand of oil called Enova that looks and tastes just like vegetable oil. It was first sold in Japan in 1999, and according to its manufacturer, it quickly became "the number one premium cooking oil in the Japanese market."

The company states that "compared to other cooking and salad oils, less Enova oil is stored in the body as fat." Technically, Enova isn't a fat substitute. It's a naturally occurring type of oil called diacylglycerol or diglyceride. Most vegetable oils are made up of triacylglycerols or triglycerides. Even though the oil is structurally different, as with all other vegetable oils, 1 tablespoon of Enova contains 120 calories and 14 grams of fat.

But will Enova melt off the pounds? Probably not. Scientists at the Chicago Center for Clinical Research fed 131 people a diet with 15 percent of their calories coming from either Enova or another vegetable oil. After 6 months, the Enova group lost 8 percent of their body fat, compared with 6 percent for the vegetable oil group.

---

besides just cutting fat, says Dr. Kantor. "Although you shouldn't depend on these foods, they do contribute small amounts of protein, which is needed for building muscle, making hormones, and fighting infection, to your diet," he says.

Other protein-based fat substitutes, called protein blends, combine vegetable or animal proteins with gums or starches and are typically used in frozen desserts and baked goods. Although these fat substitutes do supply some protein, the amount is not significant.

Into the Frying Pan

For a long time, one of the problems with fake fats was that they didn't melt and come to a boil, which meant that they couldn't be used for making fried foods such as potato chips and crackers. This changed with the introduction of a fat-based product called olestra (Olean)—the first fake fat that could stand up to the deep fryer.

Currently, olestra is found only in snack foods such as chips and crackers, but it's likely that it will eventually turn up in other products. If it's approved in other foods, olestra could wind up replacing a substantial portion of the dietary fat that now makes up some 35 percent of the calories Americans consume daily," says Rallie McAllister, MD, MPH, a board-certified family physician at Nathaniel Mission

Clinic in Lexington, Kentucky, and author of *Healthy Lunchbox: The Working Mom's Guide to Keeping You and Your Kids Trim*.

Doctor's Top Tip

Use fat substitutes judiciously, within an overall healthy diet, to gain flexibility in meal planning, suggest doctors of the American Heart Association's nutrition committee.

Olestra is made from large molecules that are held together in such a way that they cannot be broken down by digestive enzymes, which is why it has no calories. But even though olestra can be a real boon for snackers, it simply isn't healthful in large amounts.

Because olestra is made from fats, it absorbs and eliminates fat-soluble nutrients from your body. People who eat a lot of olestra may lose vitamins A, D, E, and K as well as fat-soluble phytonutrients such as the beta-carotene in winter squash or the lycopene in carrots and sweet potatoes. One study found that even small amounts of olestra reduced beta-carotene levels by 34 percent and lycopene levels by 52 percent. This is a serious problem, because low levels of carotenoids and related plant compounds may increase the risk of heart disease, eye damage, and certain cancers, says Dr. Kantor.

Olestra is now fortified, so it replaces many of the vitamins it takes out. What it doesn't replace, however, is the protective phytonutrients such as beta-carotene. "Most people don't get enough of these nutrients to begin with, and olestra may take away some of what they do get," says Dr. Kantor.

In addition, people who eat a lot of foods containing olestra may have loose stools, abdominal cramps, and other digestive complaints. Because the fake fat isn't absorbed, it remains in the digestive tract. The more olestra you eat, the more likely you are to have these side effects, says Dr. McAllister.

The bottom line? "Snack foods containing olestra are slightly more expensive than regular brands, but if spending a few extra cents saves you a few extra pounds, they're well worth the price," says Dr. McAllister.

Bear in mind that foods containing olestra, like the high-fat foods they replace, shouldn't be staples in your diet, nutritionist Stark says. "If you eat them only as an occasional indulgence, you should be able to reap the fat-reducing benefits without facing the other consequences."

Fiber

THE ULTIMATE HEALER

HEALING POWER

Can Help:

Lower cholesterol

Reduce the risk of heart disease and cancer

Prevent constipation

Over a century ago, food manufacturers began stripping away the tough outer coatings of grains, leaving behind pure white flour. The breads they made with this refined white flour had a lighter texture and more delicate taste than whole-grain breads, and people preferred them. Other technological advances soon followed, and within a few years, processed foods were on every kitchen shelf. To make room for these processed foods in their kitchens and in their stomachs, people began eating fewer fruits, vegetables, legumes, and whole grains. As a result, for the first time in history, dietary fiber was largely absent from our diets. And it didn't seem to really matter. After all, fiber contains no nutrients. It isn't absorbed by the body, and it passes out of the digestive tract almost as quickly as it goes in.

Fast-forward to the 1960s. Seemingly all of a sudden, serious conditions like heart disease, cancer, and diabetes were on the rise in the United States, England, and other industrialized countries. But in other parts of the world, where people still got a lot of fiber in their diets, these diseases were much less prevalent. The reason, researchers guessed, was fiber. It turned out that fiber *did* matter, and we simply weren't getting enough of it. Suddenly those "advances" that removed the fiber from foods didn't seem so great anymore. "Today, the average person's consumption of fiber is about 15 grams, but we need 20 to 35 grams for optimal health, so it's really missing in our diets," says Jana Klauer, MD, a New York City–based physician who specializes in the biology of fat reduction and is the author of *How the Rich Stay Thin*.

Two-Way Protection

Dietary fiber is simply the tough, structural parts of fruits, vegetables, legumes, and grains, so what makes it so good for us? The most important thing is this: We don't break fiber down during digestion. Rather, it gets swept along more or less intact from the stomach to the intestines and from the intestines into the stool. This isn't a problem. In fact, it's precisely *because* fiber isn't absorbed that it's such a powerful healer.

Although we often talk about fiber as if it were a single substance, there are actually two main types—soluble and insoluble, says Barbara Harland, PhD, RD, professor of nutrition at Howard University in Washington, D.C. Most foods from plants contain both soluble and insoluble fiber, but they usually have more of one kind than the other. Apples, for example, contain mostly soluble fiber, while grains are higher in the insoluble kind.

Both types of fiber pass through the intestine without being absorbed, but that's where the similarity ends. Soluble and insoluble fiber act in totally different ways once they get inside the body, and as a result, they help protect against different conditions, says Dr. Harland. For example, if you have high cholesterol, your doctor may advise you to eat more soluble fiber, which can help lower the amounts of this dangerous substance in your bloodstream. If you have a family history of colon cancer, however, you may want to get more of the insoluble kind. A recent Japanese study published in the *Journal of Epidemiology* found a decreased risk of colon cancer with increased intakes of insoluble fiber.

You shouldn't worry *too much* about the kind of fiber you're getting, however, Dr. Harland says. If you eat a lot of fruits, vegetables, whole grains, and legumes, you'll automatically get healing amounts of both kinds.

A 2006 study published in the *Journal of the American Dietetic Association* compared the effects of soluble fiber in the form of barley and insoluble fiber in the form of whole wheat and brown rice on blood pressure levels in 25 participants. After 5 weeks, blood pressure levels dropped in all participants, regardless of whether they were eating the soluble or insoluble fiber. This suggests that increasing all types of whole-grain foods in your diet can reduce blood pressure.

Soluble Fiber: An Essential Barrier

Many of the things that cause disease, from chemicals in the environment to too much cholesterol in the diet, make their first assault inside the digestive tract. For example, when you eat a steak, molecules of fat and cholesterol from the steak pass through your intestinal wall and into your bloodstream. Or suppose there's a harmful substance inside the stool. As it rubs against the colon wall, it can damage sensitive cells, possibly increasing the risk of cancer.

It's here, inside the digestive tract, that soluble fiber provides the most protection. When it dissolves, soluble fiber forms a sticky gel that acts like a protective coating, preventing harmful substances from doing damage, says Dr. Harland.

To continue with the example of the steak, if you accompanied it with a bowl of beans, the soluble fiber in the beans would turn into a gel, trapping molecules of cholesterol from the steak and preventing them from getting into your body, explains Beth Kunkel, PhD, RD, professor of food and nutrition at Clemson University in South

Doctor's Top Tip

"Boost your fiber intake with berries," says Jana Klauer, MD, a New York City–based physician who specializes in the biology of fat reduction. "Grains are a good source of fiber, but by eating berries, you get the fiber plus the added vitamins and minerals," she notes.

Berries are also very high in the immunity-boosting antioxidant vitamins C and E. In fact, strawberries are higher in vitamin C than oranges, she says. And blueberries are high in resveratrol, a powerful antioxidant that protects your heart and blood vessels and may increase longevity.

And as if that weren't enough, Dr. Klauer adds, berries are very low in calories—you can have a whole cup for around 80 to 100 calories!

Carolina. And because the soluble fiber itself isn't absorbed, it passes out of the body into your stool, taking the cholesterol with it.

Research has shown that people who get the most soluble fiber in their diets are at the least risk for heart disease. In one study, for example, researchers at Tulane University in New Orleans studied the relationship between total dietary fiber intake and soluble fiber intake on the risk of cardiovascular disease in 9,776 adults. After 19 years, those who ate an average of 20.7 grams of fiber a day had significantly fewer cardiovascular disease events than the people who got an average of 5.9 grams a day. That risk was even lower in men with the highest intake of soluble fiber, indicating that a higher intake of dietary fiber, particularly soluble fiber, reduces the risk of cardiovascular disease.

Soluble fiber has other benefits as well. Because it causes nutrients to be absorbed more slowly, it helps you feel more satisfied after eating, so you snack less.

Insoluble Fiber: An Intestinal Sponge

The remarkable thing about insoluble fiber, and one of the reasons it is beneficial to your health, is that it leaves the digestive system in very nearly the same condition in which it went in, which is why doctors once believed that "roughage" played little part in good nutrition.

But insoluble fiber is more than just hardy. It's also incredibly absorbent. It can soak up many times its weight in water as it passes through the intestines. As a result, it causes stools to become larger, firmer, and easier to pass, which is why doctors recommend that people with constipation and other digestive complaints eat more insoluble fiber.

Insoluble fiber helps in yet another way. Because it causes stools to become larger, the intestine is able to move them along more quickly. This is key because the more time stools and any harmful compounds they contain stay in the colon, the more likely they are to damage cells and kick off the cancer process, Dr. Kunkel says.

Research has shown a link between a low intake of fiber and an elevated risk of colon cancer. In a major study conducted by the American Cancer Society, researchers examined the whole grain, fruit, and vegetable intake of 62,609 men and 70,554 women and found that men with a high vegetable intake had a 30 percent lower risk of colon cancer, and men with very low intake of vegetables and whole grains and women with a very low intake of fruits were more likely to have developed colon cancer 4 to 5 years later.

In the past, the exact reasons *why* a low intake of fiber increases risk for colon cancer were not clearly understood. But a recent study done at the Department of Surgery of the University of Texas Medical Branch shows that the reason may be at the molecular level. The researchers showed that a substance created by the fermentation of dietary fiber in the intestines, called sodium butyrate, may act as a colon cancer tumor suppressor.

It's not only the colon that benefits from insoluble fiber. Some evidence suggests that it may help reduce the risk of breast cancer as well.

Some studies show a relationship between dietary fiber and decreased risk of breast cancer, and others do not. However, there is evidence that dietary fiber may play a role in decreasing the circulating estrogens that can raise breast cancer risk. A study done by researchers at the Keck School of Medicine at the University of Southern California and presented at the American Association for Cancer Research third annual International Conference on Frontiers in Cancer Prevention Research looked at blood hormones of 252 Latina women in relation to their intakes of dietary fiber. The researchers found an inverse relationship between dietary fiber and the two female hormones estradiol and estrone in that as the fiber intakes increased, the hormone levels sharply decreased. So the take-home message is that eating insoluble fiber can help when it comes to preventing breast cancer.

Staying Lean

Soluble and insoluble fiber may act in different ways, but they combine their talents in the one area Americans need them most: losing weight. Every year, more and more of us try to shed a few pounds, and every year, we get a little heavier.

Fiber is an incredibly powerful tool for controlling weight, says Dr. Harland. Since foods that are high in fiber are very filling, you'll naturally eat a little less. Plus, when you're eating more fiber-rich foods, you'll automatically eat less of other, more-fattening, foods. "A very important way to lose weight and keep it off is to eat more fiber," Dr. Harland says.

Making the Change

People often think of high-fiber foods as being dry, heavy, or tasteless. But in fact, many of the foods we like best, such as fruits, freshly baked breads, and baked beans,

(continued on page 246)

THE FIBER FAIR

If you asked your doctor to name the one thing you need to stay healthy, the answer would probably be dietary fiber. Because fiber is found in so many foods, it's easy to get the recommended daily amount of 25 to 35 grams. To help you get started, here is a list of 40 top fiber foods.

Food	Portion	Soluble Fiber (g)	Insoluble Fiber (g)	Total Fiber (g)
CEREALS				
Kashi Go Lean	1 cup	1.0	9.0	10.0
Kashi Heart to Heart	¾ cup	1.0	4.0	5.0
Kashi Heart to Heart Instant Oatmeal	1 packet	3.0	2.0	5.0
Kellogg's All-Bran, Original	½ cup	1.0	9.0	10.0
Kellogg's All-Bran Yogurt Bites	1¼ cups	1.0	9.0	10.0
Kellogg's Bran Buds	30 grams	3.0	10.0	13.0
Kellogg's Complete Wheat Bran Flakes	¾ cup	1.0	4.0	5.0
Quaker Oat Bran, cooked	1 cup	3.0	2.3	5.3
Quaker Oat Bran, ready-to-eat	¼ cup	3.0	1.8	4.8
FRUITS				
Apple	1 medium	0.5	2.5	3.0
Avocado	1 medium	1.3	3.9	5.2
Blackberries	½ cup	1.0	3.0	4.0
Figs, dried	2	1.5	2.0	3.5
Gooseberries	½ cup	0.7	1.2	1.9
Guava	1	0.8	3.8	4.6
Kiwifruit	1 large	0.7	1.0	1.7
Mango	½	1.7	1.2	2.9
Prunes, pitted, dried, stewed	¼ cup	1.5	1.5	3.0
Raspberries, red	½ cup	0.4	3.8	4.2

Food	Portion	Soluble Fiber (g)	Insoluble Fiber (g)	Total Fiber (g)
GRAIN PRODUCTS				
Barley, cooked	½ cup	1.0	3.0	4.0
Brown rice, long-grain	½ cup	0.1	1.6	1.7
Bulgur	½ cup	0.5	2.4	2.9
Rye flour	2½ Tbsp	0.8	1.8	2.6
Wheat germ	4½ Tbsp	1.0	4.2	5.2
Whole-wheat bread	1 medium slice	0.3	1.6	1.9
LEGUMES				
Black beans	½ cup	2.0	3.5	5.5
Black-eyed peas	½ cup	1.0	4.5	5.5
Chickpeas	½ cup	1.0	5.0	6.0
Kidney beans	½ cup	3.0	3.0	6.0
Lentils	½ cup	1.0	7.0	8.0
Navy beans	½ cup	2.0	4.0	6.0
Pinto beans	½ cup	2.0	5.0	7.0
VEGETABLES				
Artichoke	1 medium	2.2	4.3	6.5
Broccoli, chopped, cooked	½ cup	1.0	0.5	1.5
Brussels sprouts, fresh or frozen	½ cup	3.0	1.5	4.5
Carrots, sliced, cooked	½ cup	1.0	1.5	2.5
Corn	½ cup	0.3	1.7	2.0
Peas, cooked	½ cup	1.2	3.1	4.3
Spinach, cooked	½ cup	0.5	1.5	2.0
Sweet potato, mashed	½ cup	1.4	2.4	3.8

FOOD ALERT

Turning Down the Gas

Even though it's hard to say anything negative about fiber, it does have a downside. When you eat too much fiber, too quickly, it has a tendency to, ahem, talk back.

Since fiber isn't absorbed, it ferments in the intestine, often causing gas, says Barbara Harland, PhD, RD, of Howard University. "Your intestines will have to get used to it," she says.

To get the benefits of fiber without the uncomfortable and potentially embarrassing bloat, she recommends adding it slowly to your diet. Start out, for example, by eating an extra 5 grams of fiber a day (the amount in a half-cup of raspberries or a sprinkling of chickpeas). Continue eating that amount, but don't add any extra for a few days. Then, when your body has made the adjustment and feels less bloated and gassy, start eating an extra 10 grams of fiber a day, and give yourself time to get used to that, and so forth. If you do this for several weeks, Dr. Harland says, you'll get all the fiber you need without the discomfort.

are also high in fiber. So it's easy to get the Daily Value (DV) of 25 grams of fiber. Here are a few tips for getting started:

Start your day with cereal. There are some cereals that are more of a source of sugar than anything else, so breakfast cereals have gotten a bad reputation when it comes to nutrition. However, many cereals, both hot and cold, are very high in fiber. A half-cup serving of All-Bran, for example, has 10 to 13 grams of fiber, depending on the type. And Kashi Go Lean cereal has 10 grams of fiber in a 1-cup serving.

Shop for whole grains. White bread, white rice, and other processed foods contain very little fiber. Whole grains have the most. However, a lot of breads with "wheat" on the label do not contain whole grains and supply very little fiber. So when you're stocking up on high-fiber foods, look for breads, flour, and pasta that say "100 percent whole grain" on the label.

Mix up your grains. To get a good mix of soluble and insoluble fiber, it helps to eat a variety of grains, Dr. Harland says. Foods made with oats, for example, contain mostly soluble fiber, while wheat and rice contain higher amounts of the insoluble kind.

Take advantage of produce. Fruits and vegetables also contain healthy amounts of fiber. "In fact, fresh fruit typically contains twice the fiber of whole grains, and nonstarchy vegetables contain about *eight* times the fiber of whole grains, says Dr. Klauer. One unpeeled apple, for example, has 6 grams of fiber; a half-cup of Brussels sprouts has more than 3 grams of fiber; and a half-cup of raspberries has more than 4 grams. So eating several servings of produce a day will provide much of the fiber you need.

Keep the peel. Much of the fiber in potatoes, fruits, and vegetables is found in the skins—the parts that many people throw away. To get the most benefit, whenever possible, serve them with their "coats" on, advises Dr. Harland.

Save the stems. When preparing vegetables like broccoli and asparagus, we often throw away the stems, which are the most fiber-rich parts, Dr. Harland says. But even when the stems are too tough to munch on, you can salvage much of the valuable fiber by cutting them into small pieces and adding them to casseroles, soups, or stews.

Stock up on beans. Regardless of whether you buy them canned or dry, beans are among the best fiber foods you can find. A half-cup of split peas, for example, has 8 grams of fiber, while a half-cup of lima beans has 7 grams.

Chickpeas with Onions and Raisins

1 tablespoon extra-virgin olive oil

1 cup finely chopped red onions

2 tablespoons raisins

2 cans (15 ounces each) chickpeas, rinsed and drained

1 tablespoon chopped fresh cilantro

In a medium saucepan, heat the oil over medium heat. Add the onions and raisins, and cook until the onions start to soften, about 4 to 5 minutes. Stir in the chickpeas. Cook, stirring, until heated through, about 2 to 3 minutes. Remove from the heat. Stir in the cilantro.

Makes 6 servings

PER SERVING

Calories: 159
Total fat: 4.8 g
Saturated fat: 0.3 g

Cholesterol: 0 mg
Sodium: 281 mg
Dietary fiber: 7.6 g

Fibrocystic Breasts
RELIEF FROM TENDERNESS

Nothing gives a woman more relief than learning that a lump in her breast is harmless. But that relief can quickly turn to frustration when the lump grows larger and more tender, or when additional lumps begin to appear. Even though the discomfort eases after menstruation, it comes back month after month.

An estimated 60 percent of women suffer from this condition, called fibrocystic breasts, which occurs when tiny, fluid-filled sacs form in the milk-producing glands. For many women, making a few simple dietary changes can help keep it under control, says Sharon Rosenbaum Smith, MD, breast surgeon at St. Luke's–Roosevelt Hospital in New York City.

The Caffeine Connection

Some studies have shown that eliminating foods and beverages that contain caffeine, such as cola, coffee, chocolate, and tea, helps improve fibrocystic breasts. "In some women, the avoidance of caffeine does help the pain of fibrocystic breasts," says Dr. Rosenbaum Smith.

In a study at Ohio State University in Columbus, 45 women who drank an average of 4 cups of coffee a day quit cold turkey. After 2 months, 37 of the women—82 percent—reported that the lumps and tenderness were entirely gone.

And it looks like women who drink little or no coffee are much less likely to get fibrocystic breasts in the first place. Researchers at Yale University School of Medicine found that women who drank about 2 cups of coffee a day were 150 percent more likely to develop fibrocystic breasts than women getting no caffeine. Women who had four to five cups a day were 230 percent more likely to have the problem.

Lean Relief

It's not only what you drink but also what you eat that can cause tender breasts. Research has shown that women who get a lot of fat in their diets—especially saturated fat, the kind found in meats and high-fat dairy foods—are more likely to develop fibrocystic breasts than women who eat leaner fare. In one small study, 10 women with fibrocystic breasts reduced their intake of dietary fat to 20 percent of total calories. Three months later, all 10 said that their breast pain was gone.

"You need to eat a low-fat diet for about 3 months to see if it helps," says David P. Rose, MD, PhD, retired chief of the division of nutrition and endocrinology at the Naylor Dana Institute of the American Health Foundation in Valhalla, New York, and the leader of the study. "That's how long it takes for the estrogen circulating in your blood to decrease."

To get the most protection, you should limit the amount of fat in your diet to 20 to 25 percent of total calories. There are many ways to reduce the amount of fat in your diet. For example, you should avoid red meats, drink low-fat (1%) or fat-free milk instead of whole milk, and eat more fruits, vegetables, legumes, and whole grains.

The Fiber Factor

Reducing fat isn't the only way to lower estrogen levels in your body. Eating more fruits and vegetables not only reduces fat but also provides more fiber in your diet. "Fiber can help reduce swelling and tenderness of the breasts by absorbing excess estrogen and carrying it out of the body," Dr. Rose explains.

The Daily Value (DV) for fiber is 25 grams. That should be enough to reduce the estrogen and help ease the pain of fibrocystic breasts, Dr. Rose says. One of the easiest ways to get more fiber is to eat bran-containing cereals at breakfast, he says. Eating nonstarchy vegetables, fruits, legumes, and grains will also add fiber to your diet.

Soothe with Soy

There is some evidence that soy protein can combat fibrocystic breast disease. A study published in *Integrative Cancer Therapies* examined the effect of daily soy consumption on women with fibrocystic breast disease. Sixty-four women were asked to consume soy protein daily without changing anything else in their diets. After 1 year, they had significantly less breast tenderness and fibrocystic breast disease.

Get Ease with E

There isn't solid scientific evidence to prove that it works, but some women—and their doctors—say that getting more vitamin E can help reduce the pain of fibrocystic breasts. "I recommend women try vitamin E for 2 to 3 months to see if it works," says Dr. Rosenbaum Smith.

Doctor's Top Tip

"The biggest contributing factor for fibrocystic change in the breasts is caffeine," says breast surgeon Sharon Rosenbaum Smith, MD, of St. Luke's–Roosevelt Hospital in New York City. "In some women, avoiding caffeine works, but it has to be the *complete* avoidance of caffeine," she says. So totally remove caffeine from your diet for 2 to 3 months, including tea, coffee, caffeinated soda, and chocolate, and see if the tenderness in your breasts improves.

One way to get extra vitamin E is to take supplements. The Mayo Clinic recommends taking 200 to 400 IU of vitamin E a day for fibrocystic breasts. But getting more vitamin E in your diet can also help. The best sources of vitamin E are vegetable oils like sunflower and safflower oils, which can be high in calories, but you can get vitamin E from other foods as well. A quarter-cup of toasted wheat germ, for example, has 8 IU of vitamin E, or 27 percent of the DV. Almonds are also an excellent source, with 1 ounce of toasted, unblanched almonds containing 7 IU, or 23 percent of the DV.

Don't Sweat Fibrocystic Breasts

"One of the most important things I can tell women with fibrocystic breasts is that they shouldn't worry; everything is okay. Women with fibrocystic breasts are no more likely to get breast cancer than women without the condition," Dr. Rosenbaum Smith says.

Figs
A FABULOUS FIBER FIND

HEALING POWER
Can Help:

Lower high blood pressure

Relieve constipation

Control cholesterol

Prevent colon cancer

Control weight gain

Best known in this country for its role in the ever-popular Fig Newton, the fig is perhaps the most significant fruit in history. The Assyrians used figs as sweeteners as far back as 3000 BC. Figs were Cleopatra's favorite fruit. And some historians believe that figs, not apples, were the forbidden fruit of the Garden of Eden—a debate that may never be resolved, although certainly fig leaves were a convenient fashion accessory of the time.

Today, we know that the fig is a fabulous source of fiber and a significant source of potassium. Plus, figs can add some vitamin B_6 to your diet.

Figs and Fiber

The average American gets only about 12 to 17 grams of dietary fiber a day, far short of the 20 to 30 grams recommended by the American Dietetic Association. The Daily Value (DV) for fiber is 25 grams.

"Fiber is so good for so many things," says Diane Grabowski-Nepa, RD, a dietitian and nutritional counselor at the Pritikin Longevity Center in Santa Monica, California. "Because fiber builds heavier stools, it helps you eliminate waste more quickly and efficiently, which studies show helps relieve constipation and possibly prevent colon cancer." Getting more fiber in your diet also helps lower cholesterol and prevents weight gain, thus lowering the risk of heart disease.

Figs are an excellent source of fiber. Three figs, dried or fresh, provide about 5 grams of fiber, or 20 percent of the DV. That 5 grams can go a long way. A Harvard University study of 43,757 men ages 40 to 75 found that those who got the most fiber had about half the risk of having heart attacks as those who got the least. Plus, men who added just 10 grams of fiber a day to their diets dropped their risks of heart disease by almost 30 percent.

"Figs are particularly good for people who are overweight, which is another risk factor for heart disease," says Grabowski-Nepa. Because they're so high in fiber, figs stay in the stomach longer and make people feel full, which helps them eat less. "And figs are very sweet, so they satisfy those sweet cravings," she adds. Figs are fairly high

Figs, both fresh and dried, are delicious and easy to work with. Here's how:

Shop for texture. Whether fresh or dried, figs should be firm but still yield slightly to the touch. If dried figs are rock hard, don't buy them. If fresh figs seem mushy, they're probably past their prime, and you should pass them by.

Eat them fast. Fresh figs go bad very quickly, usually within a week after leaving the tree. So don't buy more figs than you plan to eat within a few days. They'll stay fresh for about 3 days when stored in the refrigerator. Dried figs will keep for months when stored in the refrigerator in an airtight bag.

Make figs less sticky. Because figs are extremely sticky, they can be difficult to cut. Chilling the figs for an hour before cutting them will help prevent them from sticking to a knife or scissors.

---

in calories, however, so pay attention to the calorie count on packages, and don't eat them without restraint.

Help for High Blood Pressure

Figs are a good source of potassium, a mineral that's crucial for controlling blood pressure. Studies have shown that people who eat plenty of potassium-rich foods not only tend to have lower blood pressures but also have less risk of related conditions like blood clots and stroke.

Potassium helps lower high blood pressure in a number of ways. For one thing, it helps prevent dangerous low-density lipoprotein(LDL) cholesterol from building up on artery walls, says David B. Young, PhD, professor emeritus of physiology and biophysics at the University of Mississippi Medical Center in Jackson. Plus, it helps remove excess sodium from inside cells, keeping the body's fluid levels in balance and blood pressure in check.

In addition, potassium helps keep your heart strong. "It appears that even moderate potassium depletion weakens heart strength in both animals and otherwise healthy humans," says Dr. Young. "My colleagues and I also uncovered that potassium helps prevent blood clotting," he says.

Three fresh figs contain 348 milligrams of potassium, or 10 percent of the DV for this mineral. Dried figs are even better, with three figs providing 399 milligrams, or 11 percent of the DV.

A Boost of B_6

In addition to the fiber and the potassium, figs can add some vitamin B_6 to your diet. While most of us get plenty of vitamin B_6, older people don't absorb it as efficiently as they did when they were younger. And since taking certain medications can also interfere with getting enough B_6, getting extra amounts can be essential. To boost B_6, eat figs every day. Three fresh figs contain 0.2 milligram of B_6, or 9 percent of the DV for this vitamin.

GETTING THE MOST

Explore the sweetness. One reason that figs are underappreciated and underconsumed in this country is that people aren't sure what to do with them. An easy way to get more figs into your diet is to add it to foods that need a touch of sweetness, like cereals, cakes, or oatmeal. You can also mash figs into foods such as mashed potatoes or chop them up and add them to rice for a tasty, healthful side dish.

Doctor's Top Tip

"If you don't particularly like figs, one good way to get them is in one of the new raw food bars, such as Rawma Bars, Life Force Energy Bars, and Perfect 10 Bars, to name just a few," says Patricia David, MD, MSPH, president of Healthy U in Columbus, Ohio. A number of raw food bars contain figs as a main ingredient, along with a lot of other healthful foods, such as almonds, pumpkin seeds, pecans, and so on. Plus, these bars taste really good.

Figs Stuffed with Orange-Anise Cream

16 dried figs

4 ounces fat-free cream cheese, at room temperature

1 tablespoon fresh orange juice

2 teaspoons grated orange zest

1½ teaspoons honey

½ teaspoon anise seed, crushed

Trim and discard the stems from the figs. Cut down through the stem ends vertically and horizontally to make an "X." Gently push each fig open. Place the figs on a platter, cut side up.

In a medium bowl, combine the cream cheese, orange juice, orange zest, honey, and anise seed. With an electric beater or a wooden spoon, beat until creamy. Spoon a dollop of the mixture into the center of each fig.

Serve immediately, or cover with plastic wrap and refrigerate for up to 2 hours.

Makes 4 servings

PER SERVING

Calories: 228
Total fat: 0.9 g
Saturated fat: 0.2 g

Cholesterol: 2 mg
Sodium: 146 mg
Dietary fiber: 7 g

Fish

HEALTH FROM THE DEEP

HEALING POWER

Can Help:

Reduce the risk of heart disease

Prevent breast and colon cancers

Promote larger birth-weight babies

Reduce inflammation

For years, Americans have wisely been reducing the amount of fat in their diets. But there's one fat you may want to get more of instead of less: the fat in fish. When it comes to healthy eating, fish swims to first place.

Cold-water fish contain a number of polyunsaturated fats, which are known collectively as omega-3 fatty acids. Omega-3s benefit the fish by helping them stay warm in chilly waters. In people, the same fats go a long way toward promoting better health.

Consider Greenland's Eskimos. They eat fish to their hearts' content, which may be why they have very low levels of heart disease. Similar benefits have been observed in fish eaters around the world. People are simply a lot less likely to die from heart disease when fish plays a role in their diets. There is compelling research that the oils in fish may do far more than protect the heart, however.

Perhaps most significant, a team of scientists at the Harvard School of Public Health reported that overall mortality was 17 percent lower among people who ate fish twice a week compared with people who ate little or no seafood.

A big reason for these protective effects is omega-3s' ability to reduce inflammation. "As we eat more processed foods, such as cookies, crackers, and fast food, we get a lot of omega-6 fatty acids," says Gretchen Vannice, MS, RD, research coordinator at Nordic Naturals, who has studied omega-3 fatty acids extensively. "Omega-6 fatty acids increase inflammation. And omega-3 fatty acids decrease inflammation, so if we don't get enough omega-3s to counteract the omega-6s, we're in a constant state of inflammation. And inflammation puts us at risk for a whole host of conditions, including heart disease, overweight, and even depression," she says. "We should get a ratio of 4:1 omega-6s to omega-3 fatty acids, but most people get an estimated 15 to 20:1, so we're way undernourished with omega-3s."

Swim Away from Heart Disease

In the 1980s, a round of studies reported that a diet high in fish could help protect against heart disease, prompting many Americans to trade some of their red meat and poultry for a couple of fish meals each week. They made the right choice.

Research has shown that people who eat fish are less likely to die from heart disease than their non-fish-eating counterparts. A recent study done at the Harvard School of Public Health reported that the death rate from heart disease was 36 percent lower among people who ate fish twice a week compared with people who ate little or no seafood.

In a study done at King's College in London, participants ages 45 to 70 increased their omega-3 intake by eating fish until their ratio of omega-6s to omega-3s was 3:1. As a result, their triglycerides went down, lowering their risk of heart disease.

The omega-3s in fish appear to work by putting the brakes on the body's production of inflammatory prostaglandins, leukotrienes, and thromboxane, naturally occurring compounds that, in large amounts, may cause blood vessels to constrict, elevating blood pressure. These compounds also may promote unwanted clotting in the bloodstream, which can lead to heart disease.

Doctor's Top Tip

"The top salmon you can buy is the Alaskan salmon from the Yukon River, the longest river in the Bering Sea," says Jana Klauer, MD, a New York City–based physician who specializes in the biology of fat reduction. "The king salmon are so big and fatty, they're chock full of omega-3 fats. It is really a spectacular fish to consume," she says. "They are in season in May and flown out on ice. You can find them at many of the larger natural foods stores and supermarkets. A bonus for eating Alaskan salmon: By buying them, you are supporting a local economy—the native fishermen," she adds.

The ability of omega-3s to prevent clotting is particularly important, says James Kenney, PhD, RD, director of nutrition research and educator at the Pritikin Longevity Center and Spa in Aventura, Florida. Clots that form in the bloodstream can block the flow of blood to the heart or brain, possibly causing heart attacks or strokes. Further, the oil found in fish appears to raise levels of high-density lipoprotein cholesterol, the good cholesterol that helps keep fatty sludge from depositing in the arteries.

Research shows that fish can offer particular benefits to people who have already had one heart attack. Having two fish meals (up to a total of 12 ounces of fish) a week may reduce the chances of suffering a second, fatal heart attack.

In addition to its favorable effects on clotting and cholesterol, the oil in fish appears to help keep the heart beating in a healthy rhythm. This is important because potentially serious heartbeat irregularities, called arrhythmias, may lead to cardiac arrest, in which the heart stops beating entirely. There is increasing evidence that the omega-3s in fish somehow fortify the heart muscle and keep it beating regularly. In one study, people getting nearly 6 grams of omega-3s a month—the equivalent of having a 3-ounce serving of salmon weekly—had half the risk of cardiac arrest as those who ate no omega-3s.

And the heart-healthy benefits seem to extend beyond adults into kids as well. A report released by the Institute of Medicine in Washington, D.C., showed that the heart benefits of seafood outweigh the risks in infants as well as in adults.

The report showed that omega-3 fatty acids found in fish promote healthy vision and brain development in infants whose mothers consume seafood while they are pregnant or breastfeeding. These healthy fats also appear to lower the risk of delivering a preterm or low-birthweight baby.

As a result of the heart-protective benefits of fish, the American Heart Association recommends that all adults eat fish at least two times a week. However, the AHA also notes that some types of fish may contain high levels of mercury, PCBs (polychlorinated biphenyls), dioxins, and other environmental contaminants. Levels of these substances are generally highest in older, larger, predatory fish and marine mammals. The benefits and risks of eating fish vary depending on a person's stage of life. Children and pregnant and breastfeeding women should follow FDA guidelines for avoiding mercury-contaminated fish. Fish with potential for the highest mercury contamination are shark, swordfish, king mackerel, and tilefish. Eating a variety of fish will help minimize any potentially adverse effects due to environmental pollutants.

In the Kitchen

While fresh fish delivers some of the most delicate flavors imaginable, it goes bad in a hurry. One day may be all it takes to turn a beautiful, flavorful fish into a dish you'd rather forget. To get the best taste from fish every time, here's what you can do:

Follow your nose. Fresh fish should smell just slightly briny. Off odors develop in the gut cavity first. When buying fish, always take a sniff in the belly area to make sure the fish is clean and fresh.

Incidentally, beware of fish that has been prewrapped in plastic. Unless the fish has been frozen, it can go bad very quickly.

Look at the eyes. When buying whole fish, look at the eyes; if the fish is fresh, they will be clear, bright, and bulging. Eyes that are slightly milky or sunken are an indication of the condition of the fish—that freshness is waning.

Check the gills. The gills should be moist and bright red, almost burgundy. If they are gray or brown, the fish is old, and you should pass it by.

Press the flesh. The flesh on fresh fish should be firm and springy. If you press it with your finger, and the indentation remains, the fish is old and won't deliver the best flavor.

Fighting Cancer

Nutritionists have long advised us to eat less fat, especially the fats in meats and dairy products, to reduce the risk of certain types of cancer. But the fat in fish is a healthy exception. "There's excellent evidence that eating fish provides protection against breast and colorectal cancers," says Bandaru S. Reddy, PhD, professor of research in the department of chemical biology at Rutgers University in New Brunswick, New Jersey.

Fish protects against cancer in much the same way that it helps prevent heart disease—by reducing the body's production of prostaglandins. In large amounts, prostaglandins act as tumor promoters—that is, they encourage cancer tumors to grow, says Dr. Reddy.

In a study of people in 24 European countries, British researchers found that people who regularly included fish in their diets were much less likely to get cancer. Indeed, they estimated that having small servings of fish three times a week, in addition to decreasing intake of animal fats, would reduce the death rate from colon cancer in men by nearly one-third.

Better Breathing

You wouldn't think that eating fish could improve breathing difficulties caused by smoking, but that's exactly what researchers have found. Consumption of fish has been linked with better lung function in adults.

There's only so much that the occasional tuna steak can do to protect you from developing lung disease if you smoke. But if you're trying to quit or if you live with someone who smokes, eating fish is one way to reduce the damage. "If you smoke, you are under big-time oxidative stress, which will increase inflammation," says Vannice. "Omega-3 fatty acids in fish help protect cell walls, which will reduce the oxidative stress. Plus, omega-3s will help your nerves and therefore lower your anxiety level—a big thing for people who are trying to quit," she says.

Multiple Protection

Here are two additional reasons to get more fish in your diet. In one study, researchers looked at the fish-eating habits of more than 8,700 expectant moms in Denmark. They found that the more fish the women ate, the less likely they were to deliver preterm, and the less likely they were to have a baby with a low birthweight. This is important because larger babies are usually healthier than those who are underweight.

Researchers speculate that the omega-3s in fish prevent preterm delivery by helping to promote bloodflow through the placenta, allowing the fetus to get more nutrients. In addition, by blocking the effects of prostaglandins, which are responsible for initiating uterine contractions, omega-3s might help prevent early labors and deliveries.

The omega-3 fatty acids in fish also help protect against autoimmune diseases, such as rheumatoid arthritis, and help prevent dementia and Alzheimer's disease, says Vannice. In addition, two studies have shown that taking fish oil in addition to exercising for 45 minutes, three times a week, leads to a lower percentage body fat, suggesting that fish oil may also aid in weight loss.

GETTING THE MOST

Shop for salmon. All fish provide some omega-3s, but salmon is perhaps the best choice, with a 3-ounce serving of Chinook (king) salmon providing 3 grams.

Don't fish for farm-raised varieties. "Farm-raised fish are often fed grains instead of their natural diets, which affects the fat in their bodies—when they are fed omega-6 fats in the grains, they become sources of omega-6 fats," says Jana Klauer, MD, a New York City–based physician, who specializes in the biology of fat reduction and is the author of *How the Rich Stay Thin*.

Look for deep colors. The more deeply colored the salmon, the more omega-3s it provides. As a rule of thumb, the more expensive varieties of salmon generally have the most omega-3s.

Shop for variety. It's not only salmon that has omega-3s. Other good sources include Spanish mackerel, tuna, sardines, anchovies, whitefish (fresh, not smoked), and herring.

Enjoy it canned. One of the easiest ways to get more omega-3s into your diet is to pick up a can of water-packed chunk light tuna (avoid albacore, which has been linked to mercury). If you're making tuna salad, choose a low-fat or fat-free mayonnaise, or skip the mayo altogether and use a mustard instead. The unhealthy fats in regular full-fat mayonnaise will more than offset the benefits of the healthy fats in the fish.

Use your microwave. The high cooking temperatures used in conventional cooking methods such as broiling can destroy nearly half the omega-3s in fish. Microwaving has little effect on these beneficial oils, however, so it's a good cooking choice for getting the most benefits from your fish.

Microwave-Steamed Salmon with Leeks

- **4 Chinook (king) salmon fillets (4 ounces each)**
- **1 large leek**
- **1 tablespoon grated fresh ginger**
- **1 tablespoon dry sherry**
- **2 teaspoons reduced-sodium soy sauce**

Rinse the salmon with cold water. Pat dry with paper towels.

Trim both the tough green part and the root end from the leek and discard them. Cut the leek in half lengthwise. Rinse thoroughly with cold water, pulling apart the layers to remove all the grit.

Cut the leek into very thin slices. Spread two-thirds of the slices evenly over a large microwaveable plate. Cover loosely with waxed paper, and microwave on high for 30 seconds.

In a small bowl, combine the ginger, sherry, soy sauce, and the remaining leek slices.

Place the salmon on the plate over the microwaved leek slices, skin side down and with the pieces arranged in spoke-fashion so the thickest parts face outward. Pour the ginger mixture evenly over the top. Cover loosely with waxed paper.

Microwave on high for 4 to 6 minutes, or until the salmon is opaque in the center. Test for doneness by inserting the tip of a sharp knife in the center of 1 fillet.

Let stand for 5 minutes before serving.

Makes 4 servings

PER SERVING

Calories: 229
Total fat: 11.9 g
Saturated fat: 2.9 g

Cholesterol: 75 mg
Sodium: 232 mg
Dietary fiber: 0.9 g

Mediterranean Tuna Wrap

2 pieces Armenian flatbread (lavash)

1 can (6 ounces) water-packed chunk light tuna, drained

4 tablespoons fat-free dill vegetable dip

1 can (2.25 ounces) black olives, drained and sliced

10 baby carrots, sliced lengthwise

1 cup mixed salad greens

Place the lavash on a cutting board.

In a small bowl, combine the tuna, vegetable dip, and olives. Spoon the tuna mixture down the middle of each lavash.

Cover the tuna mixture with the sliced carrots, then cover the carrots with the salad greens.

Tuck in one or both ends of each lavash, and roll up tightly. Slice each crosswise in half.

Makes 2 servings

Cook's Notes: *You can easily double or triple this recipe for a crowd. Use leftover dip with leftover baby carrots for healthy snacks.*

PER SERVING

Calories: 277
Total fat: 5.5 g
Saturated fat: 0.5 g

Cholesterol: 53 mg
Sodium: 794 mg
Dietary fiber: 4 g

Flavonoids

THE HEALING PIGMENTS

When tea first arrived on the shores of England, merchants sold it like snake oil. "Cure your migraines, drowsiness, lethargy, paralysis, vertigo, epilepsy, colic, gallstones, and consumption—guaranteed!" And the public bought it by the ton.

People didn't get the medical miracles they were hoping for, of course. And yet, they may have gotten something better. Tea, along with dark chocolate, cranberries, grapes, strawberries, blueberries, and other fruits and vegetables, contains tiny crystals called bioflavonoids, or flavonoids for short. These compounds, which give foods some of their colors, have been shown to help prevent a number of serious health threats, including heart and liver diseases.

HEALING POWER
Can Help:

Reduce the risk of heart disease

Treat liver disorders

Improve brain function

Possibly inhibit the growth of cancer

Scientists have speculated that what make flavonoids so powerful are their antioxidant abilities. Antioxidants help neutralize dangerous oxygen molecules called free radicals, which are found naturally in the body, thus preventing them from damaging tissue and causing disease.

"Lately, however, researchers are moving away from the theory that flavonoids act as antioxidants in the body," says Joe A. Vinson, PhD, professor of analytical chemistry at the University of Scranton in Pennsylvania, specializing in the study of these compounds. "It seems that it is not always a direct 'antioxidants trapping free radicals' story. People are finding out new mechanisms by which they work."

But the power of flavonoids to help protect the body against certain diseases and conditions—most notably, heart disease—is not in question.

There is a legion of things these compounds do, including boosting immunity, possibly inhibiting cancer, preventing hardening of the arteries, and maybe even slowing down the aging process and boosting brain power.

Help for the Heart

For years, researchers pondered how the French could drink red wine at lunch and dinner, pack away enough butter and lard to fill a Parisian pastry shop, and smoke just as much or more than Americans do, yet still have heart disease rates 2½ times lower than ours.

While the French may take delight in puffed pastries and smokes, they also eat a lot of fruits and vegetables. This is important because these foods, along with the red wines they enjoy, are good sources of flavonoids, which appear to help stop the process that allows cholesterol to stick to artery walls.

One Italian study examined more than 700 people with a history of heart attack for 8 years and looked at their intake of anthocyanidins, flavonoids found in blue/purple and red fruits such as blueberries, blackberries, cranberries, raspberries, and strawberries. They found that the men with the highest intake of anthocyanidins had the lowest rate of heart attacks, indicating that the flavonoids in these fruits seem to be protective.

In another study, Finnish researchers found that people with very low intakes of flavonoids during a 25-year period had higher risks of heart disease.

And a review published in the *Journal of Alternative and Complementary Medicine* showed that consumption of both green and black tea led to a decrease in atherosclerosis and an improvement in overall heart health.

There seems to be a common method for several kinds of foods and beverages containing flavonoids to make arteries more flexible and able to deal with the stresses of high-fat foods and exercise, says Dr. Vinson. "So after a meal or exercise, when your blood pressure naturally goes up, your arteries are nice and flexible and able to adjust to the changes in bloodflow," he says.

Much of the credit for these benefits goes to quercetin, one of the most powerful of the flavonoids, which is found in good amounts in onions and red apples. "Quercetin is a more powerful antioxidant than vitamin E, which is well known for its role in heart disease prevention," says John D. Folts, PhD, professor of medicine and director of the coronary thrombosis laboratory at the University of Wisconsin School of Medicine and Public Health in Madison.

It's not only the antioxidant action that makes flavonoids so protective, says Dr. Folts. Evidence suggests that these compounds may also act like a nonstick coating in the bloodstream, preventing platelets, the tiny disks in the blood that cause clotting, from sticking to artery walls and causing blockages.

Elixir for the Liver

In European countries, where natural plant compounds are commonly used for their curative qualities, flavonoids have been longtime favorites. For example, European clinics commonly use silymarin, a flavonoid found in certain types of artichokes, to treat alcohol-related liver disorders.

In addition, Dutch scientists have found that giving large doses of silymarin to animals prior to surgery can prevent potential liver damage from oxygen deprivation during the operation.

Hope for Cancer

Just as free radicals in the body can damage blood vessels leading to the heart, they also can damage DNA, the genetic material inside cells that tells them how to function. This DNA damage can lead to cancer. Since flavonoids help block free radicals, it would make sense that they would help prevent cancer as well.

So far, a number of large studies have failed to establish a cancer-protective link. "Unfortunately, the cancer and flavonoids story is never really satisfactory to those of us in science," says Dr. Vinson. In part, this may be because researchers have concentrated on the major flavonoids, like quercetin, rather than on some of their lesser-known kin.

It appears that some flavonoids, like silymarin and tangeretin, which is found beneath the rind of oranges, lemons, and other citrus fruits, may, in fact, play a role in preventing cancer. More research is necessary in this area, however.

In studies on rats, for example, researchers at the University of Madras in India found that silymarin helped stop the growth of a certain form of liver cancer.

> ### Doctor's Top Tip
>
> "You can never get enough green tea," says Joe A. Vinson, PhD, who specializes in the study of flavonoids. In studies, green tea appears to be particularly effective at lowering the risk of heart disease and improving cognitive function. "The only reason to worry about getting too much green tea is if you have anemia (the caffeine in green tea can worsen the problem or even bring it on), and even then, all you have to do is take your tea with vitamin C, and you solve that problem immediately," he says. So drink up!

Brain Booster

Flavonoids seem to improve our ability to think as well. A Japanese study looked at the relationship between green tea and cognitive function in humans. They studied the green tea consumption of 1,003 people ages 70 and under and found that those with a higher intake of green tea had a lower presence of cognitive impairment. So it appears that green tea may help protect the brain from age-related decline.

Finding Flavonoids

It can be a bit tricky to get enough flavonoids in your diet, not because they're scarce but because they often hide in out-of-the-way places—in the white stuff beneath an orange rind, for example, or inside an apple's peel.

The richest sources of flavonoids include green tea, onions, kale, green beans, broccoli, endive, cranberries, and citrus fruits (in the peel and white pulp). Also good are red wines, lettuce, tomatoes, tomato juice, sweet red peppers, broad beans, strawberries, apples (with the skin), grapes, grape juice, and dark chocolate.

Flaxseed

GOOD FOR THE HEART—AND MORE

HEALING POWER

Can Help:

Improve kidney function

Reduce the risk of heart disease

Prevent cancer

For centuries, flaxseed (and the plant from which it comes) was used for just about everything except food. Flax is one of the oldest sources of textile fiber and is used in making linen. Its seed, also known as linseed, is used for making paint. In the modern world, the closest it ever came to being a food was its use as a livestock feed.

Until about a decade ago, that is.

Nowadays, because of its newfound fame as a "health food," Americans are enjoying the slightly sweet, nutty taste of flaxseed. And they're getting protection from heart disease and cancer as a reward.

"Flaxseed is a rich plant source of omega-3 fatty acids. Not only are omega-3s crucial to good vision, they help fight weight gain by increasing metabolic rate, and they protect against cancer growth," says Janet Maccaro, PhD, ND, a holistic nutritionist in Ormond Beach, Florida, who is president of Dr. Janet's Balance By Nature Products and the author of *Natural Health Remedies A–Z*. "In addition, omega-3 fatty acids appear to help prevent atherosclerosis, raise good HDL cholesterol, and reduce inflammation, and they may also help lower depression," she says.

Heart and Kidney Helper

Studies show that the omega-3 fatty acids that flaxseed contains (which are also found in fish, although fish contains different omega-3 acids than flaxseed) appear to reduce the incidence of blood clotting, which can increase the risk of heart disease and stroke.

In addition, flaxseed is an incredibly rich source of a group of compounds called lignans. While many plant foods contain lignans, flaxseed has by far the most—at least 75 times more than any other plant food. (For example, you'd have to eat about 60 cups of fresh broccoli or 100 slices of whole-wheat bread to get the same amount of lignans in ¼ cup of flaxseed.) Lignans are important because they may have powerful antioxidant properties that can help block the cell-damaging effects of harmful oxygen molecules called free radicals. Foods rich in lignans have been found to lead to a lower risk of heart disease. A Finnish study of nearly 2,000 men found that those with the highest lignan intake were significantly less likely to die from heart disease than those with the lowest intake.

Flaxseed also appears to lower levels of dangerous low-density lipoprotein (LDL) cholesterol, the kind that contributes to heart disease. Three small studies showed that people who added 38 to 50 grams per day of flaxseed to their diets for 4 to 6 weeks had an 8 to 14 percent reduction in their LDL cholesterol levels.

Besides its heart-health potential, flaxseed shows some promise for reversing kidney damage caused by lupus, a condition in which the immune system produces harmful substances that attack and damage healthy tissues. When researchers at the University of Western Ontario gave flaxseed to nine people with lupus-related kidney disease, they discovered that several measurements of kidney function, including the ability to filter waste, quickly improved. The researchers speculate that the lignans and omega-3s in flaxseed fight inflammation in the tiny and very fragile arteries that supply blood to the kidneys, helping reduce the artery-clogging process that can lead to kidney damage.

Cancer Control

In addition to helping your heart, the lignans in flaxseed are thought to fight changes in the body that can lead to cancer.

"Lignans subdue cancerous changes once they've occurred, rendering them less likely to race out of control and develop into full-blown cancer," says Lilian Thompson, PhD, professor of nutritional sciences at the University of Toronto, who conducts research on flax. Lignans show some promise for battling certain types of cancer, including breast cancer and ovarian and endometrial cancers, but the research is fairly inconclusive at this point. One study of German women showed that those with the highest levels of a lignan called matairesinol were less likely to get breast cancer. The results of other studies on breast cancer and lignans have not shown a reduced risk, so the jury is still out. However, it certainly cannot hurt women to eat some flaxseed in an effort to help reduce their risk for breast cancer.

Furthermore, in the only case-controlled study of lignans and endometrial cancer risk, US women who ate the most lignans had the lowest risk of endometrial cancer, but that lowered risk was only significant in postmenopausal women. The results were similar when researchers looked at lignans and risk for ovarian cancer, so there does appear to be some promise for lignans when it comes to helping prevent these female cancers.

Flaxseed has two additional secrets that may give it cancer-fighting power as well. The omega-3 fatty acids in flaxseed appear to help limit the body's production of chemicals called prostaglandins. This is important because prostaglandins, in large

Doctor's Top Tip

"You can put flaxseeds on almost anything to get their health-promoting benefits," says holistic nutritionist Janet Maccaro, PhD, ND, a holistic nutritionist in Ormond Beach, Florida. "Sprinkle some on cottage cheese, or put them in a salad. You can even mix them into meat loaf before you bake it," she says. Ground flaxseeds add wonderful flavor and a palate-pleasing crunch.

amounts, may speed up tumor growth, says Bandaru S. Reddy, PhD, professor of research in the department of chemical biology at Rutgers University in New Brunswick, New Jersey.

In addition, flaxseed is very high in fiber. Three tablespoons of seeds contains 3 grams of fiber, or about 12 percent of the Daily Value. Fiber is very important in the diet because it can help block the effects of harmful compounds that over time may cause changes in the intestine that can lead to cancer. It also helps to move these compounds out of the intestine more quickly, giving them less time to do harm.

GETTING THE MOST

Buy it processed. Many people sprinkle whole flaxseed on salads or fresh-baked breads because they falsely think it is the better form. Whole flaxseed provides little benefit, however, because the body is unable to crack open the hard little shells surrounding the seeds. Flaxseed is the one food that provides more nutritional benefits in its processed form. So instead, buy the cracked or milled forms, which readily give up the nutritious goodness packed inside.

Pass on the oil. In an attempt to capitalize on flaxseed's healthful reputation, some manufacturers are touting flaxseed oil as a source of omega-3s. Some are even offering high-lignan oil that contains some of the seed residue.

But, there are good reasons to let the oil slide.

Most of the lignans found in flaxseed are in the meal—the non-oil part of the seed. While the oil may contain some lignans, it can't compete with the seeds. In addition, while flaxseed oil isn't without benefits, it doesn't provide as much of the other healthful compounds found in the seeds, such as fiber, protein, and minerals.

Start your day with some flax cereal. "Flax is great for elimination—it keeps you regular," says Dr. Maccaro. So eat a cereal containing flaxseed, such as Uncle Sam's or Nature's Path, and your day will be off to a good start. Don't care for the cereals that contain flax? Sprinkle the seeds into your favorite cereal for some added nutritional crunch.

Flax Banana Bread

½ cup packed light brown sugar

½ cup low-fat buttermilk

¼ cup fat-free egg substitute

3 tablespoons canola oil

¾ cup all-purpose flour

½ cup whole-wheat flour

¾ cup ground flaxseed

1 teaspoon baking powder

1 teaspoon baking soda

⅛ teaspoon salt

1 cup puréed bananas

Preheat the oven to 350°F. Coat a nonstick 8- × 4-inch loaf pan with cooking spray.

In a large bowl, combine the sugar, buttermilk, egg substitute, and oil. Whisk until smooth.

In a medium bowl, combine the all-purpose flour, whole-wheat flour, flaxseed, baking powder, baking soda, and salt. Whisk to mix.

Add to the liquid ingredients, and stir just until blended; do not overmix. Add the bananas and stir to mix.

Pour into the prepared pan. Bake for 40 to 50 minutes, or until a knife inserted in the center comes out clean. Remove the pan to a wire rack, and let the bread cool slightly. While it is still slightly warm, turn the bread out of the pan.

Makes 10 slices

Cook's Notes: *For best results, choose very ripe bananas, place them in a blender or food processor, and purée until smooth. Ground flaxseed is sold in natural food stores. Store any unused flaxseed in a tightly sealed container in the refrigerator or freezer.*

PER SLICE

Calories: 202
Total fat: 8.3 g
Saturated fat: 0.4 g

Cholesterol: 0 mg
Sodium: 227 mg
Dietary fiber: 2.4 g

Food Allergy
THE DANGERS OF DINING

A man who is allergic to shellfish orders a hamburger and fries. Minutes after his meal, he's gasping for breath. He finds out later that the oil used for his french fries was also used to fry shrimp.

When it comes to food allergies, knowing which foods will trigger an attack isn't always enough, since the offenders can appear in the most unexpected places. If you have a food allergy, you literally have to be on guard all the time and prepared to deal with an attack.

Confused Defenses

Food allergies occur when your body's immune system mistakenly identifies food proteins as enemies rather than friends. When you eat an offending food, your immune system launches an attack. Depending on the food and your individual system, the result may be congestion, digestive complaints, itchy skin, swelling of the mouth and hands, or even difficulty breathing. Even healthful foods such as low-fat milk or wheat are capable of triggering an allergy attack.

Food allergies are most common in children. Kids usually outgrow them, but some allergies, mainly those involving peanuts and shellfish, can last a lifetime, says Talal M. Nsouli, MD, clinical associate professor of allergy and immunology at Georgetown University School of Medicine and director of the Watergate Allergy and Asthma Center, both in Washington, D.C. Foods that commonly cause allergies include eggs, soy, wheat, peanuts, and shellfish, although almost any food is capable of causing allergies, Dr. Nsouli says.

Food allergies usually run in families. "Both my son and daughter have allergies," says Patricia David, MD, MSPH, president of Healthy U in Columbus, Ohio, who is also a preventive medicine specialist. In fact, if one of your parents has a food allergy, you have a 20 to 30 percent chance of developing one yourself. And if both of your parents have food allergies, your risk climbs to 40 to 70 percent.

It's not clear what causes food allergies. One theory, says Dr. Nsouli, is that infants and children who eat problem foods before their immune systems have fully matured may develop lifelong allergies to those foods. For this reason, doctors often recommend that infants should not be given solid food until they're 6 months old or

EARACHES: THE FOOD CONNECTION

Ear infections are one of the most common reasons for office visits to pediatricians, and they're also the leading reason for surgery on children in the United States. They're frustrating to treat because, despite taking antibiotics, some children get ear infections over and over again.

Food allergies may play a key role in ear infections. The reason is that children who are allergic to foods often have frequent congestion. As fluids and bacteria accumulate in the tube connecting the nose and middle ear, infections are much more likely to occur.

In a study done by Talal M. Nsouli, MD, professor of allergy and immunology at Georgetown University, and his colleagues, 81 of 104 children with recurrent ear infections were found to have food allergies. In fact, when Dr. Nsouli put the children on diets without the offending foods, most experienced significant improvements. When the children who had improved were allowed to eat the foods again, 94 percent got another ear infection.

Any child who has recurrent ear infections should go to an allergist.

cow's milk until they are at least a year. In addition, parents should refrain from giving their children eggs until they reach age 2 or fish and peanuts until they are 3 years of age.

Another way to prevent food allergies in children is to breastfeed them as infants. Breastfed babies get the intestinal flora from their mothers' milk that helps build their immune systems and therefore protects them from allergies, says Jose Saavedra, MD, medical and scientific director of Nestlé Nutrition USA, and associate professor of pediatrics at Johns Hopkins University School of Medicine and Bloomberg School of Hygiene and Public Health in Baltimore.

Little Tastes, Big Problems

People with mild food allergies may be able to eat small portions of an offending food every once in a while. But some people's allergies are so severe that even a trace of the food can lead to a potentially life-threatening condition called anaphylaxis. For those with serious allergies, the problem foods "should be avoided like poisons," Dr. Nsouli says.

Because it's often hard to know exactly what is in the foods you eat, doctors advise that people with severe food allergies carry self-injecting syringes loaded with epinephrine. This medication can stop anaphylactic attacks almost instantly.

Doctor's Top Tip

"My son has a peanut allergy, and while I was researching his allergy, I found a study done in Spain that said the probiotic lactobacillus has been shown to decrease allergy symptoms," says Patricia David, MD, MSPH, president of Healthy U in Columbus, Ohio. So I started giving him some foods containing probiotics. When I took him to the allergist a year later, he no longer had a life-threatening anaphylactic reaction—now he only gets a rash if he's exposed to peanuts," she says. "I am not advocating that everyone do this, especially when it comes to an allergy as serious as a peanut allergy, but it certainly shows that probiotics can help with food allergies. If you keep the good bacteria in your gut in full force, they may help keep milder allergic reactions at bay," she says. Rather than purchasing probiotic supplements or drinks, Dr. David recommends getting probiotics from food sources, such as yogurt, buttermilk, and soy milk. Look for products containing lactobacillus or bifidobacteria.

Eating Safely

Even though there is no cure for food allergies, there are many things you can do to prevent attacks. For starters, read labels carefully. You can't assume that a product doesn't contain the offending ingredient, Dr. Nsouli says. If you're allergic to peanuts, for example, it's obvious that peanut butter is *verboten*. But many other foods, including plain M&Ms candies, also contain hidden peanuts, in the form of peanut powder.

To make things more complicated, food companies may throw consumers a curveball by periodically changing ingredients in their products. Just because a food doesn't contain an offending ingredient today doesn't mean that it never will. So keep reading labels.

If all food labels used everyday language, such as "milk," for example, or "wheat," avoiding certain foods would be easy. But in the complex world of food processing, and with the complex names given to processed foods, it's not always easy to tell what you're getting. That's why people with food allergies often need a crash course in food vocabulary. If you're allergic to dairy foods, for example, you'll soon learn that ingredients such as casein and whey are just as dangerous as a glass of milk. Be sure to ask your doctor for a complete list of the products and ingredients—and all their odd names—that you'll need to avoid, Dr. Nsouli says.

Even when you know what foods to avoid, eating in restaurants can be tricky since you can't control what goes into each dish. To be sure you know what you're getting, ask your waiter to quiz the cook. Ask about oils, spices, and any other ingredients that you may be concerned about.

One way to make sure your dinner doesn't take you by surprise is to make it clear to the people preparing your food just how serious your food allergy is. Explain that it's not only certain ingredients that can make you ill but even what those ingredients have touched, like grills, spoons, and mixing bowls. "Warn them," Dr. Nsouli says.

Once they understand how serious your condition really is, they'll pay closer attention to what goes on your plate.

Some foods are very easy to eliminate from your diet because there are so many substitutes available. People who are allergic to cow's milk, for example, often switch to soy or rice milk, says Dr. Nsouli. (These products are often fortified with calcium, so you get the benefits of milk without the problems.) Other foods are more difficult to replace. Even though you can substitute rice flour for wheat flour, for instance, it has a noticeably different taste and texture than bread made with wheat flour. You may want to try rye, millet, or barley flour instead. You'll just have to experiment to find foods that satisfy your taste buds without upsetting your system.

Food Supplements
WHEN DIET LETS YOU DOWN

Try as you might to eat the recommended 1 to 2 cups of fruits, 2 to 3 cups of vegetables, and 3 to 4 ounces of grains every day, sometimes all you can manage is a double cheeseburger accompanied by an equally large serving of fries.

We live fast-paced lives, and we spend too many lunch hours rushing through fast-food lines or idling in drive-thrus. So we head to the supermarket or pharmacy, where we load up on vitamins, minerals, and food extracts in the hope that these pills will give us a little backup health insurance when our diets let us down.

But are these supplements really doing us any good?

"They certainly can," says Mary Ellen Camire, PhD, professor in the department of food science and human nutrition at the University of Maine in Orono. "When you're running around and skipping meals, taking a multivitamin can help you get nutrients that you may be missing."

In fact, many doctors now believe that supplements may do more than make up for shortfalls in nutrition. Evidence suggests that even when you're eating well, taking supplements will make you healthier, says Michael Janson, MD, author of *Dr. Janson's New Vitamin Revolution*. "The scientific literature is clear that people who get certain nutrients, like vitamins C and E, in higher levels than you can get from foods are going to get additional benefits," says Dr. Janson.

Beyond the Minimum

For more than 60 years, the federal Food and Nutrition Board, a committee of the National Academy of Sciences–National Research Council, which is made up of a prestigious group of nutritional scientists, has been telling us how much of various nutrients we should try to get from our food each day. The board's recommendations, called Recommended Dietary Allowances, are meant to serve as goals for good basic nutrition. (A shorthand version of these recommendations, called Daily Values, or DVs, are the numbers that you see on food labels.)

In more recent years, however, scientists have begun finding connections between vitamins and the prevention of a number of health threats that they weren't previously aware of, including links to cancer and heart disease. Even though the DVs are high enough to prevent deficiency diseases, such as rickets, scurvy, and beriberi, which used to be common problems in society, they may not be high enough to prevent other diseases that are much more prevalent today.

This deficiency is particularly true of antioxidant vitamins, such as vitamins C and E. Antioxidants are essential for blocking the effects of destructive oxygen molecules called free radicals, which damage healthy cells and are thought to be a major contributor to serious health conditions such as heart disease, cancer, and others. Because free radicals are created in enormous numbers every day, the amounts of antioxidants represented by the DVs may not be enough to stop the damage.

Another important nutrient that many Americans are lacking is omega-3 fatty acids. Omega-3s are "essential" fatty acids, meaning that our bodies don't make them—we must ingest them to get their benefits. The most powerful omega-3 fatty acids when it comes to good health appear to come from fish oils, which contain eicosapentaenoic acid (EPA) and docosahexaenoic acid (DHA).

There are plenty of benefits in making sure your diet is high in omega-3s. Research has shown that these fats, found in fatty fish, canola oil, flaxseed, and walnuts, among other foods, help prevent heart disease and cancer, improve joint health, and may even be protective against depression and dementia. Unfortunately, Americans get only about 25 percent of the omega-3 fatty acids that we need. "We should have a ratio of 4:1 omega-6 fatty acids (another essential fatty acid found in grain products) to omega-3s," says Gretchen Vannice, MS, RD, research coordinator at Nordic Naturals, who has studied omega-3 fatty acids extensively.

To get the benefits, the international agreed-upon recommendation of omega-3 fatty acids is 650 milligrams per day, which is hard to get from fish alone. Luckily, there are quality fish oil supplements available with not even a hint of a fishy aftertaste. Among them is Nordic Naturals Omega-3 capsules, which have a fresh lemony taste. Take one capsule a day to boost your omega-3s.

In addition to omega-3 fatty acids, it can be difficult to get enough of some other nutrients from food alone. About the only place you can get large amounts of vitamin E, for example, is in vegetable oils, nuts, and other high-fat foods. When people reduce the amount of fat in their diets, they may get smaller amounts of vitamin E as well. "A vitamin E supplement may help you reach your goal—without all the fat," says Joanne Curran-Celentano, RD, PhD, associate professor of nutritional sciences at the University of New Hampshire in Durham.

How High Should You Go?

The research is still fairly new, so scientists aren't sure how far above the DV you should aim. But for some nutrients, such as vitamin C, some evidence suggests that you need two to four times the DV to get maximum protection.

Some studies have shown that eating a lot of fruits and vegetables high in vitamin C can help protect against numerous forms of cancer, including cancers of the pancreas, esophagus, larynx, mouth, stomach, colon and rectum, cervix, breast, and lungs. However, the evidence is not there to support taking vitamin C *supplements* for cancer prevention. Scientists suspect the other phytochemicals in vitamin C–rich fruits and vegetables may play a role in the protection. So when it comes to cancer prevention, you may be better off sticking to foods to get your C.

Other studies have shown that getting amounts of vitamin C above and beyond the DV can boost immunity, improve lung function, and lower the risks of heart disease and cataracts. One Finnish study published in *Stroke: The Journal of the American Heart Association* showed that men with the lowest blood levels of vitamin C had more than two times the stroke risk of men with the highest blood levels of C. It seems that vitamin C may help prevent clogged arteries and lower blood pressure, making blood vessels more flexible.

The National Academy of Sciences has put an upper limit of 2,000 milligrams on vitamin C, however, because of potential toxicity. Talk with your health-care professional about how much vitamin C you should take per day.

Vitamin E is a very powerful antioxidant. Studies show that it can block the process that causes cholesterol to stick to artery walls, while at the same time preventing platelets, the blood components that are responsible for clotting, from clumping together in the bloodstream and raising the risk of heart disease. Although in the past, scientists thought people needed to get far more than the DV of vitamin E to reap the benefits, more recent studies suggest that vitamin E is safer when taken at the DV of 30 IU. For example, a study conducted by the National Cancer Institute set out to discover if higher doses of vitamin E could reduce the incidence of lung cancers and other cancers in 29,000 male smokers. The results showed no benefit for lung cancer and mixed results for other cancers.

While supplements make sense for some nutrients, the picture isn't quite so clear with beta-carotene. Even though foods rich in beta-carotene, such as carrots, spinach, and kale, have been shown to help prevent a variety of illnesses, including cancer, beta-carotene supplements haven't proven as useful and may even be harmful. The Physicians' Health Study involved 22,071 male physicians who were given either 50 milligrams of carotene, 325 milligrams of aspirin, both, or neither for 12 years. At the end of the study, there was no evidence of a significant harmful or beneficial effect of carotene on cardiovascular disease or cancer in the men studied. There was an increased risk in men who smoked, however. It appears that this nutrient may work best when it's taken in combination with other protective plant compounds—in other words, when you get it in its natural form from foods.

Besides, the amount of beta-carotene that seems to be protective, which is somewhere between 6 and 10 milligrams a day, is easy to get from foods. One sweet potato, for example, contains almost 15 milligrams of beta-carotene. Other good sources include bright orange and dark green vegetables, such as winter squash, collard greens, and broccoli, and fruits, such as cantaloupe and dried apricots.

The Incredible Shrinking Foods

The next time you're shopping for vitamins and minerals, check out the nutraceuticals section of the store. Unlike vitamin and mineral supplements, which contain isolated nutrients, the so-called nutraceutical supplements contain compounds extracted from whole foods, which are then supposedly concentrated into a Jetson-like pill. You'll find pills containing broccoli, spinach, tomatoes, mixed vegetables, fruit juices, and more. The advantage of nutraceuticals is that they supposedly contain all of the compounds naturally found in foods in the same proportions that nature intended, unlike one or two vitamins and/or minerals found in some supplements. Sounds too good to be true, right?

Well, it could be. Most researchers feel it's unrealistic to think that you can reduce foods down to pills and still get all the benefits, and most studies back this up. For one thing, even if the pills provide all of the health-protecting compounds and phytochemicals that you'd get from fruits and vegetables, they probably won't contain the fiber, says Dr. Camire. Plus, the process of making the pills may damage some of the healthful chemicals they claim to contain. "Mother Nature's chemicals are much more potent than the ones made in factories," she adds.

At the very least, however, fruits and vegetables in pill form may provide a bit of a boost for folks who aren't always able to eat as well as they'd like, or for people who dislike fruits and vegetables so much they find it impossible to choke them down. "There are a lot of people out there who simply do not or will not eat vegetables," says Dr. Camire. "For these people, the pills might be somewhat beneficial."

Dr. Camire notes that it is important to read labels carefully, however. Some products that call themselves nutraceuticals actually contain only one or a few isolated extracts—of carotenoids, for example—and not the full complement of health-promoting compounds found in the real foods.

Doctor's Top Tip

"I recommend antioxidants, but I don't think people should be chomping on vitamin C all day long," says Shawn Talbott, PhD, a nutritional biochemist and the author of *The Health Professional's Guide to Dietary Supplements*. "Instead, take an antioxidant supplement that contains a blend of antioxidants, including herbs and compounds such as turmeric, ginger, and green tea," he says. Dr. Talbott specifically recommends a product called Super Critical Antioxidants from the supplement company New Chapter. It's a nice blend of healthful and safe antioxidants, he says.

Free Radicals

A NATURAL DANGER

O h, no!" shrieked Dorothy, as she, the Scarecrow, and the Cowardly Lion looked on in horror as their metallic friend stiffened in the rain. "The Tin Man is rusting!"

The Wizard-bound bunch should have been more careful than to leave their iron-clad friend stranded in the rain. When moisture meets iron, it undergoes a chemical process called oxidation, causing the reddish coating we know as rust.

Unlike the Tin Man, we don't have to worry about rusting in the rain. But the same oxidation process that causes metal to rust is also at work inside our bodies.

As the word suggests, oxidation simply means that something has reacted with oxygen. More specifically, it means that oxygen molecules have lost an electron during their interactions with other molecules. These renegades become what scientists call free radicals—wounded, unstable oxygen molecules that are just as dangerous as their name sounds. In their quest to "heal" themselves, free radicals steal electrons from any healthy molecule they can grab, creating more free radicals in the process.

What does this have to do with us? Whenever oxygen mixes with other molecules, free radicals form as a by-product. Slice a banana, and the oxygen-exposed fruit turns brown from free-radical damage. Inhale, and you also have been exposed. In fact, every breath we take generates free radicals, which, as they seek to stabilize themselves, damage our healthy cells.

And the damage that free radicals do is significant. More and more research is showing that free-radical damage contributes to many major illnesses, including hardening of the arteries, degenerative eye diseases such as macular degeneration, certain cancers, and even the aging process itself.

Living with the Enemy

It's a mistake to think of free radicals as being foreign invaders like viruses or bacteria because most free radicals are manufactured within your own body. "People often don't realize that free radicals occur naturally," says Balz Frei, PhD, professor of biochemistry and biophysics and the director and endowed chair of the Linus Pauling Institute at Oregon State University in Corvallis. "The body produces them when it generates energy."

Normally, every cell in your body transforms the oxygen you breathe into water. But about 1 percent of the oxygen leaks from the usual production chain. It's this 1 percent that turns into free radicals, says Dr. Frei.

"White blood cells also generate free radicals purposely, in order to kill invading bacteria and microorganisms," he adds. "Unfortunately, these free radicals don't have very good aim, and they end up not just killing the foreign bacteria but also causing damage to healthy tissue."

Staying in Balance

So if every breath that we take creates a free-radical free-for-all, why don't we deteriorate soon after we suck our first breaths of air? In keeping with the laws of nature, for every force, there is a counterforce. For every villain, there is a hero. And for every free radical that our bodies produce, there is a substance called an antioxidant to control it. You've heard of antioxidants such as vitamins C and E and beta-carotene. Antioxidants literally act as a buffer between free radicals and your body's healthy molecules. By offering up their own electrons, antioxidants stabilize free radicals and therefore stop them from doing any further damage.

Luckily, nature anticipated the danger from free radicals and made preparations. Your body may create free radicals, but it also manufactures antioxidants to block their effects. And as we've seen, certain foods are loaded with antioxidant vitamins, so you can also get them through your diet.

"We have a whole orchestra of defense mechanisms to detoxify free radicals," explains Robert R. Jenkins, PhD, a retired professor of biology at Ithaca College in New York. "As free radicals are being made, our bodies are detoxifying them, either with antioxidant enzymes or vitamins."

In addition to the free radicals generated within our bodies, there are huge numbers in our environment, too. Exposure to such environmental factors as pollution, ultraviolet light, radiation, and car exhaust vastly increases free-radical production.

"Cigarette smoking, for example, is a significant external source of free radicals," says Dr. Frei. "When you're producing such an excess of free radicals, your antioxidants have a hard time keeping up." In fact, it takes one-third of the Daily Value of vitamin C—20 milligrams—to neutralize the effect of just one cigarette.

The Damage They Do

Once free radicals are running rampant, they can launch attacks and cause damage almost anywhere in the body. "The best example of the damage free radicals can cause is atherosclerosis, or hardening of the arteries," says Dr. Frei. "It's well-documented that free radicals contribute to this disease."

Doctor's Top Tip

"Gogi berries grow in the Himalayas, and they supposedly have the highest amount of antioxidants of any berry," says Patricia David, MD, MSPH, president of Healthy U in Columbus, Ohio. "In the Himalayas, gogi berries were dropping into the drinking water, and the people drinking that water were all very healthy and living to an extremely old age," she says. "The theory is that it had something to do with the high content of gogi berries in the water." Gogi berries aren't available in most local grocery stores, but you can order them online. "I throw a few of them in every glass of water I drink," says Dr. David. Or you can munch on the gogi berries themselves to get their antioxidant effects.

Cardiovascular disease often occurs when the bad low-density lipoprotein (LDL) cholesterol in your bloodstream clumps together and sticks to your artery walls, causing hardening and blockages. Scientists have found that free-radical damage is the reason that LDL cholesterol begins to stick to artery walls in the first place.

Other times, free radicals may attack your DNA. And when they damage those critical strands of genetic information, cells may undergo changes that cause them to replicate uncontrollably. In other words, they may become cancerous, says Dr. Frei.

Free radicals can also cause damage to your eyes. In a study that will send you searching for some wraparound Ray-Bans, researchers from Harvard Medical School found a strong link between macular degeneration, which is the leading cause of irreversible vision loss in people over the age of 50, and free-radical damage. Although it may be good for lifting the spirits, sunshine contains a tremendous amount of dangerous ultraviolet (UV) light—one of the leading producers of free radicals.

And your eyes aren't all that suffer under the sun's powerful UV light. So does your skin. Free-radical damage caused by UV rays is also believed to cause wrinkles, skin thickening, and other symptoms of premature skin aging.

And it appears that free radicals may also be one of the keys to unlocking mysterious neurological disorders like Alzheimer's and Parkinson's diseases. Some scientists believe that free radicals may actually poke holes in the barrier that usually shields the brain from outside invaders like viruses and bacteria. In response to the injury, the researchers believe that the immune system produces even more free radicals, which may cause damage, leading to neurological disease.

"Very often, free radicals aren't involved in initiating the disease," Dr. Jenkins adds, "but the free radicals that result from the disease keep the damage going."

Such is the case with rheumatoid arthritis. The inflammation within affected joints creates free radicals, which seem to do more damage than the actual disease itself. The same can be said for many digestive diseases. Free radicals may not be the cause of Crohn's disease, for instance, but they definitely contribute to the damage.

Fighting Free Radicals

If seemingly innocuous activities like breathing and being in the sun are such risky propositions when it comes to free-radical damage, how can you be sure that your body has sufficient antioxidant reserves to protect itself against free-radical attacks? "Aside from avoiding things you know generate excessive amounts of free radicals, like cigarette smoke, one of the best things that you can do for yourself is eat a plant-based diet rich in fruits and vegetables," advises Dr. Jenkins.

Fruits and vegetables contain an abundance of natural antioxidants, particularly vitamins C and E and beta-carotene, as well as dozens of additional free-radical-fighting compounds. "When you look at long-term population studies, people eating vegetarian diets appear to gain protection from diseases that are believed to be related to free-radical damage," says Dr. Jenkins. Compared with meat eaters, they live longer, healthier lives.

For optimum antioxidant protection against free radicals, Dr. Jenkins suggests that people increase their intake of vitamin C to between 200 and 400 milligrams and increase their daily doses of vitamin E to between 100 and 400 IU.

Some research has also shown that people with the highest intakes of carotenoids—plant compounds that are powerful antioxidants—have lower rates of macular degeneration. One study showed that people with a high intake of carotenoids had a 43 percent lower risk of macular degeneration than those getting the lowest amounts.

HEAVY BREATHING DURING EXERCISE: IS IT SAFE?

Breathe in. Breathe out. You've just generated hundreds of free radicals.

Breathe in. Breathe out. Pant. Pant. Pant. A couple of miles on your Nikes, and now you've created thousands of free radicals. So is all this exercise really good for you?

In the past, there's been some concern that exercise, which is supposed to make us healthier, may speed the production of free radicals to potentially dangerous proportions. However, new studies show that regular exercise actually bolsters the antioxidant defense system and protects the body from free radicals formed during exercise. (There is an emphasis on "regular" here because people who only exercise now and then or on weekends only do not seem to have the same protection against free-radical damage.) In addition, people who exercise also typically have healthier lifestyles, so they have more antioxidant stores. Plus, the benefits you get from exercise are enormous and very well established, so you should not stop exercising because you're worried about free radicals. And if you don't exercise often, make some time to do so.

And a Dutch study published in the *Journal of the American Medical Association* looked at the relationship between dietary intake of vitamins E and C, zinc, and beta-carotene and age-related macular degeneration (AMD) in more than 4,000 older adults at risk for the condition. A high intake of all four nutrients was associated with a 35 percent decrease in AMD risk, indicating that all four antioxidants are protective.

Some of the best food sources of antioxidant compounds include vitamin C–packed citrus fruits, broccoli, red and green bell peppers, and dark green leafy vegetables; beta-carotene–rich carrots, sweet potatoes, and spinach; and wheat germ and vegetable oils, which are loaded with vitamin E.

"You also need to keep things in perspective," adds Dr. Frei. "Even if it turns out that free radicals play a major role in disease, they are still only one player among many disease factors. You shouldn't get too panicky about them. Rather, live healthfully, eat sensibly, and exercise."

Gallstones

CLEANING UP THE CLUTTER

Even though your body needs some cholesterol, this thick, gummy substance has earned a reputation for being nothing but trouble—and with good reason. In large amounts, cholesterol not only contributes to heart disease, high blood pressure, and stroke; it also plays a role in the formation of gallstones. And although gallstones may be small nuggets, they can cause large amounts of excruciating pain. So needless to say, the more you can do to avoid these little buggers, the better.

As the name suggests, gallstones form in the gallbladder, which is simply a storage area for bile (also known as gall), which the body uses to digest fats in the small intestine. This bile is normally in a liquid state and contains small particles of cholesterol, protein, and fat.

But when you get too much fat and cholesterol in your diet, there's a tendency for these particles to come together and form gallstones, says Henry A. Pitt, MD, professor of surgery and director of the Hepatopancreatobiliary Surgery Fellowship at Johns Hopkins Hospital in Baltimore.

So it makes sense that the best advice for people who are prone to stones is to eat fewer red meats and whole-fat dairy foods and less of anything else that contains large amounts of fat and cholesterol, says Dr. Pitt.

Another way to help prevent gallstones is to eat smaller, more frequent meals. Since gallstones are caused by buildups of debris, making the gallbladder contract more often will help remove debris before it compacts into stones. The gallbladder contracts every time you eat, so having several small meals a day rather than two or three large ones will help keep it active and debris free. A group of researchers at the University of Rome watched gallbladder motion with

> ## Doctor's Top Tip
>
> Foods that come in packages, such as processed foods and fast foods, contain the bad fats and oils that contribute to gallstones, says Kaayla Daniel, PhD, a board-certified clinical nutritionist in Santa Fe, New Mexico. "The average American diet contains a lot of partially hydrogenated oils and vegetable oils (aka trans fats), and these fats cause bile to become thick and congested, which leads to gallstones," she says. "Plus, you will be doing your whole body a service because these fats aren't just bad for the gallbladder—they have been linked to diseases such as heart disease, cancer, obesity, and multiple sclerosis, just to name a few," she says.

ultrasound and found that frequent meals kept the bile turnover high, which made people less likely to form stones. Drinking a lot of water will also help keep stones from forming.

People who are overweight are much more likely to form gallstones than those who are lean, adds Michael D. Myers, MD, a physician in private practice in Los Alamitos, California. "For every pound of fat you have in your body, you produce 10 milligrams of cholesterol," Dr. Myers explains. So in addition to cutting down on high-fat foods, it's a good idea to add more fruits, vegetables, legumes, and whole grains to your diet, since these foods are the cornerstone of any weight-loss plan.

Even though losing weight can help prevent gallstones, losing too much, too fast can have the opposite effect, because it causes cholesterol in the gallbladder to rise, Dr. Myers says. And a similar reaction occurs in people on an extremely low-fat diet. What's more, if you seriously cut back on the amount of food you eat, your gallbladder will naturally be less active, permitting stone-forming sludge to accumulate.

If you're counting calories, staying in the range of 1,000 to 1,200 calories a day will help you lose weight without making you more prone to stones, says Dominic Nompleggi, MD, PhD, professor of medicine and surgery and director of the nutrition support service at the University of Massachusetts Medical Center in Worcester.

Garlic

GREAT BULBS OF POWER

Vampires may be doing themselves a disservice by running so quickly from garlic. Despite its sulfuric odor, garlic has many pleasant effects on the body.

An enormous amount of research has been done on this pungent bulb, and the results have been, quite literally, amazing. Dozens of medical benefits have been linked to garlic.

HEALING POWER
Can Help:

Ease ear infections

Lower triglycerides and cholesterol

Reduce the risk of stomach and colon cancers

Prevent heart disease and stroke

- Studies show that garlic lowers cholesterol and thins the blood, which may help prevent high blood pressure, heart disease, and stroke.
- In laboratory studies, garlic appears to block the growth of cancer cells. Population studies show that people who eat lots of garlic have fewer stomach and colon cancers than those who eat the least.
- In a study at Boston City Hospital, garlic was successfully used to kill 14 strains of bacteria taken from the noses and throats of children with ear infections.

In addition, research has shown that garlic can help boost immunity and reduce high blood sugar levels. It may also relieve asthma symptoms and keep individual cells healthy and strong, potentially delaying or preventing some of the conditions and cellular breakdown associated with aging.

Garlic's healing potential has been recognized for thousands of years. Throughout history, it's been used to treat everything from wounds and infections to digestion problems. In World War II, for example, when Russian soldiers ran out of penicillin for their wounds, they requisitioned garlic cloves, which is where garlic got the nickname "Russian penicillin." And today, in Germany, Japan, and other modern countries, garlic formulas are sold as over-the-counter treatments for a variety of conditions.

Good for the Heart

Thus far, researchers have identified two important ways in which garlic is good for the heart and circulation. First, it contains many sulfur compounds, including diallyl disulfide (DADS), which seem to help smooth bloodflow by preventing platelets from sticking together and clotting.

In a study at Brown University in Providence, Rhode Island, researchers gave 45 men with high cholesterol aged garlic extract—about the equivalent of five to six cloves of fresh garlic. When they examined the men's blood, they saw that the rate at which platelets clumped and stuck together had dropped anywhere from 10 to 58 percent.

"High platelet activity means that you're more likely to have arteriosclerosis or a heart attack or a stroke," says researcher Robert I. Lin, PhD, executive vice president of Nutrition International Company in Irvine, California. "But sulfur compounds are very potent. They thin the blood."

And in a study done at Harbor-UCLA Medical Center in Torrance, California, researchers gave half of participants aged garlic extract and half of them a placebo (dummy pill), then measured the degree of calcification in their arteries for 1 year. At the end of the study, the aged garlic extract group had calcification levels that were significantly lower (10 percent) than those in the placebo group, indicating that aged garlic extract can help prevent atherosclerosis.

Garlic is also good for the heart because it lowers the levels of cholesterol and blood fats called triglycerides in the bloodstream. In addition, garlic has some mild blood-pressure-lowering properties, and it can lower homocysteine (a protein that causes plaque buildup in the arteries), says Matt Budoff, MD, associate professor of medicine and director of the division of cardiology at UCLA. In a recent study, Dr. Budoff and his colleagues showed that aged garlic extract can reduce the buildup of plaque in the body by 66 percent.

And in a review of studies conducted over 13 years on the link between garlic and heart disease, 44 percent of studies showed a link between garlic and a decrease in total cholesterol. Overall, garlic's most profound effect was in preventing platelets from aggregating (clotting). Garlic also appears to increase the body's antioxidant status, thus lowering overall risk of heart disease.

And in a study reported by the American Heart Association, various garlic formulations/preparations led to reductions in cholesterol of between 11.6 and 24.3 milligrams per deciliter after only 3 months.

Cancer Protection

There's increasing evidence that including garlic in the diet may play a role in preventing and treating cancer. Studies suggest that garlic can help block cancer in several ways: by preventing cell changes that lead to cancer, by stopping tumors from growing, or by killing the harmful cells outright. "Garlic is an immune system booster," says Janet Maccaro, PhD, ND, a holistic nutritionist in Ormond Beach, Florida, who is president of Dr. Janet's Balance By Nature Products and the author of *Natural Health Remedies A-Z.* "So it may help the body zap cancer cells before they can grow out of control."

- A compound in garlic called s-allylcysteine appears to stop the metabolic action that causes a healthy cell to become cancerous, says John Milner, PhD, chief of the Nutrition Science Research Group in the Division of Cancer Prevention at the National Cancer Institute in Bethesda, Maryland.
- The substance called DADS, which we discussed earlier, appears to halt the growth of cancer cells by interfering with their ability to divide and multiply. "DADS chokes cancer cells until their numbers are reduced, and they start dying," says Dr. Milner.
- Another substance in garlic is diallyl trisulfide (DATS), which is 10 times more powerful than DADS at killing human lung cancer cells. "Its effectiveness is comparable to that of 5-fluorouracil, a widely used chemotherapy agent," Dr. Milner says. And since garlic is vastly less toxic to healthy cells than the chemotherapy drug, there's hope that some day, garlic could form the basis for a gentler chemotherapy.
- Garlic contains compounds that help prevent nitrites—common substances found in foods such as bacon and other cured meats, as well as in a variety of everyday pollutants—from transforming into nitrosamines, harmful compounds that can trigger cancerous changes in the body's cells.

Garlic's benefits aren't seen only in the laboratory. For example, researchers have noted that people in Southern Italy, who eat a lot of garlic, develop less stomach cancer than the people who don't eat much (if any) garlic to their north.

In a study done at the University of Southern California Norris Comprehensive Cancer Center, researchers looked at the relationship between garlic intake and stomach cancer in certain areas of China. They found that those who ate more garlic stalks had a lower risk of stomach cancer.

Closer to home, a study of 41,837 women living in Iowa found that those who ate garlic at least once a week had a 35 percent lower risk of colon cancer than women who never ate garlic.

In addition, garlic seems to help prevent skin, liver, breast, and other cancers. "If I had to take an educated guess, I'd say that eating three cloves of garlic a day might reduce your risk of many cancers by 20 percent," says Dr. Lin. "And eating six cloves could get you at least a 30 percent reduction," he adds.

In the Kitchen

Unless you have taste buds of steel, it's difficult to eat a lot of raw garlic at one sitting. Not to mention the havoc loads of garlic can wreak on some people's digestive systems. But you can substantially boost your garlic intake without hurting your tongue or your stomach in the process. By roasting it.

Unlike eating raw garlic cloves, roasting gives the bulb a sweet, caramelized taste—garlic at its most polite, in other words. It delivers just a hint of the sulfuric odor and taste rather than the full blast.

To roast garlic, cut the top from the garlic bulb to expose just the tips of the cloves. Rub the bulb lightly with a little olive oil, and wrap in a piece of aluminum foil. Leave some air space around the bulb, but seal the edges tightly. Roast in a 350°F oven for about 45 minutes, or until very tender. (You can also "roast" garlic in the microwave; use the high power setting and cook, uncovered, and without oil, for about 10 minutes, turning twice during the cooking process.)

To eat roasted garlic, simply squeeze the root end firmly to push the cloves out of their skins. You can spread the garlic on bread or toss it with cooked pasta or vegetables. If you're not eating it right away, you can refrigerate roasted garlic in a tightly covered container for up to 1 week.

Welcome "Garlicillin"

A frightening trend in recent years has been antibiotic resistance—the ability of bacteria to shrug off the effects of drugs that were once effective for killing them. Luckily, there's a new superhero when it comes to fighting bacteria. Research suggests that garlic may be effective where traditional drugs have failed or are too toxic.

In one study, researchers at Boston City Hospital swabbed 14 different strains of bacteria from the noses and throats of children with ear infections. Some of the infections had not responded to treatment with antibiotics. In the laboratory, however, garlic extract effectively killed the resistant germs.

In another study done at the School of Clinical Dentistry in England, garlic extract was shown to be effective in killing oral bacteria, suggesting that it might work to help fight gingivitis.

And in yet another study, researchers at the University of New Mexico, Albuquerque, tested whether garlic could be used to treat otomycosis, or swimmer's ear. Swimmer's ear is caused, scientists think, by a fungus called aspergillus. And normal treatments for it are less than ideal. Topical drugs can be uncomfortable and cannot be used if the eardrum has already been broken.

In the laboratory study, researchers treated swimmer's ear fungi with a mixture of garlic extract and water. Even at very low concentrations, the garlic blocked the growth of fungi just as well as available drugs. And, in some cases, it proved even better.

GETTING THE MOST

Enjoy it fresh. Crushed raw garlic contains allicin, a compound that breaks down quickly into a cascade of healthful compounds, like DADS and DATS. Not everyone enjoys the bite of raw garlic, however. To cut down on the sulfuric essence, cut a clove in half and rub it hard against the inside of a wooden salad bowl. You'll get just a hint of garlic taste in the salad without sacrificing any of the garlic benefits.

But eat for convenience. You don't have to prepare fresh garlic to get the healing benefits; each form of garlic—raw, cooked, and even powdered—has its own important compounds. By taking advantage of each of these forms, you can slip or sprinkle more garlic and its healing compounds into your menu.

Cut it fine. Whether you cook garlic or eat it raw, mincing, crushing, or pressing it vastly expands its surface area, which releases the maximum number of healthful compounds.

Cook it lightly. Overcooking garlic can destroy some of the delicate compounds it provides. It's best to cook it lightly, says Dr. Lin. Stir-fry it—with vegetables, for example, or add it to a slow-cooking stew in the last few minutes of cooking time, he suggests. "The taste of lightly cooked garlic is much gentler than raw garlic," he says.

Don't like garlic? Get it in an extract. Unfortunately, we don't completely understand the issues related to the cooking of garlic and the effect on the active ingredients, says Dr. Budoff. "Thus, I usually recommend that my patients (especially those who don't already eat a lot of natural garlic) use aged garlic extract rather than trying to increase their dietary garlic," he says. People who do not eat a lot of garlic usually will not be able to increase their garlic intake significantly, as the smell and taste may not be to their liking." He suggests following the label directions for use.

Doctor's Top Tip

"To bring out the flavor of veggies and garlic, I take a roasting pan, drizzle it with olive oil, and put every kind of cut-up vegetable I can think of in there. Then, I add lots of whole cloves of garlic, and sprinkle everything with sea salt," says Janet Maccaro, PhD, ND, a holistic nutritionist in Ormond Beach, Florida. "Then I roast the vegetables and garlic at 450°F for about 30 minutes, continuing to drizzle with olive oil once or twice as everything is cooking," she says. "Once the veggies and garlic are roasted, I toss them and serve. It's an awesome-tasting and healthful vegetable medley."

Garlicky Sour Cream Topping

3 medium cloves garlic

1 cup fat-free sour cream

2 tablespoons reduced-fat mayonnaise

1 tablespoon minced parsley

In a blender or food processor, process the garlic until minced. Add the sour cream, mayonnaise, and parsley. Process for 1 minute, or until smooth.

Makes 1 cup

Cook's Note: *Serve over baked or boiled potatoes, steamed vegetables, or fish.*

PER ¼ CUP

Calories: 91
Total fat: 2.5 g
Saturated fat: 0.5 g

Cholesterol: 3 mg
Sodium: 45 mg
Dietary fiber: 0.1 g

Garlic Bread

1 whole-wheat baguette (12 ounces)

2 tablespoons extra-virgin olive oil

4 cloves garlic, minced

1 teaspoon Italian herb seasoning

Preheat the oven to 400°F.

Split the baguette in half lengthwise. Place directly on the oven rack. Bake for 10 minutes to toast.

Meanwhile, in a small bowl, combine the oil, garlic, and Italian herb seasoning.

Remove the bread from the oven, and brush evenly with the garlic mixture. Return to the oven for 5 minutes.

Makes 8 servings

Cook's Note: *If a whole-wheat baguette is not available, a regular baguette will work fine.*

PER SERVING

Calories: 126
Total fat: 4.1 g
Saturated fat: 0.5 g

Cholesterol: 0 mg
Sodium: 231 mg
Dietary fiber: 2.9 g

Gas

EATING TO STOP THE WIND

"It is universally well known that, in digesting our common food, there is created or produced in the bowels of human creatures, a great quantity of wind."

—*Benjamin Franklin*

This was Dr. Franklin's way of saying that all of us, like it or not, will get some gas now and then. Gas, which is produced when food is broken down in the digestive tract, is a normal part of digestion. Some foods, of course, produce more gas than others. Beans and other plant foods high in carbohydrates are notorious gas producers. These foods produce so much excess air because they aren't entirely broken down during digestion. When small carbohydrate particles pass into the lower intestine, bacteria move in and begin feeding on them, producing a lot of gas in the process. This gas has to go somewhere—and out it goes, about 14 times a day.

It's not only plant foods that cause gas problems, however. Almost anything you ingest has the potential to cause gas, at least some of the time. Here are some of the most likely culprits, along with tips for keeping gas under control.

A Problem with Enzymes

Most children can drink milk and eat cheese all day long, but many adults don't produce enough of the enzyme necessary to fully digest the sugar (called lactose) in dairy foods. When undigested lactose slips into the lower intestine, it begins to ferment, causing gas, says Marvin Schuster, MD, founder of the Marvin M. Schuster Digestive and Motility Disorders Center at Johns Hopkins Bayview Medical Center in Baltimore.

Even if you can't down two or three glasses of milk anymore, you may be able to enjoy smaller amounts without having to avoid public places. Some people can tolerate up to 8 ounces of milk a day without suffering from gas. In addition, drinking milk with meals is much less likely to cause gas than having it alone.

Another way to enjoy milk without discomfort is to buy reduced-lactose milk, which has about 70 percent less lactose than regular milk. Or you can take lactase supplements, which supply the enzyme missing in people with lactose intolerance and make it easier for the body to digest the lactose in dairy foods.

Even people who cannot handle milk are often able to enjoy live-culture yogurt. "Yogurt contains bacteria that can digest the lactose for you so you don't get the symptoms," says Jose Saavedra, MD, medical and scientific director of Nestlé Nutrition USA, and associate professor of pediatrics at Johns Hopkins University School of Medicine and Bloomberg School of Hygiene and Public Health in Baltimore. Look for yogurt that says "live active cultures" on the label, which means it contains the bacteria that can help you break down the offending sugar. The more help you get with lactose digestion, the less likely you are to have gas.

Fiber Fireworks

We all know how important it is to get more fiber in your diet. Unfortunately, the same fiber that lowers cholesterol and helps protect against heart disease also produces large amounts of gas. This is especially true in people who have suddenly stepped up their intake of fiber-rich foods.

"If you add fiber too quickly, the body can't cope with it properly," says Dr. Schuster. "The average American only eats about 12 grams of fiber a day, less than half of the recommended daily amount. If you suddenly double that amount, it means a lot of gas."

To get the benefits of fiber without the gas, it's a good idea to add it slowly to your diet, says Marie Borum, MD, MPH, professor of medicine at George Washington University Medical Center in Washington, D.C. You might, for example, start by substituting whole-wheat spaghetti for your regular kind, which will provide an extra 2 grams of the rough stuff in a half-cup serving—a significant change, but not a drastic one. Then, as your body gets used to the extra roughage, add more. A half-cup of cooked artichoke hearts will deliver more than 4 grams of fiber, and the same amount of lima beans will add almost 5 grams. If you gradually introduce fiber-rich foods to your diet each day over a period of 4 to 6 weeks, you're less likely to have a problem with gas, Dr. Borum says.

How Sweet It Isn't

Sometimes you're darned if you do and darned if you don't. Many people get gas when they eat sweets like cookies or ice cream (forget the added fat and calories). But when they try to curb those cravings by substituting sugar-free candies or chewing gum, they still get gas. Why?

As it turns out, sugarless gum and candies are gas producers, says Dr. Borum. They contain artificial sweeteners like sorbitol, xylitol, or mannitol, which the body has trouble digesting. While these sweeteners help keep your calorie intake down, they can also result in large amounts of gas. And in some people, artificial sweeteners also have a laxative effect, doubling the intestinal trouble.

Mother Nature's own sweeteners aren't without their own problems, however. Fructose, for example, a sugar found in honey, fruits, and juices, frequently causes gas. It doesn't take a lot of fructose to cause problems, either. In one study, Greek researchers found that having as little as 1½ tablespoons of honey was enough to cause gas in some people.

Unfortunately, even when you try to eliminate sources of gas, it sometimes produces its ugly bubbles anyway. To fight back against a gas attack, try this gas remedy: "Add a pinch of baking soda to a glass of water and drink it down," suggests Janet Maccaro, PhD, ND, a holistic nutritionist in Ormond Beach, Florida, who is president of Dr. Janet's Balance By Nature Products and the author of *Natural Health Remedies A-Z*.

You may also want to forgo fruit at the end of a meal. "Fruit after a meal promotes gas because it causes fermentation," says Dr. Maccaro. "So if you have a salad, a main course, and then you top it off with fruit, you will have fermentation on top of all of that food, which will cause a lot of gas." This is not to say fruit isn't a wonderful alternative to other sugary desserts. "But if you suffer from gas, have your fruit first thing in the morning or at least an hour or so after a meal," Dr. Maccaro says.

Doctor's Top Tip

Consuming plants that dispel flatulence, called carminatives, can help prevent gas, says John Neustadt, ND, medical director of Montana Integrative Medicine in Bozeman. These plants include ginger, peppermint, thyme, cinnamon, nutmeg, caraway, and cardamom. "Cooking with these spices or regularly sipping teas containing them can be quite helpful for decreasing gas," he says. For best results, throw some of these spices into recipes and follow them up with a nice ginger, peppermint, cinnamon, caraway, or cardamom tea.

Ginger

THE PUNGENT HEALER

HEALING POWER
Can Help:
Prevent motion sickness
Soothe stomach upset
Relieve migraines
Reduce clotting in blood
Provide arthritis relief

Roman doctors kept it handy during military marches. Pythagoras, Greek philosopher and geometry whiz, touted it for digestive health. And King Henry VIII of England was convinced that it would protect against the plague, although there's no evidence that ginger is that good. But there's plenty of evidence that this gnarled, piquant root can help relieve dozens of conditions, from high blood pressure, motion sickness, and other digestive complaints to migraines, headaches, arthritis, high cholesterol, and even dangerous blood clots. This is why millions of people worldwide swear by ginger as a healing food.

Help for the Heaves

As anyone who has suffered from motion sickness knows, even a mild bout can derail the best-laid vacation plans. That's why nearly every thorough travel checklist, along with reminders to buy sunscreen and feed the cat, includes the notation, "Bring Dramamine."

The next time you travel, you may want to stop at the supermarket instead of the pharmacy, however. As it turns out, ginger is one of the best motion sickness remedies you can buy.

In a classic study conducted by Daniel B. Mowrey, PhD, director of the American Phytotherapy Research Laboratory in Salt Lake City, 36 motion-sickness-prone students were strapped into tilted rotating chairs and spun until they felt ill. Half were given 200 milligrams of dimenhydrinate (Dramamine) before the ride, and half were given ginger. Those who were given the Dramamine could only take the stomach-churning ride for about 4½ minutes—and most gave up even sooner. The half given ginger, however, had less nausea and dizziness than the drug-tested group and were therefore able to withstand the ride for the full 6 minutes.

In another study, Dutch researchers tested the effects of ginger on seasick naval cadets and found that ginger pills reduced the cadets' nausea and vomiting, providing relief for as long as 4 hours.

Experts aren't sure exactly why ginger suppresses a queasy stomach. But researchers in Japan have suggested that gingerols, one of the compounds in ginger, may be somehow responsible for blocking the body's vomiting reflex.

To use ginger for combating motion sickness, try taking about ¼ teaspoon of fresh or powdered ginger 20 minutes before getting in a car or on a boat. Repeat every few hours as needed.

You can also use ginger to help relieve a run-of-the-mill upset stomach, says Janet Maccaro, PhD, ND, a holistic nutritionist in Ormond Beach, Florida, who is president of Dr. Janet's Balance By Nature Products. Prepare a cup of ginger tea by adding three or four thin slices of fresh ginger to a cup of boiling water, and sip as needed. Or drink a cup after dinner to aid in digestion, she says.

Relief for Migraines

If you're one of the millions of Americans who suffer from migraine headaches, ginger may help prevent both the pain and the resulting nausea. In a small study, researchers at Odense University in Denmark found that ginger may short-circuit impending migraines without the unpleasant side effects of some migraine-relieving drugs. It appears that ginger blocks the action of prostaglandins, substances that cause pain and inflammation in blood vessels in the brain.

And in a study done at the Headache Care Center in Springfield, Missouri, 30 people with a history of migraines were given an over-the-counter combination of feverfew and ginger (called GelStat) at the early, mild pain phase of a migraine headache. Two hours after treatment, 48 percent of the participants were pain free, and 34 percent reported a migraine of only mild severity. Overall, 59 percent of the participants said they were happy with the effectiveness of the ginger-containing GelStat, indicating that its ingredients may be a good first-line treatment for migraines.

Research on the role of ginger in migraines is still preliminary, so experts are reluctant to recommend specific treatment plans for using ginger to fight migraines. If you feel a headache coming on, you may want to try taking ⅓ teaspoon of fresh or powdered ginger, which is the amount suggested by the Danish researchers.

Aid for Arthritis

Are the joints in your fingers so stiff and sore that you can't even fumble the childproof cap off the aspirin bottle in an attempt to get some relief? You may want to add ginger to your medicine chest.

In a review of various therapies for osteoarthritis, researchers at the Musculoskeletal Research Center in New York City found that ginger extract was among the experimental therapies that showed promise in being able to slow or even reverse osteoarthritis.

Whenever possible, buy ginger that is grown in Africa or India, says Stephen Fulder, PhD, a private research consultant and author of *The Ginger Book*. Studies show that varieties of ginger from these continents are more potent than the common Jamaican kind.

You can't tell the difference in gingers just by looking, though. Ask the produce manager at the supermarket or health food store. He should be able to tell you where the ginger was grown.

And in a Danish study, researchers studied 56 people who had rheumatoid arthritis or osteoarthritis and who treated themselves with fresh or powdered ginger. They found that ginger produced relief in 55 percent of people with osteoarthritis and 74 percent of those with rheumatoid arthritis.

Some experts speculate that ginger may ease arthritis pain the same way it helps block migraines, by blocking the formation of inflammation-causing prostaglandins that cause pain and swelling.

To soothe arthritis pain, brew a mild tea by putting three or four slices of fresh ginger in a cup of boiling water, suggests Charles Lo, MD, a doctor of Chinese medicine in private practice in Chicago. You can also try downing ½ teaspoon of powdered ginger or up to an ounce (about 6 teaspoons) of fresh ginger once a day.

Help for the Blood

Blood clotting can be a good thing. When you cut your finger, for example, platelets—components in blood that help it clot—help "stick" the wound together to stop the bleeding and start the healing process.

But these sticky platelets can also cling to artery walls as well as to each other. When that happens, clots stop being beneficial and start becoming something to worry about. Many people routinely take aspirin to help keep their blood clear of clots that could lead to strokes or heart attacks.

The gingerol in ginger has a chemical structure somewhat similar to that of aspirin. Research suggests that getting ginger in the diet—although at this point experts aren't sure how much—may inhibit the production of a chemical called thromboxane, which plays a key role in the clotting process.

GETTING THE MOST

Use it fresh. Ginger comes in a variety of forms, including fresh, dried, crystallized, and powdered. It's best to use it fresh, advises Dr. Lo. "Fresh ginger is more active than dried," he says. Crystallized ginger is the next best thing, he adds. To find the freshest ginger and get the most healing compounds, shop for ginger that looks healthy. "Avoid ginger with soft spots, mold, or dry, wrinkled skin," Dr. Lo advises.

Enjoy it often. To extract the most health benefits from ginger, consume it as often as possible, says Dr. Lo. But you don't need to go ginger-crazy to get the healing benefits. Less than an ounce a day will do. "Drinking a few cups of ginger tea or adding a small amount of fresh ginger to a stir-fry should be enough."

Make a ginger marinade for meats. Mix fresh ginger, minced garlic, olive oil, and light soy sauce for a marinade for chicken, beef, or fish, says Dr. Maccaro. "They use ginger for a marinade in Japan, and it's a wonderful way to get the health benefits," she says.

Double-Ginger Gingerbread

¾ **cup unsweetened applesauce**

½ **cup molasses**

¼ **cup fat-free egg substitute**

3 **tablespoons canola oil**

1½ **cups all-purpose flour**

1 **teaspoon baking soda**

1 **teaspoon ground ginger**

1 **teaspoon ground cinnamon**

⅛ **teaspoon salt**

⅓ **cup finely chopped candied ginger**

Preheat the oven to 350°F.

In a large bowl, combine the applesauce, molasses, egg substitute, and oil. Stir to mix well.

In a medium bowl, combine the flour, baking soda, ground ginger, cinnamon, and salt. Stir to mix. Add to the applesauce mixture, and stir until just mixed. Mix in all but 1 tablespoon of the candied ginger.

Pour the batter into an 8- × 8-inch nonstick baking dish. Bake until a knife inserted in the center comes out clean, 25 to 30 minutes.

Cool on a wire rack. Cut into squares. Sprinkle each piece with the remaining candied ginger just before serving

Makes 9 servings

Cook's Note: *A dollop of fat-free sour cream makes a delicious topping for the gingerbread.*

PER SERVING

Calories: 211

Total fat: 4.8 g

Saturated fat: 0.4 g

Cholesterol: 0 mg

Sodium: 192 mg

Dietary fiber: 1 g

Gout

PROTECTION AGAINST PURINES

If you're reading this, you likely either have gout, suspect that you might have it, or know someone who does. And you're probably not too happy about it. Gout is a big fraternity that nobody wants to be in.

Gout is a form of arthritis in which glasslike shards of built-up uric acid jab into joints, causing searing pain. For some, the pain is so severe that the mere weight of a blanket on an inflamed toe is too much to bear. Fever and chills can be part of the gout package, too, as the immune system attempts to fight off the assault.

About 2.1 million Americans know the pain of gout, and doctors say that it's on the rise as the population ages. Gout can occur in both men and women at any age, but most of the people with gout are overweight men over 40.

Too Much of a Bad Thing

The uric acid that causes gout is a normal part of our metabolisms. Our bodies make uric acid when they break down protein by-products called purines.

Normally, uric acid dissolves in the blood, is filtered out by the kidneys, and takes a ride out of the body in the urine. Not so in those with gout, however. Gout sufferers, perhaps through some metabolic glitch, either produce an overabundance of uric acid or have trouble getting rid of it. Over time, the excess acid condenses into sharp little crystals that lodge in joints and the connective tissues around them, resulting in inflammation and pain, says Doyt Conn, MD, professor of medicine and director of the division of rheumatology at Emory University in Atlanta. The big toe is a favorite first target of gout attacks, but gout has also been known to make its first appearance in the ankles, knees, hands, and shoulders.

Gout can be deceiving because attacks are sometimes separated by long periods with no apparent symptoms. When it does strike, it usually hits at night. Without medication, the pain of gout can persist for days or even weeks. If you get gout, you can count on getting it again. Half of those with a first attack have a second one within a year; 75 percent within 5 years.

Pain isn't the only thing you have to worry about with gout. Without treatment, gout attacks often grow more frequent and more severe. After about 10 years, lumps

CRASHING THE CLUB

What was long thought to be a men's club is now increasingly open to women. But you won't hear any cheers from the ladies. After all, who wants to join a club that involves painful, red joints?

Gout occurs in men and women at a rate of 2:1, which means that for every two men suffering with the painful condition, there is one uncomfortable woman. And chances are, she is past menopause. Why?

Doctors suspect that estrogen helps prevent a buildup of uric acid in the blood. But this shield slips at menopause, when a woman's estrogen levels fall. As the vast numbers of women in the baby boom generation age, the incidence of gout is sure to increase.

of uric acid crystals, called tophi, may begin to build up around joints and in cartilage elsewhere in the body. Tophi are sometimes visible under the skin, particularly when they park themselves in the outer ear. Left untreated, these deposits gradually grow bigger and can irreversibly cripple a joint. In addition, people with gout are more likely than others to develop uric acid kidney stones.

Unfortunately, there is no cure for gout. Drugs can keep it under control, but people with the condition have other weapons at their disposal, too. Slimming down, eating right, cutting back on alcohol, and drinking plenty of water all help lower uric acid levels and decrease the risk of gout attacks, says Dr. Conn.

Weighing the Risks

Obesity has been linked to high levels of uric acid in the blood, so weight control is especially important for people with gout. Crash diets and fasts aren't the answer, however, since these extreme weight loss measures can actually *raise* uric acid levels. Slow and steady weight loss is not only better for your general health, but also more likely to keep gout under control, says Dr. Conn.

A study conducted at Massachusetts General Hospital followed 47,150 men with no history of gout for 12 years and studied the relationship between weight change and gout flare-ups. They found that the men who gained the most weight had the highest risk of gout. Weight loss, on the other hand, was protective against gout.

As you know, it's a lot easier to keep weight off than to take it off later once you've packed on the pounds. Keeping your weight under control now will go a long way toward preventing gout in the future.

Doctor's Top Tip

The same *New England Journal of Medicine* study that pointed the finger at meat and seafood (at right) also showed that the physicians who ate the most dairy products—particularly, low-fat dairy products—had a reduced incidence of gout, says Donna Weihofen, RD, of the University of Wisconsin Hospital and Clinics in Madison. "So now there is some good news, too—eat some low-fat dairy, which is a good source of protein, and you can lower your risk of gout," she says. Specifically, the physicians who ate 2 cups or more of fat-free milk, low-fat milk, or low-fat yogurt had half the rate of gout than those who ate hardly any dairy. "So to prevent gout, aim for the same amount," Weihofen says.

Eating for Relief

In the past, the only thing to do for gout was to cut purines from the diet. And although there are a few foods you should cut down on to help improve gout, there are also some things you can add to your diet to improve the condition, says Donna L. Weihofen, RD, a senior clinical nutritionist at the University of Wisconsin Hospital and Clinics in Madison.

As far as elimination, Weihofen points to a study published in the *New England Journal of Medicine* that looked at the diets of male physicians and their rates of gout. "They found that the only foods associated with the gout were meats and seafood—the purine-rich vegetables weren't related," Weihofen says. "So the recommendation is now simpler: If you want to cut down your risk of gout, cut down on your intake of meat and seafood," she says. (And watch out for cauliflower; see opposite page.)

While you're cutting back on these foods, it's also a good idea to make sure that if you drink, you do so only in moderation, and that you drink wine instead of beer or liquor. A study published in the *Lancet* looked at the alcohol consumption of more than 47,000 men with no history of gout and measured the number who developed the condition over 12 years. They found that beer and liquor—but not wine—consumption was associated with an increased risk of gout. It seems that beer and other alcoholic beverages increase the risk for gout attacks in two ways: They increase the body's production of uric acid, and they impair the kidneys' ability to get rid of it.

Getting more water into your system will dilute the uric acid in the bloodstream and help prevent crystals from forming, Weihofen says. Both soda and fruit juices can help, but water is really the best choice, because it passes through the body quickly without adding unnecessary sugars. She recommends drinking at least 10 to 12 glasses of water a day.

Weihofen also recommends eating foods high in vitamin C. An article in *Arthritis and Rheumatism* showed that vitamin C appears to help prevent gout by lowering blood levels of uric acid. The study participants included 184 nonsmokers, half of whom took 500 milligrams of vitamin C, and half who took a placebo (dummy pill).

FRUITFUL RELIEF

The recorded use of cherries to treat gout dates at least to the 1950s, to a Texan named Ludwig W. Blau, PhD, who was crippled by a gouty big toe and forced to use a wheelchair. Dr. Blau reported in a Texas medical journal that a diet including six cherries a day soon had him up and walking. Further, he noted that his physician tried the cherry diet on 12 patients and had equally good results.

Do cherries work? A small study showed that they very well might.

In the study, after fasting overnight, 10 women ate two servings of Bing cherries. Researchers collected urine and blood samples before and after the women ate the cherries and measured antioxidant levels, urate (which contains uric acid—the substance that builds up and causes kidney stones), and the inflammatory markers C-reactive protein and nitric oxide. After the cherries were eaten, the women's plasma levels of urate fell significantly for a 5-hour period, which confirms the antigout properties of the fruit. In addition, levels of the anti-inflammatories dropped as well, suggesting that cherries help decrease inflammation.

After 2 months, the uric acid levels of the vitamin C group were lower than in the placebo group, indicating that vitamin C was effective in lowering uric acid levels. "The study results suggest that 500 milligrams of vitamin C per day can help reduce gout risk," Weihofen says. Foods high in vitamin C include strawberries, kiwifruit, oranges, and other citrus fruits, and vegetables such as peppers, broccoli, and Brussels sprouts. One vegetable high in C that should be avoided, however, is cauliflower. See "Food Alert" on page 150 to discover why this vegetable can be problematic.

Grapefruit
THE POWER OF PECTIN

HEALING POWER

Can Help:

Relieve cold symptoms

Prevent cancer

Speed wound healing

Prevent heart disease
and stroke

Grapefruit may be the biggest citrus fruit around, but in terms of popularity, it sometimes gets rolled aside. Its sour taste just isn't as appealing to some people as its sweeter kin, like oranges, tangerines, or clementines.

But in the health game, grapefruit, particularly the darker red variety, is a shining star. Grapefruit contains a number of antioxidant compounds—not just vitamin C, but also such things as lycopene, limonoids, and naringin. Together, these compounds can help reduce cold symptoms and also help decrease the risks of heart disease and cancer.

What these substances have in common is their ability to fight excess dangerous oxygen molecules in the body called free radicals. While free radicals are a natural part of metabolism, they can have dangerous effects as well. Grapefruit essentially acts as a chemical "mop" that helps clean up problems before they occur.

In addition, grapefruit contains large amounts of pectin, a type of fiber that can significantly lower cholesterol, thus reducing your risk for the health conditions high cholesterol brings on, such as heart disease, high blood pressure, and stroke.

Red with Health

One of the compounds in red (and pink) grapefruit that gives the fruit its distinctive hue is lycopene. Also found in tomatoes and red bell peppers, lycopene "is a very important, very potent antioxidant and free-radical scavenger," says Paul Lachance, PhD, executive director of the Nutraceuticals Institute at Rutgers University in New Brunswick, New Jersey. "Our cancer and heart disease situations would be a lot worse if not for the lycopene in our foods."

Grapefruit is also an excellent source of limonoids, which, like vitamin C, have been shown to have anticancer properties. A 6-ounce glass of grapefruit juice, for example, contains over 100 milligrams of various limonoid compounds. In a study conducted at the Department of Nutrition and Food Science at Texas A & M University, researchers gave rats five different diets, including one diet containing grapefruit pulp powder and one containing limonin, and then measured their rates of

FOOD ALERT

A Medical Magnifier

Sometimes the foods you eat can have an effect—good or bad—on medications that you may be taking at the same time. In a study at the University of Western Ontario in London, Canada, David G. Bailey, PhD, associate professor of medicine and physiology and pharmacology and toxicology at the university, found that when grapefruit juice was given at the same time as medication, it magnified the effects of the drug. In some cases, one dose of the drug essentially acted like 5 to 10. "The more we study, the more drugs we find that are affected by grapefruit juice," says Dr. Bailey.

It appears that furanocoumarins, naringin compounds found in grapefruit, turn off an enzyme in the small intestine that helps metabolize certain drugs. When a drug isn't metabolized as extensively, more is absorbed into the body, magnifying its effect. Thus far, more than 30 drugs have been affected by grapefruit juice. Particularly problematic are certain cholesterol-lowering statins (simvastatin, lovastatin, atorvastatin) because of their high use and the seriousness of the adverse effects (rhabdomyolysis), calcium-channel blockers (used for high blood pressure), Seldane (an allergy medication), and Halcion (an anti-anxiety drug).

To avoid problems, be sure to read the package inserts that come with your medications. Or simply substitute orange juice (which doesn't contain furano-coumarins or naringin) for grapefruit juice. Also avoid eating grapefruit itself when taking these medications.

colon cancer. The two diets that were protective against colon cancer were the grapefruit powder and limonin diets, indicating that both grapefruit and the limonoids they contain are protective against colon cancer.

Finally, grapefruit is an excellent source of vitamin C. It's one of the few foods that can provide more than the entire Daily Value (DV) for this vitamin in one serving. A cup of grapefruit sections contains 88 milligrams of vitamin C, a whopping 146 percent of the DV.

While vitamin C is a powerful antioxidant, it also helps bind skin cells together. "Vitamin C is especially important for holding collagen bundles together, which helps wounds heal," says Jana Klauer, MD, a New York City–based physician. If you don't get enough vitamin C, cuts will be slower to heal, and your gums may bleed. Vitamin C has also been shown to relieve cold symptoms by reducing levels of

Doctor's Top Tip

"Grapefruit makes a really tasty addition to a salad," says Janet Maccaro, PhD, ND, a holistic nutritionist, president of Dr. Janet's Balance By Nature Products in Ormond Beach, Florida, and author of *Natural Health Remedies A-Z*. "Toss some grapefruit halves with some dark leafy greens, throw in some walnuts for some healthful omega-3 fatty acids, and add honey for a dressing—it's a healthful mix," she says.

histamine, a naturally occurring chemical that makes your nose run.

Pectin Power

Grapefruit has received a lot of attention in recent years due to its generous supply of pectin, a type of soluble fiber that can help lower cholesterol to healthy levels. It does this by forming a gel in the intestine that helps block the absorption of fats into the bloodstream.

Research has shown that pectin can help lower cholesterol levels, as well as prevent risk of heart disease and stroke. One such study was done by the late James Cerda, MD, a former professor of medicine at the University of Florida College of Medicine in Gainesville. Dr. Cerda found that animals given a diet containing 3 percent grapefruit pectin for 9 months had more than 5 percent of their artery walls covered with plaque. In animals not given pectin, plaque covered 14 percent of the artery walls.

A 4-ounce serving (about ½ cup) of grapefruit provides 1 gram of pectin. The fibrous compound is found not only in the grapefruit flesh, but also in the peel and the thin white layer just beneath the peel.

GETTING THE MOST

Eat the sections. When you eat a grapefruit by scooping out the flesh, you leave about half the pectin behind. To get the most fiber, experts say, peel the grapefruit and eat the entire section.

Sip your juice. Grapefruit juice is a concentrated source of the antioxidant naringin. You can make your own juice, but this may be one juice variety where commercial is better; during commercial processing, parts of the healthful grapefruit peel go into the juice.

Buy it red. Both red (and pink) grapefruits contain more lycopene than the white varieties. Experts say good choices include Ruby Red, Flame, and Star Ruby.

Honey-Marinated Grapefruit

4 ruby grapefruit

2 tablespoons honey

1 tablespoon finely chopped fresh mint

Grate about 1 teaspoon of the zest from 1 grapefruit. Cut that grapefruit in half through the middle, and squeeze the juice into a small bowl; set aside.

Place the honey in a small microwaveable bowl. Microwave on medium for 20 to 30 seconds, or until warm. Add the grapefruit juice and zest. Mix well.

Peel the remaining 3 grapefruit with a sharp paring knife, cutting away most but not all of the white pith below the peel. Carefully separate the grapefruit into sections. Remove any seeds, and pierce each section in 1 or 2 places with the tip of the knife so the marinade can permeate the grapefruit.

Arrange the grapefruit sections on dessert plates. Pour the honey mixture over the sections. Let stand for at least 15 minutes to let the flavors blend. Chill, if desired. Sprinkle with the mint before serving.

Makes 4 servings

PER SERVING

Calories: 110
Total fat: 0.3 g
Saturated fat: 0 g

Cholesterol: 0 mg
Sodium: 5 mg
Dietary fiber: 3.8 g

Grape Juice

A DRINK FOR THE HEART

HEALING POWER

Can Help:

Lower cholesterol

Decrease the risk of
heart disease

Lower high blood
pressure

Grape juice made its debut in this country toward the end of the 19th century, when certain teetotaling churches decided that they needed to serve a nonalcoholic substitute for wine for Communion.

Modern-day teetotalers are still toasting the grape juice innovation. Purple grape juice provides similar benefits to red wine (both red wine and purple grape juice contain powerful compounds that can help lower cholesterol, prevent hardening of the arteries, and fight heart disease) without the unwanted health effects of alcohol.

Giving Your Heart Some Juice

Researchers might never have stumbled across the health benefits of purple grape juice and its spirited sibling, red wine, had it not been for the heart-healthy folks from the country that also brought us croissants, berets, and Brigitte Bardot.

A few years back, scientists discovered a phenomenon that they dubbed the French paradox. What they found was that while the French ate almost four times as much butter and three times as much lard, smoked just as many (or more) cigarettes, and had higher cholesterol and blood pressure than Americans, they fell victim to heart attacks 2½ times less often.

At least part of the French secret to heart health, researchers believe, is red wine. Red wine contains compounds called flavonoids, which have been linked to lower rates of heart disease.

If red wine confers protection, the researchers thought, why not the purple grape juice from where the wine comes?

As it turns out, the researchers were right. "Purple grape juice gives you most of the benefits of red wine without the alcohol," says Janet Maccaro, PhD, ND, a holistic nutritionist in Ormond Beach, Florida, who is president of Dr. Janet's Balance By Nature Products and the author of *Natural Health Remedies A-Z*. Among the most powerful ingredients in purple grape juice are flavonoids—some of the same flavonoids found in red wine. Studies suggest that flavonoids may help lower cholesterol, prevent cholesterol from sticking to artery walls, and keep blood platelets from sticking together and forming dangerous clots in the bloodstream, thus helping to prevent stroke.

Great Grapes

Scientists are still unraveling the mysteries of exactly how purple grape juice helps protect against heart disease. What they do know is that it appears to help in more than one way.

The flavonoids in purple grape juice are among the most powerful antioxidants around—maybe even better than vitamins C or E, says John D. Folts, PhD, professor of medicine and director of the coronary thrombosis laboratory at the University of Wisconsin Medical School in Madison. In your body, they help prevent bad low-density lipoprotein (LDL) cholesterol from oxidizing—the process that enables cholesterol to stick to your artery walls and create blockages.

A study published in the *American Journal of Clinical Nutrition* showed that purple grape juice has the power to reduce LDL cholesterol and triglycerides—both of which help to lower risk for heart disease.

Keeping LDL cholesterol in check is a good start against heart disease. But you also need to keep the platelets, components in blood that cause it to clot, from sticking together unnecessarily. The flavonoids in purple grape juice do that, too, Dr. Folts says. A study at the University of Wisconsin found that when purple grape juice was given to laboratory animals, abnormal clotting was significantly reduced. So drinking purple grape juice gives you two benefits for the price of one.

Actually, it's more than two.

Purple grape juice is also a fair source of potassium, with 8 ounces providing 334 milligrams, or 10 percent of the Daily Value. This is important because potassium

Doctor's Top Tip

Research shows that purple grape juice acts as a natural antioxidant. In fact, in a recent study that measured the antioxidant power of over 1,000 foods and beverages, Welch's 100 percent grape juice made from Concord grapes had the second highest antioxidant capacity overall, and the number one antioxidant capacity for a beverage.

The study, which was published in the *American Journal of Nutrition*, named blackberries as the top antioxidant food and grape juice as a close second. "Many high-antioxidant fruits and vegetables can be identified by their deep, dark coloring," says Carla McGill, PhD, RD, a nutrition scientist at Tropicana in Chicago.

To get an antioxidant boost, drink an 8-ounce serving of 100 percent grape juice each day. Throw a small bottle in your lunch box or briefcase, and keep a larger bottle in the fridge at home. No washing, chopping, or peeling required—just pour and serve.

helps control high blood pressure and protect against stroke, furthering grape juice's power to combat cardiovascular disease.

The Missing Link

While purple grape juice does contain powerful compounds, it doesn't contain a lot of them. In fact, you need about three times as much grape juice as wine to get the same protective effects, says Dr. Folts.

All of a grape's protective flavonoids are in the "must," a chunky mixture of grape skins, pulp, seeds, and stems that is used to make wine and grape juice, says Dr. Folts. When this must is fermented to make wine, a lot of the flavonoids are drawn into the liquid, he explains. Since grape juice is never fermented, you get only the flavonoids that are drawn into the juice during the heating and processing stages.

The compounds that end up in the drink are still plenty strong, though, he adds. You just need more juice to get them.

GETTING THE MOST

Pour a big glass. Since you need to drink more grape juice than wine to get the same health benefits, you'll want to down up to 12 ounces a day, Dr. Folts says.

Chill out with a nonalcoholic wine spritzer. "In the summer, I make a drink called a grape juice chiller, which is a mixture of club soda and grape juice," says Dr. Maccaro. "It's a great nonalcoholic and refreshing way to get your flavonoids," she says.

Drink it dark. "Since flavonoids are what give juice its rich purple hue, if you're looking for the grape juice with the most flavonoids, pick the darkest of the bunch," advises Dr. Folts.

Drink juice, not drink. So-called grape drink is nothing but a watered-down, sugared imitation of the original article. Nutritionally, it doesn't compare. So when you want the benefits of grape juice, be sure to buy the real thing.

Greens

NATURE'S BEST PROTECTION

HEALING POWER

Can Help:

Control blood pressure

Reduce the risk of heart disease

Reduce the risk of cancer

Protect against vision loss

Double coupons, good gas mileage, supersizing for only a dollar more—if there's one thing that Americans appreciate, it's getting more for less. That is why we really ought to love leafy green vegetables. They deliver more nutrients in fewer calories than virtually any food out there.

"You get so many important nutrients from leafy green vegetables—magnesium, iron, calcium, folate, vitamin C, and vitamin B_6—plus all the cancer- and heart disease–fighting phytochemicals," says Michael Liebman, PhD, professor of human nutrition at the University of Wyoming in Laramie. "These are the most nutrient-dense foods available."

Experts are quick to note, however, that America's favorite "salad starter"—the bland-tasting iceberg lettuce—doesn't count as a "leafy green" vegetable. Of all the foods in this powerhouse family, iceberg is the runt. Far better are such things as kale, Swiss chard, dandelion greens, beet greens, turnip greens, spinach, and chicory.

Leaves for the Heart

To some extent, the difference between people who have heart attacks and those who don't may be how many trips they make to the salad bar, provided that bar isn't stocked with iceberg lettuce only.

A review done at Harokopio University in Athens, Greece, revealed that the high consumption of wild greens and the healthful omega-3 fatty acids they provide was previously underestimated as a crucial protective part of the Mediterranean diet, which is high in olive oil, fruits, and vegetables, and low in meats and full-fat dairy products, and has been linked with a lower risk of heart disease.

And researchers from the Jean Mayer USDA Human Nutrition Research Center on Aging at Tufts University in Boston and the Framingham Heart Study in Massachusetts studied more than 1,000 people between the ages of 67 and 95 to learn what dietary factors affect heart health. In this, as in so many issues touching on food, the answer boiled down to chemistry—specifically, to an amino acid called homocysteine.

Homocysteine is a natural compound that is harmless as long as the body keeps it in check. When it reaches high levels, however, it becomes toxic and may contribute to clogged arteries and heart disease. The researchers found that among people with the most clogged arteries, 43 percent of men and 34 percent of women had high levels of homocysteine in their blood.

What's the connection with greens? The body uses folate and vitamins B_{12} and B_6 to keep homocysteine under control. Many of the people in the study were falling short of these vital nutrients—especially the B vitamin folate and vitamin B_6.

In a more recent review from Serbia, researchers looked at the relationship between homocysteine and cardiovascular disease. This research supported the findings in the Framingham Heart Study, showing that a low intake of folate, vitamin B_6, and vitamin B_{12} increases levels of homocysteine and thus increases overall risk of cardiovascular disease.

Luckily, greens can help. As it turns out, leafy greens are outstanding sources of folate, and they also provide vitamin B_6. That's why experts advise adding plenty of leafy green vegetables to your diet to counteract homocysteine levels.

In the Kitchen

With the exception of residents of the Southern states, Americans as a rule aren't all that familiar with cooking greens. Those of us who live in other areas of the country throw them in salads and maybe put them on sandwiches. But why limit yourself to raw leaves? Greens are very easy to cook once you know a few tricks.

Trim the stems. While the leaves are often surprisingly tender, the stems on leafy greens can be unpleasantly tough and should probably be discarded or used in vegetable stock. Before cooking greens, separate the leaf from the stem by running a sharp knife alongside the stem and center rib.

Make sure your greens are clean. Since the leafy greens grow close to the ground, and the frilly leaves readily capture dirt and grit, it's important to wash all parts of greens thoroughly. The easiest way is to fill the sink or a large bowl with cold water and swish the greens around, allowing any dirt or sand to sink to the bottom. When the greens are clean, transfer them to a colander to drain.

Cut thick greens into ribbons. When cooking thick greens like kale or Swiss chard, it's helpful to cut them into ribbons, or small pieces. This will help them cook more quickly and become tender.

Boil them quickly. The easiest way to prepare greens is to submerge them briefly in boiling water. Drop the greens in a cup of boiling water, cover, and cook for about 4 minutes, or until tender. You can then sauté them more quickly, if desired, for certain stir-fries and other recipes.

Cooked spinach is probably your best bet for managing homocysteine. A half-cup of Popeye's favorite snack delivers 131 micrograms of folate, or 33 percent of the Daily Value (DV) for this vitamin. It also contains 0.2 milligram of vitamin B_6, or 10 percent of the DV.

In addition to these important B vitamins, certain greens—particularly beet greens, chicory, and spinach—provide the heart-healthy minerals magnesium, potassium, and calcium. These minerals, along with sodium, help regulate the amount of fluid that your body retains. All too often, researchers say, people have too much sodium and too little of the other three, leading to high blood pressure.

Even though eating leafy greens is an excellent way to help regulate blood pressure, the calcium from spinach and beet greens isn't well-absorbed by the body. Be sure to eat a wide variety of greens to meet all your mineral needs.

Meat of the Diet

Large studies overwhelmingly show that many cancers occur least often in countries where people regard leafy greens, along with a wide variety of fruits and vegetables, as the "meats" of their meals.

In one study, researchers compared 61 men with lung cancer in Chile with 61 men of similar age and smoking habits who were cancer free. The one difference they found was that men with cancer consumed significantly fewer carotenoid-rich foods, especially Swiss chard, chicory, and spinach as well as beets and cabbage, than those without the disease.

Another study done at Banaras Hindu University in India looked at the role of

---

FOOD ALERT

When Spinach Means Stones

Popeye probably never had kidney stones, because if he had, he wouldn't have kept downing all those cans of spinach.

Spinach, along with Swiss chard and beet greens, contains high amounts of oxalates, acids that the body cannot process and that are passed through the urine. For people who are sensitive to oxalates, eating too many of these greens could contribute to the formation of kidney stones. So if you're prone to stones, says Michael Liebman, PhD, professor of human nutrition at the University of Wyoming in Laramie, choose low-oxalate vegetables such as Brussels sprouts and green peas rather than spinach, chard, and beet greens.

vegetables in protecting against gallbladder cancer. The study looked at the vegetable consumption of 153 people with gallbladder cancer and 153 people without gallbladder cancer and put them into three categories: no or rare consumption of vegetables, consumption 1 to 2 days a week, or consumption at least 3 days a week. The researchers found that the people with the highest reported intake of vegetables—particularly, leafy green vegetables—had the lowest rate of gallbladder cancer.

A similar protective benefit was found between leafy green vegetable intake and stomach cancer in a study done at the University of Occupational and Environmental Health in Kitakyushu, Japan.

And leafy green vegetables seem to be protective against prostate cancer as well. An Australian study looked at the diets of 130 men with prostate cancer and 274 men without the disease, and found that the risk of prostate cancer decreased as certain foods—one of them being spinach—increased.

The carotenoids, which are found in large amounts in most leafy greens, are like bodyguards against cancer-causing agents, explains Frederick Khachik, PhD, adjunct professor in the department of chemistry and biology at the University of Maryland in College Park. He and fellow researchers believe that certain cancers are brought on by the constant onslaught of free radicals—harmful oxygen molecules made by our bodies and also found in air pollution and tobacco smoke—which attack our bodies' healthy cells. Carotenoids counteract free radicals by acting as antioxidants, meaning that they step between the free radicals and our bodies' cells, neutralizing the free radicals before they can do damage, he explains.

"There is also plenty of evidence that carotenoids may fight cancer by activating the body's detoxification enzymes—called phase II enzymes—which are responsible for ridding the body of harmful, often cancer-causing, chemicals," says Dr. Khachik.

"Dark green leafy vegetables are among the best sources of some very important carotenoids, like lutein, alpha-carotene, and the one that everyone's familiar with, beta-carotene," he says. While all leafy greens are rich in carotenoids, the granddaddy is spinach, with a half-cup providing 1 milligram of beta-carotene.

Seeing Green

Carrots must be good for your eyes, the old joke has it, since you never see a rabbit wearing glasses. According to research, it's probably not only carrots that are good for the eyes but also all the leafy greens rabbits munch.

In one study, scientists from the Massachusetts Eye and Ear Infirmary in Boston compared the diets of more than 350 people with advanced age-related macular degeneration (AMD)—the leading cause of irreversible vision loss among older adults—with the diets of more than 500 people without the disease. They found that people who ate the most leafy green vegetables—particularly spinach and collard greens—were 43 percent less likely to get macular degeneration than those who ate them less frequently.

And a Dutch study published in the *Journal of the American Medical Association* looked at the relationship between dietary intake of vitamins E and C, zinc, and beta-carotene and age-related macular degeneration in more than 4,000 older adults at risk for the condition. A high intake of all four nutrients was associated with a 35 percent decrease in AMD risk, indicating that all four antioxidants are protective.

Experts believe that carotenoids protect the eyes in much the same way as they work against cancer, by acting as antioxidants and neutralizing the tissue-damaging free radicals before they harm the body—in this case, the macular region of the eye.

Smile and Say "Greens"

In some parts of the world, like rural China, where vegetarianism is a way of life, people meet their daily calcium needs not by drinking milk but by eating greens.

In fact, 1 cup of turnip or dandelion greens can deliver about 172 milligrams of calcium, or 17 percent of the DV for this mineral. That's more than you'd get from a half-cup of fat-free milk.

There is a catch, though. One problem with getting calcium from leafy green vegetables is that some of them contain high amounts of oxalates—compounds that block calcium absorption, says Dr. Liebman. "Spinach, Swiss chard, collards, and beet greens have the most oxalates, so don't eat these as a source of calcium," he says. "The others are fine. Research has shown that the calcium in kale is particularly well-absorbed."

Pumping Up at the Salad Bar

If you're among the many folks cutting back on meats these days, you may be cutting down on a very important mineral as well—iron. Here again, the leafy greens can help. Many green vegetables, especially spinach and Swiss chard, are good

---

Doctor's Top Tip

They may all fall under the umbrella term of "greens," but they actually come in many rich colors and textures, and you should eat the full range. One way to guarantee a nice greens buffet is with a greens mixture called mesclun. This mix may include arugula, frisée, mache, radicchio, dandelion greens, mizuna, oakleaf lettuce, and sorrel—all these greens serve up healthful vitamins and minerals, says Jana Klauer, MD, a New York City–based physician who specializes in the biology of fat reduction. "You can also make up your own batch by mixing and matching greens. Choose leaves that add interesting flavors, colors, and textures, such as endive, kale, escarole, Swiss chard, or baby spinach," she says. "Salads don't have to be boring. Get creative with your greens," she suggests.

sources of iron, a mineral your body needs to produce red blood cells and transport oxygen.

A half-cup of cooked spinach has 3 milligrams of iron, or 20 percent of the Recommended Dietary Allowance (RDA) for women and 30 percent of the RDA for men. The same amount of Swiss chard provides 2 milligrams, which is 13 percent of the RDA for women and 20 percent of the RDA for men.

Unfortunately, the iron found in plants isn't as readily absorbed by the body as the iron found in meats—unless it's accompanied in the same meal by vitamin C. Good news again. Along with their high doses of iron, leafy green vegetables also contain ample amounts of vitamin C, which substantially improves iron absorption.

But while all the leafy greens provide good amounts of vitamin C, the greens for this important vitamin are chicory (a half-cup serving has 22 milligrams, or 37 percent of the DV) and beet and mustard greens, which both provide almost 18 milligrams, or 30 percent of the DV.

In addition, beet greens and spinach are rich sources of riboflavin—a B vitamin that is essential for tissue growth and repair as well as helping your body convert other nutrients into usable forms. A half-cup of cooked spinach or beet greens provides 0.2 milligram of riboflavin, or 12 percent of the DV.

Go Deep

To get the maximum health benefits from greens, eat the darkest ones you can find. "The deeper the color of greens, the more benefits they provide," says Janet Maccaro, PhD, ND, a holistic nutritionist in Ormond Beach, Florida, who is president of Dr. Janet's Balance By Nature Products and the author of *Natural Health Remedies A-Z*. "The darker, the better. So go for spinach, kale, and other greens with a deep tone for good health," she says.

GETTING THE MOST

Cook them quickly. To cook or not to cook? That's often the question asked by people who want to maintain high levels of nutrients in vegetables. The answer with leafy greens, experts say, is yes, no, and maybe a little.

"It's always a trade-off between increasing the digestibility of nutrients when you cook foods and losing some nutrients in the cooking process," says Dr. Liebman. "But while it's great to eat them raw, you're more likely to eat more of certain vegetables if they're cooked. Just watch your cooking method. You don't want to boil them to death. Any quick-cooking method, such as blanching, is fine. One of the best cooking methods for retaining nutrients is microwaving," he says.

Steak and Spinach Salad with Pomegranate Dressing

6 tablespoons 100% pomegranate juice

2 tablepoons white wine vinegar

4 teaspoons Dijon mustard

4 teaspoons extra-virgin olive oil

1 teaspoon honey

12 cups loosely packed baby spinach leaves

1 cup juice-packed mandarin oranges, drained

½ cup pomegranate seeds

¼ cup roasted, unsalted almonds

Salt and freshly ground black pepper

12 ounces lean steak, such as top round or London broil

In a small bowl, whisk together the juice, vinegar, mustard, oil, and honey.

In a large bowl, combine the spinach, oranges, pomegranate seeds, and almonds. Add all but 3 tablepoons of the dressing and salt and pepper to taste. Toss well.

Lightly coat a large skillet with cooking spray, and heat over medium-high heat. Add the steak and cook for 5 minutes per side for medium-rare. Remove from the heat and set aside for 3 minutes.

Slice the steak thinly, and top the salad with the slices. Drizzle with the remaining dressing. Serve immediately.

Makes 4 servings

PER SERVING ⸻

Calories: 356

Total fat: 15 g

Saturated fat: 3 g

Cholesterol: 41 mg

Sodium: 238 mg

Dietary fiber: 5 g

Romaine and Watercress Salad with Anchovy Vinaigrette

½ teaspoon anchovy paste

½ teaspoon Dijon mustard

Salt (optional)

1 tablespoon balsamic vinegar

1 tablespoon red wine vinegar

6 tablespoons extra-virgin olive oil

Freshly ground black pepper

1 small head romaine lettuce

2 bunches watercress, large stems discarded

In a salad bowl, combine the anchovy paste, mustard, and salt (if using). Add the balsamic and red wine vinegars, and mix with a fork. Add the olive oil slowly while whisking constantly. Taste for seasoning, adding the pepper and more salt, vinegar, and oil to taste.

When ready to serve, add the romaine and watercress, and toss to coat.

Makes 6 servings

PER SERVING

Calories: 136
Total fat: 14 g
Saturated fat: 2 g

Cholesterol: 0 mg
Sodium: 96 mg
Dietary fiber: 1 g

Mustard Greens with Smoked Turkey

2 pounds mustard greens

1 cup finely chopped onions

¾ cup chopped smoked turkey breast

2 cloves garlic, minced

1 tablespoon white wine vinegar

Hot pepper sauce

Tear the leaves of the greens away from the stems and discard the stems. Tear the greens into bite-size pieces.

Coat a large nonstick skillet with cooking spray. Scatter the onions, turkey, and garlic evenly in the skillet, and warm over medium heat. As soon as the skillet starts to heat up,

add as much of the greens as the skillet will hold. (If necessary, add the remainder after the first batch cooks down enough to make room for them.) Cover tightly and cook until the greens wilt and soften, 7 to 8 minutes. Stir to combine. Sprinkle with the vinegar and add hot pepper sauce to taste.

Makes 4 servings

PER SERVING

Calories: 62
Total fat: 1.2 g
Saturated fat: 0.3 g

Cholesterol: 14 mg
Sodium: 304 mg
Dietary fiber: 2.6 g

Hay Fever

THE KITCHEN CONNECTION

While the usual treatment for hay fever is to stay inside and take antihistamines, there are some people with this allergy who don't want to spend the spring indoors. Now, there's some evidence that the foods you eat could make you feel even worse. So instead of shutting all the windows, take a look in your kitchen. There may be a few foods that you'll want to, well, sneeze at.

Doctors aren't sure why, but for many people with hay fever, the immune system responds not only to pollen but also to certain fruits and vegetables, especially melons and bananas, says John Anderson, MD, an allergist and immunologist at the division of allergy and clinical immunology at Henry Ford Hospital in Detroit.

If you're allergic to ragweed, for example, having a slice of watermelon or cantaloupe or eating a banana could cause your mouth to itch and swell, or you might experience additional stuffiness, says Dr. Anderson. If you're allergic to tree and grass pollens, on the other hand, eating apples, cherries, peaches, carrots, or potatoes might make your symptoms worse.

People with this type of multiple allergy (doctors call it cross-reactivity) may get hay fever symptoms in response to these foods all year long. In most cases, however, they suffer more in the spring, when pollen counts (and as a result, the body's level of histamine) are already high. There's no real solution, except the obvious one, which is a bummer if you are a fruit lover: You may have to give up the fruits and vegetables that are causing your symptoms to flare up. Or, you have another option: Cooking the offending foods will often eliminate their allergy-causing potential. But certain fruits, such as peaches and bananas, are not exactly at their tastiest after being sautéed.

In addition, people with hay fever are sometimes sensitive to the pollen in honey. "If you have honey that's loaded with the pollen you're sensitive to, you may have a reaction," says Dr. Anderson.

You probably don't have to give up honey entirely, though, he adds. Different

> ### Doctor's Top Tip
>
> "Pineapple contains bromelain, which helps block the inflammation of hay fever," says Janet Maccaro, PhD, ND, a holistic nutritionist in Ormond Beach, Florida. So when hay fever flares up, buy some fresh pineapple and munch on it for some relief, she says.

kinds of honey contain different kinds of pollen. By switching brands a few times, you'll eventually find one that doesn't make your hay fever symptoms worse.

Finally, Austrian researchers have found that for some people with hay fever, wine may cause problems. A small study found that red wine often contains histamine, the same chemical that makes people with hay fever so miserable. In someone with hay fever, pouring additional histamine into a system that's already loaded with the stuff may cause the bronchial tubes to constrict, making breathing difficult.

As far as foods that can help relieve symptoms of hay fever, go for those containing the flavonoid quercetin and vitamin C, says Janet Maccaro, PhD, ND, a holistic nutritionist in Ormond Beach, Florida, who is president of Dr. Janet's Balance By Nature Products and the author of *Natural Health Remedies A-Z*. Both quercetin and vitamin C have antihistamine properties, so they help combat the inflammation that accompanies hay fever. Quercetin is found in apples, onions, and teas, for example. Good sources of vitamin C include strawberries and citrus fruits.

Headaches

FEED YOUR HEAD RIGHT

In some ways, headaches are an unavoidable consequence of the horn-honking traffic jams, daily office politics, family squabbles, and late nights that go hand-in-hand with modern life.

Yet stress and noise aren't the only things causing heads to throb. Many of the foods we eat, from hot dogs and cheese to chocolate brownies, can cause headaches. Not eating certain foods can also cause problems. This may explain, in part, why Americans spend billions of dollars per year on over-the-counter and prescription pain relief. That's a lot of extra-strength aspirin, acetaminophen, and ibuprofen. And given the recent warnings about the link between these over-the-counter pain remedies and liver damage and stomach bleeding, you may want to think twice before you down these pills to stop your head from pounding.

While changing your diet won't eliminate headaches entirely, it can reduce their frequency and keep the pain under control. Best of all, relief won't come from a safety-sealed bottle that delivers health risks along with pain relief, but rather from the foods you eat.

Two Types of Pain

Before considering specific foods, it's helpful to understand the main types of headaches. The most common type, called muscle-contraction or tension headache, is usually caused by kinked-up neck and scalp muscles.

The second type, which includes migraines, is called vascular headache. This type of headache is caused by the expansion and contraction of blood vessels in the face, head, and neck. Vascular headaches can be extremely painful and in some cases, even disabling, as anyone who gets migraines can attest.

Both vascular and tension headaches can be caused by almost anything—stress, fluctuating hormone levels, or even changes in the weather. But substances found in foods—natural compounds as well as chemicals added during processing—are frequently to blame, says Melvyn Werbach, MD, assistant clinical professor of psychiatry at the University of California, Los Angeles, and author of *Healing through Nutrition* and *Nutritional Influences on Illness*.

Doctor's Top Tip

The best way to deal with a headache is not to get one in the first place. And the foods that cause headaches most often are those that contain tyramine, an amino acid that triggers the body to release hormones that cause blood vessels to constrict, says John Neustadt, ND, medical director of Montana Integrative Medicine in Bozeman. At some point, the blood vessels fight back and dilate, setting off the familiarly unpleasant throb. To avoid this head-pounding compound, stay away from chocolate, beer, aged dairy products, bananas, nuts, beans, and other tyramine foods if you're headache prone, he says.

Common Triggers

Although experts aren't sure exactly what causes migraines, they have identified a number of foods and additives that may set the headache process in motion.

A huge culprit is tyramine (see "Doctor's Top Tip" at left). Nitrites are another common cause of headache pain. Used to preserve cured meats such as bologna, hot dogs, and meats packaged in a can, nitrites can cause blood vessels in the head and body to dilate painfully.

And monosodium glutamate (MSG), a preservative and flavor enhancer used in a variety of foods, including lunch meats, canned and dry soups, and frozen dinners, can be a problem. It's also a common additive in Chinese cooking. The term *Chinese restaurant syndrome* was coined to describe MSG-related headaches. Luckily, a lot of Chinese restaurants have caught on to the headache side effect that sometimes goes along with their fare and have removed all MSG from their cooking processes.

There's no easy way to avoid all of these substances or to be sure which one—or which combination of them—is causing the problem. To keep track of which foods cause your head to throb, keep a headache diary, says Alan M. Rapoport, MD, cofounder and director of the New England Center for Headache in Stamford, Connecticut, and assistant clinical professor of neurology at Yale University School of Medicine. The minute you feel the first twinge of a headache coming on, make a list of everything you've eaten in the past 24 hours. Eventually, you'll gain a better understanding of which foods may be to blame so you can avoid them in the future.

The Carbohydrate Connection

Central to the headache-food equation is a feel-good brain chemical called serotonin, which transmits messages from one nerve cell to another. Low levels of serotonin in the brain are often associated with headaches, says Dr. Rapoport. Therefore, raising the levels of serotonin can ease headaches or even prevent them entirely.

One way to boost serotonin in the brain is to increase the amount of complex carbohydrates in your diet. "There's no doubt that following a diet high in complex carbohydrates and low in fat can be very helpful for some people with migraine, although we don't know exactly why," says Dr. Rapoport.

If you're prone to headaches, it might be a good idea to eat more foods that are high in fiber and complex carbohydrates, such as fresh vegetables, whole grains, and dried beans and other legumes, Dr. Rapoport advises.

But even though a high-carbohydrate diet can often ease pain, there are some people for whom it can actually make headaches worse. If you have low blood sugar, or hypoglycemia, for example, you may find that you do better if you consume fewer carbohydrates. "Having low levels of sugar in the brain can set off a headache," says Dr. Werbach. "These people may do well on a so-called hypoglycemic diet, which is usually a low-carbohydrate diet." And beyond headaches, a high-carbohydrate diet can be detrimental for people with certain health conditions, such as metabolic syndrome or diabetes.

If you've noticed that your headaches often occur after you've eaten a lot of carbohydrates, says Dr. Werbach, try eating slightly more protein in the form of lean meats, eggs, or low-fat cheese.

The Benefits of B$_6$

Vitamin B$_6$ has been shown to keep the nervous system healthy, relieve premenstrual discomfort, and bolster the immune system, and as if that weren't enough, studies also suggest that it may help relieve migraines. The brain uses vitamin B$_6$ to increase serotonin levels, explains Dr. Rapoport, "so a good intake of B$_6$ might help relieve migraines, even if you're not deficient in it."

The Daily Value (DV) for vitamin B$_6$ is 2 milligrams. One medium potato or one banana contains 0.7 milligram of B$_6$, or 35 percent of the DV. A 3-ounce serving of baked or broiled swordfish has 0.3 milligram, or 15 percent of the DV.

Your doctor may also advise getting larger amounts (up to 150 milligrams) of vitamin B$_6$ through a multiple vitamin. You shouldn't take B$_6$ supplements unless prescribed by a doctor, however, because getting too much B$_6$ can cause damage to the nervous system.

Minerals for Relief

While the exact underlying reasons aren't yet clear, certain minerals, particularly magnesium, calcium, and iron, seem to help prevent and treat both migraine and tension headaches.

People who suffer from chronic migraines often have low levels of magnesium in their brain cells. Studies suggest that correcting a magnesium deficiency may help relieve migraine, says Dr. Rapoport.

Ready-to-eat breakfast cereals are good sources of magnesium; some brands contain more than 100 milligrams of magnesium, or 25 percent of the DV, in a 1-ounce serving. Nuts, seeds, and dark green leafy vegetables are also rich in magnesium. Nuts are also loaded with fat, however, so you'll want to eat them in moderation (no more than a handful a day), and get most of your magnesium elsewhere.

Calcium is another mineral that has been linked to headache relief. One study found that women who consumed 200 milligrams of calcium a day (20 percent of the DV) had fewer headaches than women who consumed less.

Dairy foods are the best sources of calcium. Topping the list is milk, with 1 cup of fat-free milk containing 302 milligrams, or 30 percent of the DV. Other good sources of calcium include ice milk, with 176 milligrams per cup, or 18 percent of the DV, and low-fat fruit yogurt, with 312 milligrams per cup, or 31 percent of the DV. There are many nondairy sources of calcium as well, among them broccoli, with 72 milligrams in 1 cup, and Swiss chard, with 101 milligrams in 1 cup.

Last on the list of minerals that may help prevent headaches is iron. Not getting sufficient iron in the diet can lead to anemia, a condition in which the body doesn't get enough oxygen. To compensate, blood vessels dilate to admit more blood, says Dr. Rapoport. "This dilation compresses the nerves in the walls of the vessels, causing head pain," he explains. "Consuming more dietary iron may indirectly relieve headaches by treating the anemia."

It's generally easy to meet the DV of 18 milligrams for iron. A large baked potato, for example, has 7 milligrams, while 1 cup of Swiss chard has nearly 4 milligrams. Meats are even better sources; they contain heme iron, a type of iron that is more readily absorbed by the body than the nonheme iron in vegetables. A 3-ounce serving of broiled top round steak has 3 milligrams of iron, and the same amount of roasted white turkey meat has 1 milligram.

Spicy Relief

When you're searching for a drug-free form of migraine relief, you might want to try a spoonful of the popular spice ginger. "Ginger is good for headaches because it stimulates circulation," says Janet Maccaro, PhD, ND, a holistic nutritionist in Ormond Beach, Florida, who is president of Dr. Janet's Balance By Nature Products and the author of *Natural Health Remedies A-Z*.

A study done at the Headache Care Center in Springfield, Missouri, showed ginger's power at preventing headaches. Thirty people with a history of migraine were given an over-the-counter combination of feverfew and ginger (called GelStat) at the early, mild pain phase of a migraine headache. Two hours after treatment, 48 percent of the participants were pain free, and 34 percent reported a mild headache.

Overall, 59 percent of the participants said they were happy with the effectiveness of the ginger-containing GelStat, indicating that its ingredients may be a good first-line treatment for migraines.

And researchers at Odense University in Denmark believe that ginger blocks the action of prostaglandins, substances that cause pain and inflammation in blood vessels. Therefore, it might help prevent impending migraines without the side effects of some migraine-relieving drugs.

If you feel a migraine coming on, you might try taking ⅓ teaspoon of powdered ginger, the amount suggested by the Danish researchers.

When taking ginger, it's even better to use the fresh rather than the powdered form because it's more active, says Charles Lo, MD, a doctor of Chinese medicine in private practice in Chicago. He advises grating the ginger or pushing it through a garlic press; these methods release more of the potent juices than does slicing or chopping it. Or, you can make a spicy ginger tea by steeping a teaspoon of the grated root in a cup of boiling water for at least 5 minutes, says Dr. Lo.

The Coffee Cure

There's a reason some over-the-counter headache relievers can make you feel jumpy. "Caffeine is often an ingredient in pain relievers," says Fred Sheftell, MD, cofounder and codirector of the New England Headache Center in Stamford, Connecticut. For some people, sipping a cup of their favorite aromatic brew may work as well as popping an over-the-counter painkiller. The caffeine in coffee can counter a headache by temporarily constricting dilated blood vessels, which may be causing the pain, says Dr. Sheftell.

But don't overdo it with the coffee. Too much java will eventually cause the blood vessels to dilate painfully again. Dr. Sheftell recommends that people who are headache-prone drink no more than 2 cups (5 ounces each) a day, which together contain about 200 milligrams of caffeine, depending on the strength of the brew.

Heartburn

PUTTING OUT THE FIRE

If you've ever had heartburn, you know the name is appropriate. It feels as though a fire is raging in your chest. The pain can be so intense, in fact, that some people rush to the emergency room in the fear they're having a heart attack.

But contrary to its name and its sensation, heartburn has nothing to do with the heart. It occurs when acid-laden digestive juices in the stomach head in the wrong direction and surge upward into the esophagus, the tube that connects the mouth with the stomach. Normally, a tight little muscle at the base of the esophagus, called the lower esophageal sphincter (LES), prevents juices from escaping. But if that sphincter relaxes, juices splash upward and cause the "burn" that is heartburn.

There are some foods that make heartburn more likely. Likewise, there are foods that will quickly put the fire out. So before you rush to the pharmacy for an antacid, make a pit stop in your kitchen.

"Modifying the diet remains one of the first lines of treatment for people with heartburn," says Suzanne Rose, MD, professor of medical education and medicine and gastroenterology at Mount Sinai Hospital in New York City.

Inside Healing

One food that can help control heartburn is ginger, says John Hibbs, ND, a naturopathic doctor and clinical faculty member at Bastyr Center for Natural Health in Seattle. Ginger helps strengthen the holding power of the LES, which can help keep acid where it belongs. If you don't like the spiciness of fresh ginger, make a ginger tea by adding ½ to 1 teaspoon of freshly grated ginger (or ¼ to ½ teaspoon of powdered ginger) to a cup of hot water. Let it steep for 10 minutes, strain, and enjoy.

It's a good idea not to lie down soon after eating, says Dr. Rose. When your stomach is full, it's much easier for acid to rise up into the esophagus, especially when you lie down and gravity is working against you. Remain upright, whether on your feet or sitting in a chair, to help keep the acid down, she says.

Common Offenders

An estimated 60 million Americans experience heartburn at least once a month, and up to 15 million are thought to experience it daily. What's more, Americans get more calories from fat than people from any other country on the planet. A coincidence? Researchers don't think so. Studies have shown that foods high in fat, like butter and red meat, can temporarily reduce the holding power of the LES. In one study, researchers at Bowman Gray School of Medicine of Wake Forest University in Winston-Salem, North Carolina, found that people who ate high-fat meals were exposed to acid about four times as long as those eating leaner fare.

Chocolate is another offender for some people, Dr. Rose adds. Not only is it high in fat, it may contain other compounds that can relax the LES even more. In another study at Bowman Gray, researchers found that when people ate chocolate, stomach acid splashed into the esophagus for up to an hour afterward.

It's not only high-fat foods that can be a problem for heartburn sufferers, however. Onions, for example, can bring on heartburn in some people. Researchers aren't exactly sure what it is about onions that can light the fire, but for some, heartburn can flare up after only one slice of onion.

Peppermint, which is often added to candy, ice cream, and baked goods, frequently causes heartburn as well, Dr. Rose adds. In one study, researchers at the State University of New York at Buffalo found that when people ate peppermint, their esophageal muscles lost some holding power within just a few minutes.

And coffee, tomatoes, citrus fruits, and fried foods can also trigger heartburn, says John Neustadt, ND, medical director of Montana Integrative Medicine in Bozeman. So if you notice your heartburn worsens after eating one or more of these foods, try to avoid them, he says.

Finally, if you're suffering from a bout of heartburn, be careful about eating spicy foods until your esophagus has a chance to heal, says Dr. Rose. Many people don't think twice about dousing tender esophageal tissues with hot peppers or a swig of orange juice. You don't have to give up your favorite foods entirely, she says. Just avoid them for a few days until your heartburn is feeling better.

Doctor's Top Tip

The most recent development in heartburn research was a study that compared how quickly a meal was ingested rather than a type of food per se, says Donald Castell, MD, professor of medicine and the director of the esophageal disorders program at the Medical University of South Carolina in Charleston. "The study was hospital-based and probably developed originally because the interns and residents ate their meals so quickly and then ran off to see another patient," he says. "What they found was that if you took the same meal—a turkey burger, fries, and a Coke—and looked at people who ate that meal in 5 minutes versus people who ate it in 30 minutes, there was a significantly greater amount of acid reflux in the quick-eating group than in the leisurely eating group," he says. So if you have a problem with heartburn, take some time to relax and enjoy your food—no matter what you're eating—rather than scarfing it down.

Heart Disease

PRIMING YOUR PUMP

Doctors haven't always known what was best for our hearts. Only a few decades ago, little attention was paid to diet, and even smoking was thought to be acceptable by some.

Everything Has Changed

After almost 50 years of investigating what makes heart disease our worst public-health enemy, scientists have come up with some pretty simple and straightforward answers. Regular exercise is important, of course, as is staying away from cigarettes or quitting smoking if you picked up the habit. But perhaps the most important of all is having a healthy diet. Reaching for the right foods is the most effective way to lower cholesterol and high blood pressure, two of the biggest risk factors for the heart.

All too often, however, we reach for the wrong foods. So, to put confusion to rest, here are some of the best—and worst—foods for preventing heart disease, starting with fats. While there are some fats that we'd be better off avoiding, others aren't so bad, it turns out, and some might even be healthful.

The Bad Fats

We all know that saturated fat, the kind found primarily in animal foods, such as red meat, butter, and others, is incredibly dangerous for the heart. Study after study has shown that the more saturated fat people get in their diets, the higher their risks for heart disease.

Foods high in saturated fat raise levels of artery-clogging low-density lipoprotein (LDL) cholesterol, says Michael Gaziano, MD, chief of the division of aging at Brigham and Women's Hospital and associate professor of medicine at Harvard Medical School, both in Boston. What's more, foods high in saturated fat are often high in cholesterol as well.

The danger is so great that the American Heart Association recommends that we limit our intake of saturated fat to less than 7 percent of our calories each day. Suppose, for example, that you normally get 2,000 calories in a day. This means your upper daily limit for saturated fat is 14 grams. This means that in addition to eating fruits, vegetables, and other low-fat foods, you could have 3 ounces of extra-lean ground beef (which contains 5 grams of saturated fat), a serving of macaroni and cheese (6 grams), and a half-cup of low-fat frozen yogurt (3 grams).

Another type of problem fat, called trans fatty acids, has been shown to dramatically increase the amount of cholesterol in the bloodstream, says Dr. Gaziano.

Ironically, trans fatty acids (which are made when manufacturers add hydrogen to vegetable oils to turn the liquid oils into solid fats like margarine and shortening) were meant to be a healthful alternative to the saturated fat in butter. But it appears that trans fatty acids may be even more harmful than saturated fats. Trans fats raise the bad LDL cholesterol *and* lower the good HDL (high-density lipoprotein) cholesterol, increasing the risk of cardiovascular disease, heart attack, and stroke.

Trans fats appear to be so dangerous, in fact, that some US cities, including New York City, have begun banning them from being used as ingredients in french fries, doughnuts, and other foods fried in frying shortenings. And it's not only margarine and fried foods that may be a problem. Many cookies, cakes, and other snack foods contain "partially hydrogenated oil," which is also high in trans fatty acids. Because of the health risk posed by trans fatty acids, the American Heart Association recommends you limit your daily intake to less than 1 percent of your total calories.

Some Better Fats

Unlike saturated fat and trans fatty acids, some fats are relatively healthful. Here's an easy way to recognize them. Look for the "un," as in polyunsaturated and monounsaturated fats. While these "un-fats" are still high in calories, in small amounts, they play several beneficial roles.

Polyunsaturated fats (found in soy, corn, safflower, sesame, and sunflower oils, as well as nuts and seeds) help your body get rid of newly formed cholesterol; therefore, they keep cholesterol levels down and reduce cholesterol deposits on artery walls. Monounsaturated fats also appear to help lower cholesterol levels as long as the rest of the diet is very low in saturated fats. Although they are a good substitute for saturated fat, both polyunsaturated fats and monounsaturated fats should be used in moderation because their high calorie counts can lead to weight gain. No more than 30 percent of your calories should come from fat.

"Picking either polyunsaturated or monounsaturated fats over saturated fat or trans fats is a winning choice," says Christopher Gardner, PhD, assistant professor of medicine at the Stanford Prevention Research Center in Stanford, California.

Nuts are particularly good sources of these healthful fats. In a study of Seventh-Day Adventists, researchers found that those who consumed nuts at least four times a

Doctor's Top Tip

When it comes to protection against heart disease, fish is perhaps the best thing you can eat, and the fattier the fish, the better. Fish contains omega-3 fatty acids, which reduce the risk of cardiovascular disease by making platelets less sticky, says Jana Klauer, MD, a New York City–based physician who specializes in the biology of fat reduction. For optimum results, eat fatty fish, such as tuna, Spanish mackerel, herring, or salmon, twice a week.

week had almost half the risk of fatal heart attacks of those who rarely ate them.

And the famous Nurses' Health Study, which looked at the lifestyle factors of more than 86,000 women ages 34 to 59 for 14 years, found that frequent nut consumption was associated with a decreased rate of both nonfatal and fatal heart attacks. So eating nuts seems to help lower risk for cardiovascular disease.

Although the American Heart Association recommends less than 30 percent of calories from fat, many health-care professionals, including Dr. Gaziano, recommend even less. "I tell people to aim for getting about 20 to 25 percent of total calories from fat, most of which should be in the form of monounsaturated and polyunsaturated fat," says Dr. Gaziano.

There's yet another kind of healthful fat, perhaps the king of healthful fats, called omega-3 fatty acids. Found in most fish (but particularly in oily, cold-water fish) and also in flaxseed and certain dark greens, omega-3s can help prevent clots from forming in the bloodstream. In addition, they help lower triglycerides, a type of blood fat that, in large amounts, may raise the risk for heart disease.

Studies show that eating fish twice a week (salmon is a good choice, because it contains high levels of omega-3s) can help keep your arteries clear and your heart working well. In a study done at the Harvard School of Public Health, scientists found that the death rate from heart disease was 36 percent lower among people who ate fish twice a week compared with people who ate little or no seafood. The study, which was published in the *Journal of the American Medical Association,* also showed that overall mortality was 17 percent lower among the regular seafood eaters.

Feast on Folate

Almost 30 years ago, a Harvard pathologist suggested that a vitamin deficiency could be a major cause of heart disease. The theory sounded so wacky that nobody listened. Now, instead of laughing, scientists are busy researching, because evidence suggests that folate, a B vitamin abundant in beans and dark green leafy vegetables, may play a major role in preventing heart attacks.

An Italian study published in the *European Journal of Clinical Nutrition* looked at the relationship between folate intake and heart attack risk in nearly 1,000 individuals, half who had a history of one nonfatal heart attack and half who had not.

Researchers found that the individuals with a higher intake of folate were less likely to have suffered a heart attack than those with a low intake of the B vitamin.

Folate is responsible for lowering levels of an amino acid called homocysteine. While the body needs homocysteine to produce muscle and bone tissue, in large amounts, it can injure blood vessels, causing hardening of the arteries.

"High homocysteine levels are an important contributor to heart disease," says Dr. Gardner. "And it appears that homocysteine can be brought down easily with modest amounts of folate in the diet."

You don't need a lot of folate to get the benefits. The Daily Value (DV) of 400 micrograms may be plenty, says Dr. Gardner. Spinach is a good source of folate, with 1 cup of cooked spinach containing 263 micrograms, or nearly 66 percent of the DV. Lentils are even better, with a half-cup containing 179 micrograms, or 45 percent of the DV. Even a 6-ounce glass of orange juice contains 36 micrograms of folate, or 9 percent of the DV.

Aiming for Antioxidants

Doctors have known for years that the body's LDL cholesterol is bad news, and now they also understand why.

Every day, your body produces harmful oxygen molecules called free radicals, which damage cholesterol. This harmful process, called oxidation, is what causes cholesterol to stick to the lining of artery walls.

Fruits, vegetables, and other foods containing antioxidants, such as beta-carotene and vitamins C and E, are the best protection against oxidation and heart disease. In fact, one group of antioxidants, called flavonoids, is thought to be the reason that the Dutch and French have such healthy hearts, despite some unhealthy eating habits.

A study in the Netherlands, for example, found that men who ate the most flavonoid-rich foods, particularly apples, tea, and onions, were half as likely to have heart disease as those who ate the least. Flavonoids may also explain why the French, who eat more fat and cholesterol than we do, have heart disease death rates 2½ times lower than ours.

"Foods containing flavonoids, including green tea, dark chocolate, and red wine, seem to protect against heart disease by improving endothelial function, which means that arteries are more flexible and able to deal with stresses of dietary fat, exercise, and increases in blood pressure," says Joe A. Vinson, PhD, professor of analytical chemistry at the University of Scranton in Pennsylvania, who specializes in the study of flavonoids.

Doctors still aren't sure which foods—or which compounds found in foods—are the most effective. An Italian study looked at the intake of certain flavonoids and the risk of heart attack in 760 patients under age 79 with a history of nonfatal heart attack and 682 patients with no history of heart attack. Researchers found that the patients with the highest intake of flavonoids called anthocyanidins—found in cherries, blueberries, and other brightly colored fruits—had the lowest risk of heart attack.

The American Heart Association recommends eating at least five servings a day of a large variety of fruits and vegetables. One serving is equal to ½ to 1 cup of cooked or raw vegetables, ½ cup of fruit juice, or 1 medium piece of fruit.

"You just can't lose by eating plenty of fruits and vegetables," says Dr. Gardner. "Study after study shows that people who eat the most of these healthful foods have the lowest rates of heart disease."

Fortify Your Heart with Fiber

Your grandmother called it roughage. Today, we call it fiber. But whatever it's called, it's an important part of any heart protection plan.

Fiber, especially the soluble kind found in beans, fruits, and whole grains, binds with cholesterol in the body and helps remove it along with the waste, says Diane Grabowski-Nepa, RD, a dietitian and nutritional counselor at the Pritikin Longevity Center in Santa Monica, California.

Results from the Nurses' Health Study, which looked at the lifestyle factors of 68,782 women for 10 years, showed that women who consumed an average of 22.9 grams of fiber a day had a 23 percent lower risk of heart disease than women who consumed less than 12 grams a day.

The DV for fiber is 25 grams, but most Americans don't get nearly enough. "The average consumption of fiber per person is 15 grams a day, but we need 25 to 30 grams for optimum health," says Jana Klauer, MD, a New York City–based physician who specializes in the biology of fat reduction and is the author of *How the Rich Stay Thin*. Super sources of fiber include whole grains and flaxseed, beans such as chickpeas, kidney beans, and lima beans, berries such as blueberries, strawberries, and raspberries, and dried fruits like figs, apples, and peaches. Overall, Dr. Klauer recommends fruits and vegetables as the best sources of fiber. "Per 100 calories, nonstarchy fruits and vegetables typically contain about eight times more fiber than whole grains, plus they supply added vitamins and minerals," she says.

Sip a Little Health

It's a tradition in many countries to raise a glass of wine and give a toast to good health. As it turns out, what's in that glass can make the toasts come true.

Studies have shown that drinking moderate amounts of alcohol raises levels of beneficial HDL cholesterol. Plus, alcohol acts like motor oil in the blood. It makes platelets, the tiny disks that aid in clotting, a little more slippery, so they're less likely to stick together and cause heart-damaging clots in the bloodstream.

A study done at the Institut Municipal d'Investigacio Medica in Barcelona, Spain, looked at the association of nonfatal heart attack and amount and types of alcoholic beverages consumed in 244 men with a history of nonfatal heart attack and 1,270 healthy male controls. The researchers found that total alcohol consumption (beer, wine, or liquor) of up to 30 grams per day (adjusted for lifestyle and cardiovascular disease risk factors) was associated with a decreased incidence of nonfatal heart attack. Alcohol consumption of 20 grams or less per day decreased the risk even more. And alcohol consumption higher than 30 grams did not decrease risk of nonfatal heart attack. These results suggest that moderate alcohol consumption is protective against heart attack, regardless of the type of alcohol consumed, but higher amounts of alcohol are not.

That said, red wine does happen to be particularly good because it also contains heart-healthy flavonoids. A Norwegian study looked at the relationship between drinking red wine and plasma viscosity (blood plasma that is more viscous is more likely to clot and lead to heart attack or stroke). Healthy, nonsmoking volunteers were instructed to drink a glass of wine every day for 3 weeks and then to abstain from alcohol for 3 weeks. Researchers measured their plasma viscosity at the start of the study, after the first 3 weeks of wine drinking, and after the second 3 weeks of abstaining from wine. They found that viscosity levels dropped after the 3 weeks of wine drinking and remained lower through the second 3 weeks, suggesting that a daily glass of red wine helps lower plasma viscosity and, therefore, risk of heart attack and stroke.

To get the benefits of alcohol without the health problems, doctors advise drinking in moderation. For men, this means having no more than two drinks a day. Women, who are more susceptible to alcohol's effects, should limit themselves to no more than one drink a day. (A drink is defined as 12 ounces of beer, 5 ounces of wine, 1½ ounces of 80-proof liquor, or 1 ounce of 100-proof liquor.) Drinking more than one drink a day for women or two for men is counterproductive healthwise and poses dangers such as high blood pressure, obesity, stroke, suicide, and accidents. Therefore, the American Heart Association cautions people not to start drinking if they do not already drink alcohol.

Hemorrhoids

NO MORE STRAINED VEINS

Sometimes the call of nature feels anything but natural. You have to go, but it takes more effort than you'd like. So you strain. And strain. This puts a lot of stress on tiny veins in your anus and rectum, which can cause them to swell and stretch out of shape. The result is an often painful but very common condition known as hemorrhoids. Since most hemorrhoids are caused by straining to have a bowel movement, the best way to prevent them is by making stools easier to pass, says Marvin Schuster, MD, founder of the Marvin M. Schuster Digestive and Motility Disorders Center at Johns Hopkins Bayview Medical Center in Baltimore. And the best way to do this is by eating foods that are kind to your digestive system.

Bulk for Your Bowels

The reason so many Americans have hemorrhoids is that the average fiber consumption in this country is 12 to 15 grams a day, a lot less than the Daily Value of 25 grams, says Dr. Schuster. Fiber is important because it adds bulk and weight to stools, helping them to pass more easily. Studies have shown, in fact, that folks who eat a lot of fiber-rich foods have considerably fewer hemorrhoids than those who eat less fiber.

EASE THE PAIN

When hemorrhoids swell, they press against tender nerves, which is why they're often so painful. In addition, eating certain foods can make the pain even worse. So the next time hemorrhoids occur, here are a few foods that you may want to avoid.

Say *nada* to java. Drinking coffee causes the intestines to contract, which can irritate an already tender hemorrhoid. Also, coffee is a diuretic, meaning it causes the body to lose valuable water—and you need more, not less, water when hemorrhoids flare.

Take a break from alcohol. Like coffee, alcohol is a diuretic and can cause constipation. When you have hemorrhoids, abstain from drinking alcohol until they go away.

Be a little bland. The same chemicals that give spicy foods their fire can burn you in the bathroom. So when hemorrhoids are hurting, put away the hot peppers, and stick with blander foods instead.

It's not difficult to get more fiber in your diet, Dr. Schuster adds. Eating legumes and the recommended 2½ to 3 cups of vegetables, 1½ to 2 cups of fruits, and 3 to 4 ounces of whole-grain products, such as oatmeal, brown rice, or 100 percent whole-wheat bread, will provide all the fiber your digestive tract needs to work smoothly.

Another great way to add fiber to your diet is with flaxseeds, says Janet Maccaro, PhD, ND, a holistic nutritionist in Ormond Beach, Florida, who is president of Dr. Janet's Balance By Nature Products and the author of *Natural Health Remedies A-Z*. Not only will you get the benefits of the fiber content in these crunchy little guys, you will get the omega-3 fatty acids they supply as well.

More Fluid Movements

Imagine eating some saltines without drinking any water. Hard to swallow, right? Well, a similar problem occurs when the digestive tract attempts to process food without getting enough liquid, says Marie Borum, MD, MPH, professor of medicine at George Washington University Medical Center in Washington, D.C. The stools become dry and difficult to pass—and this, as we've seen, is what causes hemorrhoids.

Water does more than aid digestion. Because it's absorbed by the stools, it makes them heavier and easier to pass. This is especially true when you're adding more fiber to your diet, because fiber absorbs the water like a sponge, says Dr. Borum.

She recommends drinking six to eight glasses of water a day. This sounds like a lot, and it would be if you tried to drink it all at once. Keep water handy and sip it throughout the day. Put a bottle in your backpack, for example, or keep a plastic sipping bottle at your desk—these tricks make it easier to get the necessary amounts.

Doctor's Top Tip

Even people who eat bushels of fiber and drink water by the pitcherful will occasionally have a problem with constipation and, possibly, hemorrhoids. This is why some doctors believe that you should do everything possible to strengthen the anal veins, just in case. "With hemorrhoids, the connective tissues in the blood vessel walls within the rectum have degenerated," says John Neustadt, ND, medical director of Montana Integrative Medicine in Bozeman. To strengthen these blood vessel walls, Dr. Neustadt suggests you eat berries. "Brightly colored fruits such as blueberries, blackberries, and cherries contain anthocyanins, which can improve blood vessel strength," he says. When the walls of the capillaries and veins in the anus are strengthened, they are less likely to stretch under pressure and lead to hemorrhoids. "Eat a cup of these berries a day to help protect against hemorrhoids," he says.

While you can get the benefits of these compounds by eating whole berries, juices provide a more concentrated form to keep the veins strong. Doctors who specialize in nutritional healing recommend drinking 4 ounces of berry juice mixed with an equal amount of apple juice every day.

Herbs

HEALING THE NATURAL WAY

HEALING POWER
Can Help:

Prevent infections

Ease pain and swelling

Relieve menopausal discomfort

Lower cholesterol

Imagine marinara sauce without oregano. Baked potatoes without chives. No one who enjoys food would want to live in a world without herbs.

But herbs do more than add rich flavor to sauces or a tangy zip to potatoes and tofu. For millions of people worldwide, herbs also act as the medicines they depend on to stay healthy.

"Before the discovery of modern pharmaceuticals, both Europeans and Americans relied on herbs," says William J. Keller, PhD, vice president of health sciences and educational services at Nature's Sunshine Products in Provo, Utah. Even today, people in European nations use herbal medicines nearly every day. In this country, however, we'd pretty much cast them aside—until about a decade or so ago, says Dr. Keller.

Doctors are discovering that many herbs work as well as prescription and over-the-counter drugs for relieving common conditions, and for a very simple reason. The active ingredients in herbs are often virtually identical to the chemicals found in drugs. When you take an aspirin, for example, you get the benefit of a compound called acetylsalicylic acid, which works to ease pain, lower fever, and reduce inflammation. But before there was aspirin, people made tea from willow bark. Willow contains a compound called salicin, which has many of the same effects as aspirin.

And it's not just "simple" over-the-counter drugs that have herbal counterparts. Many prescription drugs also resemble—or are actually made from—herbs. The cancer drug etoposide, for example, is extracted from the root of the mayapple plant, and the heart drug digitalis contains compounds similar to those found in purple foxglove (do not eat the foxglove plant, however, as it is poisonous in its raw form). Researchers estimate, in fact, that up to 30 percent of the drugs we use today contain ingredients that are very similar to compounds found in plants.

From Plants to Penicillin

Today researchers use sophisticated equipment and expensive tests to discover which herbs are the most effective. For the original herbalists, however, "research" often meant watching animals in the wild to see which leaves, bark, or berries they turned

In the Kitchen

To preserve the healing powers of herbs, you have to dry and store them properly. Here's how:

- When drying leaves or flowers, tie small bunches of herbs together, and hang them upside down in a dry, well-ventilated area such as an attic or large pantry. To prevent herbs from getting dusty, hang them inside paper bags with holes punched in the sides to allow air to circulate. Be careful not to crush the herbs, which will cause the precious oils to dissipate.

- When drying roots, cut them into thin pieces, thread them on a length of string, and hang them to dry.
- To dry seeds, hang the entire plant upside down in a paper bag with holes punched in it, and allow it to dry; as the plant dries, the seeds will fall to the bottom of the bag.
- To keep dried herbs fresh, store them in tightly sealed jars in a cool, dark place. When they are properly stored, dried herbs will retain their potency for a year or more.

to whenever they were ill. Over the years, herbalists (and many doctors) became pretty knowledgeable about which herbs were best for which conditions.

By the middle of the 20th century, however, scientists were less interested in the herbs themselves than in the medicinal compounds they contained. "With the advancement of laboratory chemistry, it became possible to isolate and purify the chemical compounds from plants to make pharmaceutical drugs," says Mark Blumenthal, executive director of the American Botanical Council in Austin, Texas, and editor of the journal *HerbalGram*.

The new drugs offered a lot of advantages over their leafy predecessors. With laboratory precision, it was possible to make millions of pills, each with exactly the same strength. Drugs were also convenient. It was no longer necessary to spend hours searching for and preparing herbs—hanging them to dry, extracting their oils, or brewing them into tea—since it was possible to pop a pill that did the same thing.

"It wasn't because herbs were ineffective that people quit using them, but because there were reliable, cheaper, sexier drugs, like the sulfa drugs and later, penicillin," says Blumenthal. "So herbs fell into a kind of twilight zone."

Back to Basics

Today, of course, it's much easier to find over-the-counter drugs than herbal remedies. But more and more Americans are choosing herbs over drugs in favor of a more natural way of healing.

One advantage of herbs is that they tend to cause fewer side effects than modern drugs. Most drugs are highly concentrated, which is why taking one tiny pill or capsule can have such dramatic results. Herbs, on the other hand, are much less concentrated; you don't get as much of the active ingredients in your body at one time, so you're less likely to have uncomfortable reactions.

But the main reason that people use herbs such as garlic, echinacea, and feverfew is that they really work—which is why, in just 1 year, German physicians wrote 5.4 million prescriptions for ginkgo, an herb that has been shown to improve bloodflow to the brain. They also wrote over 2 million prescriptions for echinacea, an immunity-boosting herb that's often used for treating colds and flu.

Some evidence has shown that taking echinacea as soon as you start feeling ill shortens the duration of the infection.

Of all the healing herbs, garlic is perhaps the best-studied, and with good reason. It contains compounds that have been shown to lower cholesterol and high blood pressure, two of the leading risk factors for heart disease. In a landmark study, people in two groups were given 2½ ounces of butter for several weeks, which raised their cholesterol levels. Half of the people were also given an extract containing the equivalent of seven cloves of garlic every day. Not surprisingly, people in both groups had increases in cholesterol. The garlic eaters, however, showed less of an increase than those who did not eat garlic. What's more, they actually had a 16 percent decrease in triglycerides, another type of blood fat that has been linked to heart disease.

Feverfew is an herb that has received scientific attention because it appears to help prevent migraines. In one study, for example, researchers at University Hospital in Nottingham, England, gave migraine-prone people capsules of feverfew every day for 4 months. At the end of the study, the number of migraines in the group had dropped 24 percent.

And, in a study done at the Headache Care Center in Springfield, Missouri, 30 people with a history of migraine were given an over-the-counter combination of feverfew and ginger (called GelStat) at the early, mild pain phase of a migraine headache. Overall, 59 percent of the participants said they were happy with the effectiveness of the feverfew-containing GelStat, indicating that its ingredients may be a good first-line treatment for migraines.

Licorice root is a perfect example of an herb that may work as well or even better than its prescription counterparts. Licorice root contains compounds called phytoestrogens, which enhance the effects of the estrogen a woman produces naturally. As a result, it can be very helpful for treating a variety of menopausal symptoms and other women's problems, such as hot flashes and mood swings, says Mary Bove, ND, a naturopathic doctor and director of the Brattleboro Naturopathic Clinic in Vermont.

For some women, licorice root may work just as well as the powerful drugs used in hormone-replacement therapy, Dr. Bove adds. And better yet, licorice root doesn't appear to increase the risk of breast and uterine cancers the way the medications do. If you'd like to try licorice root, check with your doctor to see if it might work for you.

Adding Flavor to Food

In addition to their medicinal properties, some herbs add fabulous flavors to recipes and can therefore act as a healthful substitute for salt, says Jana Klauer, MD, a New York City–based physician who specializes in the biology of fat reduction and is the author of *How the Rich Stay Thin*. Instead of salt, throw fresh thyme, dill weed, peppermint, basil, rosemary, garlic, parsley, tarragon, and other herbs into your foods to make them flavorful.

Putting Them to Work

When you're used to opening a bottle and popping a neat little pill into your mouth, getting used to the various herbal remedies can take a little time. Apothecaries and natural food stores often stock hundreds of healing herbs—packed into capsules, dissolved in oils, or lying loose in covered glass jars. It's not always easy to know which form to choose or how to prepare the herbs once you get them home. Here are a few tips for getting started.

Choose the right form. Many herbal remedies come in three forms: as pills or capsules, as liquids (called extracts and tinctures), and in their natural form as leaves, bark, roots, and flowers. Each form provides healing benefits, but they act in slightly different ways, says Debra Brammer, ND, a naturopathic doctor and clinical faculty member and associate clinical dean for the naturopathic medicine department at Bastyr University Natural Health Clinic in Seattle.

When you're sick and want fast relief, herbal extracts are usually best because they're absorbed very quickly by the body, says Dr. Brammer. While they're not as convenient as taking a pill—you have to measure them, using a dropper or a teaspoon, into a glass of water or juice—they go to work almost instantly, she says.

When you're using herbs for long-term protection—to strengthen the immune system, for example—it doesn't matter how quickly they work. What does count is convenience in buying and taking them, since you're going to be using the herbs almost every day. Nothing's easier than taking herbs in pill or capsule form. Just be sure to check the label before buying them, Dr. Keller adds. Herbal pills should be standardized, which means that they contain a precise amount of the healing herb. Products that aren't standardized may contain little or none of the herb's active compounds.

(continued on page 338)

THE HEALING HERBS

There are literally thousands of herbs that are used for healing around the world. Most herbs can be taken in capsule, tablet, tea, or liquid forms. Here are some of

Herb	Benefits	How to Use
Anise	Eases hot flashes and other menopausal problems. Helps relieve gas.	Crush 1 tsp seeds, and steep in boiling water to make a tea.
Chamomile	Good for indigestion and gas, insomnia, and for easing sore throat.	Pour boiling water over 1–2 Tbsp herb, and steep to make a tea.
Echinacea	Strengthens the immune system.	Take ½ tsp tincture three times a day at the first sign of a cold. Or pour boiling water over ½ tsp coarsely powdered dried herb, and steep to make a tea.
Fennel	Eases hot flashes and other menopausal problems. Helps settle the stomach.	Crush 1–2 tsp seeds, and steep in boiling water to make a tea.
Feverfew	Helps prevent and relieve migraines.	Eat 2–3 fresh leaves a day.
Garlic	Helps lower cholesterol and high blood pressure and reduces the risk for heart disease.	Eat 1–6 cloves a day.
Gentian	Stimulates appetite and improves digestion.	Pour boiling water over ½ tsp finely cut or coarsely powdered herb, and steep to make a tea.
Ginkgo	Helps prevent blood clots and increases bloodflow to the brain. Eases anxiety.	Take a 40-milligram capsule three times a day for 1–2 months.
Horehound	A mild expectorant that's good for coughs.	Pour boiling water over 1½ tsp finely cut leaves, and steep to make a tea.
Lemon balm	A calming herb that also helps ease cold sores.	Pour boiling water over 1–2 tsp finely chopped leaves, and steep to make a tea.
Licorice root	Relieves menopausal problems such as mood swings and hot flashes. Helps heal sore throat and ulcers.	Pour boiling water over ½ tsp finely chopped root, and steep to make a tea. Do not use for more than 4–6 weeks at a time. Avoid if you have high blood pressure.
Lovage	Relieves gas and fluid retention.	Pour boiling water over ½–1 tsp finely cut root, and steep to make a tea. Repeat three times a day when using as a diuretic.

the most popular healing herbs and instructions for using them. Of course, if you are pregnant or breastfeeding or have serious health problems, be sure to talk to your doctor before using medicinal herbs.

Herb	Benefits	How to Use
Milk thistle	Good for liver problems such as hepatitis and cirrhosis.	Take a 200-milligram capsule once a day.
Nettle	Helps relieve fluid retention.	Pour boiling water over 2 tsp finely cut leaves, and steep to make a tea.
Oregano	Good for parasitic infections and for blocking the effects of carcinogens in cooked meats.	Add generous amounts of whole leaves or powdered herb during cooking.
Parsley	A digestive aid and mild diuretic.	Add generous amounts of leaves and stems during cooking.
Peppermint	Eases upset stomach and reduces gas.	Pour boiling water over 1 Tbsp dried leaves, and steep to make a tea.
Rosemary	Eases digestion and helps stimulate appetite.	Pour boiling water over 1 tsp finely chopped leaves, and steep to make a tea.
St.-John's-wort	Eases nervousness and anxiety, improves memory and concentration, and has antiviral and anti-inflammatory effects.	Take a 250-milligram capsule once a day.
Savory	Relieves gas and diarrhea and stimulates appetite.	Add generous amounts of crushed leaves during cooking.
Thyme	Eases cough and upper respiratory infections.	Pour boiling water over 1 tsp dried herb, and steep to make a tea.
Uva ursi	Helps relieve fluid retention and fights inflammation in the urinary tract.	Pour cold water over 1 tsp coarsely powdered leaves (bearberry), and let stand for 12–24 hours to make a tea.
Valerian	Good for insomnia.	Pour boiling water over 2 tsp finely cut root, and steep to make a tea.
Willow bark	Helps ease pain, fever, and headaches.	Pour boiling water over 1–2 tsp finely chopped bark, and steep to make a tea.
Yarrow	Good for indigestion and for stimulating the appetite.	Pour boiling water over 1 heaping tsp finely chopped herb, and steep to make a tea.

Doctor's Top Tip

Even though it's hard to think of herbs as drugs when you see them in their raw leafy form, they still have medicinal properties that can interact with the other drugs you're taking. "The current information on herb-drug interactions is compelling," says John Neustadt, ND, medical director of Montana Integrative Medicine in Bozeman. "Avoiding potential or negative interactions is essential to safety, and understanding which herb-drug combinations work well together may improve clinical outcomes," he says. If you are taking a combination of prescription and/or over-the-counter drugs and herbs, make sure you talk to your health-care professional about potential interactions.

You can also buy herbs in their natural form or ground into a powder. These are used for making teas, says Dr. Brammer. While herbal teas work somewhat more slowly than extracts, they're absorbed by the body faster than pills or capsules. Plus, many people enjoy the taste of freshly brewed herbal teas. "The ritual of brewing the tea and sipping it slowly is so relaxing that it often makes people feel better," Dr. Brammer adds.

Shop for freshness. The one problem with using fresh herbs is that they give up their benefits over time. "It's a bad sign if the herbs are lying in bins in the store's front window, with the sun pouring in, since herbs lose their potency when exposed to light and air," says Dr. Keller.

Before buying herbs, put your nose to work, Dr. Keller advises. Fresh herbs should smell fresh. "Don't buy herbs that smell musty or look moldy, dry, or discolored," he says. And once you get them home, be sure to store them in an airtight container in a cool, dark place, such as a kitchen cupboard away from the stove.

Shop often. Even though it's convenient to buy in bulk, dried herbs won't keep indefinitely, says Dr. Brammer. To get the most healing power, she says, it's best to buy herbs in small amounts and replenish the supply a bit more frequently.

Treat them with respect. Even though herbs are often gentler than modern medicines, they can cause side effects, such as upset stomach, says Dr. Keller. It's a good idea to take healing herbs with meals rather than on an empty stomach. And because herbs are medicine, be sure to check with your doctor before taking them, especially if you're taking other medications for serious conditions such as diabetes or heart disease, says Dr. Keller. Also, because some herbs can act as blood thinners, be sure you tell your doctor about all herbs you are taking before you have surgery.

Herpes

THE POWER OF PROTEINS

The herpes simplex virus is a master of ambush. It spends most of its virus life dormant, hidden deep within the nerves in your body and waiting for your immune system to drop its guard. When the coast is clear, herpes rushes to the surface of the skin, causing ugly, painful sores that can last a week or more. Then it retreats back into the nerves, waiting weeks, months, or even years before rearing its ugly head once again.

Contrary to the popular belief that herpes appears only on the mouth and genitals, the virus can cause sores anywhere on the body, so the last thing you want is to be infected with it. But if you already have herpes, there is some evidence suggesting that eating more of some types of foods and less of others can make the virus weaker and less likely to launch its attacks.

Take Away Its Strength

You wouldn't think that an egg or a bowl of baked beans would have much stopping power against the herpes virus. But these foods, along with meat, milk, and cheese, contain large amounts of lysine, an amino acid that can help prevent the virus from thriving.

"The herpes virus uses certain amino acids to build the protein sheath that surrounds it," explains Mark McCune, MD, a dermatologist at Kansas City Laser and Skin Surgery Center in Overland Park, Kansas. "Lysine inhibits the growth of the shield, so the virus can't flourish."

Dr. McCune recommends getting between 1,000 and 2,000 milligrams of lysine a day. In one study, researchers found that people who got 500 to 1,000 milligrams of lysine a day above their normal intake rarely had outbreaks. And when they did have outbreaks, the sores were smaller than before and in some cases lasted only half as long.

It's easy to get large amounts of lysine in your diet. An ounce and a half of provolone cheese, for example, has 1,110 milligrams. Two eggs provide 900 milligrams, and 1 cup of baked beans has 960 milligrams. Pork is a lysine powerhouse, with one broiled, center-cut loin chop providing almost 2,000 milligrams.

Doctor's Top Tip

Vitamin C is well known for its immunity-boosting, virus-fighting abilities. "People who are more prone to herpes attacks are often low in vitamin C," says Kaayla Daniel, PhD, a board-certified clinical nutritionist in private practice in Santa Fe, New Mexico. So increasing your intake by eating more fruits and vegetables rich in vitamin C may prevent herpes from rearing its ugly head. One guava, for example, has 165 milligrams of vitamin C, nearly three times the Daily Value (DV) of 60 milligrams. Orange juice is also good, with a 6-ounce glass providing 93 milligrams, or more than 150 percent of the DV. A half-cup of sliced peaches contains 118 milligrams, or nearly 200 percent of the DV, and a half-cup of raw bell peppers contains a whopping 142 milligrams per half-cup, more than 230 percent of the DV. Broccoli is also a good source; it serves up 41 milligrams of vitamin C in a half-cup, or 68 percent of the DV.

Cut Off Its Supplies

Just as foods high in lysine can inhibit the herpes virus from building its protective coat, foods high in arginine may strengthen its defenses. "Arginine is an amino acid that herpes relies on for building its protein coating," says Dr. McCune. "If your diet is very high in arginine, this might help the virus grow aggressively."

High-arginine foods include chocolate, peas, nuts, and beer. You don't have to give up these foods entirely if you have herpes, Dr. McCune explains. What you should do, however, is balance them by eating other foods that are high in lysine.

"The whole lysine-arginine system doesn't work for everybody," Dr. McCune adds. "But I've seen lots of folks have success with it. And it doesn't have the side effects of drugs."

Immune-Boosting Herbs

In addition to watching your ratio of arginine to lysine foods, eating foods with immune-stimulating properties can help protect you against a herpes outbreak. Both garlic and thyme have such properties, so eating these herbs can help prevent an outbreak or decrease the duration of an outbreak once one occurs, says John Neustadt, ND, medical director of Montana Integrative Medicine in Bozeman.

The Magic of Milk

Once a herpes sore shows up, it can seem like an eternity before it goes away. But there is one way to hurry it along, and it's probably in your refrigerator at this very moment. Doctors aren't sure why it works, but applying a milk compress to a cold sore may help it heal more quickly.

Just dip a washcloth or handkerchief in milk, apply it to the sore for 5 seconds, then remove it for another 5. Continue the process for 5 minutes, and repeat it every 3 to 4 hours, rinsing your skin between treatments.

Honey

THE BEST FROM THE BEES

HEALING POWER

Can Help:

Speed wound healing

Ease ulcer pain

Relieve constipation and diarrhea

Although most people probably wouldn't name bees as one of their favorite insects, we do have them to thank for the sweet substance they manufacture from the nectar of flowers.

Even today, when sugary foods are hardly in short supply, there's something special about pure honey. Not only is it sweeter than table sugar, ounce for ounce, but its wonderfully thick, liquid texture makes it perfect for spreading on cakes, crackers, and breads.

Although honey contains trace amounts of minerals and B vitamins, overall, it's really not much more nutritious than plain table sugar. Yet honey does several things that sugar does not. Research suggests that honey can relieve constipation, speed healing, and prevent infections. "Some people have called honey a remedy rediscovered," says Peter Molan, PhD, professor of biochemistry and director of the Honey Research Unit at the University of Waikato in Hamilton, New Zealand, who has been studying the healing properties of honey for more than 15 years.

Quicker Healing

If you saw a jar of honey in your doctor's black bag, you'd just assume that he packed in the dark. But as it turns out, doctors have been using honey for centuries. "Up until World War II, honey was used commonly to treat skin wounds," says Dr. Molan.

With the introduction of antibiotics in the 1940s, honey was taken out of doctors' bags and returned to the kitchen. But today, some doctors are trying to bring it back into circulation as a medicine. "We're finding that doctors are starting to use honey when modern medicines have been tried—and have failed—to cure skin wounds," Dr. Molan says.

Honey contains three ingredients that make it ideal for treating wounds. Because it's very high in sugar, it absorbs much of the moisture inside wounds, making it hard for bacteria to survive, Dr. Molan explains. In addition, many honey varieties contain large amounts of hydrogen peroxide, the same medicine you use at home to disinfect cuts and scrapes. Finally, some honeys contain propolis, a compound in nectar that can kill bacteria.

In the Kitchen

Even though honey and sugar can be used interchangeably in most recipes, you may have to make some adjustments. For example:

- Honey is sweeter than sugar, so you can substitute 1 cup of honey for 1¼ cups of sugar if you reduce the liquid in the recipe by ¼ cup.
- When using honey for baking, add a pinch of baking soda. This will neutralize honey's acidity and help the food to rise. (If the recipe contains sour cream or sour milk, however, you can forgo the baking soda.)
- When using honey instead of sugar in jams, jellies, or candies, increase the cooking temperature just a bit to allow the extra liquid to evaporate.

There are many different flavors of honey, and it's important to match the type to the recipe. Orange blossom honey, for example, has a light, delicate flavor and is best used for foods with mild tastes, like a honey nut cake. Honey produced from buckwheat flowers, however, has a considerably stronger flavor. It's a good choice for spreading on bread or when making whole-grain desserts.

In a laboratory study, Dr. Molan smeared honey on seven types of bacteria that frequently cause wound infections. "It very effectively killed all seven types," he says.

Sweetness Within

Just as honey can stop infections on the outside of your body, it also can help to keep your body healthy on the inside.

A type of honey called Manuka, for example, which is produced when bees feed on a type of flowering shrub in New Zealand, appears to kill the bacteria that cause stomach ulcers. In one small study, people with ulcers were given 1 tablespoon of Manuka honey four times a day. "The honey relieved ulcer symptoms in all the people who took it," says Dr. Molan.

Honey also shows promise for treating diarrhea. In children particularly, diarrhea can be dangerous because it removes large amounts of water from the body and leads to dehydration. To replace fluids and essential minerals, doctors have traditionally treated diarrhea with a sugar solution. But a honey solution may be even better because not only can honey help combat dehydration, it can kill intestinal bacteria that may be causing the problem in the first place. In fact, researchers at the University of Natal in South Africa found that when children with diarrhea caused by a bacterial infection were given a honey solution, they got better in almost half the time of those who were given a traditional sugar solution.

Honey should not be given to children less than a year old, however, because it can cause a serious type of food poisoning called infant botulism.

Honey may work against constipation as well. It contains large amounts of fructose, a sugar that sometimes arrives in the large intestine undigested. When bacteria in the intestine begin the process of fermentation, water is drawn into the bowel, which acts as a laxative, explains Marvin Schuster, MD, founder of the Marvin M. Schuster Digestive and Motility Disorders Center at Johns Hopkins Bayview Medical Center in Baltimore. Honey is higher in fructose than just about any other food, he adds.

GETTING THE MOST

Shop for raw honey. The high heats used in making processed honey will disable some of the protective compounds, says Dr. Molan. To get the most antibacterial power, raw honey is your best bet.

Make it Manuka. While most raw honeys contain some active ingredients, Manuka honey contains the most. This is particularly important when you're taking honey as a treatment for relieving ulcers, says Dr. Molan. You can often find Manuka honey in health food stores. It's important, however, to read the label to make sure that you're getting "active Manuka honey." If it doesn't contain the active compounds, the honey won't be effective for ulcers, Dr. Molan explains.

Doctor's Top Tip

"Stir some honey into your iced or green tea and get double the health benefits—in the honey and in the tea," says Janet Maccaro, PhD, ND, a holistic nutritionist in Ormond Beach, Florida. "I try to steer people away from artificial sweeteners, and honey is a wonderful healthful alternative," she says. "Honey contains all the vitamins and minerals necessary for proper metabolism and the digestion of glucose and other sugars. It's a natural sweetener with antibiotic and antiseptic properties." Dr. Maccaro recommends using a teaspoon or a tablespoon in a cup of hot tea or glass of iced tea, depending on your preferred level of sweetness. Not a tea drinker? Drizzle a tablespoon of honey over some fresh fruit for a tasty treat, she says.

Citrus Honey

1 **strip (1 × 3½ inches) orange zest**
1 **strip (1 × 3½ inches) lemon zest**
1 **tablespoon fresh orange juice**
2 **teaspoons fresh lemon juice**
1 **cup honey**

In a small saucepan, combine the orange zest, lemon zest, orange juice, and lemon juice. Bring to a simmer over medium heat. Remove from the heat, and strain through a fine sieve; discard the zests.

In another small saucepan, heat the honey until just warm. Stir the juice into the warmed honey, and serve immediately over pancakes, waffles, or French toast.

Makes 1 cup

Cook's Note: *The honey can be stored in a capped jar in the refrigerator for up to 2 weeks. Reheat gently in the microwave or on the stovetop before serving.*

PER 2 TABLESPOONS ———————————

Calories: 130   Cholesterol: 0 mg
Total fat: 0 g   Sodium: 2 mg
Saturated fat: 0 g   Dietary fiber: 0 g

Immunity
EATING FOR RESISTANCE

A co-worker sneezes and a cloud of viruses fills the air. Pick up a pen or a pair of socks, and you're exposed to thousands, possibly millions, of bacteria. Walk barefoot across a lawn, and you're picking up fungi, parasites, and still more bacteria. A dangerous world? It would be if you didn't have your immune system to protect you.

"Our bodies are constantly bombarded with bacteria, viruses, and other organisms trying to gain entry," says Thomas Petro, PhD, associate professor of microbiology and immunology at the University of Nebraska Medical Center in Lincoln. "The immune system is the one defense we have against this takeover."

It's truly a battle for survival. A mere inch of freshly washed skin may be home to more than 1 million bacteria. Without strong immunity, microbes in and on our bodies would quickly multiply to unimaginable numbers. Yet every minute of every day, our immune systems keep these microscopic invaders in check.

To a large extent, your ability to maintain a healthy immune system depends on what you eat, says Dr. Petro. Research has shown, for example, that in parts of the world where healthy, nutritious foods are in short supply, people frequently have weak immune systems, and as a result, they are much more prone to developing infections. Similarly, in people with serious illnesses such as cancer, who often have trouble eating well, immunity can take a downturn.

Having a low level of even a single nutrient may cause the immune system to pay the price. In a review done at the University of Southampton in England, researchers looked at nutrients that play a key role in immune system function and found that the essential amino acids, the essential fatty acid linoleic acid, vitamin A, folate, vitamin B_6, vitamin B_{12}, vitamin C, vitamin E, zinc, iron, copper, and selenium are all required for healthy immune system function. The researchers also found that almost all aspects of immune system health are affected by deficiencies in these nutrients and that increasing intakes of them can enhance immune system function.

And in a small study done at the department of nutrition and food management at Oregon State University, researchers looked at the relationship between an increased intake of vitamin B_6 and white blood cell counts in seven young women over 3 weeks. When the women increased their intakes of vitamin B_6 from 1.5 milligrams to 2.1 milligrams, they experienced a 35 percent increase in white blood cell counts.

And what you do eat may wreak as much havoc on your immune system as what you don't eat. Junk food and processed foods take a real toll on your immune system, says Mary Jo DiMilia, MD, an integrated medicine physician at Mount Sinai Medical Center in New York City.

"Food is powerful medicine," says Keith Block, MD, medical director of the Block Center for Integrative Cancer Care in Evanston, Illinois. In fact, eating more of certain foods and less of others can substantially boost the body's ability to fight most illnesses, from colds to cancer.

A Magnificent System

Even though people talk about the immune system, it actually consists of two very different parts. One part of the immune system is nonspecific. That is, it attacks—or simply resists—just about everything it comes into contact with. It's like a first line of defense. Your skin, for example, provides a physical barrier against bacteria, viruses, and other invaders. It also secretes sweat and oil, which, because they are acidic, help block the growth of harmful bacteria. Your stomach secretes germ-killing acids and enzymes. Your saliva and tears contain an enzyme that destroys bacteria. Even the hairs in your nose keep germs from entering your body.

Should a microbe be lucky enough to breach the nonspecific part of the immune system, it's met by the next level of defense—the specific system. This second part of the immune system is extremely selective. Depending on the type of invader it encounters, it launches customized weapons called antibodies, which are proteins specifically designed to kill one particular invader and no other.

The immune system is capable of making more than 100 billion types of antibodies, so it can attack just about anything it comes into contact with. What's more, these antibodies have a long memory. Once you've been exposed to a germ, the immune system will remember it. If that same germ comes back—months, years, or even decades later—the appropriate antibodies will quickly kill it before it can make you sick.

Foods for Defense

The most powerful protection that you can give your immune system is to eat a well-balanced diet containing a variety of fruits, vegetables, whole grains, seeds and nuts, and seafood, says Dr. DiMilia. These foods are high in nutrients that can help keep your immune system healthy. What's more, some of these nutrients are antioxidants, which may help give the immune system an added boost.

Here's why antioxidants are so important. Every second, immune cells in your body are hit by a barrage of free radicals, harmful oxygen molecules that are created in enormous numbers every day. Since free radicals are missing an electron, they rush through your body, stealing electrons wherever they can find them. And every time they grab an electron, another cell is damaged.

The antioxidants in such foods as brightly colored fruits and vegetables, however, literally come between free radicals and healthy immune cells, offering up their own electrons. This neutralizes the free radicals, stopping them from doing further harm. In the process, your body's immune cells stay protected and strong.

"When your immune system is going to fight something, it fights it by oxidizing it," says Shawn Talbott, PhD, a nutritional biochemist and author of *The Health Professional's Guide to Dietary Supplements*. "So your immune system will actually give a virus or bacteria a blast of oxidation to try to kill it. Therefore, if you are fighting off a lot of these viruses or bacteria, you will have a lot of oxidation happening in your body and will need more antioxidants," he says.

In a study at Memorial University of Newfoundland in Canada, researchers found that people who got the most of a variety of nutrients, including antioxidants such as beta-carotene and vitamins C and E, in their diets were able to produce greater numbers of natural killer cells—immune cells that search out and destroy bacteria and other invaders—than folks getting the least. Another study found that people who got large amounts of a variety of antioxidants typically got sick about 23 days a year, while those getting smaller amounts got sick about 48 days a year.

Even though vitamin C is a powerful antioxidant, it helps the immune system in yet another way. The body uses vitamin C to make interferon, a protein that helps destroy viruses in the body. Plus, vitamin C may increase levels of a compound called glutathione, which has also been shown to keep the immune system strong.

In one large study, researchers at the University of Helsinki in Finland reviewed 21 smaller studies that looked at how well vitamin C was able to beat colds. They found that people getting 1,000 milligrams of vitamin C a day were able to shorten the duration of their illnesses and reduce their symptoms by 23 percent.

And a more recent Swiss review of numerous studies revealed that 1 gram of vitamin C was effective in shortening the duration of respiratory infections including the common cold.

The Daily Value (DV) for vitamin C is 60 milligrams, but many researchers say that 200 milligrams is probably the minimum amount you need to maximize immunity. It's easy to get this much vitamin C in your diet, Dr. Block adds. Half a cantaloupe, for example, has 113 milligrams of vitamin C, almost twice the DV, while a half-cup of Brussels sprouts has 48 milligrams, or 80 percent of the DV. Of course, you can also get a lot of vitamin C in citrus fruits, broccoli, guava, strawberries, rutabagas, radishes, and rose hips tea.

Vitamin E has also gotten a lot of attention for its role in boosting immunity.

Probiotics are beneficial bacteria in your intestinal tract that can improve health. And probiotics can also help improve immune system function. Probiotics interact with a specific part of your small intestine called the pyrus patches, which directly signal your immune system to be vigilant.

"Some probiotic drink mixes out there contain beneficial probiotic organisms," says Patricia David, MD, MSPH, president of Healthy U in Columbus, Ohio. "And those are great if you're on the go. But I encourage people to obtain their probiotics directly from food sources whenever possible—these food sources include yogurt, buttermilk, goat's milk, coconut water, soy milk, miso, kim chi, and sauerkraut. For optimum probiotic exposure, look for yogurts and other probiotic products that contain bifidobacterium and/or lactobacilli.

Another way to increase your levels of beneficial immune-bolstering bacteria is to consume prebiotics—nondigestible food components that selectively stimulate the growth of "good" bacteria in the gastrointestinal tract, says Dr. David. "Natural sources of prebiotics include dandelion greens, spinach, kale, artichokes, legumes, onions, leeks, garlic, oatmeal, flaxseed, barley, and soy yogurt," she says.

The body uses vitamin E to produce a powerful immune protein called interleukin-2, which has been shown to tackle everything from bacteria and viruses to cancer cells. The DV for vitamin E is 30 IU, and good sources include dark green leafy vegetables, walnuts and pecans, wheat germ, peanut butter, and vegetable oils.

Reduce Fat, Raise Immunity

Just as eating the right foods can help keep the immune system strong, eating the wrong ones—specifically, those that are high in fat—can put it at a disadvantage. "A high-fat diet speeds up the aging of the immune system, although we don't know why," says Dr. Petro. "But we do know that it results in the production of more cell-damaging free radicals."

Studies have shown that people who cut back on fat in their diets have a rapid increase in natural killer cell activity, a sign of immune system strength. In one study, researchers at the University of Massachusetts Medical School in Worcester put men on low-fat diets for 3 months. For every 1 percent the men were able to reduce the fat in their diets, the activity of their natural killer cells went up nearly 1 percent.

It isn't necessary to go on an extremely low-fat diet to boost immunity, Dr. Petro adds. For most people, getting no more than 30 percent of calories from fat—and preferably getting between 20 and 25 percent—is probably ideal.

To cut fat from your diet, eat fewer processed foods, such as those that come in cans, packets, and boxes. With the exception of canned fruits, beans, and vegetables, many processed foods are often high in fat, not to mention salt and sugar. Eat more fresh fruits and vegetables, beans, and whole-grain breads and cereals. In addition, switching from full-fat dairy products to reduced-fat milk, yogurt, and cheese, and eating less red meat, will help bring your fat levels into the safety zone.

Infections

BACTERIA-FIGHTING FOODS

There's no way to avoid germs entirely. What you can do, however, is eat your way to better health. Eating the right foods not only helps prevent infections, but can also help fight them.

A number of plant foods, such as apples, tea, onions, and kale, contain substances called flavonoids, which can prevent germs from taking hold, says Joseph V. Formica, PhD, professor of microbiology at Virginia Commonwealth University, Medical College of Virginia School of Medicine in Richmond. It may be the flavonoids in tea, for example, that make it an effective remedy for colds and flu.

One of the most powerful flavonoids is a compound called quercetin. Found in large amounts in onions and kale, quercetin has been shown to damage genetic material inside viruses, preventing them from multiplying. Quercetin appears to be effective at blocking the herpes virus as well as one of the viruses that causes flu. The research is preliminary, so doctors can't say for sure how much quercetin (or other flavonoids) you need to block infections. For now, having several servings a day of flavonoid-rich foods will help keep germs in check, says Dr. Formica.

A Spicy Healer

The next time you have an infection, reach for the garlic. "Formerly known as Russian penicillin, garlic is great for infections," says Janet Maccaro, PhD, ND, a holistic nutritionist in Ormond Beach, Florida, who is president of Dr. Janet's Balance By Nature Products and the author of *Natural Health Remedies A-Z*. Research has shown that these cloves contain compounds that can stop infections.

Researchers at the Medical College of Virginia School of Medicine found that water extracted from garlic was able to block a fungus that can cause a type of meningitis, a serious brain infection. In laboratory studies, garlic has wiped out *Candida albicans*, the fungus that can cause yeast infections.

"It's very clear that garlic has antiviral, antifungal, and antibacterial power," says John Hibbs, ND, a naturopathic doctor and clinical faculty member at Bastyr Center for Natural Health in Seattle. "For people with infections who enjoy eating garlic, we recommend that they chew as much fresh garlic as they can tolerate. Freeze-dried or other forms of garlic may also help."

"I recommend this garlicky soup to people when they have really bad infections, and it also works as a preventative," says Melissa Wood, ND, a naturopathic doctor in private practice in San Antonio, Texas. The recipe is as follows:

   2 tablespoons olive oil

   1 head garlic, peeled, separated, and chopped

   1 box organic chicken broth, or enough to make a quart

   1 medium bunch parsley, coarsely chopped

In a large saucepan, heat the oil over medium heat. Add the garlic and cook, stirring, for 1 to 2 minutes, or until softened. Add the chicken broth and parsley, and bring to a boil. Lower the heat, and simmer for 15 to 20 minutes.

   "Drink a cup of the soup every hour," says Dr. Wood. "It's particularly good if you know something is coming—like if you feel you are getting a cold or the flu," she says. "But it's also good if you've already got an infection."

You probably need to eat about a bulb of garlic a day to get the maximum healing benefits, says Elson Haas, MD, director of the Preventive Medical Center of Marin in San Rafael, California, and author of *Staying Healthy with Nutrition*. If the very idea of eating that much raw garlic makes you cringe, you may want to try cooking it first. Baking a bulb of garlic until the cloves are soft will take away some of the sulfuric garlic sting without taking away the health benefits.

Eating for Immunity

If you think of your immune system as an army that battles infections, then two vitamins are its main generals. Vitamin A helps strengthen your body's immune defenses, while vitamin C helps the immune system go on the attack. This two-pronged approach provides powerful protection against incoming germs.

The body uses vitamin A, which you get in the form of beta-carotene from foods such as carrots, spinach, mustard greens, kale, and yellow and orange squash, to keep mucous membranes soft and moist. This is important, because these membranes, which line the nose, mouth, throat, and other parts of the body, are your first line of defense against infection. As long as they're moist, they're able to trap viruses and other germs before they get into your system.

As a form of double protection, the body also uses vitamin A to manufacture special enzymes that seek out and destroy bacteria that manage to get inside the body.

While vitamin A's role is mainly defensive, vitamin C helps the body take the offensive. Eating oranges, broccoli, and other foods high in vitamin C strengthens the "gobbling power" of the body's germ-killing cells. In a study of people with respiratory infections, for example, Japanese researchers gave two groups of participants 50 milligrams and 500 milligrams of vitamin C respectively for 5 years and found that the rate of colds was 25 percent lower in the group taking the higher doses of vitamin C.

And a review of 12 studies on the effect of vitamin C on respiratory infection revealed that about half of the studies showed a significant reduction in respiratory infections in the groups taking vitamin C.

A Mine of Health

Of all the minerals, zinc is probably the most important for keeping immunity strong. Too little zinc can lead to a drop in infection-fighting white blood cells, which can increase your risk of getting sick.

In one study, for example, researchers from Tufts University School of Medicine in Boston found that children getting 10 milligrams of zinc for 60 days were much less likely to get respiratory infections than children getting less. In fact, the children who got enough zinc were 70 percent less likely to have fevers, 48 percent less likely to have coughs, and 28 percent less likely to have buildups of mucus. (Consult with your pediatrician before giving your child zinc, however.)

And in a review done at Case Western Reserve University in Cleveland, studies from 1980 to 2003 revealed that zinc can reduce cold symptoms when administered within 24 hours of the onset of a cold.

Despite the proven powers of zinc, many Americans don't get enough of it. This is unfortunate because zinc is very easy to get in your diet. One Alaskan king crab leg, for example, has 10 milligrams of zinc, or 67 percent of the Daily Value (DV). A 3-ounce serving of lean top sirloin has 6 milligrams, or 40 percent of the DV, and 1 cup of lentils has 3 milligrams, or 20 percent of the DV.

Infertility
EATING FOR THREE

Having a baby is one of life's most exciting moments. But for an estimated 10 percent of couples trying to conceive, just getting pregnant can be a long, difficult process. While there are many physical problems that can lead to infertility, for some couples, just changing what's on the menu may put them back on the baby track.

Research has shown, for example, that a man's sperm may not be up to the job if he doesn't get enough of a few key nutrients. And for a woman, starting the day with the usual pick-me-up—or ending it with the traditional calm-me-down—can make it much harder to get pregnant. So before you start picking out baby clothes, you might want to make a few changes in the kitchen.

Trouble Brewing

Morning in America means the buzzing of alarm clocks, followed by the chugging of electric coffeemakers. But when it's your biological clock that's doing the buzzing, you may want to unplug the coffee machine.

Drinking coffee, tea, cola, or other caffeinated beverages can significantly reduce a woman's chances of getting pregnant, says John Jarrett, MD, a reproductive endocrinologist in private practice in Indianapolis.

In a study of more than 1,400 women, researchers at Johns Hopkins University School of Hygiene and Public Health in Baltimore found that nonsmoking women who consumed at least 300 milligrams of caffeine a day (the equivalent of about 5 cups of coffee) were 2½ times more likely to have delayed conception than women consuming less.

And a review done at Boston College found that caffeine use was one of the main lifestyle-related risk factors for impaired fertility, up there with smoking, a history of sexually transmitted infection, and extremes in body weight.

Researchers aren't sure why caffeine puts the stork on the slow train. They speculate, however, that caffeine could change the balance of hormones in the body, interfering with a woman's ability to ovulate. "Reducing the amount of caffeine you drink may help at least a little bit," says Elizabeth E. Hatch, PhD, assistant professor in the department of epidemiology at Boston University School of Public Health.

A Sip of Problems

Light the scented candles, pop in a Marvin Gaye CD . . . and put the cork back in the Burgundy. While a glass or two of wine may put you in the mood for love, it won't do much for your chances of making a baby.

Harvard researchers found that women who had more than one drink a day—not just wine, but also beer or liquor—were 60 percent more likely to be infertile than women who abstained. Even women who had one drink or less a day were 30 percent less likely to get pregnant than the nondrinkers.

And Swedish researchers who examined the link between alcohol use and infertility for 18 years found that women who had a high intake of alcohol were more likely to seek medical care for infertility than women with a moderate or low intake of alcohol.

Incidentally, it's not only women who should think twice about raising a glass. Even small amounts of alcohol can lower men's testosterone levels, making their sperm less hardy, says Dr. Jarrett.

Fertility-Hindering Hormones

The hormones injected into cattle can spill into dairy products and interfere with the natural hormone levels of the women who eat them. "A lot of cows are injected with growth hormone and other hormones that can mimic estrogen," says Janet Maccaro, PhD, ND, a holistic nutritionist in Ormond Beach, Florida, who is president of Dr. Janet's Balance By Nature Products and the author of *Natural Health Remedies A-Z*. These false estrogens can confuse your menstrual cycle and hinder fertility. "Reducing your intake of dairy products and red meat will help you avoid synthetic hormones that can interfere with fertility," says Dr. Maccaro.

The Zinc Link

Casanova, the legendary lover, always ate oysters before amour. History doesn't tell how many children he fathered, but he certainly had the right idea. Oysters are extremely high in zinc, a mineral that's essential for male fertility.

"Men need zinc to produce sperm and also to make those sperm healthy," says John Hibbs, ND, a naturopathic doctor and clinical faculty member at Bastyr Center for Natural Health in Seattle. "Zinc also affects sperm motility—how quickly and well sperm swim." In addition, low levels of zinc can reduce the body's production of testosterone, which can interfere with fertility.

Even though the Daily Value (DV) for zinc is only 15 milligrams, most men don't get enough, says Dr. Hibbs. By following Casanova's example, however, you'll

Doctor's Top Tip

If you're trying to conceive, just say no to soy. "Soy can have adverse effects on fertility for both men and women," says Kaayla Daniel, PhD, a board-certified clinical nutritionist in Santa Fe, New Mexico. Soy products contain plant estrogens that can cause changes in the menstrual cycle leading to infertility, says Dr. Daniel. And it only takes a little bit. "On average, a glass of soy milk contains 45 milligrams of soy isoflavones—the amount that can cause infertility," she says. So if you are having problems getting pregnant, Dr. Daniels suggests you steer clear of soy products altogether.

get all the zinc you need, and then some. Oysters are an incredible source of zinc, with 12 cooked oysters supplying up to 152 milligrams, or more than 10 times the DV. Hormone-free beef is also good, with 3 ounces of lean ground beef containing 4 milligrams, or 27 percent of the DV. And one 100-gram serving of wheat germ provides 12 milligrams of zinc, or 80 percent of the DV.

Completing the Swim

When you look at sperm under a microscope, they resemble supercharged tadpoles, all racing in the do-or-die rush to get upstream.

At least, that's what they're supposed to do. In men who don't get enough vitamin C, however, sperm lose some of their forward momentum. In fact, they get sticky and start clumping together, a problem doctors call agglutination. Once men start getting more vitamin C, however, sperm increase in number and quickly pick up speed. In one study published in the *Journal of Medicinal Food*, for example, 13 infertile men took 1,000 milligrams of vitamin C twice a day for 2 months. Results showed that the average sperm count increased by 32 percent and the average sperm motility increased by 60 percent.

Getting more vitamin C is particularly important for men who smoke. Studies have shown that smokers who get extra vitamin C in their diets will have healthier, more active sperm than those who don't.

Insomnia

RESTFUL FOODS

When life gets hectic, we've all found ourselves wishing that there were more hours in the day. Sometimes, unfortunately, we get our wish—at the expense of our sleep.

Few things are more miserable than lying awake, frustrated and tired, when everyone else is sleeping soundly. Insomnia is usually temporary, of course, caused by too much coffee, perhaps, or anxiety about tomorrow's work. But sometimes insomnia really sticks around—not just for days but for weeks, months, or even years. After a few nights spent staring at the ceiling, you may feel as if you'll never be rested again.

You're not alone. A 2003 poll by the National Sleep Foundation found that half of adults in America ages 55 and older reported at least one symptom of insomnia three or more times a week, including having trouble falling asleep, waking during the night, waking too early and not being able to go back to sleep, or not feeling refreshed in the morning. Although both men and women fall victim to insomnia, women tend to suffer from it more often than men, thanks to disturbances caused by menstruation, pregnancy, and menopause.

The next time you find yourself tossing and turning, get out of bed, put on your slippers, and head for the kitchen. There's good evidence that what you eat before going to bed can help turn out the lights on insomnia.

Nosh to Nod

Remember dear old Dad sawing logs on the La-Z-Boy after dinner? He wasn't just dodging the dishes. He was responding to one of the body's most inflexible commands: "First you eat, then you sleep."

"When you put food in your stomach at night, you should be able to sleep better," says David Levitsky, PhD, professor of nutrition and psychology at Cornell University in Ithaca, New York. "Eating draws blood into the gastrointestinal tract and away from the brain. And if you draw blood away from the brain, you're going to get sleepy."

In fact, researchers are learning more about the link between your stomach and sleep. After studying the brain activity of mice, Tamas Horvath, PhD, professor of comparative medicine, obstetrics/gynecology, and neurobiology at Yale University School of Medicine, has found that blood glucose levels are the main trigger for hypocretin, cells in the brain that keep you awake. When you go to bed on an empty stomach, and your blood glucose levels are low, hypocretin cells become active, and that keeps you from going to sleep, he says.

This doesn't mean that stuffing yourself at bedtime will send you off to dreamland. In fact, eating too much too late in the evening can leave you feeling bloated and gassy, which is more likely to keep you awake than help you sleep. But having a light snack just before bedtime will help give your body the message that it's time to nod off.

Talking Turkey

Have you ever wondered why you always nod off in front of the television after a Christmas or Thanksgiving feast? It's not because of the company. Traditional holiday foods such as turkey and chicken are very high in an amino acid called tryptophan, which has been shown to affect the part of the brain that governs sleep, says Dr. Levitsky. Dairy foods are also high in tryptophan, he adds.

The body converts tryptophan into serotonin, which is then converted into melatonin. Both serotonin and melatonin make you feel relaxed and sleepy. In fact, tryptophan may be so effective that for a long time, doctors recommended tryptophan supplements to help people sleep. Even though the pills were eventually banned (due to a tainted batch imported from Japan), doctors believe that the amino acid found in foods is safe and effective as a sleep aid.

For tryptophan to be most effective, however, it's important to get it in combination with starches, according to Judith Wurtman, PhD, a researcher affiliated with the Massachusetts Institute of Technology Clinical Research Center in Cambridge and author of *The Serotonin Power Diet*. When you eat starches—a bagel, for example—the body releases insulin, which pushes all the amino acids except tryptophan into muscle cells. This leaves tryptophan alone in the bloodstream, so it's first in line to get into the brain.

Obviously, you don't want to stuff yourself with turkey before climbing into bed at night. But having a glass of milk or a piece of cheese on a cracker at bedtime will boost your tryptophan, which will make getting to sleep a little bit easier.

A Natural Sleep Aid

Until recently, scientists thought that melatonin was only produced in the body. As it turns out, however, this sleepy-time hormone is also found in a variety of foods, such as oats, sweet corn, rice, ginger, bananas, and barley, says Russell Reiter, PhD, professor of cellular and structural biology at the University of Texas Health Science Center in San Antonio and author of *Melatonin: Your Body's Natural Wonder Drug.*

Doctors often recommend that people who have trouble sleeping take melatonin supplements. In 2004, the Agency for Healthcare Research and Quality in Rockville, Maryland, reviewed the studies showing the effects of melatonin supplements on sleep and concluded that short-term use of the supplements can help people with delayed sleep phase syndrome, or those who have trouble falling asleep before 2 a.m. However, melatonin wasn't effective for treating other sleep disorders.

When the Sandman is running late, having a banana or a bowl of oatmeal will slightly boost your melatonin levels and help prepare your body for sleep.

Sound Body, Sound Sleep

Even though scientists have identified a few key substances that help improve sleep, there's simply no substitute for having an overall healthful diet, says James G. Penland, PhD, a research psychologist at the USDA Human Nutrition Research Center in Grand Forks, North Dakota. "A deficiency of minerals or vitamins may affect your sleep," he says. "So the better your diet, the better your sleep is likely to be."

Studies have shown, for example, that when people don't get enough iron or copper in their diets, it can take longer to fall asleep, and the sleep they do get may be less than refreshing.

The easiest way to get more of these minerals in your diet is to put shellfish on the menu. Just 20 small steamed clams, for example, will provide just over 25 milligrams of iron, or 139 percent of the Daily Value (DV), and 0.6 milligram of copper, or 31 percent of the DV. Lentils, nuts, and whole-grain foods are also good sources of iron and copper.

Magnesium is another mineral that's essential for good sleep. "It's been shown that having low magnesium levels will stimulate brain-activation neurotransmitters, which leads to overstimulation of the brain," says Dr. Penland. Not getting enough magnesium is especially common in the elderly, he adds, since they may be taking medications that block its absorption. "That's a double whammy that puts them at high risk for sleep problems," he says.

Good sources of magnesium include dried beans such as pinto and navy beans and green leafy vegetables such as spinach and Swiss chard. You can also get magnesium from soybeans, pumpkin seeds, wheat germ, and almonds.

Finally, getting plenty of B vitamins in your diet may help take the edge off insomnia. The body uses B vitamins to regulate many amino acids, including tryptophan. Niacin is particularly important because it appears to make tryptophan work even more efficiently. Lean meat is an excellent source of all the B vitamins,

Doctor's Top Tip

If you're waking up at night and you don't know why, acid reflux could be the culprit. William Orr, PhD, of the Lynn Health Science Institute in Oklahoma City, studied a group of people who had poor sleep for three or four nights a week. About 25 percent had significant sleep-related reflux without heartburn, so they weren't aware that they were suffering from the condition, he says.

If you're waking in the middle of the night for unknown reasons, assume you have reflux, and treat it for a week to see if you sleep better, Dr. Orr says. Cut down on foods that create reflux, such as large, fatty meals rich with sauces and full of carbohydrates, especially if you're going to be hitting the sack soon. And adhere to a strict rule of no food for 2 hours before bed. Taking 75 milligrams of Zantac, an antacid that is sold over the counter, may also help, he says.

including niacin. Canned tuna is another good source, with 3 ounces providing 11 milligrams of niacin, or 55 percent of the DV.

In general, healthier people enjoy better sleep. Among those who reported a sleep problem to the National Sleep Foundation, 85 percent rated their health as fair or poor.

The Sleep Robbers

You know the drill. Fall into a blissfully restful sleep only to wake up once—or twice or three times—because of the urge to use the bathroom. It was the most common reason given for waking up at night by those surveyed by the National Sleep Foundation. In men, the most common reason for nightly bathroom trips is an enlarged prostate, which should be evaluated by a doctor. But if you're getting up during the night to urinate and an enlarged prostate isn't the problem, restrict your intake of liquids for 2 to 3 hours before bedtime, says William Orr, PhD, president and chief executive officer of Lynn Health Science Institute in Oklahoma City.

You already know that coffee can keep you up at night, but did you know that chocolate can also send your brain into overdrive? A serving of chocolate doesn't have as much caffeine as a cup of coffee or a cola, but it can have the same effect on your sleep, says Michael Bonnet, PhD, a sleep specialist and director of the Veterans Affairs Medical Center in Dayton, Ohio.

It's not just late-night caffeine that leaves you staring at the ceiling, Dr. Bonnet adds. Since it takes 6 to 8 hours for the body to eliminate caffeine from your system, even the coffee you had at lunch—or the chocolate bar you had in the afternoon—can keep you up at night.

Alcohol is one of the most common disturbers of sleep. A glass of wine or a drink at bedtime can very quickly turn off those hypocretin neurons that keep you awake, Dr. Horvath says, but unfortunately, the alcohol causes a rebound effect. Soon after falling asleep, the hypocretin cells in the brain are reactivated and wake you up.

When you're having trouble getting to sleep at night, it's a good idea to skip the nightcap and maybe have a little milk instead, Dr. Bonnet says.

When you choose to eat certain foods can also throw off your sleep schedule. If you've ever wondered why sleep eludes you at night while it threatens to overcome you in the middle of the afternoon, take a look at what you're eating for lunch and dinner. More solid foods, such as a hamburger, will make you more tired than a liquid meal, such as a bowl of soup and crackers, Dr. Orr says.

If you've just had a big meal and find yourself tired hours before your usual bedtime, resist it, Dr. Orr says. Giving in to sleep too early will only result in waking up in the middle of the night.

Irritable Bowel Syndrome
KEEPING YOUR INSIDES CALM

Doctors still aren't sure what causes irritable bowel syndrome (IBS), a miserable intestinal problem that often causes cramps, gas, diarrhea, and constipation. What they do know is that by eating a healthy diet—getting more of some foods and less of others—you can control IBS instead of having it control you.

Find Your Triggers

Perhaps the trickiest part of managing IBS is knowing which foods are most likely to trigger attacks. Since this varies from person to person, it takes time to learn which foods are safe and which aren't. "A lot of it is trial and error," says David E. Beck, MD, chairman of the department of colon and rectal surgery at the Ochsner Clinic in New Orleans.

Even though everyone with IBS reacts to foods differently, there are a few common denominators. Dairy foods, for example, are often a problem. Although children can usually enjoy milk and cheese to their hearts' content, up to 70 percent of adults worldwide produce insufficient amounts of the enzyme (lactase) needed to digest the sugar (lactose) found in dairy foods. For people with IBS, having dairy foods can be especially uncomfortable, Dr. Beck says.

You don't necessarily have to give up milk and cheese entirely, he adds. But you'll certainly want to try cutting back to see if your symptoms improve. Over time, you'll get a good idea of how much of a dairy food you can enjoy without having problems.

Eating beans often causes problems for people with IBS. Again, you don't have to rule them out entirely, Dr. Beck says. You may find that some kinds of beans bother you more than others, and some may not bother you at all.

Another food that's hard to digest is the sugar (fructose) found in soft drinks and apple and pear juices, says Samuel Meyers, MD, clinical professor of medicine at Mount Sinai School of Medicine in New York City. In addition, sweeteners like sorbitol, which are found in diet candy and chewing gum, can also be a problem. For many people with IBS, cutting back on juices and candies may be all it takes to ease the discomfort, he says.

NATURAL RELIEF

Just as the right foods can help calm an irritable bowel, there are also a number of herbs that will help keep the problem under control, says Daniel B. Mowrey, PhD, director of the American Phytotherapy Research Laboratory in Salt Lake City, and author of *Herbal Tonic Recipes*. Here's what he recommends:

Licorice root. This sweet-tasting herb, which you can use to make tea, is a natural anti-inflammatory that can help relieve irritation in the bowel, he says.

Peppermint. In one study, people with IBS who took peppermint capsules were able to eliminate all or most of their symptoms, Dr. Mowrey says. Peppermint tea is also effective, he adds.

Psyllium. The main ingredient in a number of over-the-counter laxatives, psyllium seeds, which are very high in fiber, have been shown to help relieve the pain of IBS as well as the diarrhea and constipation that may accompany it.

Forgo Fatty Foods, Fill Up on Fiber

A common cause of IBS flare-ups is fat. This is because the bowel normally contracts following a high-fat meal. For people with IBS, these normal contractions can be extremely painful, Dr. Meyers explains. Getting no more (and preferably less) than 30 percent of your total calories from fat will go a long way toward calming an irritable bowel, he says.

A sure way to eat less fat is to cook your own meals rather than eat out, says Paul Millea, MD, assistant professor of family and community medicine at the Medical College of Wisconsin in Milwaukee. Restaurants prepare food with their own benefit in mind, not yours. As a result, the food you eat at restaurants is loaded with fat and low in nutrients.

At the same time, high-fat food means low fiber, and fiber is key to avoiding IBS flare-ups for several reasons. Fiber makes stools larger, so the intestine doesn't have to squeeze as much to move them along, Dr. Beck says. In addition, the larger stools help sweep potential irritants from the bowel before they cause cramping, gas, or other symptoms. Getting more dietary fiber also will help relieve both diarrhea and constipation, which often occur in people with IBS, Dr. Beck says.

The Daily Value (DV) for fiber is 25 grams. As a starting point, Dr. Millea tells his patients to add a bowl of bran cereal to their diet every day and build up from there. "Most people will be surprised at how it affects their gastrointestinal system,"

Doctor's Top Tip

Because fiber has a healing effect on the bowel while fat causes the bowel to contract painfully, make the effort to eat healthier meals at home, says Paul Millea, MD, of the Medical College of Wisconsin in Milwaukee. Start with a bowl of bran cereal a day and build up to eating whole-wheat bread, whole grains such as whole-wheat pasta and brown rice, and plenty of fruits and vegetables.

he says. Although at first, the extra fiber may cause some bloating, give it time, and your body will adjust. (Avoid cereals made from corn, however, since corn tends to aggravate IBS in 20 percent of people with the problem.)

"If all Americans ate low-fat, high-fiber diets, irritable bowels would be very uncommon," Dr. Meyers says.

Stress Effects

IBS is hardly ever seen in people who are retired because its symptoms are commonly brought on by stress, says Dr. Millea. When we're under stress, we typically grab for foods that exacerbate IBS, such as coffee, soft drinks, chocolate, and fast food. That's like throwing gasoline onto the fire for most people with IBS.

"I hate to tell people to avoid stress because that essentially comes across as 'Don't live your life,'" Dr. Millea says. But it is important to be aware of the choices you make when you're under stress. Avoid stimulants such as caffeine and alcohol, add as much fiber to your diet as you can, avoid eating out, and be sure to get enough sleep and exercise.

If giving up coffee sounds impossible, try drinking less. Because both regular and decaf coffee make the bowel more sensitive, Dr. Beck recommends limiting yourself to a cup or two each day.

Swap Large Meals for Small

Finally, it's helpful to eat smaller meals. The more food you put into your body at one time, the harder the intestines have to work, and that can cause problems for people with IBS. Having several small meals is usually easier for the body to handle than having two or three big meals, says Douglas A. Drossman, MD, professor of medicine and psychiatry at the University of North Carolina at Chapel Hill School of Medicine.

Juicing
POUR A GLASS OF HEALTH

HEALING POWER
Can Help:

Prevent cancer and
heart disease

Boost immunity

Lower the risk of
Alzheimer's disease

Like disco and leisure suits, juicing became a craze in the 1970s, only to fizzle shortly thereafter. Now, as research regarding the health benefits of eating plenty of fresh fruits and vegetables mounts, people are rediscovering juicing.

In fact, juicing has been growing consistently, says Steven Bailey, ND, a naturopathic doctor in Portland, Oregon, and author of *Juice Alive*. Although he doesn't have statistics on the number of people who juice today, he estimates that 1 in 10 to 1 in 8 people are doing it. If you're not one of them, you should be. "It's one of the best ways to hedge your bets against the increasing stressors, toxins, and ever-diminishing nutrient value of our food," Dr. Bailey says.

For some, whipping fresh fruits and vegetables through a juicer and extracting glassfuls of vitamin-packed pulpy nectar ensures that they'll get the recommended five to seven servings of these foods every day. Others turn to juicing as a way to get more carotenoids and flavonoids, healing compounds that experts believe can fight major diseases like cancer and heart disease. Still others see juicing as a way to cleanse the body of toxins, boost immunity, and help treat a variety of diseases, from anemia and constipation to arthritis.

More Than a Multivitamin

For millions of Americans, a handful of vitamin and mineral pills is as much a part of their morning fare as a bowl of cereal and a tall glass of orange juice. And while this isn't a bad way to supplement your diet, there may be a better one.

"Juices are a multivitamin/mineral supplement for people who don't want to take pills and capsules," says Eve Campanelli, PhD, founder of Eve's Herbs and a holistic health-care practitioner in Beverly Hills, California. "And your body absorbs the nutrients from juices far, far better than it does from a pill."

Indeed, your body absorbs nutrients from juices better than it does from the foods themselves, says Dr. Bailey. Although plants are full of vitamins, minerals, and other healing compounds, these substances are bound to fibrous tissue and contained within cellulose walls. When you grind up vegetables or fruits to make juice, you break down the cellulose, releasing these compounds and making them available for absorption, he says.

"Unless you chew very, very well—and few people do—you won't get all the nutrients from food that you can get from juice. In fact, juice is one of the most powerful whole foods that you can put in your body," says Dr. Bailey. "It takes very little energy to digest it, so you maintain almost all of the energy and nutrients that it gives."

Plus, it takes a mountain of vegetables to get the same amount of nutrients found in one glass of juice. "To get all the vitamins you'd get from just 6 ounces of carrot juice, you'd need to eat eight carrots," says Dr. Campanelli. "Not too many people are going to eat eight carrots. But they'll drink a little glass of carrot juice."

A 6-ounce glass of carrot juice contains large amounts of beta-carotene, which, when it's converted to vitamin A in the body, delivers 948 percent of the Daily Value (DV). This same glass of juice also has 16 milligrams of vitamin C, or 27 percent of the DV; 0.4 milligram of vitamin B_6, or 20 percent of the DV; 537 milligrams of potassium, or 15 percent of the DV; and 0.2 milligram of thiamin, or 11 percent of the DV.

An added benefit: Juicing can even help control your weight. Drinking juices helps the body iron out its nutritional deficiencies, which leaves you more satisfied from a healthy diet and less likely to overeat, says Dr. Bailey.

Despite their nutritional payload, juices should be used to supplement fresh fruits, vegetables, and grains in your diet, not replace them, says Dr. Campanelli. As good as juices are, they don't contribute much toward the 20 to 35 grams of fiber that adults need each day. For example, while eight carrots provide 17 grams of fiber, a 6-ounce glass of juice has a measly 2 grams. Diets high in fiber have been linked with lower incidence of certain cancers, digestive problems, and high cholesterol.

Beyond Vitamins and Minerals

Fresh juices supply more than the necessary vitamins and minerals. They also contain a variety of phytonutrients, compounds in plants that may help prevent serious health threats like cancer, heart disease, and Alzheimer's.

Perhaps the best-known of the phytonutrients is beta-carotene, a plant pigment that puts the orange glow in sweet potatoes, carrots, and cantaloupe. Studies have shown that people who eat diets high in fruits and vegetables, particularly those containing large amounts of beta-carotene, have much lower cancer risks than those who do not.

Beta-carotene isn't the only phytonutrient found in fruits and vegetables. There are hundreds of compounds, like lutein, lycopene, and alpha-carotene, that have

DELICIOUS COMBINATIONS

There's virtually no limit to the tastes and textures that you can create by mixing a variety of fruits and vegetables in your juicer. Here are a few simple combinations you may want to try:

- Carrots and celery, which are often combined, are considered universal mixers, which means that they combine well with any other vegetable. Try juicing three carrots for every stalk of celery.
- Combining the juice from a couple of tomatoes with juice from a few slices of green bell peppers makes a refreshing, low-sodium alternative to salt-laden store-bought tomato juice.
- For a surprisingly refreshing drink, combine one large peeled cucumber and a small onion. Using different varieties of onions, from sweet Bermudas and Vidalias to the green and white parts of scallions, will create a range of interesting flavors.
- Add garlic, ginger, turmeric, and cayenne for extra flavor and heat in your juices, but keep in mind that they're potent spices. Start with small amounts.

shown disease-fighting mettle as well. Drinking the juices of carotenoid-rich foods, particularly carrots, tomatoes, and dark green leafy vegetables, gives your body a full arsenal of these compounds, says Dr. Bailey.

Fruit and vegetable juices also contain compounds called flavonoids, which show strong antioxidant powers. That is, they help prevent disease by sweeping up harmful, cell-damaging oxygen molecules called free radicals that naturally accumulate in your body.

Antioxidants help prevent low-density lipoprotein (LDL) cholesterol, the dangerous form of cholesterol, from oxidizing. This is the process that makes cholesterol stick to the lining of artery walls and contribute to heart disease. Studies show that people who eat flavonoid-rich foods such as apples and onions have lower risks of heart attack than those who do not.

In a large prospective study of more than 100,000 people, researchers found that adding one serving of fruits or vegetables to the diet each day lowered the risk of ischemic stroke, a stroke in which the artery to the brain is blocked, by 6 percent. The best protection came from citrus fruits, dark green leafy vegetables, and cruciferous vegetables, which include broccoli, cauliflower, and cabbage.

Other studies have shown that antioxidants help prevent Alzheimer's disease. In 2002, researchers studied nearly 5,500 people and found that those who ate diets rich in the antioxidant vitamins C and E lowered their risk of developing Alzheimer's disease. Citrus fruits, kiwifruit, sprouts, broccoli, and cabbage—all perfect for juicing—are packed with vitamin C, while whole grains, nuts, milk, and egg yolk contain vitamin E.

"Drinking a large variety of vegetable and fruit juices is a wonderful way to get therapeutic amounts of all of these healing compounds," says Dr. Campanelli.

For maximum healing benefits, Dr. Bailey recommends drinking about a pint to a quart of mixed vegetable juices each day.

In the Kitchen

There's more to juicing than merely dropping the pick of the day into the blender, food processor, or juicer. To get the freshest flavors while preserving the most nutrients, here's what experts advise.

Scrub it. Be sure to wash all produce thoroughly, and cut away bruised or damaged portions.

Remove the skin. While not all fruits and vegetables require peeling, many do, for a variety of reasons. The skins of oranges and grapefruits, for example, contain chemicals that can be toxic if consumed in large quantities. Waxed produce should be peeled before juicing, as should tropical fruits, which often are grown in countries where the use of pesticides isn't well regulated.

Remove the pits and seeds. Apple seeds, which contain trace amounts of cyanide, should be removed before juicing. Seeds in melons, lemons, and limes and pits from peaches, plums, and other stone fruits should also be removed. Grape seeds are safe, however, and can be placed in the juicer along with the fruit.

Use the whole vegetable. Most vegetables can be juiced in their entirety—leaves, stems, and all. Two exceptions are rhubarb and carrots; rhubarb leaves and carrot tops both contain toxic compounds.

Chunk it. The openings of most juicers are quite small, so you should cut your produce into manageable pieces. Also, small chunks put less strain on the motor, which will help your juicer last longer.

Blend your bananas. When juicing fruits or vegetables that contain little water, like bananas and avocados, it's helpful to juice other items first, then add the drier produce to produce a thick, smooth drink.

Drink it quickly. Just as juices give up their nutritional benefits soon after they are made, their flavor is also fleeting. Some juices, such as cabbage, become funky in a few hours. So it's a good idea to make only as much as you plan to drink right away.

Or freeze it. Carrot, apple, and orange juices are quite hardy and will keep for 3 to 4 weeks in the freezer when frozen in a sealed plastic container.

Get the Toxins Out

Pollution, pesticides, preservatives, artificial color-ings—these are a mere smattering of the toxic ele-ments that your body takes in every day. Your body, of course, being a good housekeeper, tries to eliminate these toxins through cleansing organs like the liver. But just as you empty vacuum cleaner bags to help the sweeper work properly, you should occasionally flush the toxins from your body, says Dr. Campanelli.

Although this theory is largely discounted by the mainstream medical community, natural-health doc-tors recommend "cleaning house" periodically with a juice fast. This means abstaining from solid food for a couple of days and getting your nourishment from fresh fruit and vegetable juices.

"When you spend a couple of days getting most of your nutrition from juices, not only do you get a higher portion of vitamins, minerals, and natural enzymes but your body doesn't have to work very hard at digestion, so you have more nutritionally rich blood with more time to clean up, heal overworked cells, and help the body regenerate," says Dr. Bailey. And it's almost impossible not to get enough nutrients from juices alone, as long as you use a good variety of organic fresh vegetables.

You could also see an enhancement of your immune system, says Dr. Bailey. As a result of juice fasting, "symptoms of chronic conditions like arthritis, sinusitis, and allergies generally decrease dramatically," he says. While natural-health doctors agree that juice fasting isn't a cure for these conditions, it may help provide temporary relief.

Although juice fasts are generally safe, certain conditions, such as type 2 (non-insulin-dependent) diabetes, can be aggravated by them. Don't do any fasting with-out first consulting your doctor, warns Dr. Bailey.

Doctor's Top Tip

When making juice, use fresh, ripe organic produce as much as possible, and choose recipes that are tasty to the palate to aid the body's acceptance of them, says Steven Bailey, ND, a naturopathic doctor in Portland, Oregon, and author of *Juice Alive*. If you're going to consume a large meal, drink juice about half an hour before eating, because the juice nutrients will be immediately absorbed if there's no other food in your stomach.

GETTING THE MOST

Sip it quickly. Once the fruit or vegetable goes through the juicer, natural enzymes in the food begin to break down the nutrients. Juice loses nutritional value quickly, says Dr. Bailey. For optimal benefits, drink juices within 30 minutes of making them, he advises.

Canned juices, of course, will keep almost forever if unopened. The trade-off is that they lack many of the nutrients found in fresh juices. The most wholesome juice, Dr. Bailey says, is always made at home.

Focus on vegetables. While a tall glass of fruit juice can be a sweet summer treat, it's better to concentrate on vegetable juices. "Fruit juices are too high in sugar and too acidic to drink in large quantities," says Dr. Bailey. "Vegetable juices are better nutritionally, and they have a higher alkaline (meaning not acidic) content."

Enjoy a variety. For maximum healing benefits, drink juices from many different vegetables, says Dr. Bailey. "The more variety you can work into your diet, the better. This is easy with juices, because you can combine several vegetables into one drink."

Wondering what a particular vegetable juice will taste like? The juice will taste like the vegetable after you've chewed it thoroughly in your mouth, Dr. Bailey says. For example, celery has a salty taste. "I like to add garlic to celery juice to give it a zing," he says. Also, while many people don't like canned beets, they often enjoy a small amount blended into another vegetable juice.

Kidney Stones
RELIEF FROM THE KITCHEN

There's pain. There's agonizing pain. And then there are kidney stones.

Actually, calling them kidney barbs would be more fitting since these stones, which consist mainly of mineral salts, are sometimes studded with sharp spikes. While it's possible to pass small stones without knowing you had them, larger stones, which can range from about the size of the tip of a pen to that of a pencil eraser, cause excruciating pain as they move from the kidney through the ureter, the long tube through which urine flows. Passing a large stone has been compared to the pain of childbirth. Some women say it's worse.

Although some think kidney stones are rare, up to 10 percent of Americans will pass at least one during their lifetime, and the number is growing. Over the past 20 years, the number of people with kidney stones has been on the rise, according to the National Institutes of Health.

There are several types of kidney stones, but the most common—in fact, 80 percent of kidney stones—are those formed from calcium. Experts aren't entirely sure what causes kidney stones to form. But one thing is certain. Diet can play a key role, says Lisa Ruml, MD, an endocrinologist in Wharton, New Jersey. What you eat affects the kinds and amounts of minerals that accumulate in your urine—minerals that, in some people, lead to the formation of stones.

Perhaps the most important point is this: If you've passed one stone, the odds are good that you'll pass another. So pay attention when your doctor tells you what kind of stones you have, since this will affect the changes you make in your diet.

The stones that respond best to dietary changes are uric acid and calcium stones. The dietary changes recommended in the next few pages are given primarily with these types of stones in mind.

Stone-Crushing Potassium

Once you've experienced the pain of a kidney stone, you don't want a repeat performance. So consider making a handful of dried apricots or a baked potato a regular part of your anti-stone diet. Along with a variety of fruits and vegetables, these foods are somewhat alkaline, which helps neutralize stone-forming acids in the body.

Here's how it works. Alkaline foods increase the level of a mineral called citrate in the urine, and citrate helps block the formation of stones, Dr. Ruml explains.

To raise your levels of citrate, Dr. Ruml says, you need to get more fruits and vegetables into your diet. "Many of the foods that are high in citrates, like citrus fruits and vegetables, are also good sources of potassium."

Studies have found that choosing orange juice over other citrus is worth your while. A 2006 study found that drinking 13 ounces of orange juice three times a day, along with a diet low in calcium, had a more positive effect on reducing kidney stones than lemonade. That's because orange juice contains potassium, which increases citrate levels, while lemonade doesn't.

In a study at the University of Texas Southwestern Medical Center in Dallas, men with histories of kidney stones were given either three glasses of orange juice a day or potassium-citrate supplements. The researchers found that the juice was almost as effective as the supplements. "We recommend drinking at least a liter (a little more than 32 ounces) a day if you have stones, because of its content of potassium and citrate," says Dr. Ruml.

Help from Magnesium

Your body is full of minerals that are constantly being adjusted for balance. Eating foods that are rich in magnesium, Dr. Ruml says, can help prevent stones by lowering the amount of another mineral, called oxalate. This mineral can be a problem because it's one of the main components of kidney stones.

Fish, rice, avocados, and broccoli all are rich in magnesium. A 3-ounce fillet of baked or broiled halibut, for example, has 91 milligrams of magnesium, or 23 percent of the Daily Value (DV). A half-cup of cooked long-grain brown rice has 42 milligrams, and a floret of cooked broccoli has 43 milligrams, or 11 percent of the DV.

Here's another easy way to get more magnesium. Drink some fortified, low-fat milk. If your doctor has recommended that you restrict dairy foods, however, don't drink more than 8 ounces a day, says Dr. Ruml.

Of course, it's also helpful to get less oxalate in your diet, Dr. Ruml says. If you're prone to kidney stones, it's a good idea to limit yourself to one serving a week of oxalate-rich foods, such as black tea, chocolate, peanuts and other nuts, spinach and other leafy greens, and strawberries.

Fiber for the Stone-Prone

If you want to leave no stone unturned, getting more fiber in your diet can be a smart strategy. In a study at the Stone Clinic at Halifax Infirmary Hospital in Nova Scotia, 21 people were put on a low-stone (low-protein, low-calcium, and low-oxalate) diet. After 90 days, they followed the same diet but also were given 10 grams (a little more than ⅓ ounce) of dietary fiber in the form of high-fiber biscuits. While the original diet helped reduce the amount of calcium in the urine, the extra fiber reduced it even more.

Doctors still aren't sure how effective fiber is at treating or preventing kidney stones, Dr. Ruml adds. "It's probably safe to say that the higher your fiber intake, the more likely you are to bind calcium and oxalate in the intestine, which will lower the urinary levels of these minerals," she says.

Doctor's Top Tip

Doctors say drinking lots of water is the most important way to prevent all kinds of kidney stones. The National Institutes of Health in Bethesda, Maryland, recommends drinking enough liquids to create 2 quarts of urine every 24 hours. That's about a gallon of water a day.

One more point about fiber: While reducing the amount of calcium in the urine may be beneficial for people with stones, it's not so good for those trying to prevent osteoporosis, the bone-thinning disease caused by low levels of calcium. "Some people with kidney stones may be prone to osteoporosis," Dr. Ruml says. The bottom line for the stone-prone: Check with your doctor before substantially increasing your fiber intake.

The Calcium Controversy

Doctors used to commonly tell patients that they could avoid kidney stones by limiting calcium intake, but more recent studies have found that getting more calcium can actually prevent kidney stones. A Harvard study of nearly 46,000 men found that those who ate the most calcium were the least likely to form stones. In another Harvard study, women who consumed at least 1,100 milligrams of dietary calcium a day had one-third the risk of developing kidney stones compared with those who consumed less than 500 milligrams a day.

A 2002 study that followed 120 men with recurrent kidney stones for 5 years found that the men who ate a normal amount of calcium but who cut down on meat and salt were less likely to have kidney stones than men who ate the traditional low-calcium diet.

While vegetables such as broccoli and turnip greens have some calcium, the easiest way to get adequate amounts is by drinking milk and eating other dairy foods. A glass of protein-fortified fat-free milk, for example, has 351 milligrams of calcium. A cup of low-fat yogurt has 414 milligrams, and 1½ ounces of mozzarella cheese made from fat-free milk has 270 milligrams.

Because calcium supplements have been associated with an increase in kidney stones, experts recommend getting calcium from your food rather than a pill.

Lactose Intolerance

DAIRY ALTERNATIVES

As we get older, milk gets harder to enjoy because we gradually start producing less of the enzyme (lactase) needed to digest the sugar (lactose) found in milk and other dairy foods. This means that undigested lactose collects in the intestine, often causing gas, cramps, and diarrhea. Doctors call this problem lactose intolerance.

Researchers estimate that about 25 percent of Americans are lactose intolerant. Its symptoms are similar to irritable bowel syndrome (IBS), which can also be caused by dairy foods, but the two conditions are quite different. IBS comes and goes, often flaring as a result of stress, but lactose intolerance consistently shows its symptoms when dairy products are consumed. If you're not sure if you're lactose intolerant, you can be tested by your doctor or easily figure it out on your own. Wait until you go on vacation, says Paul Millea, MD, assistant professor of family and community medicine at the Medical College of Wisconsin in Milwaukee. After 3 days of relaxation, drink a tall glass of milk, and pay attention to how you feel afterward. If it causes gas, cramps, and diarrhea within 2 hours, you're probably intolerant to lactose.

Lactose intolerance usually isn't serious for the simple reason that it's easy to cut back on milk, cheese, and other dairy foods, says Talal M. Nsouli, MD, clinical associate professor of allergy and immunology at Georgetown University School of Medicine and director of the Watergate Allergy and Asthma Center, both in Washington, D.C. On the other hand, giving up dairy foods means that you could risk losing out on their greatest nutritional benefit—calcium, which you can't do without. Adults should get anywhere from 1,000 to 1,300 milligrams of calcium a day, and dairy products are the main way to do it. And, in addition to calcium, dairy foods also provide other key nutrients, such as vitamin A, vitamin D, riboflavin, and phosphorus.

But there are ways to get the benefits of dairy foods without the problems. Supermarkets sell reduced-lactose milk, for example, which has about 70 percent of the lactose removed. You can also buy reduced-lactose cheeses.

Yogurt is another great food for people with lactose intolerance. Although live-culture yogurt does contain lactose, it also has beneficial bacteria that help break it down into lactic acid, which is easier to digest. Low-fat yogurt is also full of calcium, with 414 milligrams per serving.

In addition, lactose is easier for the body to digest when you have it in combination with other foods. "Many people won't have a problem when they drink milk or have cheese with a meal," says Sheah Rarback, RD, a spokesperson for the American Dietetic Association and director of nutrition in the department of pediatrics at the University of Miami in Florida.

Even if you've had trouble digesting dairy foods in the past, it's a good idea to periodically test the waters, she adds. Some people build up a tolerance to lactose over time and can increase the amount of dairy foods they can eat.

Another way to reduce problems from dairy foods is to take a lactase supplement. Available in drugstores and supermarkets, these supplements can be stirred into milk or taken as a pill or caplet along with dairy foods.

If you find it's simply too uncomfortable to have dairy foods, you'll want to find other ways to get more calcium into your diet. Rarback recommends shopping for calcium-fortified foods such as juices and cereals. "A glass of calcium-fortified orange juice is the calcium equivalent of a glass of milk."

Doctor's Top Tip

Dairy products are the obvious sources of lactose, but the sugar may be in many of the prepared foods that you eat, such as cereal, instant soups, salad dressings, milk chocolate, and baking mixes, according to the Mayo Clinic in Rochester, Minnesota. To know for sure if your foods contain lactose, read the list of ingredients included on the nutrition label. Lactose may be listed as whey, milk by-products, nonfat dry milk powder, malted milk, buttermilk, or dry milk solids.

Lemons and Limes

PUCKER POWER

HEALING POWER

Can Help:

Heal cuts and bruises

Prevent cancer and
heart disease

You may love the tartness of lemons and limes, but it's a good bet that you've never taken a big bite from the whole fruit. Back in the 19th century, however, people literally craved these colorful fruits, not for the tart blast but for the remarkable health benefits they conferred.

British sailors, for example, who typically spent months at sea without fresh fruits or vegetables, would quaff lime juice to prevent scurvy, a terrible disease caused by vitamin C deficiency. (It was because of the British Navy's dependence on limes that they became known as limeys.) And in California during the Gold Rush, when fresh fruits were equally scarce, miners paid top dollar for lemons.

A Sea of C

Of all the nutrients we're most familiar with, vitamin C is perhaps the most impressive. During cold season, it's always in hot demand, since it lowers levels of histamine, a naturally occurring chemical that can cause red eyes and runny noses. Vitamin C is also a powerful antioxidant, meaning that it helps disarm powerful

In the Kitchen

If you've ever used a box-shaped grater to remove zest from an orange or lemon, you've probably also experienced the pain of grated knuckles.

An easier way to remove citrus zest is to use a zester or a microplane grater. These inexpensive kitchen gadgets are the modern version of the old-fashioned box-shaped grater. The zester looks a bit like a bottle opener. The business end contains a strip of stainless steel lined with sharp-edged holes. As you pull the zester across the peel, it removes a thin, curly strip of zest that piles up nicely—without a single zinged knuckle. To use a microplane, which looks like a carpenter's rasp, simply hold the flat tool over a plate or cutting board and rub the fruit over the sharp holes, making sure to rotate the lemon or lime so you don't end up with the bitter white pith.

oxygen molecules in the body that contribute to cancer and heart disease. The body also uses vitamin C to manufacture collagen, the stuff that glues cells together and is needed to help heal cuts and wounds. In addition, vitamin C helps the small intestines absorb iron.

The pulp and juice from lemons and limes are rich sources of vitamin C. A large lemon, for example, contains about 45 milligrams of vitamin C, or 75 percent of the Daily Value (DV) for this vitamin. Limes are also good, with a small lime containing about 20 milligrams, or 33 percent of the DV.

There's good reason to eat lemons and limes for their vitamin C content. Studies have shown that getting 200 milligrams or more of vitamin C from fruits and vegetables may lead to a lower risk of cancer, particularly colon, lung, stomach, esophageal, and oral cancers.

Quest for the Zest

However, there's more to lemons and limes than just vitamin C. The zest of the fruits (the colorful peel part that covers the white) has essential oils that give off a scent and contain antioxidants. Two compounds found in the zest are limonin and limonene, which appear to help block some of the cellular changes that can lead to cancer.

Limonene has been shown to increase the activity of proteins that help eliminate estradiol, a naturally occurring hormone that has been linked with breast cancer. It has also been found to increase the level of enzymes in the liver that can remove cancer-causing chemicals.

FOOD ALERT

Citrus Sunburn

People who handle large amounts of citrus fruits may find themselves at risk for a curious condition that could be called lime (not Lyme) disease.

Lemons and limes contain furocoumarins, compounds that sensitize the skin and make it susceptible to sunburn. In one case, described in the *New England Journal of Medicine*, a man's left hand blistered and swelled after he squeezed about 60 limes to make margaritas. The researchers called this painful condition margarita photodermatitis.

Anytime you're squeezing or zesting large numbers of lemons and limes, be sure to wash your hands thoroughly to remove the oils, and apply a strong sunscreen before going outdoors.

There are so many healthful compounds in the zest of lemons and limes that experts haven't even identified them all, says Christine Gerbstadt, MD, RD, a spokesperson for the American Dietetic Association. So if you're squeezing the juice and throwing out the zest, you're missing out on half of the fruit's benefits.

GETTING THE MOST

Zest up your flavors. Whether you're making a lemon meringue pie or simply adding flavor to salads or store-bought lemon yogurt, be sure to add plenty of zest. The healing compound limonene makes up about 65 percent of oils in the zest, says Michael Gould, PhD, professor of oncology and medical physics at the University of Wisconsin Medical School in Madison.

Zest can be added to just about anything, Dr. Gerbstadt says, including sautéed vegetables like onions and mushrooms or as a topping for tabbouleh or rice pilaf. Zest can even be added to dry ingredients when baking. Dr. Gerbstadt adds it to zucchini and banana breads.

Use it dried. While fresh citrus zest contains the most healing compounds, dried lemon zest, which you can find in the spice rack at the supermarket, can also be used in baking and sauces, Dr. Gerbstadt says.

Store the fruits at room temperature. You'll get more juice out of them, Dr. Gerbstadt says.

Low-Carb Diet

GETTING A BETTER INSULIN RESPONSE TO LOSE WEIGHT

Some say the low-carb diet is a fad that's on its way out—destined to go wherever it is bell-bottoms and lava lamps went after they fell out of fashion. Others say it's a healthy alternative to the low-fat, high-carbohydrate diet Americans have been struggling to follow for years.

One thing is for sure, low-carbohydrate diets can help you lose weight, but don't forget that carbohydrates are a macronutrient that your body needs, so it's not a good idea to cut too many carbs out of your diet.

HEALING POWER

Can Help:

Promote weight loss

Control insulin levels and prevent type 2 diabetes

Reduce the risk of heart disease

Changing the Way We Eat

For 12 years, Americans couldn't pour themselves a bowl of cereal or open a box of crackers without seeing the icon of what was considered healthy eating stamped on the box: the USDA Food Guide Pyramid. At its base, the pyramid touted 6 to 11 servings of bread, cereal, rice, and pasta as a foundation for a healthy diet. However, it failed to distinguish between healthier carbs, and so Americans felt justified eating plenty of bread, pasta, and low-fat crackers and cookies. As a result, we gained weight. A lot of weight.

Overweight adults in the United States, or those with a body mass index (or BMI) of 25 to 29.9, and those who are obese, or have a body mass index of 30 or higher, now make up 66 percent of the population. The rate of obesity is growing so fast that it has more than doubled in the past 20 years.

The USDA recently retired the old pyramid and replaced it with a new one that emphasizes whole grains over refined carbohydrates. In the meantime, Americans are trying to lose those extra pounds. At any given time in the United States, about 45 percent of women and 30 percent of men are trying to slim down.

A low-fat diet is one way to drop the pounds, but today, many Americans—a full one-third of those trying to lose weight—are cutting the number of carbs they eat in order to slim down. And many find it's easier to jump-start weight loss on a low-carb diet.

Doctor's Top Tip

Potatoes don't have to be left out of a low-carb diet. The key is knowing how to cook them. A baked white potato, containing about ½ cup of sugar, can be a good option even for a low-carb meal because of its fiber, says Carol Forman Helerstein, PhD, a licensed clinical nutritionist in private practice in Long Island and a consultant for the Zone Diet. The fiber stops the uptake of the sugar. If you mash the potato, you break down its fiber and its glycemic index goes up.

Sweet potatoes or yams are even better choices because they're lower on the glycemic index. "If I'm choosing a potato, I'll choose a yam or half of a baked white potato instead of mashed potatoes," she says.

In one study, 63 obese men and women were assigned either to a group who ate a low-carb diet or a group who ate a traditional low-fat diet. After 6 months, the low-carb group lost 4 percent more weight and saw bigger improvements in some of the risk factors associated with heart disease. The bigger weight loss lasted for only the first 6 months, however. After 1 year, both groups had lost about the same amount of weight.

How Carbs Work

The problem with the way we eat today is that it goes against nature. In the age of the caveman, daily meals consisted mainly of fruits, vegetables, and healthy fats, such as nuts and avocados, with protein from a rabbit or other lean source once in a while, says Carol Forman Helerstein, PhD, a licensed clinical nutritionist in private practice in Long Island and a consultant for the Zone Diet. Today, too much of our food is made up of refined carbs, and that can wreak havoc on our bodies and lead to weight gain.

All carbohydrates, which include fruits, vegetables, pasta, grains, and bread, contain sugar. When you eat refined or processed carbs, such as white bread, white flour, white pasta, white rice, and many snack foods, your body will quickly convert the sugar into glucose. When you've eaten a large amount at one time, your body produces more glucose than it needs, and the excess is stored as fat.

Unrefined carbs, such as whole grains, beans, and whole fruits and vegetables, contain fiber that helps your body absorb the food more slowly with less ending up being stored as fat.

Insulin is the hormone that transports glucose into the cells. When the body stops being able to appropriately handle the glucose in the blood, it leads to type 2 diabetes.

Most of us, in fact 75 percent of the population, will have an insulin response to carbohydrates that cause us to gain weight easily when we eat too many or the wrong kinds of carbs, Dr. Helerstein says. The rest of the population is genetically blessed and can eat what they want without gaining weight.

Many Americans create a vicious cycle by eating too many refined carbohydrates—

such as soft drinks, candy, pretzels, crackers, and other snacks—that never satisfy their hunger, so they continue to gain weight.

A low-carb diet puts the kibosh on this cycle. Studies have shown a connection between lower carb intake and blood insulin levels.

In one study, researchers at Temple University School of Medicine in Philadelphia analyzed 10 people who were obese and had type 2 diabetes. After they ate normally for 7 days, the participants spent 2 weeks eating only 21 grams of carbohydrates a day while eating as much protein and fat as they wanted. On the low-carb diet, they chose to eat one-third fewer calories a day than when they ate normally, leading to an average weight loss of 3½ pounds and an average drop in blood insulin levels of 23 percent.

One reason low-carb diets seem to work is because they stave off hunger better than low-fat diets. Eating more protein and controlling blood sugar levels helps you feel fuller.

In addition to having a positive effect on blood sugar levels, low-carb diets have been shown to lower the risk of heart disease. In a study published in the *New England Journal of Medicine*, researchers looked at more than 80,000 women who filled out a food-frequency questionnaire for the Nurses' Health Study and ranked the foods according to their intakes of carbohydrates, fats, and protein.

After 20 years, the researchers found that those women who ate diets low in carbohydrates and higher in protein and fat were least likely to get heart disease. Meanwhile, those who ate foods ranked higher on the glycemic index (GI), a ranking of how much sugar a food contains and how quickly it's absorbed by the body, were more likely to get heart disease. It's important to note that the women who were protected from heart disease received their fat and protein from vegetables sources.

An even better benefit of eating fewer carbs: a flatter stomach. Insulin causes fat to be stored in the belly, and belly fat is related to heart disease and diabetes. When you eat a diet that controls your insulin levels, you'll find you'll have a slimmer middle, Dr. Helerstein says.

How Low Is Too Low?

There's a misconception that eating a low-carb diet means leaving carbohydrates out completely, Dr. Helerstein says. The reality is that we can't exist without carbohydrates. When we stop eating carbs, we starve our brain, lose concentration, feel fatigued, and experience mood swings. The brain simply needs carbohydrates.

The Institute of Medicine in Washington, D.C., which sets the recommended daily intake of nutrients, advises getting 130 grams of carbohydrates a day. Considering Americans are getting double or triple that amount, it's something to strive for.

However, the type of carbohydrates you eat is just as important as the amount, Dr. Helerstein says. "The reason we're the fattest nation in the world is because we're eating the wrong type of carbohydrates in the wrong amount," she adds.

Here's how to choose the right carbs in the right amounts to lose weight:

Limit your meals to 500 calories or fewer. Eating more than 500 calories in one sitting will create an insulin response in the body that leads to weight gain, Dr. Helerstein says.

Go for low-GI foods. To lose weight and avoid type 2 diabetes, it's better to choose foods with a lower glycemic index because they create a gradual rise in blood sugar. Reach for artichokes, peppers, apples, old-fashioned oatmeal, and kidney beans. Intermediate-GI foods include sweet corn, rice, and beets. Foods that have a high glycemic index and that will make your blood sugar spike fast include bagels, french fries, and mashed potatoes.

Look for lean cuts of meat. London broil, top round, sirloin, and T-bone steaks are good options for a low-carb diet. Pair the steak with low-GI sides, such as a baked sweet potato and broccoli rabe, and you have a perfect low-carb dinner.

Eat the way Mother Nature intended. Fat wouldn't stand a chance if we avoided processed foods and ate only the carbohydrates that Mother Nature gave us, such as fruits, vegetables, and whole grains. "Mother Nature never made white rice or white pasta," Dr. Helerstein says, so choose brown rice, whole-wheat pasta and bread, and other whole grains, such as barley and oats.

Shop the perimeter. You've probably heard it before, but it deserves repeating. The healthiest foods are found around the perimeter of your supermarket. That's where you'll find fresh produce, meat, fish, and low-fat dairy products, Dr. Helerstein says. The inner aisles are where you're more likely to find foods concentrated in sugar and calories.

Top your meal with a glass of wine or beer. Wine has only 2 to 3 grams of carbohydrates in a glass. Some experts believed beer contained maltose, a sugar with the highest glycemic index, but they've recently discovered that the brewing process eliminates the maltose. Twelve ounces of light beer actually contains only 6 grams of carbs, while a can of regular beer carries about 13 grams of carbs.

Chicken Sausage with Summer Squash

1 **medium yellow summer squash, cut on the diagonal into ¼-inch slices**

1 **medium zucchini, cut on the diagonal into ¼-inch slices**

1 **tablespoon olive oil**

¼ **teaspoon salt**

1 **package (12 ounces) fully cooked smoked chicken sausages**

Preheat a grill or grill pan to medium-high.

In a medium bowl, combine the squash, zucchini, oil, and salt. Toss well.

Place the sausages and squash mixture on the grill, and cook for about 8 minutes, turning once, or until the sausages are cooked through and vegetables are tender.

Slice each sausage on the diagonal, and serve with the grilled squash.

Makes 4 servings

PER SERVING

Calories: 156
Total fat: 7 g
Saturated fat: 1.5 g

Cholesterol: 70 mg
Sodium: 773 mg
Dietary fiber: 1 g

Low-Fat Diet

KEEPING YOUR MACHINE CLEAN

HEALING POWER

Can Help:

Reduce the risk of heart disease

Prevent cancer

Promote weight loss

Preserve good vision

A low-carb diet, as you just read in the previous section, is one way to shed extra pounds. Embarking on a low-fat diet is another, more traditional, time-tested way.

During the past 2 decades, the evidence has become overwhelming that few things are better for your health than reducing the amount of saturated fat in your diet. Fatty foods can dramatically increase your risk of heart disease, diabetes, high blood pressure, certain types of cancer, and many other conditions. Plus, eating too much bad fat has made us all, well, fatter. Today 66 percent of Americans are overweight or obese and the rate of obesity has more than doubled to 32 percent, with much of the increase happening during the past 20 years.

And it's not only adults who are carrying the extra pounds. A large percentage of children are also overweight. The National Center for Health Statistics has reported that more than three times as many young people are overweight today as in 1980. Furthermore, the incidence of type 2 (non-insulin-dependent) diabetes, a condition that is often associated with being overweight, among children has grown to the point that it's considered an epidemic in America.

To put ourselves and our children on a healthier track, researchers say, we need to switch to low-fat diets. This means not only eating lower-fat foods but also getting more fruits, vegetables, legumes, and other healthful foods.

A Weighty Issue

The key to losing weight is cutting the number of calories in our diets. And the easiest way to cut calories is to eat less fat, says Judy Dodd, RD, assistant professor in the School of Health and Rehabilitation Sciences at the University of Pittsburgh and former president of the American Dietetic Association. Gram for gram, fat packs more energy, which is measured in calories, than any other nutrient. One gram of fat delivers 9 calories, more than twice as many as the same amount of protein or carbohydrate. Plus, your body likes fat. It's much more likely to store calories from fat than calories from other sources.

In one study, Danish researchers found that those who trimmed the amount of fat in their diets from 39 to 28 percent of total calories and increased their intake of carbohydrates were able to lose an average of 9 pounds in just 12 weeks. What's more, people who stuck to lower-fat diets were able to keep the weight off long after the study ended.

If you feel as if losing weight and keeping it off is nearly impossible, a low-fat diet may be the answer. The National Weight Loss Registry reports that its members who have lost weight and kept it off for more than 5 years did so through a low-calorie, low-fat diet.

Cutting fat from your diet does more than make you thinner and healthier. Research suggests that a low-fat diet can increase your general sense of well-being as well. In a study of more than 550 women, researchers at the Fred Hutchinson Cancer Research Center in Seattle found that when the women cut their daily fat intake in half—from 40 percent to 20 percent of total calories—they felt more vigorous, less anxious, and less depressed than they had while eating their former diets.

Health for the Heart

Even if you're one of those lucky folks who can eat whatever you want and never gain an ounce, fat in the diet has to go somewhere, and all too often, that "somewhere" is inside your arteries.

There's a direct link between the amount of fat in your diet and your risk for heart disease, Dodd says. This is particularly true of saturated fat, the dangerous, artery-clogging fat found mainly in meats, full-fat dairy products, and snack foods. Research has shown that eating a diet low in saturated fat is perhaps the best way to lower this risk.

In a 2006 study, Canadian researchers looked at the weight loss and cholesterol levels of 30 obese women after they spent 6 months eating a low-fat diet and exercising for at least 40 minutes three times a week. On average, the women lost 15 percent of their body weight, and their cholesterol fell 9 percent. Artery-clogging low-density lipoprotein (LDL) cholesterol fell 8 percent, on average.

In another study, researchers put people on a very low fat diet, with only 5 percent of total calories coming from fat. After 11 days, their cholesterol levels had dropped an average of 11 percent, and their blood pressures went down an average of 6 percent. This 11 percent decrease in cholesterol may have reduced their chances of dying from heart attacks by almost 33 percent.

You don't have to go on an extremely low-fat diet to get the benefits, however. Even reducing the amount of fat in your diet just a little bit can lead to a reduction in cholesterol levels, Dodd says.

MAKING THE CUT

You can't open a magazine or tune in to late-night television without being bombarded with information about the latest new diets—weight loss guaranteed! But in fact, there's nothing complicated about embarking on a low-fat diet. Eating less red meat, for example, will automatically lower your intake of saturated fat. So will swapping full-fat yogurt for the low-fat kind and eating more fruits, vegetables, legumes, and whole grains. In addition, there are quite a few "sneaky" ways to get the drop on fat. Here are a few you may want to try.

Try some new cheeses. Even though cheese is usually one of the first foods to be labeled off-limits when you're switching to a low-fat diet, some cheeses are naturally lower in fat than others. Feta, camembert, and part-skim mozzarella, for example, have less than 10 grams of fat in a 1½-ounce serving. While not exactly fat-free, they are better choices than Cheddar, for example, which has almost 14 grams of fat per serving.

Do the napkin test. Those big, fluffy muffins at the supermarket bakery sure look healthful, but they often contain enormous amounts of fat. Before you bring home a bag of monster muffins, put them to the test. Buy one muffin, and place it on a paper napkin. If it leaves a telltale oil mark, you can bet it contains more than 3 grams of fat, and you'll want to find a lower-fat variety.

Make the good better. Pizza is one American favorite that doesn't entirely deserve its junk-food reputation. In fact, a steaming slice can be a smart choice, as long as it's not swimming in its own oil slick. To make pizza a little bit healthier, spread a napkin on top of each slice and gently blot up the excess oil.

Be wary of no-fat foods. Supermarkets seem to be bursting with fat-free versions of just about everything these days. But even though reduced-fat mayonnaise, salad dressings, and cheese can be great tools to help you stay within your daily fat budget, "fat-free" isn't the same thing as "calorie-free." Moderation is still important, says Judy Dodd, RD, assistant professor in the School of Health and Rehabilitation Sciences at the University of Pittsburgh and former president of the American Dietetic Association.

Savor a healthy soup. Broth- and vegetable-based soups are a good recommendation

A Defense against Cancer

There is a compelling reason to make the switch to a low-fat diet. "Several studies indicate that a low-fat diet offers great protection against many diseases, including cancer," says Leena Hilakivi-Clarke, PhD, assistant professor of oncology at the Lombardi Comprehensive Cancer Center at Georgetown University Medical Center in Washington, D.C.

for people eating a low-fat diet, says Lalita Kaul, PhD, a national spokesperson for the American Dietetic Association and professor of nutrition at the Medical School of Howard University in Washington, D.C. But make sure you choose the low-sodium varieties, she says, particularly if you are sodium sensitive.

Enjoy some old favorites. There's simply no reason to give up desserts just because you're following a low-fat diet. In fact, many traditional favorites like gingersnaps, vanilla wafers, and graham crackers are low in fat.

Go lean on meat. Even though a richly marbled Porterhouse steak can blow a hefty percentage of your fat budget (a 3-ounce serving has 9 grams of fat), many cuts of meat are low in fat. Meats labeled "loin" or "round," for example, can have as little as 3 grams of fat per serving. When you cook the meat, grill or broil it, and use a pan that allows the fat to drip off, Dr. Kaul says.

Make the dairy switch. Milk is a good source of protein and an excellent source of calcium. Unfortunately, it can also be a great source of fat. To get the benefits of milk without all the fat, you simply have to give up the full-fat kind, which has 8 grams of fat in an 8-ounce serving. One-percent low-fat milk is a good choice, with 3 grams of fat per serving. Better yet, drink more fat-free (skim), which has virtually no fat yet contains just as much (or even more) calcium as whole milk.

Reach for the old standbys. Americans still need to increase their intake of fruits, vegetables, and whole grains, Dr. Kaul says. Because those foods are naturally low in fat, choosing them will help you achieve that goal of having 30 percent or less of your calories come from fat. Experiment with tasty fruits and salads for lunch and dinner, and add whole grain cereal, bread, and brown rice to your diet.

Enjoy ice cream alternatives. Just a few years ago, the tastes of low-fat and fat-free frozen desserts certainly didn't compare very favorably to traditional ice cream. But today, manufacturers have gotten very good at making lean frozen desserts that have the same rich taste and creamy texture as their high-fat kin.

In a study at the University of Benin in Nigeria, researchers found that when laboratory animals were fed high-fat diets, they began producing enzymes that led to cancerous changes in their colons in just 3 weeks.

What works in the laboratory is also effective in real life. In a study of 450 women, researchers in the department of epidemiology and public health at Yale University School of Medicine found that cutting just 10 grams of saturated fat a day—the equivalent of switching from two glasses of whole milk to the same amount of fat-free milk—could reduce the risk of ovarian cancer by 20 percent.

In another study, researchers from the University of Iowa in Iowa City compared the diets of women with cancer to the diets of women who did not have the disease. They found that women who ate the most red meat were about 50 percent more likely to get cancer than women who ate the least. This is significant, since red meat is one of the major contributors of saturated fats.

A low-fat diet is protective not only because of what it doesn't contain but also because of what it does. When you cut back on fat, you generally eat more fruits, vegetables, whole grains, and legumes, all of which have been shown to keep us healthier, says JoAnn Manson, MD, professor of women's health at Brigham and Women's Hospital in Boston.

Good for the Eyes

Finally, there's some evidence that eating a low-fat diet may protect you against conditions such as macular degeneration, the leading cause of vision loss in older adults.

In a survey of more then 2,000 people, researchers from the University of Wisconsin in Madison found that those who reported getting the most saturated fat were 80 percent more likely to get macular degeneration than those getting the least.

Getting Started

Even when you're trying to reduce the amount of fat in your diet, it isn't always easy to know where to begin. For starters, you need to figure out how much fat you're actually getting each day. Ideally, you should be getting between 25 and 30 percent of your total calories from fat, Dodd says.

Suppose, for example, that you normally get 2,000 calories a day. When you're following a low-fat diet, no more than 600 of those calories should come from fat. This adds up to about 67 grams of fat a day.

If lowering your fat intake to 30 percent of your calories sounds discouraging, don't let it be. It's actually a reasonable amount of fat to get in your diet, says Lalita Kaul, PhD, a national spokesperson for the American Dietetic Association and professor of nutrition at the Medical School of Howard University in Washington, D.C. Eating low-fat means avoiding fried foods, forgoing rich, fatty restaurant meals for home-cooked fare, and searching for tasty low-fat recipes with which to replace some of your higher-fat favorites. When you're looking for at-home convenience, Dr. Kaul recommends reaching for a Lean Cuisine meal or a Lean Pocket.

Reading food labels is perhaps the easiest way to keep track of your daily fat intake, Dodd says. When you're shopping for cheese, for example, you might notice that a 1-ounce serving of Cheddar has a little more than 9 grams of fat. Since that may represent a large percentage of your daily fat budget, you may decide to choose a lower-fat cheese, instead. Now that food labels include the percentage of fat based on a 2,000-calorie diet, you can look for foods that are 30 percent or below, Dr. Kaul says.

When you're eating out or buying foods that don't have labels, you can find out how much fat you're getting by picking up a nutrition reference guide at the bookstore or supermarket. These guides list the amount of fat in most common foods, including foods that are served in restaurants. You can also visit the restaurant's Web site before leaving home. Most fast-food restaurants, including Subway and Boston Market, list the nutrition information for its menu online. Sit-down restaurants such as Applebee's and Outback Steakhouse may offer suggestions for healthier menu options online.

Doctor's Top Tip

When you're eating out at a restaurant, look for a small heart next to some of the menu options. Those dishes will be heart healthy and low in fat, says Lalita Kaul, PhD, a national spokesperson for the American Dietetic Association and professor of nutrition at the Medical School of Howard University in Washington, D.C. Restaurants and doctors across the nation are working together to provide low-fat, healthy options when eating out. Her husband, a cardiologist, has spearheaded the program in the Washington, D.C., area.

As noted above, the most important fat to watch out for is saturated fat, which is found in animal foods like meats, butter, cheese, and eggs, and some plant sources, such as coconut oil, palm oil, tropical oils, and cocoa butter. Not only is saturated fat bad for your health, but the same foods that are high in saturated fat also tend to be high in cholesterol. So when you cut one, you automatically cut the other. The American Heart Association recommends that we get less than 7 percent of our total calories from saturated fat, partly by choosing fat-free or 1% fat milk and going for leaner cuts of meat, such as sirloin and top round.

Scientists in Australia found that when people ate one slice of carrot cake high in saturated fat and drank a milk shake, their bodies had a harder time protecting against heart disease. Saturated fat lowered the ability of high-density lipoprotein (HDL) to protect the inner lining of the arteries from plaque buildup, and it reduced the arteries' ability to expand and carry blood to organs and tissues.

Although margarine and vegetable shortening have been touted in the past as healthy alternatives to saturated fat, they're not always good choices. Studies indicate that hydrogenated fats—the kinds used in making margarine and shortening—can clog the arteries just as much as saturated fats. To avoid partially hydrogenated oils, look for a spread that says "zero trans fat" on the label, and avoid store-bought cookies and other baked goods and snack foods that contain trans fats. Trans fats are now required to be listed on nutrition labels along with total and saturated fat.

Enjoy the Good Fats: In Moderation

Even though it's generally a good idea to reduce the amount of all fats in your diet, some fats, such as monounsaturated and polyunsaturated fats, aren't so bad. These fats, which are abundant in vegetable and seed oils such as olive, sesame, and safflower oils and in nuts and seeds, have been shown to actually lower cholesterol and may help prevent it from sticking to artery walls. Of course, these fats contain just as many calories as other, less healthful fats, so you don't want to eat a lot of them, Dodd adds.

There's one other kind of fat that plays an essential role in a healthful, low-fat diet. The fat found in fish, called omega-3 fatty acids, has been shown to reduce clotting and inflammation in the arteries, which can significantly lower the risk of heart disease and stroke. In fact, the American Heart Association reports that epidemiological and clinical trials have shown that cardiovascular disease incidence decreases when people consume omega-3 fatty acids, especially when the omega-3s come from fish and plant foods as opposed to supplements. You don't have to eat a lot of fish to get the benefits. When you're following a low-fat diet, having two fish meals a week will go a long way toward keeping your arteries in the swim, Dodd says.

Poached Cod with Mixed Vegetables

4 cod fillets (6 ounces each)
1 fennel bulb
2 carrots, cut into matchstick pieces
1 small zucchini, cut into matchstick pieces
2 shallots or 1 small onion, thinly sliced
1 cup apple juice
¼ teaspoon salt
   Freshly ground black pepper
2 cups water

Rinse the cod with cold water, and pat dry with paper towels.

Trim the fennel, reserving the narrow top stems and some of the feathery leaves. Cut the bulb in half lengthwise. Cut out and discard the core. Cut into matchstick pieces.

Coat a large skillet with cooking spray and heat over medium-high heat. Add the fennel, carrots, zucchini, and shallots. Cook, tossing, for 1 minute, then stir in ¼ cup of the apple juice and ⅛ teaspoon of the salt.

Cook, stirring, until the vegetables are crisp-tender, 2 to 3 minutes. Season to taste with pepper. Transfer the vegetables to a platter, and cover to keep warm.

In the same skillet, combine the water, the reserved fennel stems and leaves, and the remaining ¾ cup apple juice. Bring to a simmer over medium heat. Reduce the heat to low, and add the cod. Cook, turning once until the cod is opaque in the center, 4 to 5 minutes. Test for doneness by inserting the tip of a sharp knife into 1 fillet.

Remove the cod with a slotted spatula, and place on top of the reserved vegetables. Sprinkle with the remaining ⅛ teaspoon salt. Season to taste with pepper.

Makes 4 servings

PER SERVING

Calories: 202
Total fat: 1.5 g
Saturated fat: 0.3 g

Cholesterol: 80 mg
Sodium: 269 mg
Dietary fiber: 3.8 g

Chocolate Mint Pudding Cake

1 cup all-purpose flour

¾ cup granulated sugar

1 teaspoon baking soda

¾ teaspoon baking powder

¼ teaspoon salt

½ cup unsweetened cocoa powder

½ cup fat-free buttermilk

½ cup unsweetened applesauce

1 teaspoon vanilla extract

½ teaspoon peppermint extract

¾ cup packed light brown sugar

1 cup plus 2 tablespoons boiling water

Preheat the oven to 350°F. Coat a 12- × 8-inch baking dish with cooking spray. Set aside.

In a large bowl, combine the flour, granulated sugar, baking soda, baking powder, salt, and ¼ cup of the cocoa. Whisk to mix.

Add the buttermilk, applesauce, vanilla, and peppermint extract. Stir just until the dry ingredients are well incorporated. Do not overbeat; the batter will look like brownie batter and will be a bit lumpy because of the applesauce. Pour into the prepared pan.

In a small bowl, combine the brown sugar and the remaining ¼ cup cocoa. Mix well. Sprinkle over the batter. Pour on the water; do not stir.

Transfer carefully to the oven. Bake for 25 to 30 minutes, or until the top is set, and the cake moves away from the sides of the pan. Cool on a wire rack for 20 to 30 minutes.

To serve, scoop the cake out of the pan with a pancake turner, turning each piece upside down on a plate so the pudding is on top.

Makes 8 servings

Cook's Note: *This cake tastes best warm. If the cake has cooled, place individual pieces on a microwaveable plate, and microwave on high power for 30 seconds, or until warm.*

PER SERVING

Calories: 208	Cholesterol: 1 mg
Total fat: 1 g	Sodium: 293 mg
Saturated fat: 0.5 g	Dietary fiber: 5 g

Lupus
EATING TO FIGHT INFLAMMATION

It's a mysterious disease—a case of the body's protective forces turning traitor. Lupus erythematosus, or lupus for short, occurs when the immune system, which usually protects the body, instead turns against it, attacking and damaging healthy tissues.

After conducting two nationwide surveys, the Lupus Foundation of America estimates that about 1.5 million Americans have some form of lupus. For reasons that aren't entirely clear, lupus, which is a form of arthritis, strikes 10 to 15 times as many women as men, possibly due to the effects of female hormones on the immune system. Women of color are also two to three times more likely to be affected by the disease.

There are two types of the autoimmune disease. Discoid lupus, the less serious form, affects the skin. Systemic lupus, which is more serious, can affect the whole body, including the heart, lungs, kidneys, joints, and nervous system.

There is no cure for lupus, but there's increasing evidence that how you eat—choosing certain foods and avoiding others—can give you an edge in battling it.

Healing Yourself with Food

While you may associate linseed oil with the smell of a paint factory, the grain from which it's extracted has been shown to significantly help people whose kidneys have been damaged by lupus.

Linseed, which is also known as flaxseed, has an abundance of two compounds that may help improve kidney function. One is alpha-linolenic acid, an omega-3 fatty acid. Alpha-linolenic acid stops both inflammation and clogging of the arteries, both of which play some role in damaging the tiny and very fragile blood vessels supplying blood to the kidneys.

Flaxseed is also high in lignans, compounds that can help prevent clots from forming in the bloodstream. Such clots can damage and clog the tiny blood vessels of the kidneys.

In one study, researchers at the University of Western Ontario in Canada gave flaxseed to nine people whose kidneys were damaged by lupus. They found that the people who were given ¼ cup of raw ground flaxseed a day, which they stirred into juice or sprinkled on breakfast cereal, had better kidney function.

THE SPROUT CONNECTION

Alfalfa sprouts contain an amino acid called L-canavanine, which can stimulate the immune system and make inflammation from lupus worse, says the Lupus Foundation of America. While other legumes are safe to eat, it may be a good idea to avoid alfalfa sprouts if you have lupus. The foundation also says to check food labels because alfalfa may be an ingredient in some foods.

The omega-3 fatty acids found in flaxseed oil—and in fish, canola oil, and dark green leafy vegetables—also boost the production of anti-inflammatory compounds in the body, according to the Lupus Foundation of America. In addition, the lignans in flaxseed appear to have antibacterial and antifungal capabilities. This is significant because people with lupus are more prone to infections than people without the disease.

You can buy flaxseed in health food stores. In order to get the benefits of the lignans, however, the flaxseed must be ground before you eat it. You can buy ground flaxseed that's been vacuum-packed to preserve freshness, says Stephen Cunnane, PhD, professor of medicine and physiology at the University of Sherbrooke in Quebec. Or you can buy whole flaxseed and grind it at home. You can use ground flaxseed to replace some of the wheat flour in muffins or breads, or try sprinkling it on cereal or into stews and soups.

Cutting the Fat

We all know how important it is to eat less fat, particularly the saturated fat found in meats and many dairy products. It's particularly important for people with lupus. "Lupus patients get more artery-clogging heart disease than people in the general population, and they also get it at younger ages," says Michelle Petri, MD, director of the Lupus Center at Johns Hopkins University School of Medicine in Baltimore. Reducing fat in the diet is one of the best ways to reduce this risk.

Another reason to cut back on fat has to do with immunity, since people on high-fat diets appear to have more immunity-related problems. As you might expect, eating too much red meat, which is usually high in saturated fat, can be a problem. A Japanese study of more than 150 women, for example, showed that those who ate meat frequently were nearly 3½ times more likely to develop lupus.

It's not only meat or saturated fat that's a problem. Laboratory studies showed that when mice with lupus were given smaller-than-usual amounts of polyunsaturated fats, such as those in vegetable oils like safflower and corn oil, their symptoms were reduced.

In short, if you have lupus, it's important to cut back on all types of fat in your diet. Here are some ways to get started:

Cut back on meat. Since meat is often one of the main sources of fat in the diet, cutting back automatically reduces the total amount of fat you consume. It's a good idea to limit yourself to 3 to 5 ounces a day of baked, broiled, or grilled meat.

Put vegetables on the menu. Eating more vegetarian meals, which typically include fresh vegetables, whole grains, and legumes, is another way to keep fat levels down. At the very least, try to substitute vegetarian meals for meat meals at least twice a week.

Open the spice cabinet. Rather than automatically adding butter or margarine to your food, look for other, healthier seasonings. By using spices, fresh herbs, and a splash of lemon or flavored vinegar, you'll get all the good tastes with a lot less fat.

Choose oils wisely. Since lupus may be aggravated by polyunsaturated fats, it's a good idea to switch to oils that are higher in monounsaturated fats, such as olive and canola oils.

Doctor's Top Tip

There's no one-size-fits-all diet for people who suffer from lupus, but you can pay attention to your symptoms and shape your own diet so that it helps give you the most relief. The Lupus Foundation of America recommends keeping track of the foods that seem to aggravate your lupus symptoms so you can avoid eating them.

Aim for Vitamins C and E

Although cutting out fat and getting omega-3 fatty acids may help people with lupus in more ways than one, the largest study to date of the relationship between the disease and diet didn't find a connection between dietary fat and the activity of systemic lupus, the Lupus Foundation of America says. The study of 216 women with lupus in Japan found no association between total fat, the type of fat consumed, or the intake of omega-3 fatty acids and the activity of the disease over 4 years.

However, those in the study who had higher levels of antioxidants in their diets, such as vitamins C and E, saw less of an occurrence of systemic lupus over the time period. Vitamin C can be found in citrus fruits, kiwifruit, broccoli, and cabbage. Vitamin E is found in whole grains, nuts, milk, and egg yolks.

Meat

A MINE OF MINERALS

HEALING POWER

Can Help:

Prevent iron-deficiency anemia

Boost the immune system

Prevent pernicious anemia

Americans are back in the saddle again. After a decade of searching for greener pastures, we've decided that the grass was actually pretty tasty back at the ranch. So we're stampeding back, steaks in hand, ready to hit the backyard barbecue.

Does this latest swing back to red meat mean that we're headed straight for imminent health disaster? Not at all. In moderation, lean meats—not just beef but also pork, venison, and other meats with less than 25 to 30 percent of calories from fat—can provide significant health benefits, from preventing vitamin and mineral deficiencies and boosting immunity to building stronger blood.

"People read these reports that red meat causes cancer and heart disease, so they think that they have to stop eating meat altogether," says Susan Kleiner, PhD, RD, owner of High Performance Nutrition in Mercer Island, Washington, and author of *The Good Mood Diet*. "What they don't realize is that the people in these studies are eating 10 ounces of red meat a day."

"Moderation is the key," urges Dr. Kleiner. "When it comes to red meat, you should have no more than 3 to 5 ounces a day. That's about the size of a deck of cards. For a lot of people, that looks like a garnish. But if you use just enough meat to accent a meal, you'll be able to get all the benefits without the potential detriments."

To know what a true 3-ounce serving of meat is, you may want to weigh it on a kitchen scale, says Christine Gerbstadt, MD, RD, a spokesperson for the American Dietetic Association. It's an eye-opener for people because they often don't know what a healthy serving of meat looks like.

Ironing Out Anemia

Iron deficiency is the most common nutritional deficiency in the United States. Maybe that's why fatigue, the main symptom of iron-deficiency anemia, is the number one reason that people drag themselves to see their doctors.

Meat is an important source of iron, a mineral that's essential for boosting the oxygen-carrying capability of blood. Once you've depleted your iron stores, your red

LIKE BEEF? CHOOSE LEAN CUTS

If you like eating beef, there's good news. Your favorite meat is getting leaner. In fact, many cuts of beef are 20 percent leaner than they were in 1990, according to the National Cattlemen's Beef Association, which lists 19 cuts of beef from the USDA Nutrient Database that meet government guidelines for being lean. The cuts, beginning with the leanest, include:

- Eye round roast
- Top round steak
- Mock tender steak
- Bottom round roast
- Top sirloin steak
- Round tip roast
- 95% lean ground beef

- Brisket (flat half)
- Shank crosscuts
- Chuck shoulder roast
- Arm pot roast
- Shoulder steak
- Top loin (strip or New York) steak

- Flank steak
- Ribeye steak
- Rib steak
- Tri-tip roast
- Tenderloin steak
- T-bone steak

blood cells get smaller. This makes it difficult for your lungs to send enough oxygen to the rest of your body. Without enough oxygen, you start feeling worn out.

"Women especially don't get enough iron," says Dr. Kleiner. "Mostly because, unlike men, they deny themselves foods that are rich in this mineral, like red meats." This is especially troubling, she says, because women generally need more iron than men to replace what is lost each month during their menstrual cycles.

In addition, women who exercise are at higher risk for anemia, says Dr. Kleiner. That's because the body uses more iron during exercise to meet the increased demand for oxygen. If you don't have enough iron to begin with, it's easy to run out while you're working up a sweat.

In one study, researchers had 47 inactive women step up the pace in a 12-week moderate-intensity aerobic exercise program. After just 4 weeks, all of them had significant dips in their iron stores. If you're active, it's particularly important to keep an eye on your iron intake.

What's so special about meat when you can also get iron from nonmeat sources like fortified breakfast cereals, tofu, and beans? Or, for that matter, when you can take an iron supplement?

For one thing, meats are unusually rich in iron. A 3-ounce serving of top round, for example, contains 3 milligrams of iron, or 20 percent of the Recommended Dietary Allowance (RDA) for women and 30 percent of the RDA for men. A 3-ounce serving of pork tenderloin has 1 milligram of iron.

Even though some plant foods are rich in iron—a baked potato, for example, contains 3 milligrams—it comes in a form that's harder for your body to absorb than the iron found in meats.

Meats contain a type of iron called heme iron, which is up to 15 percent more absorbable than nonheme iron, the kind found in plant foods. Plus, when you eat heme iron from meats, it helps your body absorb nonheme iron, so you get the maximum iron absorption from all your food, says Dr. Kleiner.

Zinc Immunity

Your immune system's duty is to keep your body from falling down on the job. Zinc's duty is to keep your immune system from doing the same. Not getting enough of this important mineral means that your immune system will have a harder time fending off infections, colds, and other health invaders.

As with iron, you can get zinc from foods besides meats, such as whole grains and wheat germ. But again, your body has a harder time retrieving zinc from plant sources, whereas the zinc in meats is readily absorbed, explains Dr. Kleiner.

By including a little meat in your diet, it's easy to meet the Daily Value (DV) of 15 milligrams of zinc. Three ounces of top round steak, for instance, provides 5 milligrams, or about a third of the DV for this essential mineral.

In the Kitchen

Lean meats like top round steak and pork loin have all but supplanted their high-fat predecessors in healthy kitchens. To be truly good, however, they do require special handling.

To ensure that your lean meat meals are moist and flavorful, try the following cooking tips:

Start with a marinade. Marinating lean meats in the refrigerator several hours prior to preparation will infuse them with flavor and add extra liquid to help keep them moist during cooking. There are so many options for healthy marinades, says Christine Gerbstadt, MD, RD, a spokesperson for the American

Dietetic Association. One easy marinade is to use ¼ cup of lemon juice, ¼ cup of vinegar, ¼ cup of a healthy oil such as canola or olive oil, and your favorite seasoning, such as fresh garlic, freshly ground black pepper, or dried herbs.

Add fat-free flavor while cooking. People tend to add fat to meat when they're cooking it to give it more flavor, Dr. Gerbstadt says, but it's just as easy and even more delicious to flavor your meat with healthier options. When grilling or broiling, add a fat-free salsa or sauce or fresh herbs to the meat near the end of cooking.

The Best of the Bs

For most of us, getting enough vitamin B_{12} (the DV is 6 micrograms) isn't a problem. If you eat meats, fish, eggs, poultry, or dairy products on a regular basis, you're almost certainly getting enough.

But if you don't eat these foods, and many strict vegetarians don't, you could be headed for trouble. Low levels of vitamin B_{12} can result in a rare and sometimes fatal blood disorder, called pernicious anemia, which causes fatigue, memory loss, and other neurological problems. And worse, you may not even know that there's a problem until it's already well advanced.

"Pernicious anemia comes on very slowly and can take up to 7 years to develop," says Dr. Kleiner. "And because one of the symptoms of the illness is deteriorating mental function, lots of people aren't even aware that there's anything wrong with them. It can take a long time to straighten this problem out, and the damage can be irreversible, especially in children."

Including small amounts of meats or other animal foods in your diet on a regular basis makes it easy to get enough vitamin B_{12}, says Dr. Kleiner. If you're a strict vegetarian who doesn't get vitamin B_{12} from animal foods, it's essential that you take a daily supplement or eat soy foods such as tempeh and miso, which are high in this nutrient. In addition, many cereals, pastas, and other packaged foods have been fortified with vitamin B_{12}, she points out.

Most meats are full of other B vitamins as well. They generally provide 10 to 20 percent of the DV for B-complex vitamins: riboflavin (essential for tissue repair),

(continued on page 400)

SAFER GRILLING

Grilled foods taste great, but for a long time, researchers have worried about their safety. The problem is that grilling causes certain compounds in meats to change into other compounds called heterocyclic amines, which may increase the risk for cancer. Charring or burning your meat on the grill carries the biggest risks to health.

What's a grill-chef to do? The answer, some researchers say, can be summarized in one word: marinade. In one study, researchers found that when medallions of chicken breast were marinated (or even dipped) in a mixture of olive oil, brown sugar, mustard, and other spices before being grilled, they contained 90 percent less of the dangerous compounds than nonmarinated meat that was cooked the same way. Another good rule of thumb: Don't eat the blackened or burned parts of the meat.

THE BEST CUTS

While meats can play a valuable role in a healthful diet, it's important to shop only for those items that are suitably low in fat—preferably with no more than 25 to 30 percent of calories coming from fat. In the following table, we've listed a few meats (and a variety of

Cut	Calories	Fat (g)	Calories from Fat	Vitamin B$_{12}$ (mcg)	Zinc (mg)
Beef—eye round	143	4	26%	2 (33% of DV)	4 (27% of DV)
Beef—top round	153	4	25%	2 (12% of DV)	5 (11% of DV)
Pork tenderloin	141	4	26%	—	3 (20% of DV)
Lamb foreshank	159	5	29%	2 (33% of DV)	7 (47% of DV)
Venison	134	3	18%	—	2 (13% of DV)
Elk	124	2	12%	—	3 (20% of DV)
Veal leg	128	3	20%	1 (17% of DV)	3 (20% of DV)
Moose	114	1	6%	—	3 (20% of DV)
Bison/ Buffalo	122	2	15%	—	2 (13% of DV)
Emu	103	3	23%	—	—

cuts) that you may want to try. Only prominent nutrients—those providing more than 10 percent of the DV—are mentioned. All nutritional information is based on 3-ounce servings.

Iron (mg)	Niacin (mg)	Vitamin B$_6$ (mg)	Potassium (mg)	Riboflavin (mg)	Thiamin (mg)
2 (20% of RDA for men and 13% for women)	3 (15% of DV)	0.3 (15% of DV)	—	—	—
3 (30% of RDA for men and 20% for women)	5 (25% of DV)	0.5 (25% of DV)	376 (33% of DV)	0.2 (33% of DV)	—
1 (10% of RDA for men and 7% for women)	4 (20% of DV)	0.4 (20% of DV)	457 (13% of DV)	0.3 (18% of DV)	0.8 (53% of DV)
—	14 (70% of DV)	—	—	—	—
4 (40% of RDA for men and 27% for women)	6 (30% of DV)	—	—	0.5 (29% of DV)	0.2 (13% of DV)
3 (31% of RDA for men and 21% for women)	—	—	—	—	—
—	9 (45% of DV)	0.3 (15% of DV)	—	0.3 (18% of DV)	—
4 (40% of RDA for men and 27% for women)	5 (25% of DV)	—	—	0.3 (18% of DV)	—
3 (30% of RDA for men and 20% for women)	—	—	—	—	—
4 (40% of RDA for men and 27% for women)	—	—	—	—	—

Doctor's Top Tip

Exploring the health food aisles of your supermarket may help you uncover some new meat options. Many grocery stores now have natural foods sections that stock tasty turkey sausage that's 98% lean, low-fat lunch meat, and other healthy meat choices, says Christine Gerbstadt, MD, RD, a spokesperson for the American Dietetic Association. If your supermarket doesn't carry these products, a natural foods store or gourmet grocery in your area surely will.

And if you're inclined, making a healthy sausage at home is not as hard as you think, Dr. Gerbstadt says. Deer meat, turkey breast, chicken breast, veal, lean pork loin, or a lean piece of beef can all be ground alone or in combination for a delicious and healthy alternative to the higher-fat store varieties.

vitamin B_6 (needed for immunity), niacin (vital for skin, nerves, and digestion), and thiamin (which helps the body convert blood sugar into energy).

GETTING THE MOST

Buy free-range. For the best healing meats, some experts advise, look for "free-range" meats or "grass-fed" beef. These are meats that come from livestock that is allowed to roam free instead of being restricted in close quarters. Because the animals aren't crammed together, the ranchers generally use fewer antibiotics and skip the growth hormones, explains Dr. Kleiner.

"Although I recommend organic, chemical-free meat, if the higher price is going to keep you from eating it, don't worry about the chemicals, and get the nutrients," recommends Dr. Kleiner. "In the long run, that's more important."

Add some variety. Although much of the research on the health benefits of meats has been done in studies with lean beef, experts are quick to note that you shouldn't limit yourself to eating beef alone. Other meats such as pork and lamb can also play a role in a healthful diet. "In the same way that you should eat a wide variety of whole grains and vegetables, you should also eat a variety of meats to ensure that you get all the nutrients they have to offer," advises Dr. Kleiner.

You might also want to take a walk on the wild side and go with game. Many people believe that game meats such as venison are tastier than more pedestrian meats such as beef. In addition, game is generally much leaner—deriving less than 18 percent of its calories from fat—while delivering the same powerhouse of B vitamins and minerals. To compare: A lean cut of beef, such as top round steak, has 34 percent calories from fat.

Horseradish-Spiked Pork and Apples

12 ounces pork tenderloin, trimmed of fat

2 medium apples

2 tablespoons all-purpose flour

1 cup apple cider

1 tablespoon extra-hot horseradish

Cut the pork crosswise into ¼-inch-thick slices. Core the apples and cut into thin slices.

Coat a large nonstick skillet with cooking spray, and heat over medium-high heat. Add the pork and cook until lightly golden on the bottom, about 2 minutes. Turn and cook until lightly golden on the second side and cooked through, 2 to 3 minutes longer. Test for doneness by inserting the tip of a sharp knife in a piece of the pork. Remove the pork to a clean plate, and set aside.

Reduce the heat to medium. Add the apples and cook, stirring occasionally, until they begin to turn light golden, 3 to 4 minutes. Sprinkle with the flour, and continue cooking, tossing to coat evenly with the flour.

Stir in the cider. Cook, stirring, until the sauce thickens, 3 to 4 minutes. Stir in the horseradish. Spoon the apples and sauce over the pork.

Makes 4 servings

PER SERVING

Calories: 218
Total fat: 6.3 g
Saturated fat: 2.2 g

Cholesterol: 52 mg
Sodium: 38 mg
Dietary fiber: 1.6 g

Beef and Spinach Stir-Fry

1 pound beef eye of round, trimmed of fat

1 tablespoon cornstarch

2 teaspoons canola oil

2 teaspoons grated fresh ginger

1 small onion, thinly sliced

1 bag (6 ounces) spinach, washed and trimmed

⅓ cup defatted beef broth

2 tablespoons ketchup

Freshly ground black pepper

Cut the beef across the grain into very thin slices. Place in a medium bowl. Add the cornstarch, and toss to coat.

In a wok or large skillet, heat the oil over medium-high heat until it is nearly smoking. Add the beef and ginger. Stir-fry until the beef is no longer pink on the surface, about 2 minutes. Transfer to a plate.

Add the onion to the pan, and stir-fry until softened, 1 to 2 minutes. Add the spinach, and stir-fry until just wilted, about 30 seconds.

In a small bowl, combine the broth and ketchup. Add to the pan. Add the beef. Stir-fry until the sauce is heated through and coats the beef and vegetables, 2 to 3 minutes. Season to taste with pepper.

Makes 4 servings

Cook's Note: *Serve over rice or noodles.*

PER SERVING

Calories: 207	Cholesterol: 61 mg
Total fat: 7.6 g	Sodium: 263 mg
Saturated fat: 2.1 g	Dietary fiber: 1.6 g

Mediterranean Diet

A MODEL FOR GOOD HEALTH

D uring the early 1960s, when the rate of heart disease in the United States was skyrocketing, people in Greece had some of the lowest heart disease rates in the world.

Here's the curious part. They were enjoying this robust good health even though their diet racked up nearly 40 percent of its calories from fat, plus they generally washed down their meals with a glass or two of wine.

Scientists wanted to know more. So they searched the shores of the Mediterranean Sea and discovered that it wasn't only in Greece that people were living longer and healthier but also in neighboring nations like France, Italy, and Spain. Clearly, these folks were onto something.

But what?

"For one thing, the traditional Mediterranean diet includes a lot of vegetables and legumes, along with fruits, fresh whole-grain breads, dates, and nuts," says Christopher Gardner, PhD, assistant professor of medicine at the Stanford Prevention Research Center in Stanford, California. "Meats like lamb and chicken are consumed infrequently and in small portions, and the main source of fat in the diet is monounsaturated fat from olives and olive oil rather than the saturated fat from animal foods. In addition, physical activity is a big part of the daily routine," he adds.

HEALING POWER

Can Help:

Reduce the risk of heart disease and cancer

Lower cholesterol

The Heart of the Matter

Just how healthful is traditional Mediterranean fare? In one study, French researchers looked at 600 men who had recently had a heart attack. They put half of the men on a traditional Mediterranean diet and half on a low-fat, low-cholesterol diet that people with heart disease are typically told to follow. Those following the traditional Mediterranean diet had a 70 percent lower rate of recurrent heart problems than those following the prudent low-fat diet.

Other studies had similar results. When researchers examined the diets and disease rates of people in seven different countries, for example, they found that while heart disease accounts for 46 percent of deaths of middle-aged men in America, only 4 percent of men in Crete, an island in the Mediterranean, had similar problems. In fact, the death rate from all causes in Crete during this 15-year study was lower than that of the other countries.

In 2006, researchers reviewed 35 experimental studies of the Mediterranean diet and found that the diet had a positive effect on cholesterol and insulin resistance. Researchers also learned that the diet lowers the risk of metabolic syndrome, heart attack and heart disease, and the risk of cancer in obese patients and patients who have had a heart attack.

In addition to its health benefits, one study found that people have an easier time sticking to a Mediterranean diet compared with a low-fat diet. A group of 772 older adults in Spain who had diabetes or three or more risk factors for heart disease were assigned to one of three groups. Two groups followed a Mediterranean diet, and the third followed a low-fat diet. In addition to the Mediterranean diet contributing to lower blood pressure, cholesterol, and blood sugar levels after 3 months, it also made it easier for the study participants to maintain the diet, researchers say.

The Fat Factor

There are many reasons the Mediterranean diet is good for the heart, but perhaps most important is where it gets its fat. Olive oil is the principal fat used in a Mediterranean diet, with total fat intake ranging from 25 percent to 35 percent of total calories.

Even though people in Mediterranean countries eat as much fat as we do (or more), they eat relatively little meat. Red meat is eaten only a few times a month, while fish and poultry are eaten every week. This means that they consume only minuscule amounts of artery-clogging saturated fat. "The biggest bang for the buck comes from limiting saturated fat and replacing it with monounsaturated fat, like olive oil," says Dr. Gardner. Olive oil is not only a monounsaturated fat, it also contains antioxidant compounds that help prevent chemical changes in the body that can cause the dangerous low-density lipoprotein (LDL) cholesterol to stick to the lining of artery walls.

The second-most common source of fats in the Mediterranean diet is nuts and seeds. Nuts contain alpha-linolenic acid, which the body converts to the same kind of heart-healthy fats found in fish (which people in the Mediterranean also eat). Studies show that people who get the most of these fatty acids are the ones least likely to have heart disease.

"This doesn't mean people should run out and start adding tons of olive oil and nuts to their diets," warns John A. McDougall, MD, medical director of the McDougall Program in Santa Rosa, California, and author of *The McDougall Program for a Healthy Heart*. It's not only diet that makes people in Mediterranean countries so healthy. They also tend to walk a lot, do hard physical labor, and generally stay active. So even though they take in a lot of calories from fat, they're usually able to keep their weight under control.

"If Americans got all that fat from olive oil, they would just get fat, which itself is a major heart disease risk," Dr. McDougall says. But some olive oil is good, particularly when you use it to replace the less-healthy saturated fats in your diet.

Meanwhile, the fish that people in the Mediterranean eat provide omega-3 fatty acids, which have been shown to reduce clotting and inflammation in the arteries and thus significantly lower the risk of heart disease and stroke. In fact, the American Heart Association reports that epidemiological and clinical trials have shown that cardiovascular disease incidence decreases when people consume omega-3 fatty acids, especially when it comes from fish and plant foods as opposed to supplements.

Five-a-Day Protection

The folks at the American Heart Association would be delighted if they could get us to eat the five servings (or more) of fruits and vegetables that people in the Mediterranean region eat every day. The Mediterranean diet emphasizes seasonally fresh and locally grown fruits and vegetables over highly processed foods that don't contain as many micronutrients and antioxidants. On most days, fresh fruit serves as dessert, while sweeter desserts made with sugar and saturated fat are consumed no more than a few times a week.

Studies have shown that people who eat the most fruits and vegetables have fewer problems with heart disease. Presumably this is due to the antioxidant vitamins and other healing compounds in these foods.

In addition, fruits, vegetables, and beans, which are another Mediterranean staple, are among the best sources of folate, a B vitamin that may work hard in the fight against heart disease, says Dr. Gardner.

Folate helps decrease levels of an amino acid called homocysteine. There is a link between too much homocysteine and heart disease. Research has shown that healthy people who have high levels of homocysteine are about 14 times more likely to have heart disease than those with low or moderate levels.

In addition, the Mediterranean diet is extremely high in fiber. High-fiber foods not only help keep your weight down by filling you up without a lot of fat and calories, they also help block the absorption of certain fats and cholesterol. This means that some of these harmful substances are flushed away before making it into the bloodstream.

So powerful are the effects of fiber that a study of nearly 44,000 men ages 40 to 75 found that men who added just 10 grams of fiber a day to their diet decreased their risk of heart disease by almost 30 percent.

Doctor's Top Tip

Americans love eating out, and one of our favorite types of restaurant food is certainly Italian. However, many Italian dishes filled with cheese and meat don't qualify as heart-healthy Mediterranean meals. Before you order another plate of greasy Chicken Parmesan, look for a restaurant that makes authentic southern Italian dishes, suggests the American Cancer Society. Traditional dishes from that area of the Mediterranean are mainly made up of pasta, bread, beans, vegetables, fruit, and olive oil.

A Drink for Health

It's not only olive oil and fruits and vegetables that make the Mediterranean diet so good for the heart. Another factor appears to be the wine, especially red wine, that people in these countries drink with almost every meal.

Wine contains compounds called phenols that help prevent LDL cholesterol from sticking to artery walls. It also keeps platelets in blood from sticking together and causing clots. "In moderation, wine can be a nice addition to a healthy diet," says Robert M. Russell, MD, director and senior scientist at the Jean Mayer USDA Human Nutrition Research Center on Aging at Tufts University in Boston.

Beyond the Heart

Although the Mediterranean diet is most renowned for its role in helping to keep the heart healthy, it also appears to reduce the risks of other health threats, among them cancers of the breast and colon.

Studies show that compared with women elsewhere in the world, women in some Mediterranean countries have half the risk (or less) of getting breast cancer. This could be due to their low intake of saturated fat and high intake of monoun-saturated fats, fruits, and vegetables.

Indeed, Italian researchers have found that people in the Mediterranean region who follow the traditional diet—that is, those who eat lots of fruits and vegetables and not much fat and protein—are less likely to get cancer than those who eat more-modern, less-healthful diets.

"The message here is simple," says Dr. Gardner. "For optimal health, choose a plant-based diet, which is naturally high in vitamins, minerals, fiber, and anti-oxidants, and low in fat, cholesterol, and sodium."

THE MEDITERRANEAN PLAN

Unless you've been living on popcorn and Twinkies for the past 10 years, you should know that the USDA uses a Food Guide Pyramid to give Americans guidelines on how they should eat for their health. For 12 years, the USDA used a pyramid with bread and cereal at its base, but recently, the USDA revised the pyramid to give out more individual advice based on a person's nutritional needs, including advising Americans to make half of their grains whole.

In this country, the pyramid is considered the optimal eating plan.

However, the USDA's isn't the only pyramid going. There's also a Mediterranean Pyramid, based on the traditional diet of southern Europe. Unlike our pyramid, which includes meats as a way of getting enough protein every day, the Mediterranean Pyramid depends instead on legumes, fish, and nuts to supply the necessary protein. Red meat is reserved for a few times a month.

The Mediterranean Pyramid also calls for large amounts of olive oil and daily doses of cheese and yogurt, all washed down with a healthy splash of red wine. Regular physical activity is also an essential part of the plan.

To the right is the traditional Mediterranean Pyramid. You should choose most of your foods from the base of the pyramid and save those at the top for special occasions.

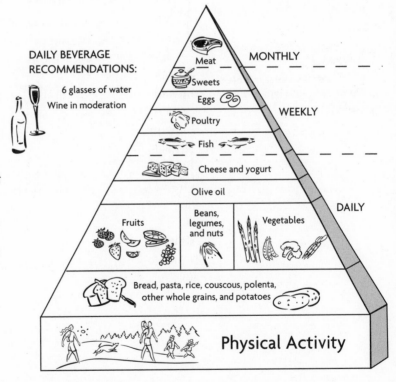

DAILY BEVERAGE RECOMMENDATIONS:

6 glasses of water
Wine in moderation

Meat — MONTHLY
Sweets
Eggs
Poultry — WEEKLY
Fish
Cheese and yogurt
Olive oil
Fruits | Beans, legumes, and nuts | Vegetables — DAILY
Bread, pasta, rice, couscous, polenta, other whole grains, and potatoes

Physical Activity

Greek Lemon Chicken

4 each skinless, fat-trimmed chicken legs and thighs (about 1½ pounds total)

1 medium red bell pepper, cut into 8 wedges

1 medium orange bell pepper, cut into 8 wedges

2 medium Yukon Gold potatoes, each cut into 8 wedges

1 medium red onion, cut into 8 wedges

2 tablespoons extra-virgin olive oil

Grated zest and juice of 1 lemon

1 tablespoon minced garlic

1 teaspoon dried oregano

¼ teaspoon salt

¾ teaspoon freshly ground black pepper

¾ teaspoon paprika

8 pitted kalamata olives, each quartered lengthwise

Chopped fresh mint or parsley, grated lemon zest, and lemon wedges, for garnish (optional)

Preheat the oven to 400°F. Tear off 2 sheets of nonstick foil, each 24 inches long. Put the dull sides (nonstick sides) together, and fold the edge on 1 side over twice, to make a seam. Open up, and line and cover the edges of a 17- × 12-inch rimmed baking sheet (face the dull side of the foil up).

Place the chicken on one side of the pan and the bell peppers, potatoes, and onion on the other side.

In a small bowl, mix the oil, lemon zest and juice, garlic, oregano, salt, black pepper, and paprika. Drizzle over the chicken and vegetables, and toss to coat.

Roast for 40 to 45 minutes, turning the chicken and stirring the vegetables halfway through cooking, until the chicken is cooked through and the vegetables are lightly browned and tender. Sprinkle with the olives. Garnish, if desired.

Makes 4 servings

PER SERVING

Calories: 290
Total fat: 13 g
Saturated fat: 2 g

Cholesterol: 80 mg
Sodium: 530 mg
Dietary fiber: 3 g

Mediterranean-Style Penne

8 **ounces penne**

½ **cup dry-packed sun-dried tomatoes, cut into 3 or 4 strips each**

2 **tablespoons olive oil**

2 **cloves garlic, minced**

1 **can (15 ounces) cannellini or Great Northern beans, rinsed and drained**

2 **tablespoons minced fresh sage**

¼ **teaspoon salt**

Freshly ground black pepper

In a large pot of boiling water, cook the pasta according to the package directions. About 1 minute before the pasta is done, add the tomatoes to the pot.

Scoop out ¼ cup of the cooking water and set aside. Drain the pasta and tomatoes. Place in a large bowl. Add the reserved cooking water, and toss to mix.

In a medium saucepan, heat the oil over medium heat. Add the garlic, and cook until fragrant, about 30 seconds. Stir in the beans, sage, and salt. Cook, stirring, until the beans are heated through, 1 minute longer. Season to taste with pepper.

Pour the bean mixture over the pasta, and toss gently to combine.

Makes 4 servings

PER SERVING

Calories: 394

Total fat: 11.8 g

Saturated fat: 1.5 g

Cholesterol: 0 mg

Sodium: 413 mg

Dietary fiber: 7.6 g

Melons

HEALTH FROM THE VINE

HEALING POWER

Can Help:

Prevent birth defects

Reduce the risk of cancer and heart disease

Keep blood pressure low

Summer picnics don't really come alive until the barbecue is cold and the potato salad has been put away. That's when it's time to pick up a knife and cut into the tough green rind of an ice-cold watermelon, revealing the sweet red flesh within.

There's always something exciting about cutting open a watermelon, crenshaw, or honeydew. For one thing, they come encased in protective rinds, so what's inside always comes as a surprise. And even before you cut, most melons whet your appetite by releasing a rich, penetrating scent, which is why they're sometimes called the "perfumy fruits."

Here's another reason melons are so marvelous. Researchers have found that they contain a number of substances that are very good for your health. Both watermelons and muskmelons—which include honeydews, crenshaws, and a few other melons— provide folate, a B vitamin that has been shown to lower the risks of birth defects and heart disease. Melons also contain potassium, which is essential for keeping blood pressure at healthy levels. And because melons are low in calories and fat, they're the perfect food for waist watchers.

Cantaloupes are especially healthful, and they contain certain nutrients that other melons don't, which is why they're discussed in a separate chapter (see page 135).

Melons for Moms—and More

In what has been called one of the most critical discoveries of the 20th century, researchers found that if all women of childbearing age consumed at least 400 micrograms of folate a day, the incidence of brain and spinal cord birth defects (called neural tube defects) could be cut in half or even more. For a long time, doctors weren't sure what folate did. They suspected that it played a role in preventing birth defects, but there wasn't strong evidence one way or the other.

Then a study of almost 4,000 mothers revealed that those who got enough folate were 60 percent less likely to have children with brain and spinal cord defects than women who got smaller amounts.

Folate, a B vitamin, is an essential ingredient when cells are dividing rapidly. It serves as the shuttle bus that carries fragments of proteins. When folate levels are low, these fragments, lacking transportation, may be left behind. As a result, the newly forming cells may have defects that can lead to birth defects. (Later in life, the same problem can lead to cellular changes that could lead to cancer.)

So before you start shopping for pickles, put a few melons in your cart because they're very good sources of folate. A cup of honeydew, for example, contains 11 micrograms of folate, or 3 percent of the Daily Value (DV) for this vitamin. Casaba melons are even better, with the same 1 cup providing 29 micrograms of folate, or 7 percent of the DV.

If 7 percent doesn't sound like a lot, remember that a cup of melon is the equivalent of about five good bites. Most people eat two or more cups of melon at a time, making it a very good folate find.

Incidentally, it's not only moms-to-be who should be making the most of melons. The same nutrient that protects against birth defects is also good for the heart.

The body uses folate to control levels of a chemical in the blood called homocysteine. "Although small amounts of homocysteine are normal, too much of it somehow contributes to the artery-clogging process that leads to heart disease," says Killian Robinson, MD, associate professor of medicine at Wake Forest University Baptist Medical Center in Winston-Salem, North Carolina, and author of *Homocysteine and Vascular Disease*. "We know that low levels of folate are related to too-high homocysteine levels," he says.

MELONS WITHOUT MOTION

There's a good chance that whoever invented the wheel was a watermelon fan. As you've probably noticed, a watermelon's smooth, cylindrical shape gives it a tendency to roll—usually off a table or the seat of your car—creating instant melon purée.

There's another problem with the shape of watermelons. Since they can't be stacked, they take a lot of room to store, which is expensive for melon growers. In Japan, where space is at a premium, growers have hit upon an ingenious solution: the square watermelon.

When melons are young and still on the vine, Japanese growers sometimes place them in boxes. As the melons grow to fit the space, they develop flat bottoms and sides, making them perfect for stacking. Square watermelons aren't yet available in this country, but just for fun, if you have a backyard garden, you may want to try growing your own.

Finally, folate has been shown to reduce the risk of polyps, precancerous growths in the colon that sometimes progress to full-blown cancer. Researchers at Harvard Medical School found that people getting the most folate were 33 percent less likely to develop polyps in the colon than those getting the least.

The Fiber Fix

One thing that your digestive tract needs is a steady supply of dietary fiber. Fiber is so important, in fact, that people who don't get enough have higher risks for cancer as well as for a variety of digestive problems, says John H. Weisburger, MD, PhD, vice president for research and director of the Naylor Dana Institute for Disease Prevention at the American Health Foundation in Valhalla, New York.

The type of fiber that is found in melons, called soluble fiber, is tremendously important for helping to keep the colon healthy, Dr. Weisburger explains. Because soluble fiber absorbs water as it moves through the digestive tract, it causes stools to get heavier and larger. As a result, they move more quickly through the intestine, reducing the amount of time that harmful substances in the stool are in contact with the colon wall.

Most fruits, including melons, have soluble fiber, says Christine Gerbstadt, MD, RD, a spokesperson for the American Dietetic Association. Soluble fiber is like a

In the Kitchen

Unlike most fruits and vegetables, which are easy to check for ripeness, melons hide their succulence—or their toughness—behind a protective rind. To get the best taste every time, here are a few tips you may want to try:

Check the bottom. A watermelon that's pale yellow or beige on the bottom was allowed to ripen on the vine and will probably be at the peak of freshness. If the color is uniform, however, it may have been picked early and won't deliver its full flavor.

Take a sniff. Most melons (with the exception of watermelon) release a rich, fragrant odor when they're fully ripe. If you can't smell it in the store, don't take it home.

Check the stem. When muskmelons are allowed to ripen in the field, the fruit slips off the vine, leaving the stem behind. So if you see a muskmelon with the stem attached, you'll know that it was picked early and isn't fully ripe. It's okay, though, if watermelons still have their stems.

Give it a slap. Although thumping is the time-honored method for testing a watermelon's ripeness, a slap works better. If the melon sounds hollow rather than solid, it's ready to go.

policing agent. As fiber moves through the gastrointestinal (GI) tract, it absorbs pollutants such as excess cholesterol and other trace minerals along the way and moves it out of the body. At the same time, it will increase the movement of the GI tract and help with constipation. "It normalizes you," Dr. Gerbstadt says. "If your system is moving too fast (and you have diarrhea), soluble fiber will slow you down. If your system is moving too slow, it will speed you up."

"Getting more fiber can reduce the number of polyps in the gastrointestinal tract and also the risk of colon cancer," says Dr. Weisburger. All melons contain some fiber, although honeydews beat out watermelon by quite a bit. Half a honeydew has nearly 3 grams of fiber, or 12 percent of the DV.

More Melons, Less Pressure

If you have high blood pressure, you're probably already getting less salt and more minerals in your diet. It's a good idea to get more melons as well. All melons, especially honeydews and crenshaws, are good sources of potassium, which is perhaps the most important mineral for keeping blood pressure down.

Doctor's Top Tip

Mango salsa may be the first thing you think of to dress broiled or grilled fish, but there are literally hundreds of ways to make melon salsa. "I use a cup of finely diced melon, a minced red onion, chopped chile peppers, and lemon or lime juice," says Christine Gerbstadt, MD, RD, a spokesperson for the American Dietetic Association. You can also add garlic, chopped cilantro, chopped yellow or green bell peppers, diced tomatoes, other fruit such as blueberries, or anything you have in your fridge to enhance melon salsa, Dr. Gerbstadt says. If salad is on the menu for the day, add the salsa to your greens as well.

The potassium in melons acts as a natural diuretic, removing excess fluids from the body. This is important because when fluid levels are high, blood pressure can rise, says Michael T. Murray, a naturopathic doctor in Bellevue, Washington, and author of *Natural Alternatives to Over-the-Counter and Prescription Drugs*. Plus, potassium keeps the artery walls relaxed.

Relaxed arterial walls do not contract as strongly as more "taut" or rigid walls. This means that the blood pressure created with each heartbeat is not as great. The result, of course, is lower blood pressure—which can reduce the risk of stroke, heart disease, and other serious conditions.

People with high blood pressure are often advised to get at least the DV of 3,500 milligrams of potassium a day. Melons make it easy. Half a honeydew, for example, has about 1,355 milligrams of potassium, or more than a third of the DV. Watermelons also contain potassium, but only about half as much as honeydews or crenshaw melons.

GETTING THE MOST

Make it a honey. Even though watermelon is a decent source of nutrients, it contains so much water that the nutrients are very diluted. Ounce for ounce, honeydews have over twice the potassium and almost three times more folate than watermelons.

Try new varieties. Although honeydews are rich in nutrients, don't stop there. If you look at your supermarket or gourmet food store, you may find some melon varieties you've never tried, such as casaba, Persian, Santa Claus, and Galia. Cutting them open to see what's inside can be a pleasurable treat, Dr. Gerbstadt says. "You may find one that you like better than honeydew," she says.

Buy them whole. Supermarkets often sell watermelons, honeydews, and other melons cut into halves or slices. This can save space in your refrigerator, but it won't save much in the way of nutrients. When the flesh of melons is exposed to light, the nutrients start to break down. So it's a good idea to buy melons whole. And once you've cut them, keep them covered in the refrigerator to prevent the vitamins from breaking down.

Keep them cold. Folate is readily destroyed by heat, so it's important to store melons, whole or cut, in a cool, dark place.

Watermelon Smoothie

2 **cups chopped watermelon**

¼ **cup fat-free milk**

2 **cups ice**

In a blender, combine the watermelon and milk, and blend for 15 seconds, or until smooth. Add the ice, and blend 20 seconds longer, or to your desired consistency. Add more ice, if needed, and blend for 10 seconds.

Makes 2 servings

PER SERVING

Calories: 50
Total fat: 0 g
Saturated fat: 0 g

Cholesterol: 1 mg
Sodium: 20 mg
Dietary fiber: 1 g

Honeydew and Blueberry Salad

1 honeydew melon

1 cup fresh blueberries

2 strips lemon zest (1 × 3½ inches each)

¼ cup berry vinegar (see Cook's Note)

2 teaspoons sugar

Cut the honeydew in half, scoop out the seeds, and remove the flesh from the rind; discard the rind. Cut the flesh into ¾-inch cubes. Place in a large glass bowl. Add the blueberries and lemon zest.

In a small bowl, combine the vinegar and sugar. Whisk until the sugar is dissolved. Pour over the fruit and toss gently. Cover and refrigerate for 1 to 2 hours.

Toss gently to mix. Discard the lemon zest. To serve, remove the honeydew and blueberries with a slotted spoon.

Makes 8 servings

Cook's Note: *Raspberry vinegar is available in some large supermarkets. Blueberry vinegar, sold in some specialty shops, is especially good in this salad. The juice left from marinating the salad can be served with the salad or drained and refrigerated for a refreshing drink.*

PER SERVING

Calories: 71
Total fat: 0.2 g
Saturated fat: 0 g

Cholesterol: 0 mg
Sodium: 18 mg
Dietary fiber: 1.5 g

Memory Problems
EATING FOR RECALL

Like a Dick Tracy decoder ring, sometimes the answers to life's most perplexing memory problems are found inside a cereal box. Just ask William Regelson, MD, professor of medicine at the Virginia Commonwealth University College of Medicine in Richmond.

"What we sometimes assume is the onset of 'senility' may be caused by marginal nutritional deficiencies," says Dr. Regelson. "When people say that they're losing their mental functions, one of the first things I tell them is that they should eat Total cereal. It has varying amounts of all the vitamins and minerals they need. You'd be surprised how many people are fine once they meet their nutritional needs."

Many researchers are discovering the same thing. When people are low in certain nutrients, their mental performance dips. Even not getting enough water can cause the mind to get fuzzy, says Susan A. Nitzke, PhD, RD, professor in the nutritional sciences department at the University of Wisconsin in Madison. "The thirst mechanism slows down as we age, so we're not always aware right away that we need water," she says. "One of the symptoms of severe dehydration is mental confusion."

In addition, the body begins absorbing some nutrients a little less efficiently over time. So even though your need for calories doesn't change, you may need additional nutrients to keep your mind sharp, says Dr. Regelson.

Not all memory problems are caused by diet. But when nothing else is amiss, it may be what you're eating—or not eating—that's slowing you down.

B Is for Brains

The B vitamins are perhaps the most essential nutrients for helping to keep your mind sharp. Your body uses B vitamins to turn food into mental energy and to manufacture and repair your brain tissue. "Deficiencies in thiamin, niacin, and vitamins B_6 and B_{12} can all cause mental dysfunction," says Vernon Mark, MD, author of *Reversing Memory Loss*. "In fact, pellagra, a niacin deficiency, used to be a leading cause for admissions into state mental hospitals," he explains.

Research has shown, in fact, that when children are given 5 milligrams of thiamin instead of the Daily Value (DV) of 1.5 milligrams, they achieve substantially higher scores when given tests of mental functioning, Dr. Mark adds.

Today, many breads, cereals, and pastas are enriched with thiamin and niacin, so most people get enough of these nutrients. Niacin deficiencies have become extremely rare, especially in this country. But in older folks or in people who frequently drink alcohol, levels of thiamin can dip low enough to cause memory problems, says Dr. Mark.

The easiest way to make sure you get enough brain-boosting B vitamins is to eat foods containing enriched grains. One cup of enriched spaghetti, for example, has 0.3 milligram of thiamin, or 20 percent of the DV, and 2 milligrams of niacin, or 10 percent of the DV. Meat is also a good source for getting these nutrients. Three ounces of pork tenderloin, for example, provide 0.8 milligram of thiamin, or 53 percent of the DV. For niacin, 3 ounces of chicken breast deliver 12 milligrams, or 60 percent of the DV.

It's not as easy to get additional amounts of vitamins B_6 and B_{12}, because it's harder for the body to absorb them as we get older. "After the age of 55, it's pretty common to be low in these vitamins, because the lining of the stomach is changing," says Dr. Regelson.

As you get older, it's a good idea to get more than the DV of both of these nutrients. Vitamin B_6 is abundant in baked potatoes, bananas, chickpeas, and turkey. One baked potato provides 0.4 milligram of vitamin B_6, or 20 percent of the DV, and one banana provides 0.7 milligram, or 35 percent of the DV. For vitamin B_{12}, meat and shellfish are good choices. Three ounces of lean ground beef will provide 2 micrograms of vitamin B_{12}, or about a third of the DV. Clams are an incredible source, with 20 steamed clams providing 89 micrograms, or 1,483 percent of the DV.

Maintaining the Flow

One way to alleviate memory problems is to get more blood to the brain, says Dr. Regelson. When adequate bloodflow isn't maintained, the brain and memory begin performing poorly.

The lack of blood to the brain is often caused by the same thing that leads to heart disease: a buildup of cholesterol and fat in the arteries. "This condition is not only preventable through diet," says Dr. Regelson, "it's at least partially reversible."

A primary cause of cardiovascular disease—clogged arteries in the heart and the brain—is too much fat, especially saturated fat, in the diet, says Dr. Nitzke. "Keep your intake of saturated fat low by cooking with small amounts of liquid oils, such as olive or canola oil, instead of butter or margarine and by minimizing your intake of fatty foods, such as full-fat mayonnaise, rich desserts, and fatty meats," she says.

Just as important, she adds, is getting more fruits and vegetables. Fruits and vegetables are packed with antioxidants—compounds that block the effects of harmful oxygen molecules called free radicals. This is important because when free radicals damage the harmful low-density lipoprotein (LDL) cholesterol, it becomes stickier and is more likely to stick to artery walls.

Studies have shown that antioxidants in fruits and vegetables can help prevent Alzheimer's disease. In 2002, researchers studied nearly 5,500 people and found that those who ate diets rich in the antioxidant vitamins C and E lowered their risk of developing Alzheimer's disease. Citrus fruits, kiwifruit, sprouts, broccoli, and cabbage are packed with vitamin C, while whole grains, nuts, milk, and egg yolks contain vitamin E.

The combination of reducing fat in your diet and eating more fruits and vegetables will help keep your arteries, including those leading to your brain, clear. In fact, it may even help restore bloodflow through arteries that have already begun to close up, says Dr. Regelson.

The Coffee Conundrum

Millions of Americans jump-start their brains each morning with steaming cups of coffee, and for good reason. The caffeine in coffee has been shown to improve mental functioning, including memory.

In one study, researchers from the Netherlands used a chemical to block short-term memory in 16 healthy people. They found that giving these folks 250 milligrams of caffeine—about the amount in 3 cups of coffee—quickly restored their powers of recall.

Getting too much coffee, of course, can be more of a bane than a boon, if only because the java buzz wears off within 6 to 8 hours. For some people, at least, the after-coffee slump can result in mental fogginess.

"Everyone has different reactions to caffeine," says Suzette Evans, PhD, assistant professor at Columbia University College of Physicians and in New York City. For people who rarely drink coffee, having a cup or two can definitely improve performance and memory, she says. But if you drink coffee throughout the day, you quickly build up tolerance and won't get the same benefits. In fact, too much caffeine can make you jittery and reduce your concentration.

Doctor's Top Tip

If you're not sure if you're deficient in vitamin D, which plays an important role in brain function, pay attention to your mood. People who are deficient in vitamin D are more likely to be depressed or have a low mood, says Stanley Birge, MD, of Washington University School of Medicine. Fixing the deficiency will not only improve your brain function, it will improve your spirits as well.

Avoiding the Brain Drain

Killing brain cells is not the best way to get a high score in the memory department. Yet that's exactly what many of us do to our gray matter every day, says Dr. Mark.

"Alcohol is a brain poison," says Dr. Mark. "Even if you're doing everything else right, drinking too much alcohol can cause a significant decrease in memory function." In fact, even small amounts of alcohol can damage cells in the part of the brain responsible for memory.

Many doctors recommend abstaining from alcohol entirely to keep your mind at its sharpest. At the very least, it's a good idea to limit yourself to one or two drinks—meaning 12 ounces of beer, 5 ounces of wine, or 1½ ounces of liquor—a day. When you do drink, choose red wine. It contains resveratrol, a compound that may keep the brain young.

Your Brain's Optimal Diet

You can't prevent Alzheimer's disease and dementia altogether, but you can keep them at bay longer with a heart-healthy diet that focuses on the nutrients that have been found to be critical for brain function and aging, says Stanley Birge, MD, associate professor of medicine in the division of geriatrics and nutritional sciences at Washington University School of Medicine in St. Louis. Here's what he advises:

Aim for a body mass index of 23 to 25. Being overweight increases your risk for diabetes, metabolic syndrome, and hypertension, which leads to vascular disease and brain damage. "It's just like the water pipes in an old house," Dr. Birge says. "The flow—in this case of blood to the brain—gradually decreases to a point that cells in small regions of the brain begin dying."

Grab dairy. Eat one serving of low-fat, low-sugar dairy once a day, such as milk, plain yogurt, cottage cheese, or ricotta cheese. Epidemiologic studies show that people who drink milk are less likely to develop Alzheimer's disease.

Toast to a young brain. Drink one glass of red wine or 4 ounces of purple grape juice or pomegranate juice a day. They contain resveratrol, a compound that doctors believe activates a gene associated with longevity.

Buy berries. Eating 1 cup of berries a day also gives your brain resveratrol and other flavonoids that make you less likely to develop the chronic diseases associated with aging.

Sip some juice. Drink 8 ounces of fruit juice high in vitamin C, such as orange or apple, or take 500 milligrams of vitamin C a day. Three times a week, substitute a glass of vegetable juice that you buy or make on your own for the fruit juice, Dr. Birge says. Antioxidants and other compounds in both types of juice help protect the brain from dementia.

Figure in the fish oil. Omega-3 fatty acids are power agents for a healthy heart and arteries. Eating oily cold-water fish such as salmon or Spanish mackerel two or three times a week will ensure you get enough omega-3s, but you can also take 2,000 to 3,000 milligrams a day of fish oil or flaxseed oil, Dr. Birge says. Walnuts also are rich in omega-3s. Eating 8 to 10 walnuts a day or using walnut oil (sold along with olive oil and other oils in most supermarkets) in salads of dark green leafy vegetables will help protect your brain.

Drink green tea every day. Green tea is rich in antioxidants and has been associated with reduced risk of dementia, Dr. Birge says. Experts recommend drinking one to two cups a day.

Make time for a multivitamin. This is particularly important for older, inactive adults whose caloric intake doesn't supply the micronutrients that they need, Dr. Birge says. Choose a multi without iron or reduced iron if you're not anemic or menstruating, he says.

Consider supplementing vitamin D. Vitamin D is a new shining star in the role of brain development and function, Dr. Birge says, and many people are deficient without knowing it. We get about 95 percent of our vitamin D from sunlight, but younger people who work long hours and elderly adults who are homebound or institutionalized often don't get enough sunlight to fill their vitamin D requirements, especially in northern regions between October 1 and April 1. Taking an over-the-counter vitamin D_3 supplement of 2,000 IU is sufficient for most people, he says, but the frail and homebound may need 4,000 IU. Dr. Birge recommends the Carlson Laboratory brand to ensure you're getting the amount of vitamin on the label.

Avoid omega-6 fats. The omega-6 fatty acids in corn, safflower, and sesame oils aren't as healthy as omega-3s found in olive and canola oil, so use those oils sparingly.

Nourish your brain. An overall brain-healthy diet is low in refined carbohydrates (found in sugars, baked goods, candy, and other sweets, for example), red meat, and trans fats. It's high in fatty fish, poultry, soy protein, fruits, vegetables, and legumes.

Menopausal Problems
FOODS FOR MIDLIFE—AND BEYOND

For many women, menopause is a time of great exuberance. Unfettered by monthly periods, concerns about pregnancy, or the anxiety of starting a career, it's natural to feel a sudden sense of freedom—as though the rest of your life is truly your own.

"There is no more creative force in the world than the menopausal woman with zest," said anthropologist Margaret Mead, who did some of her most exciting work when she was well past her fifties.

Still, the body does undergo a number of physical changes during menopause that can take the zest from the best. Hot flashes, mood swings, and insomnia are just a few of the symptoms many women experience around this time. For years, women (and their doctors) assumed that the discomfort of menopause was an inevitable part of the process. But it doesn't have to be that way. Many of the problems of menopause can be controlled or even eliminated by eating the right foods, says Isaac Schiff, MD, chief of obstetrics and gynecology at Massachusetts General Hospital in Boston and author of *Menopause*.

Now that many women worry about the risks of treating their menopausal symptoms with hormone replacement therapy (HRT), diet is even more important.

Hormonal Shifts

As a woman approaches menopause, her ovaries begin producing less of the female hormones estrogen and progesterone. At some point, they begin producing so little of these hormones that menstrual periods stop, and the physical problems, such as hot flashes and mood swings, begin.

Even more serious are some of the long-term changes in the body caused by low hormone levels. Estrogen, for example, regulates a woman's cholesterol levels. When estrogen dips, cholesterol rises, which is why women have higher risks of heart disease after they have passed menopause. Estrogen also plays a role in keeping a woman's bones full of calcium. When estrogen levels drop, the bones lose calcium at a very fast rate. Unless women take care to get extra calcium in their diets, their bones may become thin and weak, a condition called osteoporosis.

For years, many women replaced their estrogen levels with synthetic hormones, thinking it was a cure-all for everything from hot flashes to high cholesterol. But in

2002, new research found that the hormones may actually increase the risk of heart disease, which led the National Institutes of Health and the American Heart Association to advise women not to take HRT to lower cholesterol or prevent a heart attack.

According to the Nurses' Health Study, postmenopausal women who have had a heart attack or have been diagnosed with heart disease and have been on HRT for less than a year have a 25 percent higher risk of another heart attack or dying of heart disease than similar women who have never been on hormone therapy.

Researchers at the Duke Clinical Research Institute in Durham, North Carolina, reviewed the records of 1,857 female heart patients and found that those who began HRT after a heart attack had a higher risk of a second heart attack than those who didn't start therapy.

Although HRT still has advantages, such as protecting bones and easing problems in menopause, many women are looking for alternatives, and they're finding them in their own kitchens. Even women who do take HRT may find that making small adjustments to their diet will give them additional relief.

Soy's Protection

Since many of the problems of menopause are caused by low levels of estrogen, it makes sense that replacing some of the estrogen will make women healthier. Scientists have found that a number of foods—most notably soy foods such as tofu and tempeh—contain large amounts of phytoestrogens, plant compounds that act very much like the natural hormone.

Consider this: In Asian countries, where women eat a lot of soy foods, only about 16 percent have a problem with menopausal discomfort. In fact, there isn't even a word in Japanese for "hot flash." In this country, however, where soy foods are used much less often, 75 percent of menopausal women complain of hot flashes or other uncomfortable symptoms.

Of course, it's always better to reach for the food rather than the supplement, says Mary Jane Minkin, MD, clinical professor of obstetrics and gynecology at Yale University School of Medicine and author of *A Woman's Guide to Menopause and Perimenopause*. Dr. Minkin recommends getting two servings of soy a day, such as a glass of soy milk and a serving of tofu. Or you could have a bowl of miso soup, which is flavored with a condiment made from soybeans and salt.

Soy is also particularly important for protecting the heart, since a woman's risk for heart disease rises after menopause. Research has shown that eating more soy foods can help bring down cholesterol levels and the risk for heart disease. In a study at the University of Kentucky in Lexington, people eating just under 2 ounces of tofu a day were able to reduce total cholesterol by more than 9 percent and harmful low-density lipoprotein (LDL) cholesterol by nearly 13 percent.

Of course, when you're eating more soy foods, you're automatically eating less saturated fat, and this can also help keep cholesterol levels down. "Women approaching menopause and those who are already menopausal should concentrate on having the heart-healthiest diet," adds Wulf H. Utian, MD, PhD, chairman of the department of reproductive biology at Case Western Reserve University in Cleveland. "It's one of the most important issues they face because of menopause."

There's some concern that soy may increase risk for breast cancer and hypothyroidism, but Dr. Minkin says you'd have to eat quite a bit to see negative effects. After all, soy-loving Asian women are diagnosed with breast cancer much less often than American women. It's important to eat soy in moderation, however, Dr. Minkin says, by sticking to the two servings a day. And if you see an oncologist, it's a good idea to talk with the doctor before you add soy to your diet.

For an alternative to soybeans, try eating black beans to reduce your hot flashes. They contain about the same amount of phytoestrogens, and they can be cooked into great-tasting soups or sprinkled into salads.

Feel Better with Flaxseed

In addition to getting a little soy in your diet, it's a good idea to add flaxseed, Dr. Minkin says. Another phytoestrogen, flaxseed seems to help relieve hot flashes and sleep problems, the two complaints Dr. Minkin hears the most from her patients going through menopause.

Flaxseed contains a large amount of lignans that may have antioxidant properties, which means they'll help menopausal women fight cancer. Of all the plant foods that contain lignans, flaxseed contains the most, at least 75 times more than other foods.

In one study that looked at flaxseed's effects on breast cancer, 16 women ate about 1 tablespoon of flaxseed every day for 2 months. At the end of the study, the women had a 31 percent improvement in the ratio of chemicals that protect against breast cancer over chemicals that promote breast cancer in their blood.

Add a tablespoon of ground flaxseed to your cereal or on top of your salads, or bake it into bread and muffins. You don't need a lot of flaxseed to get the benefits, Dr. Minkin says.

Herbal Relief

Dr. Minkin has found that taking 20 milligrams twice a day of the herb black cohosh helps her patients with menopausal symptoms. Because the United States doesn't regulate herbal products, she recommends buying the German brand Remifemin.

Doctor's Top Tip

Menopausal symptoms such as hot flashes and sleep problems are certainly bothersome, but they're small potatoes compared with the heightened risk of breast cancer and cardiovascular disease menopausal women face, says Jay Kenney, PhD, RD, director of nutrition research and educator at the Pritikin Longevity Center and Spa in Aventura, Florida.

Luckily, doing all of the things that protect you from cancer and heart disease will also help with your menopausal symptoms, so add some soybeans to your diet, and eat more whole grains, fruits and vegetables, and legumes. "The more, the merrier," he says. "You can certainly eat beans every day. Have chili one day, black bean soup the next, a salad with garbanzo beans the next."

Herbal products are regulated in Germany, and you'll know that you're actually getting what's on the label.

However, not all experts agree that black cohosh will ease menopause symptoms. A December 2006 study of 351 menopausal and postmenopausal women didn't find that taking 160 milligrams of black cohosh a day relieved symptoms. But in another 2006 study conducted in Germany, researchers gave 62 women 40 milligrams of black cohosh a day for 12 weeks. At the end of the trial, the women saw an improvement in their symptoms and said they were sleeping better. The bottom line? While the jury is still out on whether or not black cohosh is an effective treatment for menopausal symptoms, it wouldn't hurt to try the herb and find out if it works for you.

Turn Down the Heat

There are classic triggers for hot flashes. Here's how to avoid them and stay cool.

Pass on hot foods. When it comes to temperature and spiciness, hot foods are likely to bring on a hot flash, Dr. Minkin says. It's a good idea to avoid hot beverages such as coffee or hot soups. The same goes for spicy foods, such as Chinese or Mexican food.

Avoid red wine. If you're going to drink, keep in mind that red wine is a classic trigger of hot flashes, says Dr. Minkin. White isn't as bad, so it may be a better choice.

Dress for indulgences. If you really want to indulge in a spicy meal or drink a glass of red wine, prepare for a hot flash by dressing in layers. Wear a cardigan over something light so you can take off the top layer and cool off, Dr. Minkin suggests. If you're at a restaurant, you may want to look for a table near a cool air vent or ask to sit away from the hot kitchen.

Take Charge of Your Bones

One of the most critical issues facing women is keeping their bones strong after menopause. "Getting enough calcium before, during, and after menopause is one of the most important things a woman can do to prevent possibly disastrous bone fractures," says Dr. Utian.

Here, too, soy foods can make a difference, because there's some evidence that the phytoestrogens in soy play an active role in helping bones hang on to their calcium. A laboratory study found, for example, that animals given small amounts of genistein (a phytoestrogen found in soy) were able to maintain healthy, calcium-filled bones even when they were no longer producing estrogen.

Holding on to calcium is important because many women don't get anywhere near enough of this important mineral. On average, women ages 20 to 50 get about 600 milligrams a day, and women past menopause get only about 500 milligrams a day.

Scientists at the National Institutes of Health recommend that women in their childbearing years get at least 1,000 milligrams of calcium a day. Women past menopause should aim for 1,500 milligrams a day.

Most women can get plenty of calcium in their diets. For example, 1 cup of fat-free milk contains 302 milligrams of calcium, or 30 percent of the Daily Value (DV). An 8-ounce serving of yogurt has 415 milligrams, or 41 percent of the DV, and 3 ounces of salmon has 181 milligrams, or 18 percent of the DV.

Easy Tofu Salad

2 tablespoons extra-virgin olive oil

1 tablespoon balsamic vinegar

1 teaspoon Dijon mustard

½ teaspoon freeze-dried chives

Salt and freshly ground black pepper

1 pound firm tofu, drained and blotted dry, cut into ¾-inch cubes

1 package (6 ounces) mesclun or spring mix

4 marinated sun-dried tomatoes, drained and chopped

4 anchovy fillets (optional)

In a small bowl, whisk together the oil, vinegar, mustard, and chives. Add salt and pepper to taste, and whisk again.

Place the tofu in a medium bowl. Add about 1 tablespoon of the dressing, and toss gently.

In another medium bowl, toss the mesclun with the remaining dressing. Arrange the greens on 4 plates, and scatter the tofu and tomatoes over the greens. Top with the anchovies (if using).

Makes 4 servings

PER SERVING

Calories: 180
Total fat: 14 g
Saturated fat: 3 g

Cholesterol: 0 mg
Sodium: 50 mg
Dietary fiber: 2 g

Milk

A GLASSFUL OF GOODNESS

HEALING POWER

Can Help:

Keep bones strong and prevent osteoporosis

Lower blood pressure and cholesterol

Reduce the risk of stroke

Reduce cancer risk

Even people who love milk often feel guilty about indulging. Despite its old-time reputation as being the perfect food, milk is extremely high in fat. A cup of whole milk is 49 percent fat. Reduced-fat (2%) milk isn't much better. It contains 34 percent fat. Worse, most of this fat is saturated, the kind that clogs your arteries. Not exactly what you'd call "perfect."

Before you wipe away your milk mustache forever, though, consider the lighter side: low-fat and fat-free milk. A cup of low-fat (1%) milk gets only 23 percent of its calories from fat. Fat-free milk (also called nonfat or skim) is the ultimate, with virtually no fat. Both fat-free and low-fat milk are two of the cheapest, easiest ways to help fulfill your daily requirements for a variety of important nutrients. Best of all, fat-free milk isn't the thin, gray, watery stuff it used to be. Several manufacturers, wise to the fact that consumers want the flavor of fat without the fat itself, now offer richer, creamier versions. Chances are, you won't be able to tell the difference.

"Once you get the fat out, milk is a highly nutritious food," says Curtis Mettlin, PhD, chief of epidemiologic research at Roswell Park Cancer Institute in Buffalo, New York. The nutrients that milk contains can help prevent high blood pressure, stroke, osteoporosis, and maybe even cancer—all for 85 calories, less than 5 grams of cholesterol, and less than 1 gram of fat per glassful of fat-free milk.

Skim Past Heart Disease

If you're concerned about cholesterol, you're probably already eating foods like apples, oats, and beans. Milk is another food that can send cholesterol south.

Researchers at Kansas State University in Manhattan, Kansas, and Pennsylvania State University in University Park had 64 people drink a quart of fat-free milk a day. After a month, the people with the highest cholesterol levels saw their cholesterol drop almost 10 points. That's almost a 7 percent reduction. Since every 1 percent drop in cholesterol translates into a 2 percent reduction in death from heart disease, milk helped these folks reduce their risks of heart attacks or strokes by nearly 14 percent.

Researchers in Quebec have also found that getting at least 1,000 milligrams of calcium a day improves total and good high-density lipoprotein (HDL) cholesterol, and lowers bad low-density lipoprotein (LDL) cholesterol.

Here's another great thing about milk. Its abundance of calcium may help reduce blood pressure as well as cholesterol. In the University Park study, people drinking milk were able to lower systolic blood pressure (the top number), on average, from 131 to 126 after 8 weeks, while diastolic pressure (the bottom number) dropped from 82 to 78.

Researchers aren't sure how much milk you should drink when trying to lower cholesterol or blood pressure. However, a good place to start would be with four glasses a day—the amount used in the study. If you think that's a lot, try drinking an 8-ounce glass of fat-free milk with each meal, then have another one as a snack.

Research also suggests that dairy in the diet may lower the risk of developing metabolic syndrome, aka syndrome X, a set of risk factors that includes obesity (which can lead to prediabetes), diabetes, high blood pressure, and heart disease. One study looked at adults over a 10-year period and found that those who were overweight and included dairy foods in their diets were less likely to develop syndrome X.

The Best Bone Builder

Milk is best known for its ability to help strengthen bones. There's good reason for this. Milk is an excellent source of calcium, with 1 cup of fat-free milk containing more than 300 milligrams, almost a third of the Daily Value (DV) for this mineral. That's why drinking milk is often recommended as a great strategy for preventing osteoporosis, the bone-thinning disease that affects more than 28 million people in the United States, most of them women.

In a study of 581 women past menopause, researchers at the University of California, San Diego, found that those who drank the most milk in their teens and early twenties had stronger bones than those who drank less.

The DV for calcium is 1,000 milligrams. But the amount that you need depends on your age, sex, and other factors. While men between the ages of 25 and 65 and women between the ages of 25 and 50 need 1,000 milligrams of calcium a day, men and women over 65 need 1,500 milligrams. Women who are postmenopausal and taking estrogen need 1,000 milligrams, and women over 50 who are not taking estrogen need 1,200 milligrams a day. Pregnant women or those who are breastfeeding need 1,200 to 1,500 milligrams a day.

A Strike against Stroke

Milk not only does the body good, research suggests it's also good for the brain. In one study, men who drank 16 ounces or more of milk a day had 50 percent lower risks of thromboembolic stroke (which occurs when a clot blocks bloodflow to the brain) than those who did not drink milk.

It's not certain why milk showed such impressive results. Calcium didn't appear to have anything to do with it since people who took calcium supplements without accompanying dairy foods didn't show the same benefits, says study leader Robert Abbott, PhD, professor of public health sciences at the University of Virginia School of Medicine in Charlottesville. "But milk contains all kinds of nutrients besides calcium, and it did appear to be protective," he says. The benefits weren't due only to the milk, he adds. "The milk drinkers tended to be leaner, more physically active, and to eat healthier foods than the men who didn't drink milk."

Help for Cancer

Fruits and vegetables have gotten the most glory as cancer-fighting foods, and rightly so. Still, drinking fat-free or low-fat milk may also play a protective role.

Researchers at Roswell Park Cancer Institute, led by Dr. Mettlin, asked more than 4,600 people with and without cancer how many glasses of whole milk, fat-free milk, or reduced-fat milk they drank a day. They found that those who drank fat-free or reduced-fat milk had lower risks of developing several types of cancers, including cancers of the stomach and rectum, than those who drank whole milk. "These reduced risks were most likely due to their consuming less dietary fat from the milk as well as from other foods," says Dr. Mettlin.

Another study, sponsored by the American Cancer Society, found that women who drank either fat-free or reduced-fat milk were three times less likely to develop ovarian cancer than women who drank more than a glass of whole milk a day.

Since a high intake of dietary fat is linked to cancer, it's not surprising that people who drank whole milk had the highest risks of cancer. But what did surprise was that in both studies, people who didn't drink milk had higher risks of cancer than those who drank fat-free or reduced-fat milk. So there may be something in milk that helps protect against this disease, says Dr. Mettlin.

A Possible Partner in Weight Loss

There's debate about whether or not milk and dairy products can aid in weight loss. Some research suggests that calcium and other substances in milk help regulate weight loss, and scientists have speculated that the calcium in dairy products helps the body metabolize calories and burn fat faster. However, other studies have failed to find a connection between dairy and weight loss.

Studies by the University of Tennessee suggest that calcium blocks fat storage in

RICHNESS WITHOUT THE FAT

With a name like "buttermilk," you would expect this thick, creamy, and delectably tart drink to be very high in fat. But despite the name, buttermilk is lower in fat than regular milk, making it a healthful alternative to milk, cream, and mayonnaise in everything from salad dressings to baked goods.

A cup of buttermilk made from fat-free milk has about 2 grams of fat. Buttermilk made with reduced-fat (2%) milk contains 5 grams of fat. By contrast, 1 cup of regular milk has approximately 8 grams of fat. Making this one simple change—replacing some of the milk in your diet with buttermilk—can cut substantial amounts of fat from your diet. Just be sure to check the label before putting buttermilk in your shopping cart, since some brands are quite a bit lower in fat than others. You can buy buttermilk in fat-free, low-fat (1%), and reduced-fat versions.

Buttermilk is good in yet another way. As with low-fat and fat-free milk, it's among the best calcium sources you can find. A cup of buttermilk made from fat-free milk has more than 285 milligrams of calcium, or about 29 percent of the Daily Value.

cells that add inches to the stomach, hips, and thighs. In one Tennessee study, researchers put 32 obese adults on a low-calorie diet that included either 400 milligrams of calcium from dairy foods a day, an additional 800 milligrams of calcium from supplements, or 1,200 milligrams of calcium from food. After 6 months, the group getting 1,200 milligrams of calcium from dairy foods dropped 24 pounds, while the group taking supplements lost 19 pounds, and the group getting the least amount of calcium dropped 15 pounds.

But other studies have not proven this. Mayo Clinic scientists conducted a study in which 72 overweight men ate a low-calorie diet with 800 milligrams or 1,400 milligrams of calcium. Both groups, regardless of whether they took in more or less calcium, lost about 20 pounds over the course of a year.

In another study, researchers at the University of Vermont in Burlington studied 54 overweight women. Half of the women received 500 milligrams of calcium a day from dairy foods, while the other half received 1,200 to 1,400 milligrams a day. Both groups lost an average of 22 pounds.

The bottom line is that low-fat dairy foods will probably help you lose weight. Many dieters get as little as 200 milligrams of calcium a day, so increasing that amount may help with weight loss. In the meantime, it's absolutely clear that calcium protects your heart and bones, so aiming for three servings of low-fat and/or fat-free cheese, yogurt, or milk a day is always a healthful choice.

Doctor's Top Tip

Looking for a new way to add low-fat dairy to your meals? Purée fat-free or low-fat cottage cheese, fat-free evaporated milk, lemon juice, and rosemary to make a light sauce to serve over pasta, suggests the Mayo Clinic in Rochester, Minnesota.

Liquid Nutrition

We've been talking about milk's role in preventing disease. Yet even for healthy, day-to-day living, milk is a truly nutritious food. Apart from its high calcium content, 1 cup of milk also contains 100 IU of vitamin D, or 25 percent of the DV. Just as your bones need calcium to stay strong, they also need vitamin D, which helps the calcium be absorbed.

In addition, 1 cup of fat-free milk supplies about 400 milligrams of potassium, or approximately 12 percent of the DV. Potassium is a key mineral for protecting against high blood pressure, stroke, and heart trouble. Milk also contains 0.4 milligram of riboflavin, or more than 23 percent of the DV.

GETTING THE MOST

Buy it in cartons. While those translucent plastic jugs are a convenient way to carry milk home from the store, they also admit light, which destroys riboflavin and vitamin A. In fact, milk stored for 1 day in a translucent plastic jug loses 90 percent of its vitamin A and 14 percent of its riboflavin. Further, the action of light can give milk an off-taste that many people find unpleasant. So you may want to buy the cartons instead.

Give your taste buds time to adjust. While some people take to fat-free milk right away, others loathe the taste, at least at first. To make fat-free milk part of your diet without shocking your taste buds, make the switch slowly. Try mixing a carton of whole milk with a carton of reduced-fat milk and drink that for a few weeks. Slowly reduce the amount of whole milk you add to the mix until you're drinking straight reduced-fat milk. When you're used to that, add fat-free milk to the reduced-fat. Eventually you'll be drinking—and enjoying—pure fat-free.

Add some thickening. One of the things people dislike about fat-free milk is its rather thin consistency. To make it thicker and creamier, try adding 2 to 4 tablespoons of nonfat milk powder to each cup of fat-free.

Try a new brand. If you're not happy with the milk you've been drinking, try one of the creamier versions. For example, Borden makes a product called Lite Line that's fat-free but tastes like reduced-fat. Lite Line is available in Texas and other selected regions. Or look for fat-free milk that's fortified with nonfat milk solids. It's labeled "protein fortified."

Work it into your diet. Even if milk isn't your favorite beverage, there are other ways to get it into your diet. Using fat-free milk instead of water when preparing oatmeal, for example, will boost your breakfast's calcium content from 20 to 320 milligrams.

Creamy Potato Soup

3½ cups fat-free milk

½ cup water

2 cloves garlic, halved

4 medium boiling potatoes, peeled and cut into 1-inch chunks

¼ teaspoon salt

3 tablespoons chopped parsley

¼ teaspoon freshly ground black pepper

⅛ teaspoon ground nutmeg

2 teaspoons unsalted butter

In a Dutch oven, combine 3 cups of the milk, the water, and garlic. Cook over medium heat until the mixture almost starts to simmer.

Reduce the heat to low. Add the potatoes and salt. Cover and cook, stirring occasionally, until the potatoes are tender, about 30 minutes. Stir in the parsley, pepper, nutmeg, and the remaining ½ cup milk. Remove from the heat, and let cool for 5 minutes.

Transfer the soup to a blender or food processor and purée, in batches if necessary. Return the soup to the Dutch oven and reheat briefly. Stir in the butter.

Makes 4 servings

PER SERVING

Calories: 212
Total fat: 2.5 g
Saturated fat: 1.5 g

Cholesterol: 9 mg
Sodium: 253 mg
Dietary fiber: 1.9 g

Millet

A GRAIN FOR WOMEN'S HEALTH

HEALING POWER

Can Help:

Ease premenstrual
discomfort

Speed wound healing

In many parts of the world, millet, a nutritious, mild-tasting grain that looks like a tiny yellow bead, has been a staple for about 6,000 years. In Ethiopia, for example, it's cooked into a porridge. And in India, millet is used to make bread.

In this country, though, millet is eaten more by birds than people. When you pour out a tray of bird feed, you'll see pale little pellets filling the spaces between sunflower seeds. Those pellets are grains of millet.

We would do well to take a hint from our feathered friends, since millet is a very nutritious grain. It contains magnesium, an essential mineral that may help ease premenstrual discomfort. In addition, millet is higher in protein than most other grains, which is good news for those folks who eat little or no meat. And, like all grains, millet contains dietary fiber, although much of the fiber is lost during processing. Still, a half-cup of cooked millet contains more fiber than an equal amount of cooked brown rice.

Doctor's Top Tip

You can find millet in natural food stores and many general markets. Use it as a cereal base, cooking it the same way you would barley or oatmeal, says Jeannie Gazzaniga Moloo, PhD, RD, a Sacramento, California-based spokesperson for the American Dietetic Association. Or you can add the grain to a soup, and allow it to simmer the same way you would rice or barley in a soup.

Help for Monthly Discomfort

Magnesium takes part in controlling more body functions than just about any other nutrient. It regulates the heartbeat, helps nerves function, and keeps bones strong. In addition, it may even play a role in easing women's premenstrual discomfort.

Research has shown that women with premenstrual syndrome (PMS) often have low levels of magnesium. "A marginal magnesium deficiency could make certain women more susceptible to PMS," says Donald L. Rosenstein, MD, chief of the psychiatry consultation service at the National Institutes of Health.

A half-cup of cooked millet contains nearly 53 milligrams of magnesium, which is about 13 percent

Unlike brown rice, millet doesn't take forever to go from pot to plate. And it's very easy to make.

In a large saucepan, mix 1 cup of whole millet with 2½ to 3 cups of water, bring to a simmer, and cook, covered, until the grains are tender, usually about 30 minutes. Although millet is usually cooked plain, here are some ways that you can customize the taste and texture.

- Cooking millet in apple juice instead of water will add a bit of sweetness to the dish.
- If you want millet to have a fluffy texture that's more like rice than cereal, let it cook undisturbed for about 20 minutes.
- For a creamier texture, stir millet frequently while it cooks, which causes the grains to absorb more water.

of the Daily Value (DV) for the mineral. Eating more millet, along with various other magnesium-rich foods like tofu, avocados, spinach, bananas, and peanut butter, could help ease the irritability, sadness, and other emotional ups-and-downs that some women experience every month, says Dr. Rosenstein.

Essential for Repairs

The body uses protein for building and repairing muscles, connective fibers, and other tissues. Getting more protein in your diet is particularly important when you've cut yourself, been burned, or had surgery, says Michele Gottschlich, PhD, RD, director of nutrition services for the Shriners Burns Institute in Cincinnati. "Without plenty of protein in the diet, wound healing can be delayed," she explains.

A half-cup of millet contains nearly 4 grams of protein, or more than 8 percent of the DV. Compare that to a similar amount of brown rice, which supplies only 2.5 grams of protein.

While meat is also a potent source of protein, it also can be high in cholesterol-raising saturated fats, adds Lynne Brown, PhD, associate professor of food science at Pennsylvania State University in University Park. One cup of cooked millet provides about as much protein as an ounce of beef, making it a low-fat, cholesterol-free alternative.

GETTING THE MOST

Shop for the whole grain. While cracked millet cooks more quickly than whole millet, it loses some of its nutrients during processing. So to get the most value, it's a good idea to shop for the whole grain.

Fit in some flour. Using millet flour in place of wheat or corn flour is an easy way to pack more of this healthful grain into your diet. However, since millet lacks gluten, the protein in wheat flour that allows yeast breads to rise, it's best used for quick breads and other recipes that don't call for yeast.

Store it carefully. Millet can go rancid rather quickly, giving up both its good taste and some of its essential nutrients. To keep millet fresh, be sure to store it in an airtight container in a cool, dry place.

Millet Pilaf

1 cup millet

1½ cups water

1 cup chicken broth

¼ teaspoon salt

½ cup golden raisins

2 tablespoons dry sherry

1 tablespoon extra-virgin olive oil

⅓ cup natural almonds

1½ teaspoons chopped fresh rosemary

2 tablespoons chopped flat-leaf parsley

In a medium saucepan, cook the millet over medium-high heat, stirring frequently, until the grains are fragrant, browned in spots, and just beginning to crackle, about 4 minutes.

Add the water, broth, and salt. Bring to a boil over high heat. Reduce the heat to low, cover, and simmer until the millet is tender, some grains have burst, and the water has evaporated, about 25 minutes. Remove from the heat and let stand, covered, for 10 minutes.

Meanwhile, in a small bowl, soak the raisins in the sherry.

In a small skillet, heat the oil over medium heat. Add the almonds, and cook, stirring frequently, for 4 minutes, or until lightly toasted. Stir in the rosemary and raisins, and cook, stirring, for 30 seconds. Remove from the heat.

Fluff the millet with a fork. Stir in the almond mixture, and sprinkle with the parsley.

Makes 4 servings

PER SERVING

Calories: 342	Cholesterol: 0 mg
Total fat: 10 g	Sodium: 389 mg
Saturated fat: 1 g	Dietary fiber: 6 g

Motion Sickness

KEEPING YOUR STOMACH CALM

Food is the last thing you want to think about when your stomach is turning upside down. But if you're among the 90 percent of Americans who occasionally suffer from motion sickness, you may want to make food the first thing on your list, even before you get on the boat or climb into the car. Research has shown that what you put—or don't put—into your stomach can have a big impact on how you feel.

Motion sickness happens when the feeling of being moved in a car, boat, or plane and the visual cues that tell your brain that you're apparently standing or sitting still confuse your brain. As a result, you'll feel dizzy, tired, and nauseous, which could lead to vomiting. Feeling anxious about these symptoms only exasperates them.

Even worse, some foods you ate before your trip may stimulate your body to produce more gas and acids, and that won't make for a pleasant ride. Other foods, by contrast, can help keep your stomach calm, either by blocking the effects of natural toxins or by preventing "nausea signals" from even reaching your brain.

One of the best ways to prevent motion sickness is to have a little ginger. This spice acts as a sponge, absorbing a lot of the acid that your stomach pumps out as a natural reaction to motion. In addition, it helps block nausea signals that sometimes travel from the stomach to the brain, says Daniel B. Mowrey, PhD, director of the American Phytotherapy Research Laboratory in Salt Lake City, and author of *Herbal Tonic Recipes*. Dr. Mowrey has studied the calming effects of ginger on thousands of motion sickness sufferers. What's more, he has firsthand knowledge of how well it works. He gives it to his own kids. "When we get in the car to take a trip, if they forgot their ginger root, they're out of it," he says. "When they have it, they're fine."

For minor motion sickness, having some ginger ale, ginger snaps, or ginger tea before and during the trip can help settle your stomach, Dr. Mowrey says. For those who need more relief, he recommends taking two 940-milligram capsules of fresh ginger (or an equivalent amount of smaller capsules) about

Doctor's Top Tip

If you don't want your stomach turning and twisting during your next ride, eat light before traveling, avoiding spicy foods and alcohol, says the Mayo Clinic in Rochester, Minnesota. You may also want to try eating dry crackers or drinking a carbonated drink to settle your stomach.

DESPERATE MEASURES

People have been getting seasick for as long as there have been boats. The rolling waves make many people feel so sick that they'll try—or eat—anything to make the churning go away. In *Heave Ho! My Little Green Book of Seasickness*, Charles Mazel, PhD, an ocean engineer and marine biologist in Andover, Massachusetts, has chronicled some of the more unusual strategies that people have used through the ages to cope with this miserable condition. Here are just a few:

- Poke your finger in a loaf of bread, and fill the hole with Worcestershire and hot pepper sauces. Enjoy.
- Try rice covered with horseradish sauce, herrings, and sardines.
- Eat cold stewed tomatoes with saltines.
- Take a handful of salted peanuts with breakfast each morning.

20 minutes before leaving and again every half-hour during the trip. If you tend to get really ill, Dr. Mowrey recommends increasing the amount to six capsules before leaving and six to eight capsules every half-hour during the trip. "You know you've taken enough of it to do the job when you get an aftertaste," he adds. "If you don't get that aftertaste, you can take more."

Since stomach acid can play a role in causing motion sickness, it's a good idea to eat something before traveling. Foods that are high in carbohydrates, like breads and crackers, are particularly good because they soak up large amounts of stomach acid, says William Ruderman, MD, a gastroenterologist in Orlando, Florida. In a study of 57 pilots, researchers at the University of North Dakota in Grand Forks found that those who ate carbohydrate-rich foods such as breads and cereals before their flights tended to experience less motion sickness than those pilots who ate foods high in protein, sodium, or calories.

It's not only what you eat that can ease motion sickness but also what you drink. It's a good idea to drink plenty of water before and during your trip, says Dr. Ruderman. It's particularly important to drink more fluids when you're flying, because the air in airplane cabins is extremely dry.

However, don't use coffee, soda, or alcohol as substitutes for water, he adds. Both caffeine and alcohol are diuretics, which means that they take away more fluids than they replace.

Muscle Cramps
A MATTER OF MINERALS

Whether you're on a treadmill, writing a letter, or even lying in bed at night, your muscles are constantly contracting and relaxing. As a result, they need a lot of nourishment. When they don't get it, they'll sometimes contract into tight, painful spasms known as muscle cramps. Cramps are a muscle's way of telling you it's tired, hungry, and in need of rest.

Muscle cramps are painful, but they play a protective role, says Leslie Bonci, RD, a dietitian at the University of Pittsburgh Medical Center and a spokesperson for the American Dietetic Association. Essentially, they force the muscle to remain inactive until it has time to recover, usually within a few minutes.

While you can't prevent muscle cramps entirely, choosing the right foods will make them less likely to return. Here's how it works.

Help from Electrolytes

Muscles don't move without orders from the brain. Before you can stand up, blink an eye, or turn the pages of this book, the brain sends electrical messages to the appropriate muscles, telling them when (and how much) to contract or relax. Minerals such as calcium, potassium, sodium, and magnesium, which are known as electrolytes, play a role in helping the messages get through, says Joel Press, MD, medical director of the Spine and Sports Rehabilitation Center at the Rehabilitation Institute of Chicago.

If you haven't been getting enough of these minerals or have sweated them out during vigorous exercise, a muscle may not get the message to relax. This can cause it to contract in a painful cramp.

Of all the electrolytes, magnesium is one of the most important, because it helps other electrolytes do their jobs, says Robert McLean, MD, associate clinical professor of internal medicine and rheumatology at Yale University School of Medicine. When you don't eat enough magnesium-rich foods, minerals such as calcium and potassium can't get into muscle-fiber cells. So even if you have an abundance of other electrolytes, without magnesium, they may be locked out and ineffective. "People who are depleted of magnesium tend to have greater irritability of the muscles and nerves," says Dr. McLean. "This irritability may cause muscle cramping."

Doctor's Top Tip

Water will go a long way toward keeping your muscles healthy during exercise, but you'll need more help if you're exercising vigorously or for an hour or more. In this case, reach for a sports drink, such as Gatorade. The electrolytes and carbohydrates in such drinks get into the bloodstream quickly and help keep muscles from cramping, says Leslie Bonci, RD, a dietitian at the University of Pittsburgh Medical Center and a spokesperson for the American Dietetic Association.

Here are a few tips for improving your electrolyte balance:

Get magnesium from tofu, spinach, and Spanish mackerel. A serving of tofu has 128 milligrams of magnesium, or 32 percent of the Daily Value (DV). A serving of spinach has about 44 milligrams, or 11 percent of the DV, and a serving of mackerel has 82 milligrams, or 20 percent of the DV.

Include dairy in your diet. Calcium helps regulate the muscles' ability to contract. Dairy foods are the best sources. A cup of fat-free milk, for example, has nearly 302 milligrams of calcium, or 30 percent of the DV, while a serving of low-fat yogurt has 77 milligrams, or 7 percent of the DV.

Choose potassium-rich bananas and potatoes. Getting enough potassium in your diet may also be helpful for preventing cramps, says Dr. Press. Bananas are a good source of potassium, with one banana supplying 451 milligrams, or 13 percent of the DV. Potatoes are also a good source, with a half-cup containing 114 milligrams, or 3 percent of the DV.

Say no to sodium. For most people, the problem isn't getting enough sodium, it's getting too much, since this mineral is found in large amounts in many foods, particularly processed foods. And for those who are sensitive, sodium can lead to fluid retention and high blood pressure. So even if you have been getting cramps, leave the sodium alone—you're almost certainly getting enough.

Hydrate, hydrate, hydrate. Whenever you perspire, you lose fluids from the muscle cells, which can result in cramping, Bonci says. And you're more likely to get muscle cramps when you exercise in hot weather because you'll be sweating more and losing fluid, salt, and minerals that keep your muscles working optimally. Sipping water frequently throughout the day will help keep electrolyte levels in balance. When you're planning on being active, it's a good idea to drink at least 16 ounces of water or juice to prime your body with the necessary minerals.

Dodge cramps with carbs. Muscles need more than electrolytes and water to function well. They also need glycogen, a sugar that comes from carbohydrates. Getting plenty of carbohydrates in your diet will help keep muscles working well. Good sources include potatoes, rice, bananas, and bread.

Mushrooms

THE HEALING FUNGUS

HEALING POWER

Can Help:

Inhibit tumor growth

Boost the immune system

Lower cholesterol levels

Mushrooms are so popular in Asian countries that they're sold by streetcart vendors, just as we sell corn dogs and Italian ices. Those Asian buyers are following in ancient traditions. The use of mushrooms as medicine has been recorded in ancient Chinese manuscripts, and the earliest records of humans using psychotropic mushrooms date as far back as the Paleolithic period. Today, there are about 35 species of mushrooms available to us, and most are edible and have medicinal properties.

But while Americans have been slow to embrace these meaty morsels, they're becoming increasingly commonplace, both in the kitchen and in numerous research laboratories.

Scientists are discovering what natural healers have known for ages. Mushrooms not only are important sources of nutrients but also stimulate the immune system. Researchers say that they possibly can help fight cancer and high cholesterol, and perhaps even AIDS.

A Cap on Cancer

Not long ago, scientists thought America's favorite mushroom, the white button mushroom, had little medicinal value, but more recent studies have found that the mushrooms actually pack quite a punch, especially when it comes to preventing breast cancer.

Researchers at City of Hope, a Duarte, California, cancer research and treatment center, have found that the mushrooms suppress estrogen production, particularly in postmenopausal women. They conducted several studies on mice and found that these animals had a 58 percent reduction in the growth of breast tumors when they were fed mushroom extract.

The mushrooms contain a phytochemical called conjugated linoleic acid that inhibits aromatase, the protein in the body that makes estrogen, says Shiuan Chen, PhD, director of the department of surgical research at City of Hope. About 60 percent of premenopausal women and 75 percent of postmenopausal women with breast cancer have a hormone-dependent cancer, which means estrogen helps tumors grow,

In the Kitchen

Although you can buy fresh shiitake mushrooms at specialty markets, you're more likely to find them in their dehydrated form. Here's how to use them:

Soften them. To reconstitute dried mushrooms, place them in a saucepan, cover with water, and bring them to a rolling boil. Reduce the heat and simmer for 20 minutes. Then drain, slice, and add them to your recipe. You may want to reserve the mushroom water, which adds a rich taste to soups and sauces.

Cut them fine. Reconstituted mushrooms don't look as pretty as their freshly picked brethren. Also, they have a slightly pungent flavor that in large amounts may be objectionable to some diners. Chefs usually chop them, using them sparingly for stir-fries, meat and vegetable casseroles, soups, pasta, and grain dishes.

---

so controlling estrogen levels can limit or prevent tumors. Postmenopausal women have smaller amounts of estrogen in their bodies, so the mushrooms provide even greater protection for them.

Other forms of mushrooms were also found to help prevent breast cancer. White stuffing mushrooms had the strongest protection but white button, shiitake, portobello, cremini, and baby button mushrooms all showed a significant effect, whether eaten raw or cooked.

Eating only about 3½ ounces of mushrooms a day could help prevent breast cancer, Dr. Chen says. He is now researching these compounds and their effects on prostate cancer.

This isn't the first time mushrooms have been in the spotlight for their cancer-fighting abilities. Shiitake mushrooms have long been used in Japan to shrink tumors. These large, meaty black mushrooms contain a polysaccharide, or complex sugar, called lentinan. Polysaccharides are large molecules that are similar in structure to bacteria, explains Robert Murphy, ND, a naturopathic doctor in Torrington, Connecticut. When you eat shiitake mushrooms, your immune system starts amassing an army of infection-fighting cells. "In essence, they fool the immune system into kicking into action," he says. Researchers have found that when they feed lentinan in the form of dried mushroom powder to laboratory animals with tumors, they can inhibit tumor growth by 67 percent.

Researchers are also looking at the maitake mushroom, also known as hen of the woods or the dancing mushroom. Like shiitakes, maitake mushrooms have a centuries-old reputation for being helpful in treating people with cancer. Only recently are they getting the attention that they deserve in Western nations.

The active polysaccharide in maitake mushrooms, which is called beta-glucan or D-fraction, has been highly effective in shrinking tumors in laboratory animals—maybe even more effective than lentinan, say experts.

"You definitely get some of these polysaccharides that activate the immune system when you eat a healthy serving—about ½ cup—of these mushrooms," says Dr. Murphy. "I tell people that they can go to the market and buy shiitake and maitake mushrooms and include them in their diets." Both types are usually found in Asian food stores and some supermarkets.

Immunity Boosting and AIDS

Because the shiitake and maitake mushrooms have proven so effective in bolstering the immune system, some scientists have tested their mettle, with some success, against HIV, the virus that causes AIDS.

In laboratory studies, an extract of the maitake mushroom's beta-glucan was able to prevent HIV from killing T cells, the immune system's crucial white blood cells. "Eating these mushrooms on a regular basis seems to be a very good way to keep your immune system up and running," says Dr. Murphy.

Cutting Cholesterol

If your cholesterol levels are hovering near the danger zone—200 and above—you might want to consider making mushrooms a regular side dish on your table.

During the 1970s and 1980s, human and animal studies in Japan showed that one of the compounds in shiitake mushrooms, eritadenine, could effectively lower cholesterol levels. More recently, researchers from Slovakia have found that by feeding mice 5 percent of their diets in dried mushrooms, particularly oyster mushrooms, they could reduce blood cholesterol by 45 percent, even when the mice were given high-cholesterol foods.

FOOD ALERT

Raw Dangers

Raw sliced mushrooms are a salad bar favorite. But you don't want to make a habit of eating too many uncooked mushrooms, warn experts.

Raw mushrooms contain hydrazines, toxic chemicals that studies show can produce tumors in laboratory animals. Though nobody really knows how many raw mushrooms people have to eat to have that happen, experts recommend eating your mushrooms cooked because hydrazines are eliminated during heating.

Doctor's Top Tip

Mushrooms are a good filler in the dishes you make because they so often take on the taste of what they're prepared with, says Jeannie Gazzaniga Moloo, PhD, RD, a Sacramento, California-based spokesperson for the American Dietetic Association. Sauté firm mushrooms such as cremini with other vegetables and seasonings. Or dice any kind of mushroom you like into small pieces, and add to soups and sauces.

If you don't like the taste of mushrooms but you want to reap the nutritional benefits they offer, cut them very small, and add them to a marinara sauce. Then, just before you serve the sauce, use an immersion blender to incorporate the mushrooms right into the sauce, Dr. Moloo says. You'll forget they're even there.

Researchers still can't say how many mushrooms people have to eat to get the same effect. But experts agree that adding a couple of these large, meaty morsels to your plate each day certainly can't hurt, and it may help play a role in bringing your cholesterol levels down.

A Boost of Bs

Mushrooms offer two important B vitamins, niacin and riboflavin, that are not often found in vegetables. For once, the common white button mushroom may be a key player. While dried shiitake mushrooms have a higher nutrient concentration, they also have a strong flavor; most people won't use them in large quantities. But white mushrooms, with their mild taste, can be eaten with virtually every meal.

Niacin is important because it helps your body form the enzymes needed to convert sugars into energy, to use fats, and to keep your tissues healthy. White button mushrooms are a good source, containing 4 milligrams of niacin, or 20 percent of the Daily Value (DV).

Like niacin, riboflavin is a "helper nutrient." It's needed to convert other nutrients, like niacin, vitamin B_6, and folate, into usable forms. If you're low on riboflavin, you could also be low on these other nutrients. A half-cup of boiled white mushrooms contains 0.2 milligram of riboflavin, or 12 percent of the DV.

GETTING THE MOST

Cook 'em up. For both taste and nutrition, mushrooms are better cooked than raw. This is because they are mostly water. When you cook them, you remove the water and concentrate the nutrients as well as the flavor. See "Food Alert" on page 441 for more on why cooked mushrooms are better for you.

Eat the exotic. To get optimal healing power from mushrooms, stick to Asian varieties, particularly shiitake and maitake, say experts. Other mushrooms that may provide therapeutic benefits are the enoki, oyster, pine, and straw varieties.

Pan-Cooked Cremini Mushrooms

2 tablespoons olive oil

2 shallots, minced

1 pound cremini mushrooms, stems removed

1 tablespoon unsalted butter

1 tablespoon fresh thyme leaves

½ cup white wine

   Salt and freshly ground black pepper

In a large skillet, heat the oil over medium-high heat. Add the shallots, and cook until golden. Add the mushrooms, top side down, and cook them for 5 minutes. Turn them over, and add the butter, thyme, wine, and salt and pepper to taste. Reduce the heat to medium, and cook until the liquid has evaporated, about 10 minutes.

Makes 4 servings

PER SERVING ─────────────────────

Calories: 139	Cholesterol: 8 mg
Total fat: 9.9 g	Sodium: 145 mg
Saturated fat: 2.8 g	Dietary fiber: 1 g

Nuts

A SHELL GAME YOU CAN WIN

HEALING POWER
Can Help:
Lower cholesterol
Protect against heart disease
Prevent cancer
Help prevent gallstones

The ancient Persians believed that eating five almonds before drinking alcoholic beverages would prevent intoxication, or at least the hangover that might follow. They also believed that almonds would ward off witches and stimulate milk production in nursing mothers.

As nutty as this seems today, it's not surprising that ancient civilizations took their nuts seriously. Not only are nuts a compact source of energy, they also are easily stored through cold winters and hot summers, making them available throughout the year. What's more, nuts contain a number of compounds that may help prevent heart disease and cancer.

The Fat Factor

Before we talk about the health benefits of nuts, it's important to discuss one of their potential drawbacks. While nuts are high in nutrients, they're also high in fat. One-third cup of nuts typically contains anywhere from 240 to 300 calories and 20 to 25 grams of fat.

Not all types of nuts are loaded with fat, but most are. The coconut, for example, contains a lot of fat, and most of it is the dangerous saturated kind. "On the other end of the spectrum is the chestnut, which is extremely low in fat, and almost all of it is unsaturated," points out Joan Sabaté, MD, DrPH, chairman of the department of nutrition and associate professor of nutrition and epidemiology at Loma Linda University School of Public Health in California.

"It's very unfortunate that people shun nuts just because they're high in calories," Dr. Sabaté adds. "The trick to eating nuts is not overdoing it—fitting them wisely into a healthy eating plan."

If you're worried about gaining weight from eating nuts, consider this. A review of top studies by researchers at Loma Linda University found that eating nuts is not associated with obesity. For instance, people who live in the Mediterranean eat twice as many nuts as Americans, but their rates of obesity are much lower. In one study, 81 people were given raw and dry-roasted almonds to add to their diet. After 6 months, the women in the study saw no significant weight gain, and the men gained less than 2 pounds. The study authors suggest that the protein and fiber in nuts may help us feel full so that we eat less of other foods.

As you add nuts to your diet, be sure to get less of other, less healthy fats, such as butter, hydrogenated margarines, and nutrient-empty snack foods such as chips and cookies, Dr. Sabaté says.

Here are some easy ways to make a healthy substitution. Choose 2 tablespoons of slivered almonds over ⅔ cup of a low-fiber cereal, or have 4 tablespoons of pistachios instead of 1 cup of cooked pasta, or add 1 tablespoon of chopped walnuts to your salad instead of ¼ cup of seasoned croutons.

Good for the Heart—and the Gallbladder

One great thing about nuts is that they contain a number of compounds that help keep the arteries open and blood flowing smoothly.

It was quite by accident that researchers at Loma Linda University discovered that eating nuts seems to protect against heart disease. They asked 26,000 members of the Seventh-Day Adventist Church, an extremely health-conscious bunch, to indicate the frequency with which they ate 65 food items.

As it turns out, the Adventists are very fond of nuts. Twenty-four percent ate nuts at least five times a week. In the population at large, by contrast, only 5 percent of people eat them that often. As the researchers discovered, this difference in nut consumption made a colossal difference in heart disease risk. Eating nuts just one to four

In the Kitchen

Blending your own peanut butter is a lot of fun. Not only does it taste good, depending on the amount of oil you add, it also has a bit less fat than the store-bought kind. Plus, it's very easy to make. Here's how:

- Buy roasted peanuts, the kind that come in a vacuum-sealed can or jar. You can also use roasted peanuts in the shell, but shelling them requires more work.
- For each cup of peanuts you use, add 1½ to 2 tablespoons of canola or another light-flavored oil. Some people will add ½ teaspoon of salt per cup of peanuts, but this is optional.
- Put the peanuts and oil in a blender, and purée until you get the texture you want—extra-chunky, chunky, or creamy.
- Transfer the peanut butter to a jar, and store in the refrigerator. It will stay fresh for 3 to 4 months. However, the oils in "natural" peanut butter will separate, so be sure to stir it well before using.

Doctor's Top Tip

An ounce, or one handful, a day of nuts is a healthy amount, suggests Andrew Weil, MD, clinical professor of medicine and director of the integrative medicine program at the University of Arizona in Tucson. To get the benefits of omega-3 fatty acids, choose cashews, almonds, and walnuts.

times a week reduced the risk of dying from artery-clogging heart disease by 25 percent. People who ate them five or more times per week slashed their risks in half.

Researchers aren't sure which nuts made the most difference. Among the most popular choices were peanuts, almonds, and walnuts. (Even though peanuts are technically a legume, they're nutritionally similar to nuts and, in fact, are sometimes referred to as groundnuts.)

What is it about nuts, which are practically dripping with oil, that amazingly defats arteries? "With a few exceptions, most nuts are high in monounsaturated and polyunsaturated fats," says Dr. Sabaté. "When these types of fats replace saturated fats in the diet, they can help lower total cholesterol as well as the unhealthy low-density lipoprotein (LDL) cholesterol." At the same time, nuts don't affect levels of the heart-healthy high-density lipoprotein (HDL) cholesterol.

A study in the journal *Circulation* found that bad LDL cholesterol levels fell 4 percent and good HDL cholesterol levels rose 5 percent in people who ate 25 almonds a day.

Another thing that makes nuts healthy for the heart is an amino acid called arginine. Some arginine may be converted in the body to nitric oxide, a compound that helps expand the blood vessels. In fact, it acts much like the drug nitroglycerin, which is used to rapidly dilate arteries to permit more blood to reach the heart. Nitric oxide also appears to help keep the platelets in blood from clumping, which can further reduce heart disease risk.

"Nuts are also high in vitamin E, which may keep LDL cholesterol from oxidizing," says Dr. Sabaté. This is the process that makes cholesterol more likely to stick to artery walls and block bloodflow. Nuts have more vitamin E than any other food, with the exception of oils. Almonds and walnuts are particularly good choices. One-third cup of either nut contains about 12 IU, or 40 percent of the Daily Value (DV) for this vitamin.

Nuts also contain generous amounts of heart-healthy copper and magnesium. Magnesium appears to regulate cholesterol and blood pressure as well as heart rhythms, while copper may play a role in lowering cholesterol.

Interestingly, in the same way that nuts help keep arteries clear and free of blockages, they also help prevent gallstones, which block the release of bile from the gallbladder. Researchers at Harvard Medical School followed 81,000 women over 20 years and found that women who ate 5 or more ounces of peanuts, peanut butter, or other nuts a week were 25 percent less likely to need gallbladder surgery.

Preventing Cancer

Just as nuts contain compounds that may help prevent heart disease, they also contain compounds that may help stop cancer.

Walnuts, for example, contain a compound called ellagic acid that appears to battle cancer on several fronts. "Ellagic acid is a good antioxidant, disabling harmful oxygen molecules, called free radicals, that are known to instigate the cancer process," says Gary Stoner, PhD, professor and cancer researcher at Ohio State University in Columbus. Ellagic acid also helps detoxify potential cancer-causing substances, while at the same time helping to prevent cancer cells from dividing.

In one study, laboratory animals given ellagic acid as well as a cancer-causing substance were 33 percent less likely to develop esophageal cancer than animals given only carcinogens. In another study, laboratory animals were 70 percent less likely to develop liver tumors when they were given purified ellagic acid.

The vitamin E in nuts also appears to help in cancer prevention. In 2004, researchers at Purdue University in West Lafayette, Indiana, found that gamma-tocopherol, a form of vitamin E in walnuts and pecans, killed human prostate and lung cancer cells in the laboratory, while leaving healthy cells untouched.

A Nutritional Payload

All nuts are richly endowed with protein, and most contain a generous supply of vitamins and minerals as well as dietary fiber.

While the plain old peanut doesn't hit the charts for healing potential, it's the highest in protein of any nut, with ⅓ cup containing more than 11 grams, or 22 percent of the DV. That's more protein than you'll get from the same amount of beef or fish. Better yet, the protein in peanuts is a complete protein, meaning that it contains all the essential amino acids we can't do without. Brazil nuts, cashews, walnuts, and almonds also are good sources of protein, each containing at least 6 grams in ⅓ cup, or 12 percent of the DV.

In addition, all nuts are a good source of fiber, with ⅓ cup typically containing 1 to 2 grams—about the amount in a similar amount of Cheerios. Among the most fiber-rich nuts are pistachios (nearly 5 grams per ⅓ cup, or almost 20 percent of the DV), and almonds (just over 6 grams, or about 24 percent of the DV).

Spiced Almond Cereal Snack Mix

1 egg white
1½ teaspoons Cajun seasoning blend
1 teaspoon Worcestershire sauce
½ teaspoon garlic powder
1 teaspoon water
2 cups whole-wheat cereal squares
1½ cups whole almonds

Preheat the oven to 300°F. Coat a rimmed baking sheet with cooking spray.

In a large bowl, combine the egg white, Cajun seasoning, Worcestershire sauce, garlic powder, and water. Whisk to thoroughly mix. Add the cereal and almonds. Toss well to coat.

Spread the mixture out evenly on the prepared pan. Bake for 30 minutes, or until golden and crisp. Allow to cool. Store in an airtight tin or jar.

Makes about 3⅓ cups

PER ⅓ CUP

Calories: 139	Cholesterol: 0 mg
Total fat: 11 g	Sodium: 146 mg
Saturated fat: 1.1 g	Dietary fiber: 2.9 g

Walnut and Red Pepper Pasta Topping

⅔ cup chopped walnuts
⅔ cup chopped roasted peppers
2 cloves garlic, minced
2 tablespoons minced parsley
⅛ teaspoon salt
⅛ teaspoon crushed red pepper flakes

In a large nonstick skillet, heat the walnuts over medium heat, shaking the pan frequently, until toasted and fragrant, 1 to 2 minutes.

Stir in the roasted peppers, garlic, parsley, salt, and red pepper flakes. Cook, stirring frequently, until heated through, about 3 minutes. If the mixture starts to stick to the pan, add a little water.

Makes 1⅓ cups

PER ⅓ CUP

Calories: 149	Cholesterol: 0 mg
Total fat: 13 g	Sodium: 240 mg
Saturated fat: 1.2 g	Dietary fiber: 1.4 g

Oats

MOPPING UP CHOLESTEROL

HEALING POWER
Can Help:

Lower cholesterol and blood sugar

Improve insulin sensitivity

Control appetite

Reduce the risk of heart disease and cancer

If it weren't for horses, we probably wouldn't even know about oats, to say nothing of the great health benefits they provide. When horses were introduced in various parts of the world, oats went along as their feed. Not surprisingly, however, humans were a bit reluctant to take a taste. Samuel Johnson's 1755 *Dictionary of the English Language* defined oats as "a grain which in England is generally given to horses, but which in Scotland supports the people." It seems that the Scots were ahead of their time.

Oats are a very healthful grain. For one thing, unlike wheat, barley, and other grains, processed oats retain the bran and germ layers, which is where most of the nutrients reside. In addition, oats contain a variety of compounds that have been shown to reduce heart disease, fight cancer, lower blood sugar, improve insulin sensitivity, and help with dieting.

Help for High Cholesterol

All you have to do is watch some television before you come across a commercial that says oatmeal can help lower cholesterol, a critical move in reducing the risk of heart disease. In fact, studies show that getting more oats in the diet not only lowers total cholesterol but, more encouragingly, lowers the bad low-density lipoprotein (LDL) cholesterol while leaving the beneficial high-density lipoprotein (HDL) cholesterol alone.

A Tufts University study compared a low-calorie diet that included oats to one that didn't. Although both diets helped the study participants lose weight, those who ate oats experienced a bigger drop in blood pressure, total cholesterol, and bad LDL cholesterol.

Oats contain a type of soluble fiber called beta-glucan, which traps dietary cholesterol within a sticky gel in the intestine. Since this gel isn't absorbed by the body, it passes through the intestine, taking unwanted cholesterol with it. Americans get only about half of the recommended 25 grams of a fiber a day, and oats have more soluble fiber than any other grain.

Studies have shown that people with high cholesterol benefit from eating oats and other foods high in fiber. Weight loss helps lower cholesterol, but data from 13 studies found that the fiber from two servings of oats a day helped lower cholesterol an additional 2 to 3 percent more than modifying fat did.

Soluble fiber isn't the only thing doing the trapping. Oats also contain compounds called saponins, which in preliminary animal studies appear to bind to cholesterol and usher it out of the body. Saponins also glom onto bile acids. This is good because high levels of bile acids can cause cholesterol levels to rise.

"We used to think that saponins had only negative effects on the body," says Joanne L. Slavin, PhD, professor of nutrition at the University of Minnesota in St. Paul. "In fact, we call them anti-nutrients because they inhibit the absorption of various nutritional substances. But their positive health benefits are clearly stronger than their negative attributes."

It doesn't take a loaf of oats to lower cholesterol. Having about ¾ cup of dry oatmeal (which cooks up to about 1½ cups) or just less than ½ cup of dry oat bran (which cooks up to about 1 cup) a day can help lower total cholesterol by up to 5 percent.

A Stable of Protection

Like all plant foods, oats contain a variety of compounds that provide different kinds of protection. Three of these compounds—tocotrienols (related to vitamin E), ferulic acid, and caffeic acid—are antioxidants. That is, they help control cell-damaging particles called free radicals, which, when left unchecked, can contribute to heart disease, cancer, and certain eye diseases.

Tocotrienols, which are richly abundant in oats, pack at least two punches against heart disease. They're very effective at stopping oxidation, the process that causes LDL cholesterol to turn rancid and stick to artery walls. Indeed, tocotrienols are 50 percent more powerful than vitamin E, says David J. A. Jenkins, MD, DSc, PhD, professor of nutritional sciences at the University of Toronto. In addition, tocotrienols act on the liver, which might turn down the body's own production of cholesterol.

Battling Cancer

Some of the same compounds in oats that protect against heart disease may also help prevent cancer, says A. Venket Rao, PhD, professor of nutrition at the University of Toronto.

We've already discussed how the saponins in oats bind to bile acids. This is important because, while bile acids are necessary for the absorption and digestion of fat, they also cause problems. In the large intestine, they get converted by bacteria

---

FOOD ALERT
The Fat Factor

When you're trying to reduce the fat in your diet, reading the label on a container of oats may give you a moment's hesitation. Although all grains contain a little fat, oats contain quite a bit. For example, a half-cup serving of oatmeal has a little more than 1 gram of fat, while the same amount of farina has 0.1 gram.

Much of a grain's fat is found in the bran and germ layers. In most grains, these layers are stripped away during processing, but in oats they're retained. So when you're trying to limit the amount of fat in your diet, a bowl of oatmeal may not be your best choice.

On the other hand, while oats are somewhat high in fat, almost 80 percent of the fat is the heart-healthy, unsaturated kind.

---

into a form called secondary bile acids. Secondary bile acids can damage intestinal cells, possibly setting in motion the events that lead to cancer. "By binding up bile acids and reducing the amount that can be transformed into a toxic version, saponins may help lower cancer risk," says Dr. Rao.

In addition, saponins appear to strengthen the immune system, making the body better able to detect and deactivate foreign invaders such as bacteria, viruses, and cancer cells. "In animal experiments, the addition of saponins to the diet increased the number of natural killer cells, which translates into a stronger immune surveillance system," says Dr. Rao.

Other compounds in oats protect against cancer in much the same way that they help prevent heart disease—by neutralizing cell-damaging free radicals before they cause harm.

Oats also contain generous amounts of a compound called phytic acid, says Dr. Slavin. "Although we haven't identified the exact mechanism, there's some evidence that phytic acid binds up certain reactive minerals, which may be important in preventing colon cancer."

In addition, the fiber in oats helps this food fight cancer. In 2001, 54 cancer experts wrote in a public letter that they agreed that high-fiber diets offer protection from cancer. They found more than 200 studies that said so, compared with only three studies that don't show a connection between high-fiber diets and lower risk for cancer.

In the Kitchen

Oats are among the easiest foods to cook. Just add one part oatmeal to two parts water, cover, simmer, and serve. Here are a few ways to change both the texture and the taste of oats to suit your personal preference.

Cream them with milk. Cooking oats in milk instead of water yields a much creamier porridge, which some people prefer to the firmer, water-cooked variety. Choose low-fat or fat-free milk to avoid additional fat.

Make them coarser. If you prefer your oats with a firm, slightly coarse texture, chefs advise adding the oats to water that's already boiling rather than mixing them with cold water and then raising the heat.

Change the taste. To add extra flavor to oats, you can eliminate the water or milk altogether and cook them in apple, pear, or peach juice. Since the sugars in fruit juices can readily scorch and give the cereal a slightly burnt taste, make sure that you use a heavy-bottomed pan or use a double boiler over a slow, steady heat, and watch the time carefully.

Keeping Blood Sugar Steady

Another benefit of oats is that they appear to help keep the body's blood sugar levels in balance. This is important for the estimated 21 million Americans with impaired glucose tolerance, a condition that is similar to diabetes and that increases the risks of heart disease and strokes.

In people with this condition, blood sugar levels are higher than they should be, but not so high that the people are actually diabetic. Yet even slightly elevated blood sugar levels may be cause for concern because they cause the body to pump out larger amounts of insulin to bring them down.

The soluble fiber in oats lays down a protective gummy layer in the intestine. This slows the rate at which carbohydrates are absorbed by the body, which in turn helps keep blood sugar levels stable. In addition, soluble fiber appears to reduce the output of hormones in the digestive tract, which indirectly lowers the body's production of insulin.

Here's an additional benefit of the soluble fiber in oats. Because this type of fiber soaks up lots of water, it creates a feeling of fullness. This means that when you eat oats, you feel satisfied longer and so are more likely to eat less, which is good news for anyone who's trying to lose weight.

In one study by the New York Obesity Research Center at St. Luke's–Roosevelt Hospital in New York City, 60 people who ate oatmeal for breakfast instead of corn-flakes had 30 percent fewer calories at lunch.

Help for HIV

Although the evidence is still preliminary, the saponins in oats may be effective in disabling HIV, the virus that causes AIDS.

It's long been a puzzling fact that while some people infected with HIV develop AIDS relatively quickly, others don't become sick for years. Scientists are working to discover what makes HIV stronger, or more virulent, in some people.

It could be that various compounds found in food, including the saponins in oats, may play a role in squelching HIV. "Although this research is in its very early stages, it certainly is something to pursue," says Dr. Rao.

Doctor's Top Tip

If you're looking for more ways to reap the health benefits of oats, slip them into the dishes you're already making, such as meat loaves and patties, pancake batter, homemade granola, or into a breading to coat chicken, suggests the American Diabetic Association.

GETTING THE MOST

Look for 3 grams or more. Cereal and bread that contain oats are considered a good source of fiber if they have at least 3 grams per serving, so check the nutrition label to make sure you're getting the best health benefit from your food. An excellent source of fiber contains 5 grams or more a serving.

Eat for convenience. Unlike many foods, in which the processed versions are often the least nutritious, oats retain their goodness in different forms. So when time is an issue, go ahead and enjoy quick oats. They provide just as many vitamins and minerals as the traditional, slower-cooking kind. Keep in mind, however, that quick oats do contain more sodium than their slower-cooking kin.

For protein, take your pick. Both rolled oats and oat bran are good sources of protein. One cup of cooked oat bran contains 7 grams, or 14 percent of the Daily Value (DV), while a serving of rolled oats has 6 grams, or 12 percent of the DV.

Cut calories with bran. When you're trying to eat lean, oat bran is often a better choice than oatmeal. A 1-cup serving of cooked oat bran contains 87 calories, whereas the same amount of oatmeal has 145.

Oatmeal-Apricot Cookies

⅔ cup dried apricots, coarsely chopped

⅓ cup boiling water

1 cup packed light brown sugar

¼ cup unsalted butter, at room temperature

¼ cup fat-free egg substitute

1½ teaspoons vanilla extract

½ cup all-purpose flour

1 teaspoon ground cinnamon

1 teaspoon baking soda

¼ teaspoon salt

2½ cups quick-cooking rolled oats

Preheat the oven to 350°F. Coat two baking sheets with cooking spray.

In a food processor, combine the apricots and water and process until well blended (some small chunks may remain).

Transfer to a large bowl. Add the brown sugar and butter. Beat with an electric mixer until well blended. Add the egg substitute and vanilla extract. Beat to mix.

Add the flour, cinnamon, baking soda, and salt. Beat just until well mixed. Sprinkle with the oats. Stir with a large spoon to mix.

Drop by tablespoonfuls onto the prepared baking sheets. Bake one sheet at a time until the cookies are golden, about 10 to 12 minutes. Transfer the cookies to a wire rack to cool. Store in a cookie jar or other covered container that's not airtight.

Makes 28 cookies

PER COOKIE ——————————————

Calories: 78
Total fat: 2.1 g
Saturated fat: 1.1 g

Cholesterol: 4 mg
Sodium: 70 mg
Dietary fiber: 1 g

Okra

A FOOD FOR HEALTHY CELLS

Even in the Deep South, where gumbo is eaten all the time, okra isn't everyone's favorite vegetable. It can be tough. It can be slimy. It has an unusual, tart taste that's described as being somewhere between that of eggplant and asparagus. No wonder it's usually hidden inside a bowl of this thick, aromatic broth.

But okra's status as a secondary player should be changed to that of a powerful partner in fighting disease. A study from Emory University in Atlanta found that it contains a powerful compound that shows promise for fighting cancer and heart disease. In addition, okra contains a variety of healthful nutrients, including vitamin C, calcium, and potassium.

"Okra does have a little bit of everything," says Belinda Smith, RD, research dietitian at the University of Kentucky College of Medicine in Lexington. "And it's very low in calories."

HEALING POWER

Can Help:

Prevent cancer

Ease cold symptoms

Reduce the risk of heart disease

Prevent constipation

Promising Protection

A key compound in okra, called glutathione, attacks cancer in two ways. It's an antioxidant, which means that it hampers the effects of free radicals, unstable oxygen molecules that can damage healthy cells and cause them to become cancerous. In addition, glutathione prevents other cancer-causing chemicals called carcinogens from damaging DNA, the chemical blueprint that tells cells how to function. It does this by ushering chemicals away from cells, into the urine, and eventually out of the body.

In a study of more than 1,800 people, researchers at Emory University discovered that those who had the highest intake of glutathione, which is found not only in okra but also in watermelons, avocados, and grapefruit, were 50 percent less likely to develop oral and throat cancers than those with low levels of the compound.

Okra isn't the highest source of glutathione, but it isn't the lowest, either. A study at the University of Louisville in Kentucky that measured glutathione levels in food found that okra scored in the medium range, according to Calvin A. Lang, ScD, professor of biochemistry at the University of Louisville School of Medicine.

In the Kitchen

When people are asked to describe okra, the words you often hear are "tough" and "slimy." Here are a few ways to find the true taste in this Southern treat.

Buy it fresh. Old okra is tough and stringy. Linda Eck, RD, assistant professor at the University of Memphis in Tennessee, recommends doing the fingernail test when buying okra. If you can't easily push your fingernail through the outer skin of the pod, it's probably too tough to eat. The pods should snap easily. And look for small- to medium-size pods with a deep green color.

Although fresh okra is available in the South all year long, in the rest of the country, the best time to buy it is from May to October. Okra can be stored in a plastic bag in the refrigerator for up to 3 days.

Boil it whole. Wash okra just before cooking, or else it will become slimy. If it has a lot of fuzz on its surface, rub it with a towel. To cook, boil or microwave the vegetable just until it's tender. You may want to flavor it with lemon juice and ground pepper. Other ways to prepare okra include stewing or sautéing it with tomatoes (see page 458).

Turn up the heat. To reduce the amount of slime produced by okra, it's important to cook it quickly, which will help keep the juices from thickening.

But don't overcook it. When okra is overcooked, the juices get extremely gooey. So cook it just until it's tender, then remove it from the heat, and serve. Okra is a fast-grilling vegetable, so if you're going to throw it on the fire, cut the vegetable into pieces that are about ½-inch thick, baste with a light dressing, and cook for only 5 to 7 minutes.

Cut it up. When making gumbo, soup, or stew that contains okra, cut the stems or slice the pod into pieces to thicken the dish. To cut down on the thickening, throw the whole pod in during the last 10 minutes of cooking.

Combine it with curry. Okra is often found in Indian dishes. When you're in the mood for Indian cuisine at home, add the vegetable to curries, or sauté it with cumin, coriander, turmeric, or curry powder.

Researchers aren't sure how much glutathione people need to stay healthy, but they know one thing. It's better to have more than less. "If you keep your glutathione at a high level, you lower your risk of getting a serious illness," Dr. Lang says.

A Mixed Pod of Nutrients

Okra's nutritional benefits come from a hodgepodge of ingredients. Topping the list is vitamin C. A half-cup of cooked okra contains more than 13 milligrams, or 22 percent of the Daily Value (DV). A powerful antioxidant, vitamin C has been shown to help fight cancer, prevent heart disease, and even help calm the common cold.

Okra provides a good amount of magnesium as well. A half-cup of cooked okra has about 46 milligrams, or 11 percent of the DV. This mineral may help you avoid heart disease, fight chronic fatigue syndrome, lower blood pressure, ward off diabetes, and slow bone loss.

The vegetable also contains calcium. A half-cup cooked has 50 milligrams of calcium, or 5 percent of the DV.

In addition, okra is a good source of fiber, Smith says. Whether frozen or cooked, a half-cup serving of okra has about 2 grams of fiber, or 8 percent of the DV. That's about the same amount as a half-cup of raw carrots or apples.

The two kinds of fiber in okra help in different ways. The soluble fiber lowers cholesterol and helps control symptoms of diabetes. In addition, it can help with weight control because it forms bulk in the stomach, making you feel full. Insoluble fiber (what used to be called roughage) has been shown to help prevent colon cancer and digestive disorders such as constipation.

Doctor's Top Tip

Some people don't care for okra because of its tendency to become slimy, but it actually has a nice, natural thickening property that adds a pleasant texture to stews and gumbos, says Jeannie Gazzaniga Moloo, PhD, RD, a Sacramento, California–based spokesperson for the American Dietetic Association. In addition to adding it to stews, consider chopping it and adding it to your marinara sauce.

GETTING THE MOST

Put water to work. Okra is traditionally served fried, which adds a tremendous amount of fat to the diet. A better way to prepare it is by steaming, Smith says. Cooking with moist heat requires no added fat. Plus, it has the added advantage of preserving more of the nutrients than other cooking methods.

Savor the slime. When cooked, okra releases a thick, slimy fluid that's a rich source of nutrients. Rather than discarding the juice, you can use it as a natural thickening ingredient for gumbos, stews, and soups.

Creole-Style Okra

1 pound fresh okra

1½ cups chopped onions

1 can (16 ounces) reduced-sodium tomatoes (with juice)

½ teaspoon dried basil

½ teaspoon hot pepper sauce

½ teaspoon packed light brown sugar

¼ teaspoon dried thyme

⅛ teaspoon salt

Trim the okra, and cut the pods into ½-inch slices.

Coat a large saucepan with cooking spray. Add the onions, and cook over medium heat, stirring frequently, until lightly golden, 7 to 8 minutes.

Meanwhile, drain the tomatoes through a fine sieve set over a medium bowl; set aside the juice. With a spoon, lightly crush the tomatoes.

Add the tomatoes to the pan. Stir in the basil, hot pepper sauce, brown sugar, thyme, salt, and ¼ cup of the reserved tomato juice. Cook, stirring, for 2 minutes.

Add the okra. Cook, stirring frequently, until the okra is tender, 10 to 15 minutes. Add the remaining tomato juice, if needed, to keep the okra from sticking.

Makes 4 servings

Cook's Note: *If fresh okra is unavailable, substitute frozen. Do not thaw before using. Add 2 to 3 minutes to the cooking time.*

PER SERVING

Calories: 81	Cholesterol: 0 mg
Total fat: 0.6 g	Sodium: 92 mg
Saturated fat: 0.1 g	Dietary fiber: 5.7 g

Olive Oil

AN ELIXIR FOR YOUR HEART

HEALING POWER

Can Help:

Lower cholesterol

Reduce the risk of heart disease, breast cancer, and rheumatoid arthritis

Researchers were amazed more than 40 years ago when they first started studying Greeks living on the island of Crete. Even though the traditional Greek diet is very high in fat, people had exceptionally low rates of heart disease. "They have to be doing something right, and olive oil seems to play a critical role," says Dimitrios Trichopoulos, MD, professor of epidemiology and cancer prevention at the Harvard School of Public Health.

We would do well to follow their example. Olive oil, which is made from crushed olives, not only appears to lower the risk of heart disease, it may reduce the risk of breast cancer as well.

A Better Fat

All fats, from butter and margarine to olive oil, contain almost the same number of calories. But they behave quite differently inside the body. Saturated fats, for example, which are found mainly in meats and dairy foods, are incredibly destructive because they make it difficult for the body to rid itself of harmful low-density lipoprotein (LDL) cholesterol, the kind that blocks arteries and raises the risk of heart disease.

Olive oil, however, is a monounsaturated fat. With no more than 2 grams of saturated fat per tablespoon, olive oil is recommended by the American Heart Association for your food preparation. Replacing saturated fats in the diet with olive oil lowers levels of LDL cholesterol while leaving the beneficial high-density lipoprotein (HDL) cholesterol alone.

Compared with butter, olive oil also seems to make us more satisfied, which means we won't overeat later. Researchers at the University of Illinois at Urbana-Champaign gave 341 restaurant diners bread and either olive oil or butter. Those who dipped their bread in olive oil tended to put 26 percent more fat on each bread slice, but those who had butter ate more bread, which added up to 17 percent more calories overall.

The olive oil–loving Greeks eat very little butter or margarine, Dr. Trichopoulos adds. What's more, their main meals usually consist of vegetables or legumes instead of meats. So even though they use a lot of olive oil, they get very little saturated fat.

One scientific project, called the Seven Countries Study, found that while 46 percent of deaths among middle-aged American men were due to heart disease, the number in Crete was a mere 4 percent—more than 10 times lower.

In addition to offering protection from heart disease, olive oil may help prevent many cancers by protecting cells in the body from oxidation. In a 2006 Denmark study, 182 European men included ¼ cup of olive oil in their diets every day. After 2 weeks, their DNA cells showed less oxidation, and, therefore, had more cancer protection.

Extra-virgin olive oil may also help lower the risk of rheumatoid arthritis, according to a Greek study published in the *American Journal of Clinical Nutrition*. The study authors examined the diet of 145 people with rheumatoid arthritis and 188 control subjects. They found that those who took in the lowest amount of extra-virgin olive oil over their lifetime were 2½ times more likely to develop rheumatoid arthritis than those who had the highest intake of the oil. Experts believe extra-virgin olive oil reduces the risk of rheumatoid arthritis because of its anti-inflammatory effects. One study found that the oil was similar to ibuprofen in reducing inflammation.

Chemicals for the Heart

It's not only the monounsaturated fat that makes olive oil good for the heart. It also contains other disease-fighting compounds that can prevent damage in the arteries before it starts.

In the Kitchen

Some olive oils are quite rare and exquisitely flavored—and exquisitely priced. Others are much more affordable and, of course, the flavors reflect that. Many cooks keep two (or more) kinds of olive oil in the kitchen—a gourmet oil for drizzling on salads or pastas and a heartier oil to use for cooking.

Extra-virgin is the Cadillac of olive oils. It's usually used as a flavoring oil and not for cooking. When buying extra-virgin olive oil, look at the color. The deeper the color, the more intense the olive flavor.

Pure (also called virgin) olive oil is paler than extra-virgin and has a milder flavor. It's usually used for low- to medium-heat frying.

Light olive oil is often used by people who want the heart-healthy benefits of monounsaturated fats but don't want the strong olive taste. It stands up to heat well, so you can use it for high-heat frying.

Here's why. The body naturally produces harmful oxygen molecules called free radicals. These molecules damage LDL cholesterol in the bloodstream, making it more likely to stick to the linings of artery walls. But several of the compounds in olive oil, such as polyphenols, are powerful antioxidants. This means that they're able to disable free radicals before they do damage, Dr. Trichopoulos explains. As a result, getting more olive oil in your diet can help keep your arteries clear.

But it doesn't have to be a lot. Getting just 2 tablespoons of olive oil every day has been associated with a lower risk for heart disease in studies.

Doctor's Top Tip

Before you bring home another bottle of olive oil, check the label and make sure it says "cold pressed," says Jeannie Gazzaniga Moloo, PhD, RD, a Sacramento, California–based spokesperson for the American Dietetic Association. When the oil is cold pressed it means that it was extracted without heat and chemicals that can break down the healthy fats and take away some of the oil's health benefits.

A Woman's Best Friend

Even though olive oil is best known for protecting the heart, evidence suggests that it may play a role in protecting the breasts as well. In a study of more than 2,300 women, researchers from the Harvard School of Public Health and the Athens School of Public Health in Greece found that women who used olive oil more than once a day had 25 percent lower risks of breast cancer compared with those who used it less often. And in fact, women in Greece are much less likely to die of breast cancer than their American counterparts.

"We're still not certain what accounts for this apparent protective effect," says Dr. Trichopoulos. Olive oil is rich in vitamin E, which has been shown to stop cellular damage that can lead to cancer. And of course, the same polyphenols that help prevent free radicals from damaging the heart may play a role in preventing cancer as well.

GETTING THE MOST

Look for extra-virgin. All olive oils are high in monounsaturated fats, but they don't contain equal amounts of disease-fighting polyphenols. To get the most of these compounds, look for olive oil labeled "extra-virgin." This type of oil is made from the first pressing of perfectly ripe olives, which leaves the polyphenols in and the bitter acids out.

Although it's a little more expensive, studies have shown that it's worth your money to buy extra-virgin olive oil. Researchers in Spain asked 24 men to use refined olive oil for 3 months and extra-virgin olive oil for 3 months. They found that the antioxidants in the extra-virgin olive oil kept their LDL, or bad, cholesterol from oxidizing and slowed the formation of plaque in the arteries, while the refined oil didn't offer the protection.

Keep it cold. Because people don't always use a lot of olive oil, it tends to go bad on the shelf, giving up both its good taste and its protective compounds. To keep olive oil fresh, store it in the refrigerator or another dark, cool place. Bringing it to room temperature will quickly restore its pourable nature. Or look for an olive oil that comes in a dark bottle to keep the light from adversely affecting it.

Buy only what you need now. Unless you'll finish the bottle of olive oil within 2 months, buy a smaller size. Oxygen fills the container when it empties, which begins to deteriorate the oil and cause it to taste stale.

Lemon-Rosemary Dressing

1 sprig fresh rosemary

1 small clove garlic

1 strip lemon zest (1 × 3½ inches)

¾ cup extra-virgin olive oil

¼ cup fresh lemon juice

Place the rosemary and garlic on a cutting board. Lightly crush both with the side of a heavy knife.

Place the rosemary, garlic, and lemon zest in a bottle or jar with a tight-fitting cap. Pour in the oil and lemon juice. Cap the bottle and shake well. Refrigerate if not using right away. Shake again before serving.

Makes 1 cup

Cook's Notes: *The dressing can be stored in the refrigerator for up to 1 week. Drizzle over steamed vegetables, fish, or seafood. Or use as a dressing for pastas, potato salads, or other salads.*

PER TABLESPOON

Calories: 90	Cholesterol: 0 mg
Total fat: 10.1 g	Sodium: 0 mg
Saturated fat: 1.4 g	Dietary fiber: 0 g

Onion Family
ROOTS OF GOOD HEALTH

HEALING POWER
Can Help:

Raise beneficial HDL cholesterol

Lower blood pressure

Decrease the risk of cancer

Relieve congestion

Reduce inflammation

Scene: The Civil War, 1864. The Union soldiers are ailing with dysentery. General Ulysses S. Grant wires a directive to the War Department to save his troops.

"I will not move my army without onions!"

Three trainloads are shipped the next day. The rest, as they say, is history.

It's a stretch to say that onions won the war between the states. And scientists haven't proven that onions can stave off dysentery. But onions and other members of the allium family—such as leeks, shallots, and scallions—contain dozens of compounds that provide protection from other conditions, including cancer, high blood pressure, heart disease, high cholesterol, and asthma.

So grab an onion, a sharp knife, and a hanky, and start chopping your way to better health.

Onion Rings and Heart Strings

Don't be offended the next time your honey suggests you "go Dutch" when you go out to dinner. He may be suggesting you take a cue from a group of heart-healthy men who ate their fill of onion-laden delights as part of a groundbreaking study in the Netherlands.

In this much-acclaimed study, researchers found that men who ate ¼ cup of onions a day, along with an apple and 4 cups of tea, had one-third the risk of dying from heart attacks compared with those who ate the least amounts of these foods.

What's so important about onions? Wrapped beneath their papery skins are dozens of compounds that help lower cholesterol, thin the blood, and prevent hardening of the arteries—all of which can go a long way toward preventing heart disease.

The first family of heart-healthy compounds in onions is the flavonoids. These are substances in plants that have potent antioxidant powers, meaning that they help prevent disease by sweeping up harmful, cell-damaging oxygen molecules called free radicals, which accumulate naturally in your body.

One particular onion-dwelling flavonoid called quercetin has been shown to

FOOD ALERT

A Problem with Pickling

Even though eating raw or cooked onions may help fight the airway inflammation that accompanies asthma attacks, eating certain pickled onions may have the opposite effect, warn researchers.

In a study in Spain, scientists found that some people with asthma experienced attacks after eating Spanish pickled onions (but not the Dutch variety), presumably because high levels of sulfites are added as preservatives.

If your doctor has told you that you're sensitive to sulfites, the best advice is to get your onions out of the ground. Or if you do buy pickled onions, check the label to make sure they're made without sulfites.

help prevent heart disease in two ways. One, it helps keep the dangerous low-density lipoprotein (LDL) form of cholesterol from oxidizing, which is the process that makes it stick to the lining of artery walls. Two, it helps prevent platelets in the blood from sticking together and forming harmful clots.

A second group of protective compounds in onions are the same ones that make you cry—the sulfur compounds. Experts say that these compounds can raise your levels of beneficial high-density lipoprotein (HDL) cholesterol, which helps keep plaque from sticking to artery walls. At the same time, they can lower levels of dangerous blood fats called triglycerides, which helps make blood thinner, keeping your blood pressure in the safety zone.

You don't need a lot of onions to keep your pump primed with protective compounds. In fact, studies show that you can reap the benefits by eating just one medium onion, raw or cooked, a day.

Cancer Protection

You can hold the pickles if you like, but when you're looking for cancer protection, don't skimp on the onions. They may be a key player in cancer prevention, especially cancers of the gastrointestinal tract, say experts.

"The primary flavonoid found in onions—quercetin—actually halts the progression of tumors in the colons of animals," says Michael J. Wargovich, PhD, professor of pathology and microbiology at the University of South Carolina School of Medicine and director of the chemoprevention program at the South Carolina Cancer

Center, both in Columbia. This means that onions do double duty in suppressing tumors, because the sulfur compounds also fight cancer, he adds.

In a large study in the Netherlands, researchers looked at the diets of nearly 121,000 men and women. The more odoriferous bulbs these onion-loving Hollanders included in their daily diets, the lower their risks of stomach cancer.

Scientists suspect that onions prevent cancer not only by putting the brakes on tumor development but also by stomping out harmful bacteria that may get stomach cancer started.

Onions have been shown to protect against other forms of cancer as well. After studying a group of 471 men in China, researchers found that the men who ate the largest number of onions had a much lower risk of prostate cancer than those who ate the least amount of onions.

In addition, eating onions has been found to reduce the risk of cancers of the oral cavity and pharynx, esophageal cancer, colorectal cancer, laryngeal cancer, breast cancer, prostate cancer, and renal cell cancer in southern Europe.

The sulfur in onions helps protect against cancer by damaging cancer cells and slowing their growth, according to the National Cancer Institute. Researchers at Cornell University have discovered that four types of onion—shallots, western yellow, pungent yellow, and northern red—are filled with more anticancer chemicals than other varieties.

A Good Kind of Onion Breath

Putting a few layers of raw onions on your turkey burger can give you industrial-strength breath, but those very same onions also may give people with asthma or other respiratory ailments clearer airways.

"There are sulfur compounds in onions that inhibit the allergic, inflammatory response like that seen in asthma," says Eric Block, PhD, professor of chemistry at the State University of New York at Albany.

Although more research needs to be done on onions' asthma-attacking abilities, you can see the anti-inflammatory effect for yourself. The next time you have an insect bite or other type of minor inflammation on your skin, rub a cut onion on it. This should help reduce the inflammation, says Dr. Block.

You only need to eat a few servings of onions a day to keep your breathing passages free and clear. "Unlike some foods, where it's just not conceivable that you could eat enough to produce a significant effect, you can with onions," says Dr. Block. "If you like onions, you can consume them in pretty large quantities. And there's good evidence that you should."

Doctor's Top Tip

A wonderful way to enjoy onions is to put them on the grill. The Mayo Clinic in Rochester, Minnesota, recommends putting chunks of sweet onions on a skewer along with other vegetables, such as eggplant and squash, and grilling until they're lightly browned and tender. Brush the onions and veggies with heart-healthy olive oil before adding to the grill.

Combined Benefits

Whether you're eating for health or good taste, there's no reason to limit yourself to onions. Scallions, shallots, and other allium vegetables not only pack the same sulfur compounds and flavonoids as their bigger brothers, they also have a few of their own nutrients that can help fight disease and boost immunity.

Scallions, also called spring or green onions, are actually just young, underdeveloped onions. But they are higher in nutrients, particularly in the B vitamin folate and vitamin C, than their adult counterparts.

A half-cup of chopped raw scallions provides 32 micrograms, or 8 percent of the Daily Value (DV) of folate, a nutrient that's essential for normal tissue growth and that may protect against cancer, heart disease, and birth defects. In that half-cup, you'll also get more than 9 milligrams (almost 16 percent of the DV) of vitamin C, an immunity-boosting antioxidant nutrient that helps vacuum up tissue-damaging oxygen molecules in the body.

Shallots, another miniature member of the allium family, have their own benefits. Just 1 tablespoon of chopped shallots contains 600 IU of vitamin A, or 12 percent of the DV. This essential nutrient helps keep immunity strong and also guards against vision problems associated with aging, like cataracts and night blindness.

GETTING THE MOST

Add some color. To get the most nutrients from your daily dose of onions, eat several different kinds. Red and yellow onions and shallots have the highest flavonoid content, while white onions have the least.

Save your breath. If the fear of having horrific halitosis is keeping you from enjoying the health benefits of onions, here's a freshening tip. Eat a sprig of fresh parsley. This will help neutralize the sulfur compounds before they turn into offending breath. A breath freshener made with parsley seed oil can also help.

Keep your eyes peeled. Even if you like onions, you may not love them enough to eat a half-cup or so a day. That's why scientists are trying to develop new onion strains with high concentrations of flavonoids like quercetin. Experts aren't sure when these new onions will be on the market, but keep your eyes open for special displays at your supermarket.

Stuffed Vidalia Onions

4 **Vidalia onions**

½ **teaspoon olive oil**

3 **medium zucchini, shredded**

3 **cloves garlic, minced**

1 **teaspoon dried basil**

1 **teaspoon dried thyme**

3 **tablespoons unseasoned dried bread crumbs**

1 **tablespoon plus ½ teaspoon chopped toasted pine nuts**

3 **teaspoons grated Parmesan cheese**

Salt and freshly ground black pepper

Preheat the oven to 400°F. Line a baking sheet with foil.

Leaving the peels on, cut about ½ inch off the top of each onion. Slightly trim the bottoms so the onions stand upright. Place the onions, cut side up, on the baking sheet, and coat each onion lightly with cooking spray. Bake for 1 hour, or until soft. Set aside for 15 minutes, or until cool enough to handle.

Reduce the oven temperature to 350°F.

Remove and discard the onion peels. With a spoon, scoop out the onion centers, leaving a ½-inch shell. Chop the centers, and reserve 1 cup for the stuffing; save the remainder for another use.

In a large nonstick skillet, heat the oil over medium heat. Add the zucchini, garlic, basil, thyme, and chopped onion. Cook until the zucchini is softened and most of the liquid has evaporated, about 6 minutes.

Remove from the heat, and stir in the bread crumbs, pine nuts, and Parmesan. Season with salt and pepper to taste. Mix well. Divide the filling among the onion shells.

Coat the baking sheet with cooking spray. Place the onions on the baking sheet, and bake until golden, about 20 minutes.

Makes 4 servings

PER SERVING

Calories: 144
Total fat: 4 g
Saturated fat: 1 g

Cholesterol: 3 mg
Sodium: 267 mg
Dietary fiber: 5 g

Oranges

THE SWEET TASTE OF CITRUS

HEALING POWER

Can Help:

Lower the risk of heart disease and stroke

Fight cancer

Promote regularity

The orange is nearly the perfect fruit. Not only is it high in vitamin C and fiber; it's also rich in natural sugars for quick energy. And because it comes ready-wrapped in its own protective skin, you can eat it anywhere, anytime.

Yet oranges are more than just a wholesome (and convenient) food. They also contain a quartet of compounds—limonin, limonene, limonin glucoside, and hesperidin—that show promise for blocking cancer. Plus, they contain compounds that may be able to stop heart disease even before it starts.

Help for the Heart

Studies have shown that the vitamins and other compounds in oranges are surprisingly effective antioxidants. That is, they're able to block free radicals, corrosive oxygen molecules in the body that can damage cells, before they do harm. This is important because free-radical damage can set the stage for clogging of the arteries, a key risk factor for heart disease and stroke.

Vitamin C has long been recognized as a powerful antioxidant. Yet there appear to be other compounds in oranges that are even more powerful.

"We measured the total antioxidant capacity of oranges and found that vitamin C only accounted for maybe 15 to 20 percent of the total activity," says Ronald L. Prior, a senior investigator for the Arkansas Children's Nutrition Center in Little Rock and a scientist and liaison for the USDA. "The other compounds in oranges turned out to be very strong antioxidants—anywhere from three to six times as potent as vitamin C."

In one study, researchers gave rats an extract from the peel and pith of oranges. The extract, which contained the compound hesperidin, significantly raised the animals' levels of healthful high-density lipoprotein (HDL) cholesterol, while at the same time lowering the dangerous low-density lipoprotein (LDL) cholesterol. If hesperidin works the same way in human tests, oranges could be used to help temper high cholesterol, which is one of the main risk factors for heart disease.

Hesperidin may have other benefits as well. In laboratory studies, for example,

Brazilian researchers found that hesperidin was able to help stop inflammation. And since it doesn't damage the delicate stomach lining the way aspirin can, it someday could be used to help relieve swelling in people who are sensitive to other anti-inflammatory drugs such as ibuprofen.

In a large prospective study of more than 100,000 people, researchers found that adding one serving of fruits and vegetables to the diet each day lowered the risk of ischemic stroke, a stroke in which the artery to the brain is blocked, by 6 percent. Oranges and other citrus fruits were one of the foods that showed the best protection in the study.

Cancer Control

Laboratory studies have shown that the limonene found in oranges can help block lung and breast cancers, says Bill Widmer, PhD, a research scientist with the Florida Department of Citrus Research Center in Lake Alfred.

In a study at Duke University Medical Center in Durham, North Carolina, laboratory animals given a diet consisting of 10 percent limonene showed a 70 percent reduction in cancerous tumors. Among the tumors that remained, 20 percent shrank to less than half their former size.

In another study, researchers at Cornell University in Ithaca, New York, fed animals with early stages of liver cancer an extract of orange juice concentrate from which the vitamin C had been removed. The incidence and size of precancerous lesions dropped 40 percent.

"The rats were drinking the human equivalent of a gallon of orange juice a day for 4 months," adds Robert S. Parker, PhD, professor of nutritional and food sciences at Cornell. "That's an unrealistic amount for humans, but since we fed the animals only certain components of the juice, the actual protective effect of whole juice may be greater than the results suggested. Humans may be able to obtain protective effects at lower levels, particularly if they consume the juice regularly over a long period of time."

The research on limonene has been so promising that researchers in England are testing its effects on breast cancer.

"The way that limonene acts on tumor cells or lesions is really interesting and unique," says Michael Gould, PhD, professor of oncology and medical physics at the University of Wisconsin Medical School in Madison. Essentially, the compound gets cancer cells to self-destruct. It assists them in their own suicides.

Seize the Cs

Oranges are best known for their vitamin C, and with good reason. One orange contains about 70 milligrams of vitamin C, or almost 117 percent of the Daily Value (DV).

FOOD ALERT

Citrus Stings

One of the nicest things about oranges is their pleasant, citrusy zing. But for some people these natural acids can deliver a painful bite.

While few people have severe allergic reactions to oranges, some may have a condition called oral allergy syndrome, which causes itching and burning in the mouth or throat. It can happen by handling or eating oranges and other raw fruits and vegetables, especially in people who have hay fever.

While reactions to citrus fruits are rare in adults, they occur more often in young children. "Infants may get a rash around their mouths because of the natural acid in foods like oranges," says Marianne Frieri, MD, PhD, director of the allergy and immunology training program at Nassau County Medical Center–North Shore University Hospital in East Meadow and Manhasset, New York.

She adds, however, that in most cases, the discomfort is only temporary. Healing quickly occurs once the offending food is taken away.

Vitamin C is critical not only for controlling harmful free radicals but also for aiding healing and boosting immunity. It's vitamin C's immune-boosting power that gives it its reputation for fighting the symptoms of a cold.

The vitamin also helps the body absorb iron from food, which is particularly important for women, who lose a little bit of iron (and blood) each month during menstruation.

In one large study, Gladys Block, PhD, professor of epidemiology and public health nutrition at the University of California, Berkeley, reviewed 46 smaller studies looking at the effects of vitamin C. Most of those studies found that people who got the most vitamin C had the lowest risks of cancer.

A Finnish study also found that vitamin C reduced the risk of stroke. The researchers examined the eating habits of nearly 2,500 middle-aged men over 10 years and found that those with low plasma vitamin C levels were 2.4 times more likely to have a stroke. Among overweight men or those who had high blood pressure, consuming less than 40 milligrams of vitamin C, the equivalent of a half glass of orange juice, made them three times more likely to have a stroke. To boost your vitamin C, drink two 8-ounce glasses of orange juice a day.

Filled with Fiber

An orange contains 3 grams of fiber, or about 12 percent of the DV. Because insoluble fiber adds bulk to the stool, it can help relieve a host of intestinal problems, from constipation and hemorrhoids to diverticulosis. By speeding digestion, it can also help reduce the risk of colon cancer by moving the stool and any harmful substances it might contain through the colon more quickly. Insoluble fiber also keeps you regular, helping with both diarrhea and constipation.

Oranges also contain a second form of fiber, called soluble fiber. This type of fiber, which includes pectin, breaks down to form a gel-like barrier in the small intestine. Studies show that it can help lower cholesterol as well as help control changes in blood sugar, critical for those with diabetes.

If you were to eat more than seven oranges a day, you could lower your total cholesterol by about 20 percent. Of course, it's unlikely that anyone likes oranges that much. But by eating a variety of fruits and vegetables, including oranges whenever possible, you can do a lot to keep your cholesterol levels down.

GETTING THE MOST

Don't shy away from pulp. The easiest way to get the benefits of oranges is to drink its juice, which holds almost all of the health benefits of fresh oranges, says Christine Gerbstadt, MD, RD, a spokesperson for the American Dietetic Association. Orange juice makers use the whole fruit to make the juice, so all of the nutrients

In the Kitchen

Whether you're making juice or adding sections to a salad, there's a certain type of orange—and a way of using it—that's right for the specific job. Navel oranges from California are often considered the best eating oranges. They're easy to peel, have no seeds, and are sweet and juicy. Florida Valencia oranges, which often have a slightly greenish tint, are juicier than navels and are usually used for making juice. Here are some tips for getting the best from oranges.

- When cooking navel oranges, add them at the last minute. Cooking them too long can cause them to turn bitter.
- Don't freeze juice made from navel oranges because the cold, like heat, can cause it to turn bitter.
- To get the most juice out of an orange, warm the fruit to room temperature, then roll it on the counter with your palm before squeezing.

Doctor's Top Tip

Add oranges to your meals for an unexpected and sweet surprise. "I use orange wedges in about everything," says Christine Gerbstadt, MD, RD, a spokesperson for the American Dietetic Association. Add orange slices to your salads, on top of stir-fry dishes, and even to cakes.

from the oranges' sweet flesh, white pith, and rind end up inside your glass, albeit with a little pulp. When you buy OJ from the store, choosing orange juice with the pulp rather than the low-pulp or no-pulp versions may give you a little more of the nutrients in oranges, she says.

Stock your freezer. Fresh juice is delicious, but it's also a bother to make. Fortunately, frozen orange juice retains most of the nutrients.

Eat the sections. Half of an orange's pectin is contained in the albedo, the inner white spongy layer that lies right under the colorful part of the skin. "Some people painstakingly take off the white part of the orange, but it's really nutritious," Dr. Gerbstadt says. So don't be too neat when you eat. Enjoying a little of this spongy layer with each section will provide more fiber and biotin, an important B vitamin that keeps the skin healthy.

Quick Apple-Orange Compote

1 Granny Smith apple, cored and chopped

1 navel orange, peeled and chopped

1 teaspoon ground cinnamon

½ cup fat-free vanilla yogurt

2 tablespoons pecan or walnut pieces

In a medium microwaveable bowl, combine the apple, orange, and cinnamon. Cover with plastic wrap, and microwave on high for 4 minutes, or until the fruit is hot and soft. Divide among 2 bowls, and spoon the yogurt evenly over each. Sprinkle with the nuts, and serve warm.

Makes 2 servings

PER SERVING

Calories: 180
Total fat: 5 g
Saturated fat: 0.5 g

Cholesterol: 0 mg
Sodium: 35 mg
Dietary fiber: 4 g

Osteoporosis

DAIRY FOR BETTER BONES

For years now we've been trying to reduce the fat in our diets in order to control weight and reduce the risk of high cholesterol and heart disease. But in the rush to save our hearts, we may be losing our bones.

While milk, cheese, and other dairy foods can be very high in fat, they're among the best sources of calcium, the nutrient that's essential for keeping bones strong, says Daniel Baran, MD, professor of medicine, orthopedics, and cell biology at the University of Massachusetts Medical Center in Worcester. But by forsaking these foods for fear of fat, you're at risk for developing osteoporosis, a condition in which bones become thin and brittle.

After age 50, one in two women will suffer a bone fracture as a result of osteoporosis. It's no mystery why osteoporosis is so prevalent in this country. The average American woman only gets 450 milligrams of calcium a day—nowhere near the 1,000 to 1,500 milligrams that's needed to ward off the disease, says Susan Broy, MD, director of the Osteoporosis Center at the Advocate Medical Group in Chicago. Ironically, women, who need calcium even more than men do, are more likely to turn away from calcium-rich foods because they're more worried about their waistlines than their bones, she says.

Getting enough calcium is especially important for women approaching menopause, when estrogen levels decline. Estrogen helps bones absorb and keep calcium. When estrogen levels fall, in many cases, the bones become weaker. In fact, the highest rate of bone loss occurs in the first 5 to 7 years after menopause.

Meanwhile, men aren't immune to osteoporosis, but they're often overlooked for being at risk and even go undiagnosed when they do develop it. Two million American men have osteoporosis, and 12 million more are at risk for the disease. Taking steroids, anticonvulsants, certain cancer treatments, and antacids that contain aluminum put men at higher risk. Also, chronic diseases that alter hormone levels, such as diseases of the kidneys, lungs, stomach, and intestines, put men at higher risk. And, as with women, men's risk for osteoporosis increases with age.

The sad thing about osteoporosis, says Dr. Broy, is that it's often preventable—if you get enough calcium. In one study, for example, researchers in the Netherlands found that women who got at least 1,000 milligrams of calcium a day—about the

BONING UP ON SOY

In an effort to turn back the clock, it may be possible to restore estrogen without taking drugs—just by eating a little more soy.

Research has shown that tofu, tempeh, and other soy foods contain compounds called isoflavones, which are very similar to (although weaker than) the estrogen women produce naturally, says Jeri W. Nieves, PhD, a nutritional epidemiologist at Columbia University in New York City and director of the bone density testing center at Helen Hayes Hospital in West Haverstraw, New York. There's some evidence that getting enough isoflavones in the diet may play a powerful role in keeping bones strong.

In a study at the University of Illinois, women were given either 55 milligrams or 90 milligrams of isoflavones a day. (A half-cup of tofu contains 35 milligrams, a cup of soy milk has 30 milligrams, and a cup of roasted soy nuts has 60 milligrams.) After 6 months, women getting the larger amount had an increase in bone density of 2 percent.

Animal studies that show a positive effect of isoflavones on bones have been consistent, but it's only been fairly recently that researchers began looking at using phytoestrogens in delaying or preventing osteoporosis, according to a review of the research in *Alternative Medicine Review*. Further research is needed, but the studies so far have shown promise that soy can improve bone health.

Not all soy foods contain the beneficial compounds, though. Soy sauce, soybean oil, and soy hot dogs, for example, may share the name, but don't provide the benefits.

amount in three glasses of milk—were able to reduce their bone loss by 43 percent. Another study, this one done by researchers at Radcliffe Infirmary in Oxford, England, found that women who drank the most milk had bone densities 5 percent higher than those who did not drink milk.

Men should make sure they're getting the recommended 1,000 milligrams of calcium a day until age 50. After age 50, they need 1,200 milligrams a day.

Thanks to low-fat dairy foods, it is easy to get more calcium without having to worry about weight, adds Dr. Baran. A glass of whole milk, for example, has more than 8 grams of fat, while a glass of low-fat (1%) milk has 3 grams—almost three times less. A glass of fat-free milk has barely 0.5 gram per serving.

Low-fat doesn't mean low in calcium, adds Dr. Broy. Low-fat dairy foods have just as much calcium as their full-fat counterparts. In fact, fat-free milk has even more calcium, because manufacturers replace some of the fat with the calcium-rich portions of whole milk. So while a glass of whole milk has about 290 milligrams of calcium, a glass of fortified fat-free has nearly 352 milligrams.

Even if you're not a milk drinker, you can still get plenty of calcium by adding nonfat milk powder to cereals or baked goods, like muffins and cakes, says Edith Hogan, RD, a spokeswoman for the American Dietetic Association. A half-cup of fat-free milk powder contains almost 420 milligrams of calcium, and it has little effect on the texture or flavor of foods, Hogan says.

Of course, you can also add milk powder to foods that already contain milk. When Hogan makes her morning oatmeal, for example, she substitutes 1 cup of low-fat milk for the cooking water, then adds a half-cup of milk powder to the finished cereal. This one-two punch provides 720 milligrams of calcium—twice as much as many Americans get in an entire day.

Putting more cheese on the menu is an excellent way to get more calcium, Hogan says. A half-cup of ricotta cheese has 337 milligrams of calcium, more than you'd get in an 8-ounce glass of low-fat milk.

It's very easy to work more cheese into your diet, she adds. Ricotta, for example, can be added to casseroles, lasagnas, enchiladas, and other dishes that call for a little cheese. Or you can simply sprinkle a little low-fat Parmesan on pastas or salads. One tablespoon provides almost 70 milligrams of calcium and very little fat.

Even though dark green leafy vegetables don't contain as much calcium as dairy foods, they can still help you get the calcium you need. A half-cup serving of kale, for example, has nearly 47 milligrams of calcium, while the same amount of broccoli provides 36 milligrams. And you don't have to eat salads to get the benefit, Hogan adds. Mixing a cup of chopped kale into a soup, for example, will add great taste, and with it an extra 94 milligrams of calcium.

While dairy foods and produce are the best natural sources of calcium, many packaged foods, such as orange juice, have been fortified with calcium, says John Bilezikian, MD, professor of medicine in the division of endocrinology and director of the metabolic bone diseases program at Columbia University College of Physicians and Surgeons in New York City. Fortified orange juice has as much calcium as a glass of milk. So when you're at the supermarket, read the labels on packaged breads, juices, and breakfast cereals to be sure that you're getting all the calcium that you can.

Beyond the Basics

While calcium is *the* mineral for strong bones, it doesn't work alone. In fact, it can't even get into your bones without help from other nutrients, especially vitamin D. "Without vitamin D, you absorb very little of the dietary calcium," Dr. Baran says.

You can get some vitamin D by eating salmon and other fatty fish, but fortified foods such as milk and breakfast cereals are often the best sources, says Dr. Baran.

Spending 15 minutes a day in full sunlight without sunscreen, with only your face and hands exposed, would provide all of the vitamin D you need. However, where you live makes a big difference in how likely you are to get enough direct sunlight all year long.

"Vitamin D in the diet isn't so important here in Florida," says Jay Kenney, PhD, RD, director of nutrition research and educator at the Pritikin Longevity Center and Spa in Aventura, Florida. But if you live north of Atlanta, it's a good idea to take a vitamin D_3 supplement of 1,000 IU a day for bone health during the winter, he says. It's also important to take a look at your lifestyle. If you have a job that keeps you indoors for long hours, you may not be getting enough vitamin D, no matter what time of the year.

"Lack of vitamin D is clearly linked to increased risk of breast cancer and colorectal cancer," Dr. Kenney says. "And low levels of vitamin D weaken the bones and reduce calcium absorption. There's also good evidence that low levels of vitamin D can weaken muscles."

And while most men and women already know that calcium and vitamin D are important, few know that vitamin K, which promotes bone formation, is also essential for fighting osteoporosis. If you have at least one serving a day of dark greens, such as spinach, kale, or broccoli, and then eat a fair amount of fruits and vegetables,

STRENGTHEN WITH SUPPLEMENTS

In today's fast-paced, eat-on-the-run world, it's not always easy to get all the calcium your bones need. When your diet falls short, taking a calcium supplement makes good sense, says Daniel Baran, MD, of the University of Massachusetts Medical Center in Worcester.

Women who are past menopause, when bone loss is greatest, need 1,200 milligrams of calcium a day. (Postmenopausal women taking estrogen need less, about 1,000 milligrams a day.) All calcium supplements, whether they're made from bone meal, oyster shells, or calcium citrate, are effective, says Dr. Baran. But the best supplements, as well as the least expensive, are those containing calcium carbonate, which is the same ingredient found in many antacids.

Beware of bogus claims about coral calcium supplements, however. Various companies producing coral calcium were charged by the government in 2003 for making outrageous, unsubstantiated claims about the supplements, including that their product could cure cancer, heart disease, and multiple sclerosis; provide the same amount of calcium in 2 gallons of milk; and allow your body to absorb significantly more calcium at a faster rate. None of those claims are supported by science.

you should be getting the 75 micrograms of vitamin K you need, Dr. Kenney says.

Stop the Bone Robbers

When trying to prevent osteoporosis, what you eat is generally more important than what you avoid. A number of foods and beverages can prevent calcium from being absorbed, however, so it's important to cut back on the worst offenders.

Coffee and colas, for example, contain caffeine, which can substantially reduce the amount of calcium you're able to absorb. To keep bones strong, doctors often advise having no more than two or three servings of coffee or soda a day, says Elaine Feldman, MD, professor emeritus of medicine, physiology, and endocrinology at the Medical College of Georgia in Augusta.

Doctor's Top Tip

Many women don't know about the detrimental effects salt can have on their bone health. Because salt is added to a host of foods, check the nutrition labels, and look for low-salt bread and cereal, says Jay Kenney, PhD, director of nutrition research and educator at the Pritikin Longevity Center and Spa in Aventura, Florida. Women get about twice as much of the recommended amount of salt a day.

When you do have coffee, it's a good idea to pour in a bit of milk, adds Jeri W. Nieves, PhD, a nutritional epidemiologist at Columbia University in New York City and director of the bone density testing center at Helen Hayes Hospital in West Haverstraw, New York. Milk essentially blocks the effects of caffeine, preventing it from pulling calcium from your bones.

You may also want to make a cup of green tea instead. Women who drink tea get less osteoporosis, Dr. Kenney says, and that's probably partly because tea is a good source of vitamin K.

Getting too much salt in your diet can also be bad for bones. Not only does it decrease the amount of calcium your body is able to absorb, it also increases the amount of calcium that's excreted from the body. "The more salt in your diet, the more calcium ends up in your urine," Dr. Kenney says.

Unfortunately, it's all too easy for Americans to get an excess amount of salt. Foods like potato chips and french fries are obvious sources, but many people don't realize that their whole-wheat bread or whole-grain cereal may contain even more salt than the junk food. Calorie for calorie, wheat bread can have more than double the amount of sodium of potato chips, he says.

And because certain medications—such as steroids, anticonvulsants, some cancer treatments, and antacids with aluminum—can cause bone loss, it's important for both men and women to ask their doctors about the risks associated with these or other medications and get their bone mass tested if their doctor is concerned about their bone health.

Overweight
EATING AWAY THE POUNDS

"Lose a pound a day—without dieting!" "Burn fat—while you sleep!" Yeah, right. When it comes to diets, most of us have swallowed enough snake oil to float a tanker. The only miracle about so-called miracle diets is that we keep trying them.

Losing weight and keeping it off doesn't take a miracle. It rests on one simple premise: "Energy in equals energy out," says Simone French, PhD, professor of epidemiology at the University of Minnesota in Minneapolis. "If you take in more energy than you expend, you gain weight. If you take in less energy than you expend, you lose weight." In other words, calories count. The number of calories you take in has to be less than the number of calories you burn. Exercise also counts because it helps you burn more calories.

Moreover, researchers are finding that what you eat is just as important as how much of it you eat. For example, the body doesn't process the calories in a high-fat chocolate-chip cookie the same way it does the calories in a potato or in a plate of carbohydrate-loaded pasta. Further, studies show that while some foods fuel the impulse to eat, others seem to "switch off" the appetite.

So the real miracle may be that certain foods can actually help, rather than hinder, your efforts to lose weight. Most people trying to lose weight can count calories in their sleep. But calories, while important, are just part of the weight-loss equation. Intriguing weight-loss research from major universities is revealing that when you pack a reduced-calorie diet with high-satisfaction foods, you can lose weight more easily. The magic foods: fruits, veggies, whole grains, lean protein, and good fats.

The High-Satisfaction Solution

Green beans and fresh-from-the vine tomatoes; juicy peaches and luxurious raspberries; stick-to-your-ribs whole grains. These nutrient-dense foods form the backbone of the most effective healthy-eating plans that control your weight. Why? They satisfy. All that fiber means food digests slowly, warding off hunger pangs and crazy food cravings by keeping your blood sugar low and under control—something refined carbs like white bread, white rice, and pasta just can't deliver.

Today, many overweight Americans are insulin-resistant—meaning that their cells "ignore" signals from the hormone insulin to absorb blood sugar. Insulin levels

SATISFACTION GUARANTEED

Controlling appetite is perhaps the key to successfully losing weight, according to a study at the University of Sydney in Australia. Researchers there have identified a number of "high-satisfaction" foods that help keep you feeling full longer. In the accompanying table, anything with a rating of 100 or better (the score given to white bread) is considered satisfying. Foods that scored less than 100 tend not to stick around, so you'll probably wind up eating more of them—and gaining weight.

Food Rating

Potatoes: 323	Bran cereal: 151	Jelly beans: 118
Fish: 225	Eggs: 150	French fries: 116
Oatmeal: 209	Cheese: 146	White bread: 100
Oranges: 202	White rice: 138	Ice cream: 96
Apples: 197	Lentils: 133	Potato chips: 91
Whole-wheat pasta: 188	Brown rice: 132	Yogurt: 88
Steak: 176	Crackers: 127	Peanuts: 84
Baked beans: 168	Cookies: 120	Candy bar: 70
Grapes: 162	White pasta: 119	Doughnut: 68
Grain bread: 154	Bananas: 118	Cake: 65
Popcorn: 154	Cornflakes: 118	Croissant: 47

rise extra high after meals if you're insulin-resistant. It's your body's way of forcing blood sugar into cells. So, if you've just eaten lots of refined carbs, your body's got a huge dose of blood sugar to dispose of. Insulin resistance throws up an extra weight-loss obstacle as well: Researchers think high insulin levels keep fat "locked" in fat cells, where it cannot be burned as readily. When you eat foods that keep your blood sugar low and steady, however, your body pumps out less insulin, and this doesn't happen.

Studies back this up. In a Tufts University-New England Medical Center study of 39 overweight women and men, those with high insulin levels lost an average of 22 pounds in 6 months on the "steady blood sugar" plan—compared with 13 pounds on a diet with more refined carbs. Other research suggests that this eating strategy keeps your metabolism from downshifting dramatically, as happens on most weight-loss diets. Researchers from Children's Hospital Boston found that adult dieters who ate low-glycemic index (GI) foods burned 80 more calories per day than those on a higher-GI, lower-fat diet. They also felt more energetic.

Don't Be Afraid of Protein . . . or Fat

Two scrambled eggs for breakfast. Chicken salad (made with a smidgeon of canola oil mayo) on whole-wheat bread for lunch. A grilled tenderloin steak for dinner. We bet you're feeling satisfied just reading about these healthy weight-loss-friendly entrées!

It used to be that dieters were told to steer clear of liquid fats (no salad dressings, no cooking in oil) and fatty protein (watch out for those well-marbled steaks). After all, conventional wisdom said, fat's got 9 calories per gram, more than twice what you'd find in carbs like bread or a low-fat cookie. Fat on your plate . . . fat on your hips . . . was the mantra. But researchers now say that we actually need good mono- and polyunsaturated fats, like those found in seafood, olive oil, and canola oil, to maintain a healthy cardiovascular system and nervous system. And it's now been shown that good fats and good protein both have the unique power to satisfy hunger as well.

Protein makes you feel full after eating and keeps you feeling full for hours. A new study from the Rochester Center for Obesity Research in Michigan found that 30 women who started their day with two eggs and toast felt so much more full and satisfied than those who had a bagel and cream cheese that they ate 274 fewer calories the rest of the day. The egg eaters even ate fewer calories the following day. Eggs, noted the researchers, are simply more satisfying than breads and bagels. In a Danish study of 25 women and men, those who ate a bit more protein lost 10 percent more belly fat than those on a higher-carb plan—and what they lost was dangerous fat tucked around internal organs that raises risk for diabetes and heart disease.

A moderate amount of good fat—the kind in nuts and nut butters, olive and canola oils, and oily, cold-water fish—has weight-loss advantages, too. When 65 overweight women and men followed a 1,000-calorie-a-day diet for 24 weeks, those who ate almonds at snack time lost 18 percent of their body weight, while those whose treats were carbohydrate-based (such as wheat crackers or baked potatoes) lost just 11 percent. The nut eaters whittled their waists 14 percent; the carb snackers, 9 percent. Other research shows that eating a moderate amount of peanut butter every day also aids weight loss.

High-Satisfaction Foods

If your idea of a weight-loss plan is to "eat light," you may want to consider doing just the opposite. Research suggests that controlling appetite and weight gain may be as simple as choosing "high-satisfaction" foods.

Researchers at the University of Sydney in Australia had volunteers eat 240-calorie portions of a variety of foods, including fruits, baked goods, snack foods, high-carbohydrate foods, high-protein foods, and cereal. After eating, the participants rated their feelings of hunger every 15 minutes. The goal was to see which foods kept them feeling satisfied the longest.

White bread was assigned an automatic score of 100 points, and all other foods were measured against that. Here's how the menu lined up. A potato topped the list, receiving a score of 323 and making it more than three times as satisfying as white bread. It was followed by fish (with a score of 225), oatmeal (209), oranges (202), apples (197), and whole-wheat pasta (188). Surprisingly, baked goods got the least satisfactory ratings. Even more surprising, the more fat a food contained, the less likely it was to rank high on the scale. A croissant, for example, received a score of 47, which meant that it was less than half as satisfying as a piece of white bread. Foods containing more protein, fiber, and water received higher scores.

To put the results of this study to work, always select satisfying foods like vegetables and fruits over their higher-fat, lower-fiber counterparts, recommends Barbara Rolls, PhD, professor in the nutrition department at Pennsylvania State University. For example, choose a baked potato over a serving of french fries. Between meals, snack on a cup or two of air-popped popcorn, which is more likely to satisfy you than the same amount of potato chips. Better yet, grab an apple or an orange. The idea is to satisfy your hunger immediately and help control your appetite for the next few hours, without loading you up with unwanted calories.

Doctor's Top Tip

Filling your plate with high-fiber fruits, veggies, and whole grains plus generous portions of lean protein may be the smartest weight-control strategy ever, says Donald K. Layman, PhD, professor of nutrition in the department of food science and human nutrition at the University of Illinois at Urbana-Champaign. In a 4-month study of 48 overweight women, those who ate more protein and fewer refined carbs lost 20 percent more weight than those on an equal-calorie, higher-carb plan—and most of their loss was body fat, not muscle.

Protein foods like eggs and lean meat contain an amino acid that seems to protect muscle, Dr. Layman says. And study volunteers in the high-protein group ate about 9 ounces per day.

Parkinson's Disease

FOODS THAT EASE SIDE EFFECTS

Every move you make, from turning the pages of this book to swallowing a sip of water, is controlled by a brain chemical called dopamine, which transmits signals to muscles throughout your body. But in people with Parkinson's disease, the cells that make dopamine are damaged or destroyed. As dopamine levels decline, the simplest movements become increasingly difficult.

There isn't a cure for Parkinson's disease yet. But research shows that what you eat can help your medications work more effectively (and may even augment them). Eating right can also ease uncomfortable and even dangerous "side effects" of this condition, such as constipation, unwanted weight loss, and risk of bone fractures.

Balancing Protein and Levodopa

The drug levodopa is the first-line treatment for Parkinson's disease; early on, this dopamine-increasing medication works so well, you may forget you have a medical condition at all. But people with Parkinson's often quickly notice a food-related double-whammy when they take it: On an empty stomach, levodopa can cause nausea and even vomiting; but on a full stomach, absorption of this important drug can be so delayed that Parkinson's symptoms return. Taking it with a meal that contains protein can also interfere with effectiveness because levodopa enters the brain by piggybacking on the same carrier molecules that transport protein molecules (amino acids) across the blood/brain barrier. These molecules grab amino acids first, leaving levodopa with no way to get inside.

It's a catch-22. But experts at the Parkinson's Disease Foundation have an answer: Take levodopa on an empty stomach a half-hour to an hour before a meal. If nausea's a problem, have your medication with a slice of bread or some crackers. Sipping 4 to 5 ounces of water with your medication can speed absorption, too. Then eat moderate amounts of protein at mealtime.

Smart Food Strategies

So far, researchers have not found any food or supplement that protects against the progressive brain-cell destruction that happens in Parkinson's disease. But these food strategies can help ease side effects.

Calcium for fracture prevention. Up to 68 percent of people with Parkinson's experience falls due to muscle stiffness, frozen movement, shuffling, balance problems, or stooped posture. Falls raise the risk for broken bones. Be sure to include three servings of milk, cheese, or yogurt in your diet every day to maintain bone density. Add a 500-milligram calcium supplement with vitamin D for each serving you miss.

Fiber and fluids to counter constipation. Digestive slowdowns can lead to constipation in Parkinson's disease. Fight back by sipping plenty of fluids (aim for eight 8-ounce glasses of water or herbal tea per day) and by including fruits, veggies, and whole grains at each meal.

Small meals for slower eaters. Movement problems can make feeding yourself, then chewing and swallowing, a surprisingly slow affair. The result: The food's cold before you can eat it all, and you may end up not eating enough to maintain a healthy weight. Eating smaller, more frequent meals can help.

Food adjustments for levodopa-induced nausea. If your medications make you feel sick, these steps can help: Choose cold drinks that contain a little bit of sugar to calm your tummy; avoid orange and grapefruit juice, as well as fried or greasy foods. If the smell of hot food triggers nausea, eat food cold or at room temperature. Rest, with your head elevated, after a meal. If you feel sick when you wake up in the morning, keep crackers on your bedside table. Munch a few before you get up.

The Fava Bean Story

For years, people with Parkinson's disease have traded stories about getting relief by eating fava beans. Research now suggests that they might be on to something. One study even found that people eating huge amounts of favas—approximately 10 ounces a day—got about the same benefits as they did when taking medication, says Christine Tangney, PhD, associate professor of clinical nutrition at Rush-Presbyterian–St. Luke's Medical Center in Chicago.

It makes sense, but read this before you dig in. Fava beans (also known as broad

> ## Doctor's Top Tip
>
> Something to smile about when you pour that second cup of morning coffee: A study from Duke University has found that drinking two cups of joe a day could cut your lifetime risk for Parkinson's by 40 percent. The link? Possibly dopamine. Levels of this message-carrying brain chemical plummet in Parkinson's, but research shows that coffee seems to increase it. (Smoking cigarettes also cut risk, but we won't recommend that!) "Caffeine may modify underlying genetic susceptibilities that exist in families with Parkinson's disease, but further work is needed to see how this interaction ultimately plays out," says researcher Mark A. Stacy, MD, associate professor of medicine and director of the Duke Movement Disorders Center in Durham, North Carolina.

beans) contain levodopa—the same active ingredient in Parkinson's disease medicines like Sinemet, Madopar, Dopar, Larodopa. (Cool fact: The whole fava plant, including leaves, stems, and pods, contains levodopa.) The body converts the levodopa in fava beans into dopamine, the chemical the brain needs to communicate with muscles, Dr. Tangney says. Three ounces (about 84 grams or ½ cup) of fresh green fava beans, or 3 ounces of canned green fava beans, drained, may contain about 50 to 100 milligrams of levodopa.

A few small research studies suggest the beans can help control Parkinson's symptoms—but not for everyone. Some people report no benefits, others have side effects such as stomach upset, and still others get the same serious side effects that come from long-term use of levodopa drugs such as dyskinesia, or difficulty controlling your body's movements.

Fava beans aren't risk-free. Each batch may have a different levodopa concentration, depending on the species of fava beans used and growing conditions, including location and rainfall levels. Favas can also cause allergic reactions in some people. And if you have a rare, inherited condition called favism—meaning that you lack an enzyme called glucose-6-phosphate dehydrogenase (G6PD)—eating fava beans can lead to kidney failure. People who take monoamine oxidase inhibitor (MAOI) drugs should talk with the prescribing doctor before trying favas—some of these drugs react with high-dopamine foods to raise blood pressure to dangerous levels.

Now that you know the risks, if you still want to add fava beans to your treatment plan, do talk with your doctor. You will probably be asked to begin with an ounce—about 2 tablespoons—a day. If the beans ease your symptoms, the doctor may adjust your medications. If there's no effect, you may be able to raise your intake slightly.

Parsley

MORE THAN A GARNISH

There's probably no other green as universally recognized as parsley. Each year, tons of this aromatic leaf are placed upon dinner plates worldwide, only to be scraped away with the leftovers. To most, parsley's purpose is merely to garnish, along with a slice of orange or lemon, an otherwise brown-looking entrée. But parsley's original intent upon the dinner plate was for a much nobler cause. Parsley is nature's original breath freshener, and its bracing taste deliciously cleanses the palate.

Today, the strength of these sprigs supersedes sweet-smelling breath. Eaten as a food rather than a garnish, parsley has earned a reputation as a natural healer.

HEALING POWER

Can Help:

Relieve urinary tract infections

Ease premenstrual discomfort

Bolster heart health

Urinary Relief

Parsley's healing magic can be found in two compounds it contains, myristicin and apiol, which can help increase the flow of urine. Passing more urine helps remove infection-causing bacteria from the urinary tract. This same diuretic action can also help prevent premenstrual bloating. Nibbling parsley in the days before menstruation can help increase urine flow, thus removing excess fluids from the body before they cause discomfort.

Leafy Medicine Chest

Even though parsley is generally used in small amounts, it has as much healing power, tablespoon for tablespoon, as many of the more widely known healing foods. For example, a half-cup of fresh parsley contains 40 milligrams of vitamin C, or 66 percent of the Daily Value (DV) for this vitamin. That's more than half the amount found in a whole orange. A diet rich in vitamin C can help protect against rheumatoid arthritis and osteoarthritis, recent research suggests.

> ### Doctor's Top Tip
>
> Many of us add salt to boiling water when cooking pasta. If you're trying to cut back on salt to reduce water-weight gain or control blood pressure, call on parsley. Omit the salt when cooking noodles, and instead flavor the water, or the cooked pasta, with chopped parsley, suggests dietitian Alice Henneman, MS, RD, an extension educator with the University of Nebraska Cooperative Extension in Lincoln.

In the Kitchen

Even though fresh parsley is readily available in supermarkets, it's often in short supply at home. The reason for this is that parsley is somewhat perishable and doesn't always last long enough to use for a second meal.

To keep parsley fresh and available, here's what you need to do:

Keep it cold. Parsley will wilt within hours when stored at room temperature, so it's important to get it into the refrigerator as soon as possible.

Store it right. Parsley comes in big bunches. To store it for up to a week, wrap the leaves in a moist paper towel, and keep it in a loosely closed plastic bag in the crisper drawer of the refrigerator.

For long-term storage of extra from the farmers' market, grocery store, or your own garden, dry flat-leaf parsley in a single layer on a clean dish towel. Store it in a sealed container in a cool, dark, dry spot. Freeze curly-leaf varieties in single-serve portions in a freezer-safe container or a small zip-top bag. Toss, unthawed, into soups, stocks, or stews.

Let it drink. Another way to keep parsley fresh is to stand the bunch in a drinking glass filled halfway with water, with a moist paper towel wrapped around the leaves to prevent them from wilting.

Wash only what you'll use. Fresh parsley is fragile, so only clean what you'll use in the meal you're making. Let it soak in a bowl of cold water. Swish, then drain. Repeat until all dirt is gone.

Parsley is also a good source of folate, with a half-cup containing 46 micrograms, or more than 11 percent of the DV. You need folate, a B vitamin, for producing red blood cells and helping to prevent birth defects. Folate may also cut your risk for heart disease and cancers of the colon and cervix.

GETTING THE MOST

Make it a main ingredient. Even though parsley is best known as a culinary garnish, you'll get more of its healing benefits by using it as a main ingredient. The Lebanese salad called tabbouleh, for example, typically calls for one or more cups of chopped fresh parsley. Or you can add half a bunch to a green salad. Using whole sprigs will provide a pleasant texture, along with a celery-like flavor. Italian flat-leaf parsley has a stronger flavor than curly parsley.

Store it well. Since it's easier to store dried parsley than fresh, most cooks have a small bag or bottle in the kitchen pantry. To prevent dried parsley from giving up its benefits, store it in a cool, dry place, in an airtight opaque container.

Parsnips

A PARTNER AGAINST STROKE

Parsnips might as well be called Pursed Lips for the reaction that these strong-tasting, oddly sweet vegetables often get. And they certainly won't win any awards for Best-Looking Vegetable in Show. They look like carrots that have seen a ghost.

But despite parsnips' strong flavor and pale appearance, their nutritional profile is attractive. A member of the parsley family, parsnips are good sources of folate, fiber, and phenolic acids, which have been shown in laboratory studies to help block cancer.

HEALING POWER

Can Help:

Prevent colon cancer

Lower the risk of heart disease

Stabilize blood sugar levels

Decrease the risk of stroke

Protect against birth defects

Fabulous Fiber

Whenever experts compile their "A" lists for healing substances, they put dietary fiber near the top. And parsnips are an excellent source. One cup of cooked parsnips contains nearly 7 grams, or 28 percent of the Daily Value (DV) for fiber.

A little more than half of the fiber in parsnips is the soluble kind, which means that it becomes gel-like in the digestive system. This helps block the intestine from absorbing fats and cholesterol from foods. At the same time, it dilutes bile acids in the intestine, which can prevent them from causing cancer. Parsnips also contain insoluble fiber, which speeds the rate at which stools move through the intestine. This is important because the less time bile acids are present in the intestine, the less likely they are to damage cells, causing changes that could lead to cancer.

In a review of more than 200 scientific studies, researchers found that getting more dietary fiber can protect against a wide variety of cancers, including cancer of the stomach, pancreas, and colon. Fiber has shown similarly impressive ability to relieve or prevent many other conditions as well. Researchers have found that getting enough fiber in the diet can help prevent hemorrhoids and other intestinal conditions. Fiber can also curb the blood sugar swings that occur with diabetes.

Stroke Prevention

Some nutrition experts say that too little of the B vitamin folate is our number one nutritional deficiency, particularly among younger folks, who often eat large amounts of fast food that's largely devoid of vitamins. Parsnips are a good source of folate, with 1 cup containing 91 micrograms, or 23 percent of the DV.

Getting enough folate has been shown to prevent certain birth defects. It's also strongly suspected of reducing the risk of heart attack and stroke. Folate decreases blood levels of homocysteine, an amino acid that may promote blockage of blood vessels.

Researchers in the Framingham Heart Study found that men who ate the most produce had a 59 percent lower stroke rate than those who ate the least. Even those who ate just a little more produce reaped substantial benefits. The study found that folks who helped themselves to an extra three servings of fruits and vegetables a day lowered their risk of stroke by 22 percent.

Obviously, unless you truly have a passion for parsnips, it's unlikely that you'll ever eat three or more servings a day. But eating just a half-cup will provide not only fiber and folate but also 280 milligrams of potassium, or 8 percent of the DV for this mineral. This will go a long way toward keeping your arteries in the swim.

The Acid Test

Along with carrots and celery, parsnips are members of the umbelliferae family. Foods in this family contain a number of natural compounds called phytonutrients, which have been shown in laboratory studies to block the spread of cancer cells. Chief among these are compounds called phenolic acids. What phenolic acids do is attach themselves to potential cancer-causing agents in the body, creating a bigger molecule—so big that the body can't absorb it.

Research has shown that members of the umbelliferae family can also fight cancer by inhibiting tumor growth.

In the Kitchen

Parsnips cook up like carrots, except they don't take as much time. What's more, they're prepared in similar ways—that is, they can be mashed, puréed, or served in chunks.

To a greater degree than carrots, however, parsnips are a vigorous vegetable. It's not uncommon for them to grow quite large, sometimes up to about 20 inches long. Large parsnips tend to have a strong flavor that many people find disagreeable. "Look for small or medium parsnips," advises nutrition specialist Marilyn A. Swanson, PhD, RD, adjunct associate professor of pediatrics at Baylor College of Medicine in Houston, Texas. "They have a better flavor and texture." Parsnips measuring about 8 inches in length are the tenderest. You can accentuate their sweetness by adding ginger, cinnamon, nutmeg, allspice, or mace to mashed or steamed parsnips.

The research is still preliminary, so it's not yet certain how effective parsnips themselves are at blocking cancer—though there's plenty of data proving that a diet rich in a variety of veggies does protect against cancer. And the American Institute for Cancer Research gives parsnips' nutritional profile (lots of fiber and health-promoting phytochemicals) high marks. So go ahead and enjoy this vegetable for all the fiber and folate it contains.

GETTING THE MOST

Buy them after the first frost. Look for locally grown parsnips at farmers' markets after a cold snap. After the first frost, the starches in parsnips begin converting to sugar—lending them a surprisingly sweet, dense flavor.

Look for handsome young ones. Select medium-size roots with uniform creamy beige skin. Avoid limp, pitted, or shriveled roots. And avoid those with lots of little hair-like rootlets—they tend to be tough. Extra tip: Make sure you've really got parsnips—often, they're displayed next to look-alike parsley root. But while parsley root is sold with greens attached, parsnips are more often sold without their leafy tops.

Trim the greens. If your parsnips come with greens on top, snip the greens before storing in the fridge. Otherwise, the greens will draw moisture and nutrients from the root itself, according to nutritionist Densie Webb, PhD, RD, coauthor of *The Dish on Eating Healthy and Being Fabulous.*

Keep them cold. Although some root vegetables keep well at room temperature, parsnips should be kept in the refrigerator—or a root cellar, if you have one. "Keeping them cold and humid will prevent them from drying out and losing some of their nutritional value," says dietitian Susan Thom, RD, a nutrition consultant in Brecksville, Ohio.

Stock up ahead of time. Parsnips will keep for a couple of weeks when stored in the refrigerator. Wrap unwashed roots in a paper towel, then store them in a perforated or loosely closed plastic bag. "The longer you keep them in storage, the sweeter they get," says Thom.

Boil before peeling. Some of the nutrients in parsnips are water-soluble and are quickly lost during cooking. "They're fragile in boiling water—some of those vita-

> ## Doctor's Top Tip
>
> High oven temperatures intensify the flavor of the natural sugars in parsnips. Experts at the Centers for Disease Control and Prevention in Atlanta suggest roasting parsnips with other root vegetables such as carrots or sweet potatoes in a 400°F oven with a drizzle of olive oil and your favorite herbs. A variation recommended by the American Institute for Cancer Research: Roast parsnips with sweet potatoes and apple chunks, then flavor with reduced-sodium soy sauce and honey.

mins float away," says Anne Dubner, RD, a nutrition consultant in Houston, Texas. In fact, you can lose almost half the water-soluble nutrients by cooking peeled parsnips. The solution, of course, is to cook them unpeeled. Once they're tender, let them cool, then scrape or peel the skin away.

Mashed Parsnips with Sour Cream

1 pound parsnips
⅓ cup fat-free sour cream
⅛ teaspoon ground allspice
⅛ teaspoon salt

Trim about ½ inch from the top and bottom of each parsnip. Scrub the parsnips well but do not peel.

Bring a large saucepan of water to a boil over high heat. Add the parsnips. Cover, reduce the heat to medium-low, and cook until very tender, 25 to 30 minutes. Test for doneness by inserting the tip of a sharp knife into a parsnip.

Remove the parsnips with tongs, and place on a clean work surface. Set the cooking water aside.

Using a paper towel to protect your fingers, hold each parsnip by the end, and scrape off the skin with a small paring knife or vegetable peeler. Discard the skin. Place the parsnips in a large bowl.

Add the sour cream, allspice, salt, and 2 tablespoons of the reserved cooking liquid. With a potato masher or fork, coarsely mash the parsnips. Add 1 to 3 more tablespoons of cooking liquid if necessary to make the mixture smooth and creamy.

Makes 4 servings

PER SERVING

Calories: 99	Cholesterol: 0 mg
Total fat: 0.3 g	Sodium: 91 mg
Saturated fat: 0 g	Dietary fiber: 4.3 g

Pears

THE CHOLESTEROL-FIGHTING FRUIT

The tender, juicy pear—once extolled as "the fruit of the gods"—got a headline-grabbing nutritional upgrade recently. Once thought to contain a respectable 4 grams of fiber, this sweet treat was reclassified by the FDA as a fiber superstar in late 2005, when new research revealed that a medium pear actually packs a whopping 6 grams. A single pear, we now know, provides one-quarter of your daily fiber needs.

That's good news for your heart, since 41 percent of the fiber in a medium-size pear is pectin—a type of water-soluble fiber that whisks cholesterol out of your body.

Soluble fiber acts like Velcro, trapping cholesterol molecules in bile acids—one of the body's digestive fluids—in the intestine before they get absorbed into the bloodstream. And because pectin can't pass through the intestinal wall, it goes into the stool, taking cholesterol along with it, explains Mary Ellen Camire, PhD, professor in the department of food science and human nutrition at the University of Maine in Orono. When your body needs more bile acids, it must pull more bad low-density lipoprotein (LDL) cholesterol out of your bloodstream to manufacture them—and in the process, lowers levels in your blood. "Eating pears on a regular basis can have a big impact on lowering cholesterol," Dr. Camire says. "There aren't many fruits that measure up."

The other type of fiber in pears—insoluble fiber—has its own health benefits. Insoluble fiber, as the name suggests, doesn't dissolve in the intestine. What it does, however, is absorb large amounts of water. This causes stools to pass more easily and quickly through the digestive tract, which helps prevent constipation and hemorrhoids and also reduces the risk of colon cancer.

HEALING POWER
Can Help:
Lower cholesterol and blood pressure
Boost immunity
Improve memory and alertness
Keep bones strong

Mineral Magic

With 190 milligrams of potassium, or 5 percent of the Daily Value (DV) for this mineral, a fresh pear can help fight high blood pressure. Experts say getting a total of 3,500 milligrams of this important mineral each day could cut blood pressure enough to lower stroke risk by 22 to 40 percent.

Pears also provide 11 percent of the vitamin C and 9.5 percent of the copper you need each day. Both function as antioxidants in your body, disarming cell-damaging free radicals, while vitamin C also bolsters immunity by stimulating infection-fighting white blood cells.

But that's not all. The presence of the trace mineral boron in pears plays a role in keeping bones strong—good news for postmenopausal women at risk for osteoporosis, the brittle-bone disease that can lead to debilitating fractures. Boron is also brain food: In one study by USDA scientists, reflexes and mental alertness improved when people were given additional boron.

GETTING THE MOST

Pears are usually harvested just before they're ripe—the flesh spoils easily once they're completely ready to eat. That means the pears you find in most stores need to sit for a few days in a bowl or paper bag in a warm spot outside of the fridge, suggests Cristie Mather of the Pear Bureau Northwest—the marketing group that represents American farmers in Oregon and Washington who grow more than 80 percent of the nation's pears.

To test for ripeness, press near the stem. It will "give" under gentle pressure when it's sweet, juicy, and ready to munch. Pears ripen from the inside out—don't wait until the flesh around the middle is soft—the rest may be overripe by then.

In the Kitchen

With more than 5,000 varieties of pears worldwide, you could eat a different one every day for years and never have the same taste twice. Here are a few of the pears you're most likely to find in neighborhood markets.

Anjou. These pears have a yellow-green skin and are usually available in winter. They're sweet and very juicy and make a pleasant addition to salads.

Bartlett. Available during the summer and early fall, Bartletts have yellow-green skin and a sweet and juicy flesh. They can be eaten raw as a snack and are also delicious poached or in cobblers.

Bosc. Bosc pears have a slender neck, russeted yellow skin, and a sweet-tart flavor. The flesh is firm, making them a good choice for poaching. They can even be grated, adding a sweet accent to oatmeal or dry cereal.

Comice. Comice pears have melt-in-your-mouth texture and a sweet fragrance and a color ranging from greenish yellow to yellow brushed with red. Because they're so soft and lush, they're frequently served as a dessert fruit.

Once ripe, store in a zip-top bag in the coldest part of your fridge. Keep away from cabbage, carrots, celery, onions, and potatoes—all absorb pear odors. Onions can also impart their own odors to pears.

Keep it clothed. Most of a pear's fiber is in the peel. By eating pears with the skin on, you'll get the full complement of fiber, along with the cholesterol-lowering benefits, Dr. Camire says.

Fresh is better. While canned pears are convenient, they don't provide anywhere near the benefits of fresh, says Donald V. Schlimme, PhD, professor emeritus of nutrition and food science at the University of Maryland in College Park. For one thing, canned pears have been peeled, so they have lost most of their healing fiber. In addition, they may lose large amounts of nutrients during the canning process.

This isn't to say that you don't gain anything from canned pears. You do, although you probably don't want it. A serving of canned pears packed in heavy syrup delivers 25 percent more calories than its fresh counterpart, Dr. Schlimme says.

Doctor's Top Tip

Got a chronic cough? Munch a pear. In a study of 49,140 men and women, National Institutes of Health (NIH) researchers found that those who ate the most pears (as well as apples and grapes) had the lowest rates of coughing problems, notes researcher Lesley M. Butler, MD, of the NIH's Epidemiology Branch in Research Triangle Park, North Carolina. Antioxidants in pears and other fruits may protect against lung damage, he suspects.

Pear and Smoked Turkey Salad

- 4 **Anjou or Bartlett pears**
- 2 **ounces thinly sliced smoked turkey breast**
- 2 **tablespoons rice vinegar or white-wine vinegar**
- 4 **teaspoons olive oil**
- 1 **tablespoon honey**
- 2 **tablespoons minced fresh basil**
  Freshly ground black pepper

Quarter the pears lengthwise, and remove the cores. Cut each quarter in half lengthwise. Arrange the pears decoratively on a platter, alternating occasionally with strips of smoked turkey.

In a small bowl, combine the vinegar, oil, and honey. Whisk until smooth. Add the basil and stir to mix. Spoon the dressing evenly over the pears and turkey. Season lightly with pepper.

Makes 4 appetizer servings

PER SERVING

Calories: 193	Cholesterol: 6 mg
Total fat: 5 g	Sodium: 175 mg
Saturated fat: 0.7 g	Dietary fiber: 7 g

Peas

LITTLE GREEN CANCER TRAPS

HEALING POWER

Can Help:

Relieve cold symptoms

Prevent cancer and
heart disease

Thanks to peas and an Austrian monk named Gregor Johann Mendel, we now have the science of genetics. Mendel found that when he bred two different types of peas together, their offspring had the features of both "parents." He concluded that physical characteristics could be passed from generation to generation—not only in plants but in people as well.

Peas are more than an interesting scientific footnote, however. Researchers have found that they contain a powerful compound that can help prevent healthy cells from becoming cancerous. In addition, peas contain substances that can help lower cholesterol and ease symptoms of the common cold.

It's Healthy Being Green

The cancer-fighting compound in peas is called chlorophyllin, which is the pigment responsible for giving them their shiny green hue. Chlorophyllin (which is related to chlorophyll, the substance that allows plants to convert sunlight into food) has a special molecular shape that allows it to grab cancer-causing chemicals in the body. "When you eat peas, the chlorophyllin attaches to carcinogens and helps prevent them from being absorbed," says Mary Ellen Camire, PhD, professor in the department of food science and human nutrition at the University of Maine in Orono.

Researchers haven't pinned down exactly how many peas you'd have to eat to get the most benefits from chlorophyllin, Dr. Camire says. You can't go wrong, however, by including them on your menu as often as possible, along with other bright, green vegetables. After all, the greener a vegetable is, the more chlorophyllin it contains.

Helping Your Heart

Doctors have known for a long time that getting more dietary fiber is one of the best ways to lower cholesterol, and with it the risk for heart disease and other serious conditions. Green peas are an excellent source of fiber, with more than 4 grams in each half-cup serving.

Research suggests that eating peas can also bring down levels of triglycerides,

In the Kitchen

Nature couldn't have made shucking peas more convenient. Pea pods come with their own strings, which work like zippers. Give a quick pull, and the peas tumble out. It only takes about 7 minutes to shuck enough peas to get 1 cup.

To shuck peas quickly and easily, here's what you need to do.

1. Pinch off the blossom end of the pod, so the string dangles at the end.

2. Grip the string and pull it down the length of the pod.

3. Using your thumb, nudge the pod open while pushing out the peas into a waiting bowl or cup.

blood fats that play a role in heart disease. A study in Denmark, for example, found that when people were given small amounts of pea fiber in addition to their usual diets, total triglyceride levels fell almost 13 percent within 2 weeks.

These tasty green orbs are packed with the B vitamins folate and B_6, nutrients that help your body keep levels of homocysteine under control. High levels of homocysteine are associated with a higher risk for heart disease and stroke and with weaker bones, too.

Pods of Good Health

Peas have always been a favorite in school cafeterias—not because they're fun to flip off a fork but because they contain an abundance of disease-fighting vitamins. A half-cup of green peas, for example, contains more than 11 milligrams of vitamin C, or almost 19 percent of the Daily Value (DV). This is important because getting enough vitamin C in the diet has been shown to reduce the risk of cancer and heart disease. And when you have a cold, getting extra vitamin C can make the symptoms just a little more bearable.

Peas are also loaded with vitamin K, which helps keep levels of the bone-building protein osteocalcin high. Like a carpenter nailing together the sturdy frame of a well-built house, osteocalcin "anchors" calcium molecules within bone.

GETTING THE MOST

Fresh is finer. Peas shucked right out of the pod have more vitamin C than those that come in a can because canned peas lose many of their nutrients during processing, says Donald V. Schlimme, PhD, professor emeritus in the department of

Doctor's Top Tip

Peas are actually a legume—a half-cup has as much protein as a tablespoon of peanut butter (minus the fat!), say experts at the Mayo Clinic. Studies show that getting adequate protein at each meal cuts cravings and boosts satisfaction longer after eating—making peas perfect for weight loss. Steam the peas, then mix them with a touch of olive oil, some chopped fresh mint, and salt and pepper to taste for a fast, height-of-summer side dish.

nutrition and food science at the University of Maryland in College Park.

Go for the greenest. The pods of green peas should be firm, smooth, and a medium, grassy-green color. Skip darkened pods or those that look pale or dotted with specks of mildew. Pass up any that look water-soaked, too. The peas inside won't be very tasty. The sugar in peas converts swiftly to starch in heat—buy from supermarkets and farm stands that keep their peas refrigerated.

Visit the freezer case. Fresh peas can be hard to come by at certain times of the year, but frozen peas are always available. While they lack some of the crispness of fresh, they're just as good for you because freezing keeps most of the nutrients, especially vitamin C, intact.

Crunch an early summer snack. Farm stands and backyard gardens overflow with snow peas and sugar snap peas—some of the first garden veggies to ripen. Enjoy them in the pod—their sweet, refreshing crunch is great as a snack with fat-free dip, or add the peas to stir fries. Choose small, firm snow peas and snap peas—they're sweeter than the bigger ones.

Shuck the pods for more fiber. Even though edible-podded peas (such as sugar snap peas) contain large amounts of vitamin C, the peas themselves contain most of the fiber, folate, niacin, phosphorus, riboflavin, thiamin, and vitamin A. To get the most nutritional bang for your buck, it's better to eat a half-cup of shelled peas than an equal serving of peas in the pod, Dr. Camire says.

Turn on the steamer. Whether you're using fresh or frozen peas, it's best to heat them by steaming rather than boiling. Boiling leaches nutrients out of peas into the cooking water. In addition, the high heat used in boiling may destroy some of the nutrients, particularly the vitamin C. If you don't have a steamer, heating peas quickly in the microwave is a good alternative.

Pectin

STAY WELL WITH GEL

The next time you sit down to breakfast, spread a little jam on a piece of toast. Then take a bite from a succulent pear. Even though their tastes and textures are totally different, these foods actually have something in common, and that something is very good for your health.

Jellies and jams, along with legumes, fruits, vegetables, and a variety of grains, contain pectin, a type of dietary fiber that acts as a natural thickener. Food manufacturers often use pectin as a binding agent in jellies and jams. Nature, as it turns out, uses pectin in much the same way.

Because pectin is a water-soluble fiber, it dissolves in the body, creating a sticky gel inside the intestine. The gel binds to potentially harmful substances, preventing them from being absorbed. At the same time, it causes nutrients to be absorbed a little more slowly. Both of these factors make pectin a key player in preventing a number of conditions, from heart disease and diabetes to weight gain.

Protection from Heart Disease, Diabetes . . . and Cancer, Too

The biggest health threat that Americans face is heart disease, and one of the leading causes of heart disease is high cholesterol. The danger from cholesterol is so great, in fact, that doctors estimate that for every 1 percent that you lower your cholesterol, you reduce the risk of heart disease by 2 percent.

Getting more pectin in your diet is an excellent strategy for lowering cholesterol, says nutrition researcher Beth Kunkel, PhD, RD, professor of food and nutrition at Clemson University in South Carolina. Because pectin dissolves into a gel, molecules of fat and cholesterol get trapped before they make it into your bloodstream. And because pectin itself isn't absorbed, it goes out of the body in the stool, taking the fat and cholesterol with it.

Pectin helps lower cholesterol in yet another way. Because it isn't digested, bacteria in the intestine start gobbling it up. In the process, they release chemicals that travel to the liver, interrupting the production of cholesterol, says cardiologist Michael H. Davidson, MD, executive medical director of Radiant Research in Chicago. In fact, research has shown that people who get about 6 grams of pectin a

Doctor's Top Tip

Eat a smart mix of high-fiber foods for the best heart disease protection strategy, says Arja Erkkila, PhD, a researcher in the department of clinical nutrition at the University of Kuopio in Finland. That means pectin-rich fruits such as apples, blackberries, boysenberries, grapefruit, plums, and oranges—as well as vegetables and whole grains packed with insoluble fiber. Together, studies show, they lower levels of cholesterol and cut your risk for heart attack.

day—approximately the amount in 3 cups of grapefruit sections—can lower their cholesterol by at least 5 percent. While grapefruit is a good source of pectin, with 1 gram in a 4-ounce serving of sections, it's not the only one. Apples, bananas, and peaches are good sources, as are beans.

Pectin also helps lower insulin resistance—a serious health threat often linked with obesity—say nutrition researchers from the University of Kuopio in Finland. Less insulin resistance means your cells easily "obey" signals from the hormone insulin to absorb blood sugar—lowering sugar levels and reducing your body's need to produce extra insulin. Less sugar and less insulin cut your risk for diabetes and for cardiovascular disease.

Getting more pectin can be especially important for people with diabetes, who must do everything they can to keep their blood sugar levels steady. Since pectin slows the rate at which sugars are absorbed, it can prevent the sudden surges of glucose (blood sugar) that can damage the nerves, eyes, and organs in people with diabetes.

There's emerging evidence that pectin fights cancer, too. Researchers at Taiwan's Taipei Medical University say pectin seems to protect cells from damage that can lead to cancer, and it can also slow the proliferation of cancer cells. It may work by cooling off damaging inflammation in the body.

Smoother Digestion

People who are trying to lose weight are often advised to eat more fruits, legumes, and other pectin-rich foods. There's a good reason for this. When pectin dissolves in the stomach, it gradually expands, taking up more room. At the same time, it slows the absorption of sugars and nutrients into the bloodstream. This helps you feel more satisfied even when you haven't had a lot to eat.

"Pectin helps to give you that feeling of fullness, so you don't need to eat as much," says researcher Barbara F. Harland, PhD, professor of nutrition at Howard University in Washington, D.C. "One of the most important things for losing weight and keeping it off is getting more fiber, including pectin."

In the Kitchen

Pectin, whether it comes in a plastic package or ready-wrapped in nature's own fruit, is what makes it possible for jellies, jams, and preserves to gel. An easy, fun, and fast way to watch pectin at work is to make your own cranberry sauce for Thanksgiving. Simply heat a cup of water and a cup of sugar to a boil, then dump in a bag of cranberries. Bring back to a boil, then simmer. Within minutes, the berries begin to break down, releasing pectin and causing the mixture to rapidly thicken.

Here are a few pectin pointers for the next time you're making your own jam, jelly, or sauce.

- Some fruits, like apples and gooseberries, are naturally high in pectin and will gel without the addition of commercial pectin.
- Blueberries and peaches contain very little pectin. To help them gel, you'll probably need to add liquid or powdered pectin.
- Another way to promote gelling is to combine low-pectin fruits with those that are higher in pectin. Apples are a common addition to jams, not just for their flavor but also because of their high pectin content.

Phytonutrients
BEYOND VITAMINS AND MINERALS

Somewhere in China, a 12-year-old girl sits down to her evening meal of tofu-scallion soup, a bowl of rice, green tea, and a stir-fry containing bok choy, snow peas, and eggplant.

Across the globe in the United States, a girl the same age dines on a burger and fries and washes it down with a frosty cola.

If both girls continue their culinary courses, the girl in China will be about half as likely to get cancer during her lifetime as her American counterpart.

Now let's sail across the ocean to Finland, where two men are sitting down to their dinner of meat, potatoes, and good beer. One of the men routinely eats an apple a day, along with ⅛ cup of onions and 4 cups of tea. As a result, he's less likely to die of heart disease than his fellow Finn, who sticks to the main course.

What Is Going On Here?

That is a question scientists have asked themselves since Hippocrates first proclaimed, "Let food be thy medicine." What does diet have to do with disease?

More than we ever imagined. We've known for a long time that we need vitamins and minerals from foods to maintain good health and to prevent malnutrition and diseases such as rickets and scurvy. But research is revealing that the essential nutrients we all know about, such as vitamins A through E, are just the beginning: Hidden within plant foods are thousands of compounds that are taking the diet-disease connection to an exciting new level. It appears likely that some of these previously unknown compounds will fight not only deficiency-type diseases such as anemia but also elusive, age-related illnesses such as arthritis, cancer, diabetes, heart disease, high blood pressure, and stroke.

Health from the Garden

Researchers call these compounds phytochemicals or phytonutrients, terms that mean chemicals or nutrients found in plants. They're not there accidentally—they're Mother Nature's way of helping her garden survive and thrive. Potent sulfur compounds in garlic and onions, for instance, act as bug repellents to keep the vegetables healthy. Vibrant pigments like beta-carotene, found in acorn squash and cantaloupe, are natural advertisements, luring animals to eat up—and disperse the plant's seeds. Other compounds protect plants from bacteria, viruses, and other natural enemies.

We aren't Bermuda onions or acorn squashes, so should we care? A convincing stack of research says yes. Nature recycles its precious resources. When we eat plant foods, these compounds protect us, too—not from bugs but from the forces that wreak havoc in humans.

And the research has only begun. Scientists are discovering new phytochemicals all the time and also ways in which these compounds fight disease.

Neutralizing Free Radicals

The family of phytonutrients is a large one, and each member of this family works in several different ways. Their most common weapons against disease, however, appear to be their antioxidant abilities.

Every day, your body is under attack by harmful substances known as free radicals. These are oxygen molecules that, due to pollution, sunlight, and everyday wear and tear, have each lost an electron. As they attempt to regain their missing electrons, they careen through your body, stealing electrons wherever they can. The molecular victims of these raids are your cells themselves—and sometimes even your DNA. Unless this chain reaction is stopped, the result is huge numbers of damaged molecules and, over time, irreparable damage and disease.

Here's an example. Normal cholesterol is a benign, helpful substance. But when cholesterol molecules are damaged by free radicals, they begin sticking to the lining of artery walls, causing hardened arteries and heart disease. Another example: When free radicals attack molecules in your body's DNA, the genetic blueprint that tells your cells how to function, the blueprint is damaged. This can spark dangerous cell changes that lead to cancer and other diseases. Even aging, many scientists believe, is caused by free-radical damage.

The phytonutrients in plants, using their antioxidant powers, can quite literally save your life. Essentially, they step between the marauding free radicals and your body's cells, offering up their own electrons. When free radicals grab these "free" electrons, they become stable again and do no further damage. Most phytonutrients are potent antioxidants.

Eliminating Toxic Wastes

Another way phytonutrients keep us healthy is by neutralizing and flushing toxic chemicals from our bodies before they make us sick. They do this by manipulating enzymes known as phase-1 and phase-2 enzymes, explains Gary Stoner, PhD, professor and cancer researcher at Ohio State University in Columbus.

Phase-1 enzymes are like double agents. They're created by your body and are important for normal cell function. But they have the ability to work against you, too. When cancer-causing toxins enter your system, phase-1 enzymes help make them active. Phase-2 enzymes, on the other hand, are real good guys. They seek out carcinogens and detoxify them before they do damage.

When you eat broccoli or other vegetables, some of the phytonutrients begin stomping out the enemy phase-1 enzymes while increasing the production of helper phase-2 enzymes. This process helps neutralize various cancer-causing toxins that naturally accumulate in the body.

Regulating Hormones

A third way in which some phytonutrients fend off disease is by keeping certain hormones—most notably the female sex hormone estrogen—at healthy levels.

Estrogen is a good news–bad news kind of hormone. When it's produced at normal levels, it helps control everything from menstruation to childbirth. At the same time, it helps keep artery-clogging cholesterol in check, thus preventing heart disease. When estrogen levels rise, however, they can fuel hormone-stimulated cancers like those of the breast and ovaries, researchers say.

There are several ways in which phytonutrients keep estrogen at proper levels. For example, a class of phytonutrients called isoflavones is extremely similar to natural estrogen. When we eat foods containing isoflavones, these faux hormones bind to the body's estrogen receptors, leaving the real hormone with nowhere to go but out.

Although estrogen is often referred to as if it were one hormone, in fact there are different forms. One kind of estrogen, called 16-alpha-hydroxyestrone, has been linked to breast cancer. Another form, 2-hydroxyestrone, appears to be harmless. Certain phytonutrients are able to increase levels of the harmless form of estrogen while decreasing levels of the dangerous kind.

Eating Your Medicine

As you can see, phytonutrients put up a variety of powerful defenses. Indeed, their potential is staggering. As with vitamins and minerals before them, scientists foresee a day when many of these compounds will be used for treating disease in the hospital and for preventing it at home.

In the meantime, researchers stress that there is only one way to get the phytonutrients your body needs: You must eat them in the packages Mother Nature provides, that is, fruits, vegetables, and grains, getting at least nine servings a day.

Researchers are learning more every day about this huge class of compounds hiding in the glass of orange juice you have at breakfast, in that lunchtime side salad, in the sauce on your pizza, and in the baked sweet potato and green beans at dinner-time. Let's take a look at some of the emerging stars.

CAROTENOIDS

Carotenoids are the phytonutrients you can thank for the brilliant red, orange, and pink hues in salads, pumpkin pie, cranberry sauce, berry smoothies, and more. This class of about 600 red and yellow plant pigments, which includes beta-carotene, gives the deep reds to tomatoes and the vibrant oranges to carrots and cantaloupes. Carotenoids are also prevalent in dark green leafy vegetables like spinach—but you can't see them because the green chlorophyll in these plants overpowers the lighter carotene pigments.

Carotenoids are powerful antioxidants, making them prime fighters against heart disease and certain forms of cancer. "There are good, clear associations between eating a lot of beta-carotene-packed foods and low levels of heart disease and cancer," says carotenoid researcher Dexter L. Morris, MD, PhD, an associate professor in the department of emergency medicine at the University of North Carolina School of Medicine at Chapel Hill. "But some of those benefits may be from some other carotenoid in fruits and vegetables that we have not even begun to study yet."

Research has shown promising results for a number of carotenoids, particularly lycopene (also found in tomatoes), lutein (found in vegetables such as spinach and kale), and zeaxanthin (found in dark green leafy vegetables). All three play powerful roles in cancer prevention. Researchers in the Tufts University Carotenoids Health Laboratory say skipping fruits and veggies is part of the classic "profile" of people who develop cancers of the head and neck, but that increasing your produce intake may actually cut your risk for recurrence of these cancers.

In one study, researchers found that people in northern Italy who ate seven or more servings of raw tomatoes every week had a 60 percent lower chance of developing colon, rectal, and stomach cancer than those who ate only two servings or less. And German researchers have found that cooked tomato products containing some oil—such as spaghetti sauce—boost lycopene absorption dramatically. They suspect that crushing and heating releases more lycopene, and that the body needs substances in oil to aid absorption.

Finally, Harvard researchers looking at dark green leafy vegetables, especially spinach, had quite an

Doctor's Top Tip

Eat your greens every day. Harvard School of Public Health researchers report that people who eat at least 6 milligrams a day of lutein and zeaxanthin—carotenoids that give greens their dark color—significantly cut their odds for cataract surgery. One cup of cooked kale, collards, spinach, or turnip greens supplies a whopping 12 to 25 milligrams of these two nutrients.

eye-opener. They found that people eating the most lutein and zeaxanthin—two carotenoids found in these vegetables—had a 43 percent lower risk of macular degeneration than those eating the least. Macular degeneration is the leading cause of irreversible vision loss in people over 50. Lutein and zeaxanthin concentrate in your retinas and protect them by absorbing harmful blue-wavelength light found in sunshine.

FLAVONOIDS

You've probably heard of the French paradox—the unfair fact that even though our butter-, cream- and lard-loving French allies chow down on cuisine loaded with culinary no-nos, they die of heart disease 2½ times less often than we do.

The reason, researchers believe, may lie in a group of phytonutrients called flavonoids. Like carotenoids, flavonoids add color—specifically reds, yellows, blues . . . and shades of brown—to the foods we eat and drink. (Also as with carotenoids, these colors often are masked by chlorophyll in the plants.)

Present in the largest quantities in apples, celery, cocoa (and dark chocolate), cranberries, grapes, broccoli, endive, onions, green and black teas, and red wines, flavonoids are powerful antioxidants, and sturdy defenders against heart disease and cancer.

But experts are beginning to suspect that these compounds do more. Some flavonoids make the linings of blood vessels more supple, lowering blood pressure and protecting against a buildup of heart-threatening plaque. (In one study, grape juice and chocolate had this effect.) Flavonoids also act like Teflon coating for the millions of tiny disks in your blood called platelets. They keep the platelets from clumping together in the bloodstream and forming clots, which helps prevent heart attacks and stroke. A recent Harvard Medical School lab study has found that one magical flavonoid found in wine and grapes, resveratrol, also lowers blood sugar levels and boosts liver function. In fact, in a group of lucky mice, it increased longevity 31 percent. And, in one recent University of Virginia lab study, resveratrol—found in grape skins, raspberries, mulberries, and peanuts—literally starved cancer cells by interfering with a protein called nuclear factor-kappa B that helps feed them.

Doctor's Top Tip

Double your flavonoids with cocoa. Cornell University scientists say cocoa has twice as many flavonoids as red wine and three to nine times more than a cup of green tea. The results surprised the researchers, who expected green tea to win. (Wisely, however, lead researcher Chang Y. Lee, PhD, professor of food science and technology at Cornell University–New York State Agricultural Experimental Station in Geneva, suggests you use this strategy to get the widest variety of flavonoids possible: "Personally, I would drink hot cocoa in the morning, green tea in the afternoon, and a glass of red wine in the evening. That's a good combination," says Dr. Lee.

In one Dutch study that examined the eating patterns of 805 men ages 65 to 84, researchers found that those who got the least flavonoids in their diets were 32 percent more likely to die from heart attacks than those who ate the most. It didn't take many flavonoids to get the benefits. The high-flavonoid group had the equivalent of 4 cups of black tea, ½ cup of apple, and ⅛ cup of onions a day.

When it comes to cancer prevention, flavonoids may help out by influencing cell-signaling pathways—the way cells turn genes on and off in order to perform thousands of everyday maintenance activities. Flavonoids may help turn on genes that stop cancer cells from dividing or invading healthy tissues, or even help activate genes that make cancer cells commit suicide, say experts from the Linus Pauling Research Institute at Oregon State University in Corvallis.

Intriguing proof: In a recent study at the University of California, Los Angeles, those prostate-cancer survivors who drank 8 ounces of pomegranate juice daily increased by nearly four times the period during which their levels of prostate-specific antigens, a cancer biomarker, stayed stable. The study surprised even the researchers, who say the combination of flavonoids, anti-inflammatory compounds, and antioxidants in pomegranate juice may be responsible. (The juice isn't a substitute for medical treatment, but researchers say its worth sipping as extra insurance.)

INDOLES

Broccoli, cabbage, and other cruciferous vegetables have a bitter taste that bugs don't like. The phytonutrient responsible for this clever bit of plant protection is called indole-3-carbinol—known to researchers by the nickname I3C. In humans, this compound plays a role in regulating hormones, which may be useful in preventing breast cancer.

Indole-3-carbinol has been shown to knock down levels of harmful forms of estrogen while increasing more benign forms of the hormone. Researchers at the Strang Cancer Prevention Center in New York City found that when women took 400 milligrams of I3C a day—about the amount found in half of a head of cabbage—their levels of the harmless estrogen increased dramatically. In fact, they had the same levels as those found in marathon runners, which is quite a feat, since vigorous exercise has been shown to have a strong positive effect on estrogen

Doctor's Top Tip

Get your kids or your grandkids into the habit of eating a half-cup serving of an indole-rich veggie from the brassica family—such as broccoli, Brussels sprouts, cabbage, cauliflower, kale, or turnips—several times a week. (A dash of salt, even a sprinkle of Parmesan may help!) Harvard Medical School researchers suspect that these veggies work best at cutting *early-stage* cancer risk in young men and women—in essence, stopping cancer before it starts.

levels. Why it matters—and why you should say yes to broccoli and cabbage: The form of estrogen that I3C helps deactivate promotes tumor growth, notably in estrogen-sensitive breast cancer. I3C also helps stop tumor cells from spreading to other parts of the body. But indoles aren't for women only. Studies also show that I3C may also slow the growth and reproduction of prostate-cancer cells.

ISOFLAVONES

Can the plant estrogens—isoflavones—hiding in soy milk, tofu, and many meatless cheeses and hot dogs *really* cut your cholesterol, slash your risk for breast cancer, and protect against brittle bones? For many years, experts thought so—and health food stores championed soy foods and soy supplements as super-healthy alternatives to fat-clogged, isoflavone-deficient Western foods.

But that was then; this is now. A decade of careful study is setting the record straight on isoflavones. (The good news: If you never loved soy, you don't have to feel guilty anymore about not eating it!) Linus Pauling Institute nutrition experts who analyzed hundreds of isoflavone studies say that while the isoflavones called genistein, daidzein, and glycitein do have weak estrogenic activity in the body, their effect is less profound than originally believed.

Isoflavones may lower bad low-density lipoprotein (LDL) cholesterol by a modest 3 percent (that's six points if your LDL is now at 150 milligrams per deciliter), they've found—not the 13 percent drop shown in early studies. There's no evidence that soy isoflavones cut breast cancer risk, either. (It's true that women in Asia have traditionally enjoyed lower breast cancer rates than American women, but experts now think lifestyle and genes account for the difference.) Nor do isoflavones seem to cut prostate-cancer risk. And while soy isoflavones may protect bones slightly, the evidence isn't strong for this either. Moreover, research shows that soy doesn't even ease menstrual cramps.

Bottom line? Soy foods are safe for most people (see "Doctor's Top Tip" at left for some cautions), but experts say the jury's still out on the safety of high-dose isoflavone supplements.

Doctor's Top Tip

Eat soy because you like it, not because the isoflavones will have a dramatic impact on your health. According to the American Heart Association, the best use of soy may be simply to replace less-healthy foods in your diet. Having soy crumbles in your chili instead of ground beef packed with saturated fat, for example, gives you extra fiber and heart-healthy unsaturated fats. If you're at high risk for breast cancer or are a breast cancer survivor, be cautious about soy. Soy experts from the National Cancer Institute say there's not yet enough evidence to say whether soy foods or supplements increase risk for developing breast cancer, or having a recurrence.

ISOTHIOCYANATES

Isothiocyanates, sometimes called mustard oils, protect cruciferous vegetables by leaving invading insects with a bitter taste in their mouths. Like indoles, isothiocyanates, which are found in broccoli, Brussels sprouts, and cabbage, show promise for helping to prevent cancer.

So far, sulforaphane, a compound abundant in broccoli, has been crowned the leading isothiocyanate for its cancer-blocking ability in laboratory tests. In one study, researchers at Johns Hopkins University in Baltimore exposed laboratory animals to a powerful cancer-causing agent. In animals given high doses of sulforaphane, only 26 percent developed breast tumors, compared with 68 percent of the group that didn't get the compound.

Isothiocyanates may be particularly effective against the damaging effects of cigarette smoke, says Stephen Hecht, PhD, professor of cancer prevention at the University of Minnesota Cancer Center in Minneapolis.

In a laboratory study, a compound called phenethylisocyanate, found in watercress, was able to reduce by 50 percent the rate of lung cancer in rats exposed to carcinogens found in tobacco smoke. Human trials have revealed similar results, says Dr. Hecht.

> ### Doctor's Top Tip
>
> Protect against cancer by sprinkling tangy broccoli sprouts on your salads. Cute little broccoli seedlings—marketed as BroccoSprouts—contain 20 to 50 times the amount of the leading isothiocyanate, sulforaphane, found in mature heads of broccoli, says world-renowned cancer researcher Paul Talalay, PhD, of the Laboratory for Molecular Pharmacology at the Johns Hopkins University School of Medicine.

LIGNANS

Like isoflavones, lignans are plant estrogens that may help keep levels of human estrogen in check. Flaxseed is an especially rich source of lignans, which are also found in sesame seeds, curly kale, broccoli, apricots, cabbage, and strawberries. How do they work? Beneficial bacteria in your intestinal tract convert lignans into compounds called enterolactone and enterodiol, which may function as weak estrogens in the body.

The effect of lignans on the body is the subject of lively debate. Some experts say these compounds help protect against breast cancer. But while some studies have found higher cancer risk in women with the lowest levels of these lignan-based compounds in their bloodstream, other studies have not. Different researchers argue over whether lignans play a role in protecting heart health: For example, a 12-year study of 1,889 guys from Finland showed that those with the highest levels of enterolactone (a sign of a high lignan intake) in their bloodstream slashed their risk for fatal heart

Doctor's Top Tip

Pat yourself on the back if you include lignan-rich ground flaxseed, sesame seeds, kale, or broccoli in your diet on a regular basis. Recent research from the University of Kuopio in Finland suggests that the lignans in these foods may work as cell-protecting antioxidants.

disease. But other studies have found that lignans don't have any effect on cholesterol levels.

But don't give up on this phytonutrient yet. Lignans may not be a solo magic bullet, but there's an important reason to keep them in your diet. Increasingly, researchers respect lignans as team players that, like a skilled second baseman or a tough fullback, work with other phytonutrients in food to protect against heart disease, cancer, diabetes, and other health conditions. Experts think the lignans are just part of the story. Foods that are rich in lignans, such as flaxseed, are also packed with heart-smart omega-3 fatty acids and fiber.

MONOTERPENES

If you've ever polished furniture with lemon oil, you've likely smelled the citrusy aroma of limonene, a phytonutrient that scientists say may be yet another important warrior in the battle against cancer.

Large doses of limonene, which is found primarily in orange peels and citrus oils, have actually shrunk breast tumors in laboratory animals. This fragrant phytonutrient has also prevented tumors from developing when breast tissue is exposed to high doses of cancer-causing chemicals. In laboratory studies, limonene has been shown to reduce tumor production by 55 percent.

Unlike other cancer-preventing phytonutrients, limonene works by blocking proteins that are known to promote cell growth in various cancers. Limonene may be the reason that people who eat a lot of oranges and other citrus fruits appear to have a reduced risk of cancer.

Doctor's Top Tip

Grate organic orange zest into salad dressings, baked goods, and fruit medleys. Ninety percent of the compounds in orange peel oil are monoterpenes, say Purdue University biologists, making this "throwaway" part of the fruit a cancer-prevention treasure. Use a microplane grater or zester to gently scrape orange bits from a freshly-washed, organic orange (avoid nonorganic varieties, which may contain agricultural chemicals, dyes, and wax).

A monoterpene that is found in cherries, called perillyl alcohol, has been shown to prevent cancers of the breast, lung, stomach, liver, and skin in preliminary animal studies at Indiana University School of Medicine in Indianapolis. But more research needs to be done before scientists know how effective this compound is in people.

"Perillyl alcohol has been very promising in clinical trials," says Charles Elson, PhD, professor emeritus of nutritional sciences at the University of Wisconsin in Madison. "We're not just showing that this compound fights cancer, meaning that it neutralizes cancer-causing toxins. We're also showing that it is effective in animals with existing tumors."

ORGANOSULFUR COMPOUNDS

Take a sharp knife to a fresh onion, or peel a clove of garlic, and you'll be introduced to some of nature's most potent phytonutrients—organosulfur compounds called allylic sulfides. These compounds can make your eyes water and your nose run as you chop away. Other members of the allium family, such as chives and leeks, can be less pungent, but they boast similar powers to cut your risk for heart disease and possibly even cancer.

Allylic sulfides are a class of phytonutrients that stimulate toxin-eliminating enzymes. According to sulfide researcher Michael J. Wargovich, PhD, professor of pathology and microbiology at the University of South Carolina School of Medicine in Columbia, these compounds are particularly effective against cancers of the gastrointestinal tract.

In a study of more than 120,000 men and women in the Netherlands, researchers looked at the amounts of sulfide-containing onions these Hollanders ate and compared them with the incidences of stomach cancer. The more onions people put on their plates, the lower their risks of stomach cancer.

In another study, garlic, which like onions is a member of the *Allium* genus, showed equal tumor-squelching promise. Researchers gave one group of mice large amounts of garlic every day for 2 weeks; another group received no garlic. When the animals were exposed to cancer-inducing chemicals, the group that received the garlic developed 76 percent fewer tumors than those given only their normal food. Studies even show that a garlic compound called ajoene can shrink tumors—probably by promoting the body's healthy, natural efforts to make cancer cells self-destruct, a process called apoptosis.

Allylic sulfides also have the unique ability to keep cholesterol and other blood fats known as triglycerides from causing health-threatening blood clots and hardening of the arteries.

In one study, researchers loaded volunteers' diets

Doctor's Top Tip

Grill your steak with plenty of garlic. Studies presented at a recent Frontiers in Cancer Prevention conference hosted by the American Association for Cancer Research suggest that diallyl sulphide in garlic cuts cancer risk by inhibiting the effects of carcinogens called heterocyclic amines, which can develop when meat is charred during grilling.

with more butter and lard than you'd find in a French bakery, then watched their cholesterol climb and their blood coagulate. Then they gave the same volunteers a sulfide-packed onion extract. Not only did it prevent the fat-induced rise in cholesterol; it also increased the volunteers' ability to dissolve clots.

In lab studies, the compounds allicin (believed to be the most potent compound in garlic) and diallyl disulphide also made blood vessels relax, reducing blood pressure and improving bloodflow. Garlic's organosulfur compounds may also help lower cholesterol levels by turning down the liver's production of cholesterol. In test-tube studies, these compounds discouraged blood platelets from clumping together. Researchers suspect that in the human body, they can discourage the formation of heart-stopping blood clots.

Allicin also has potent germ-killing powers. Studies show that it can kill microbes responsible for colds, the flu, tummy viruses, yeast infections, and possibly even tuberculosis. Researchers from the University of California Irvine Medical Center even found that garlic juice could kill antibiotic-resistant strains of highly infectious staph bacteria.

Other studies have shown that as few as two or more servings of garlic a week may help protect against colon cancer. Substances found in garlic, such as allicin, have been shown to not only protect colon cells from the toxic effects of cancer-causing chemicals, but also to stop the growth of cancer cells once they develop. While more research is needed, recent animal research has also suggested that garlic may confer protection against the development of stomach cancer through its potential ability to decrease *H. pylori*-induced gastritis (acute inflammation of the stomach lining).

PHENOLIC COMPOUNDS

Almost all fruits, vegetables, cereal grains, and green and black teas are rich in phytonutrients called phenolic compounds, or polyphenols. These compounds fight cancer on two fronts. They stimulate protective enzymes while squelching harmful ones, and they're also heavy-duty antioxidants.

Particularly active polyphenols include ellagic acid from strawberries, green tea polyphenols, and curcumin, the yellow coloring in the spice turmeric, says Dr. Stoner.

In one study, researchers at the University of Scranton in Pennsylvania found that of 39 antioxidants found in food, polyphenols from tea showed the greatest prowess at controlling free radicals. Meanwhile, lab studies suggest curcumin may play a role in cancer prevention because it acts as an antioxidant and also, in test tubes, seems to inhibit the spread of cancer cells and helps cut off the efforts of cancer cells to grow blood vessels. And curcumin is also being studied as a potential way to prevent, or help treat, Alzheimer's disease and arthritis.

SAPONINS

Perhaps the most common phytonutrients are the molecules called saponins. You can find saponins in a wide variety of vegetables, herbs, and legumes, including beans, spinach, tomatoes, potatoes, nuts, and oats. Soybeans alone contain 12 different kinds of saponins.

Studies show that people who eat saponin-rich diets have consistently lower rates of breast, prostate, and colon cancers, says A. Venket Rao, PhD, professor of nutrition at the University of Toronto.

Unlike other cancer-fighting phytonutrients, however, saponins possess a unique array of weapons. One way that they help prevent cancer is by binding with bile acids, which over time may metabolize into cancer-causing compounds, and eliminating them from the body, says Dr. Rao. They also stimulate the immune system so that it's better able to detect and destroy precancerous cells before they develop into full-blown cancer.

Perhaps most important, saponins have a special ability to target the cholesterol found in cancer cell membranes. "Cancer cells have a lot of cholesterol in their membranes," Dr. Rao explains, "and saponins selectively bind to these cells and destroy them."

Not surprisingly, this ability to bind to cholesterol is helpful for lowering total cholesterol as well. Saponins bind with bile acids, used for digestion, in the intestinal tract. The bile is then excreted, instead of being reabsorbed. Since bile acids are made of cholesterol, getting rid of some of these acids means your body will have to use up cholesterol to make more, effectively lowering cholesterol levels in the process.

> ### Doctor's Top Tip
>
> Get curcumin the old-fashioned way—by using more turmeric, the ancient Indian spice packed with curcumin. Integrative medicine expert Andrew Weil, MD, suggests adding curry (which contains turmeric) to cauliflower soup. He also recommends taking a curcumin supplement such as Zyflamend. Talk with your doctor first if you take anticlotting drugs such as aspirin, Plavix, or heparin. Too much curcumin could raise bleeding risk.

PHYTONUTRIENTS AT A GLANCE

Here's a guide to the most potent phytonutrients and the foods with the highest amounts, plus the best ways to prepare the foods to unlock their healing potential.

Phytonutrient	Food Source	Disease Prevention	Preparation Hints
Carotenoids	Broccoli, cantaloupes, carrots, greens, tomatoes	Antioxidant action; prevent heart disease and certain cancers	Eat with meat or foods that contain oil. Your body absorbs carotenoids better with a little fat.
Flavonoids	Apples, broccoli, citrus fruits, cranberries, endive, grape juice, kale, onions, red wines	Antioxidant action; prevent blood clotting and heart disease	Eat pulpy parts of citrus fruits, and keep the skin on apples for the most flavonoids.
Indoles and isothiocyanates	Broccoli, cabbage, cauliflower, mustard greens	Stimulate cancer-preventing enzymes; lower levels of harmful estrogen	Microwave or steam lightly to preserve the phytonutrients.
Isoflavones	Chickpeas, kidney beans, lentils, soybeans	May slightly reduce cholesterol levels	Isoflavones hold up through processing; save time and buy canned beans.
Lignans	Flaxseed	Antioxidant action; lower levels of harmful estrogen; may prevent certain cancers	The recommended amount for optimum benefits is 1 to 2 heaping tablespoons of flaxseed.
Monoterpenes	Cherries and citrus fruits	May work with other nutrients to cut cancer and heart risks	Though most of the monoterpenes are found in the citrus peel, you can get them in the juice.
Organosulfur compounds	Garlic and onions	Raise good HDL cholesterol; lower blood fat levels; prevent heart disease; stimulate enzymes that suppress tumors	Chop or crush to release the phytonutrients.
Phenolic compounds	Almost all cereal grains, fruits, green and black teas, vegetables	Antioxidant action; activate cancer-fighting enzymes	Just eat a wide variety of fresh fruits and vegetables.
Saponins	Asparagus, chickpeas, nuts, oats, potatoes, soybeans, spinach, tomatoes	Bind with and flush out cholesterol; stimulate immunity; help cut risk of heart disease and cancers	The richest sources are soybeans and chickpeas.

Pineapple
A TROPICAL CHAMP

When King Louis XIV of France was first presented with a pineapple—the most exotic and sought-after fruit in 17th-century Europe—he immediately took a huge bite. Unfortunately, His Greediness hadn't given his servants a chance to peel it, so he cut his royal lips on the prickly rind. This episode put an end to the royal cultivation of pineapple in France until Louis XV took the throne in 1715.

The pineapple-punctured potentate didn't know what he was missing. Stripping a pineapple of its spiny hide (or at least opening a can of the stuff) is well worth your time. Not only is pineapple a rich source of vitamin C, it also contains substances that keep bones strong and promote digestion.

HEALING POWER
Can Help:

Keep bones strong

Improve digestion

Ease inflammation

Relieve cold symptoms

Lower the risk of cancer and heart disease

Tropical Inflammation Soother

In lab studies and in human studies, the bromelain extracted from pineapple has eased swelling and inflammation associated with rheumatoid arthritis, tendonitis, bursitis, soft tissue injuries, inflammatory conditions in the colon, and even chronic pain. In a recent University of Connecticut lab study, researchers found that bromelain reduced the level of eosinophils, the main inflammatory cells associated with asthma, by half. "Maybe it could cut down on steroid use—the standard treatment for asthma patients—and thus decrease the side effects sometimes seen with long-term steroid use," says lead researcher Eric Secor, ND, a naturopathic physician and National Institutes of Health (NIH) postdoctoral fellow in immunology at the university. But don't give up your asthma meds just yet. "Asthma is a very serious disease. It can be life-threatening," he says. "I don't want people throwing away their inhalers."

Bromelain may even speed up healing time and decrease pain and bruising after surgery. In Germany, the government agency that regulates herbs and other supplements has approved bromelain for healing after injuries and surgical procedures—and for easing swelling in the nose and sinuses after operations involving the ears, nose, and throat.

A Juicy Bone Builder

You know that you need calcium to prevent osteoporosis, the bone-thinning disease that primarily affects postmenopausal women. What you may not know is that your bones need the trace mineral manganese as well.

The body uses manganese to make collagen, a tough, fibrous protein that helps build connective tissues like bone, skin, and cartilage. Research has shown that people deficient in manganese develop bone problems similar to osteoporosis. One study found that women with osteoporosis had lower levels of manganese than women who did not have the disease.

"Eating fresh pineapple or drinking pineapple juice is a good way to add manganese to your diet," says Jeanne Freeland-Graves, PhD, professor of nutrition at the University of Texas in Austin. A cup of fresh pineapple chunks or pineapple juice will give you more than 2 milligrams of manganese, or more than 100 percent of the Daily Value (DV).

Sweeten Your Digestion

Pineapple has a centuries-old reputation for relieving indigestion, and there may be good reasons for that. Fresh pineapple contains bromelain, an enzyme that helps digestion by breaking down protein. This might be important for some older people who have low levels of stomach acid, which is needed for protein digestion.

Even if you love pineapple, of course, it's unlikely that you'd eat it after every meal. But if you are older and have frequent indigestion, adding a few pineapple slices to your dessert plate might help keep your stomach calm, says Joanne Curran-

In the Kitchen

With its tough skin and sharp edges, the pineapple doesn't give up its sweetness easily. To choose the best fruit and get to the "heart of gold" inside, here's what you need to do.

Buy it firm. Find a fruit that's plump and firm. Avoid pineapples that are bruised or have soft spots. Surprisingly, shell color is not always a reliable indicator of ripeness. The stem end should have a sweet, aromatic fragrance and not smell fermented.

Look for freshness. The leaves on pineapple should be crisp and deep green, without yellowed or browned tips. Don't bother testing the fruit by pulling a leaf from the crown. Contrary to popular wisdom, a leaf that comes off easily doesn't indicate that the fruit is ripe.

Reveal the fruit. When you get the pineapple home, cut off the top and bottom ends, then place the pineapple in a shallow dish to catch the juices as you slice off the spiny skin vertically. You can then cut it into rounds and remove the tough center core.

Celentano, PhD, RD, associate professor of nutritional sciences at the University of New Hampshire in Durham.

A Great Source of Vitamin C

Few nutrients get as much attention as vitamin C, and for good reason. This vitamin is a powerful anti-oxidant, meaning that it helps thwart free radicals, unstable oxygen molecules that damage cells and contribute to the development of cancer and heart disease. In addition, the body uses vitamin C to make collagen, the "glue" that holds tissue and bone together. And when you have a cold, the first thing you probably reach for is vitamin C. It reduces levels of a chemical called histamine, which causes such cold symptoms as watery eyes and runny noses.

While pineapples aren't as rich in vitamin C as oranges or grapefruits, they're still excellent sources. One cup of pineapple chunks, for example, contains about 24 milligrams of vitamin C, or 40 percent of the DV. Juice is even better. A glass of canned pineapple juice contains 60 milligrams, or 100 percent of the DV.

Doctor's Top Tip

For anti-inflammatory benefits, make pineapple a between-meals snack. The bromelain in pineapple has powerful anti-inflammatory properties, says bromelain researcher Eric Secor, ND, an NIH postdoctoral fellow in immunology at the University of Connecticut. Studies show it can sooth irritated sinuses and swollen sore throats, ease arthritic inflammation, and even help cuts and scrapes heal faster. Eat pineapple alone to get the most benefit; otherwise, the bromelain will be de-activated as it helps digest protein in the other foods that you eat.

GETTING THE MOST

Buy it fresh. Canned pineapple is convenient, but when you're eating it to soothe an upset stomach, the fresh fruit is best because the intense heat used in canning destroys the bromelain.

Try a new variety. The next time you're at the store, look for a "Gold" pineapple. Imported from Costa Rica, this variety is exceptionally sweet, and it has more than four times the vitamin C found in other varieties.

Have some juice. Canned pineapple juice is an excellent way to get your DV of vitamin C. In fact, 4 ounces of pineapple juice contains more vitamin C than the same amount of apple, cranberry, or tomato juice.

Pineapple with Almond Cream Topping

1 **large pineapple, peeled**
⅔ **cup 1% cottage cheese**
1 **tablespoon sugar**
¼ **teaspoon vanilla extract**
¼ **teaspoon almond extract**

Cut the pineapple crosswise into 8 slices. Use a knife or small cookie cutter to remove the center core from each slice, and discard. Place 4 of the slices on dessert plates. Cut the remaining slices into small chunks.

In a blender or food processor, combine the cottage cheese, sugar, vanilla extract, and almond extract. Process until smooth and creamy.

Place a dollop of the cream topping in the center of each pineapple slice. Scatter the pineapple chunks around the sliced pineapple and serve.

Makes 4 servings

Cook's Note: *Some supermarkets sell pineapples already peeled, with or without the center core still in place. If the core is there, simply slide it out and discard before using.*

PER SERVING

Calories: 98
Total fat: 0.9 g
Saturated fat: 0.3 g

Cholesterol: 2 mg
Sodium: 153 mg
Dietary fiber: 1.4 g

Plantains

ULCER PROTECTION IN A PEEL

HEALING POWER
Can Help:

Lower blood pressure

Prevent and treat ulcers

Prevent constipation

Decrease the risk of heart disease

It looks like a banana. It feels like a banana. But peel back the skin and take a bite, and you'll know it's no banana.

Though people often bunch them in the same category, comparing bananas and plantains is a bit like comparing, well, apples and oranges.

First, you can't eat plantains raw—it would be like taking a bite of uncooked potato. (Plantains are often called cooking bananas or even "potatoes of the air.") Popular in Latin America, Africa, Asia, and India, these close relatives of bananas are longer and thicker-skinned and are usually treated as vegetables—they're cooked first—rather than eaten out of hand as a fruit.

But taste isn't all that separates bananas from plantains. Plantains also pack different nutrients inside their green peels.

Keeping Your Pump Primed

Ounce for ounce, plantains contain more potassium than their yellow-skinned cousins, the bananas. That means that if your blood pressure has been climbing to new heights, and you need to bring it down, a plateful of plantain is a step in the right direction.

One cup of sliced, cooked plantain delivers a potassium lode of 716 milligrams, or about 20 percent of the Daily Value (DV). Potassium has been well-established as a key mineral for heart disease prevention.

Studies have shown that people who don't get enough potassium in their diets are at much higher risks of high blood pressure, heart attacks, and strokes. A study conducted by scientists at the University of Naples in Italy found that eating three to six servings a day of potassium-rich foods such as plantains allowed many people to reduce or even eliminate their need for blood pressure medication.

At the same time, a potassium-rich diet reduces the risk of stroke significantly—by up to 40 percent in some cases, say researchers from the University of California, San Diego, and the University of Cambridge School of Medicine in England.

Plantains can also keep your ticker in tip-top shape by helping to keep your arteries plaque-free, according to researchers. This is because potassium-rich foods like plantains appear to help prevent the body's low-density lipoprotein (LDL) cholesterol from oxidizing, the process that makes it stick to the artery walls. This may be a good defense against atherosclerosis, or hardening of the arteries, says David B. Young, PhD, professor emeritus of physiology and biophysics at the University of Mississippi Medical Center in Jackson.

"Studies show that you can get a significant impact from relatively small changes," says Dr. Young. "But you can never eat too many potassium-rich foods, especially since so much of our modern diet is overprocessed and high in sodium and depleted of potassium."

One last word about blood pressure: One cup of cooked plantains delivers about 49 milligrams of magnesium, or more than 12 percent of the DV. This is another mineral that can help keep blood pressure in check, especially among people who are sensitive to sodium.

Quenching the Flames

In India, if you go to a doctor's office clutching your stomach, you're more likely to walk out with a bag of plantain powder than a bottle of Tagamet.

Experts aren't sure how they do it, but plantains are known for their ability to both prevent and treat ulcers, as well as to quell digestive upset such as flatulence and indigestion.

In fact, there may be more than one magic, protective factor inside the plantain

In the Kitchen

Like potatoes, plantains are extremely easy to work with. In fact, you can use plantains in almost exactly the same ways you use potatoes—mashed, sautéed, or baked. Their mild flavor works well in omelets, soups, and stews.

Here's some expert advice on the easiest ways to choose and prepare your plantains:

Peel and simmer. When cooking plantains, first peel them as you would a banana. Remove and discard the long, fibrous strings that run alongside the fruit. Cut into 1- or 2- inch pieces, then steam for 10 minutes. When the plantains are tender, they can be mashed or sautéed. Or simply drizzle them with a little extra-virgin olive oil and serve.

Cook them gently. While plantains must be cooked until tender, you don't want to cook them too long. When overcooked, they release a compound that causes a bitter taste. In fact, when adding plantains to stews, omelets, or other dishes, it's best to add them late in the cooking process to prevent the taste from turning.

that guards the walls of the gastrointestinal tract. Researchers are currently studying whether soluble fiber from the plantain can ease the painful inflammation of Crohn's disease and ulcerative colitis. Gastroenterologists at the University of Liverpool, England, have found that compounds from plantain soothe inflammation in the digestive tract. Now, a British company is working on a food that would use plantain's fiber to protect the fragile inner lining of the intestines from damage caused when the immune system tries to fight off bacteria. And a flavonoid called leucocyanidin, also discovered in unripe plantains,

Doctor's Top Tip

Latex allergy? Skip plantains. People with latex allergies often react when they eat bananas, say researchers at France's Pasteur Institute. What's the culprit responsible for this "latex-fruit syndrome"? Compounds called chitinases, which are also found in plantains.

seems to protect the lining of the stomach from damage caused by aspirin. Researchers at the University of Birmingham, England, think it works by thickening the natural mucous barrier that protects the stomach lining.

More Filling, Fewer Calories

Although they're not one of the best food sources of fiber, plantains have the distinction of being among the top foods to offer a gram of fiber for the fewest calories. To get about 1 gram of fiber, all you need is ⅓ cup of boiled, mashed plantain, for the small price of about 46 skinny calories.

Serve yourself 1 cup of this starchy fruit, and you'll have almost 5 grams of fiber, or nearly 20 percent of the DV. Fiber has been shown to help reduce cholesterol and prevent a variety of digestive problems such as constipation and hemorrhoids.

Immunity Booster

On top of all its other disease-fighting abilities, the plantain is also filled with nutrients that strengthen the immune system. This means you'll be better able to stave off whatever illnesses come your way.

For example, 1 cup of cooked, sliced plantain contains almost 17 milligrams of vitamin C, or more than 28 percent of the DV. Vitamin C is perhaps the best known of the infection-fighting, immunity-building vitamins.

That same cup of sliced plantain also delivers 40 micrograms of folate, or 10 percent of the DV for this B vitamin; 0.4 milligram of vitamin B_6, or 20 percent of the DV; and 1,400 IU of vitamin A, or 28 percent of the DV.

The benefits? Folate promotes normal tissue growth and may protect against cancer, heart disease, and birth defects. Vitamin B_6 is essential to keep your nervous system working in peak condition and to increase immunity. Vitamin A also bolsters immunity and safeguards against impaired night vision and vision problems associated with aging, such as macular degeneration.

GETTING THE MOST

Get the best quality. When completely ripe, plantains should feel firm but not rock-hard. Skip any that are mushy or moldy. Store the plantains on the kitchen counter until they've reached the stage of ripeness you desire; the coldness of the fridge halts ripening.

Experiment with ripeness. You can use plantains unripe, when they're green and slightly ripe, when they're yellow and nearly ripe, or even when they're black and totally ripe. Here's how each can be used:

- **Green for your tummy.** When you're eating plantains to prevent ulcers or to speed the healing of an ulcer you already have, experts advise choosing those that are green and unripe because they're thought to contain more of the healing enzymes than fruits that are a ripe yellow or black. Green plantains can be boiled, fried, or dropped into a soup or stew.
- **Yellow for creaminess.** Yellow plantains are softer and a bit sweeter. They're good mashed, baked, or grilled.
- **Black for sweetness.** Fully ripe black plantains can be cooked like yellow, but this is the stage when they taste sweetest and smell more like a banana.

Plantains with Garlic and Thyme

2 large green plantains

2 cups water

1½ teaspoons dried thyme

1 teaspoon paprika

¼ teaspoon salt

4 teaspoons olive oil

3 cloves garlic, minced

Cut the tips off both ends of the plantains and discard. Run a knife lengthwise down a "seam" of each plantain. Peel off and discard the skin. Cut into ⅛-inch-thick slices.

In a large nonstick skillet, bring the water to a boil over medium heat. Add the plantains. Cover and simmer until tender, about 15 minutes. Test for doneness by inserting the tip of a sharp knife into a slice.

With tongs or a slotted spoon, remove the plantains to paper towels to drain. Pour off the liquid from the skillet, and wipe the skillet with paper towels.

In a large bowl, combine the thyme, paprika, and salt. Add the plantain slices, and toss with your hands to coat.

Add the oil to the skillet, and heat over medium-high heat. Add the plantain slices, and spread them evenly in the skillet. Cook until the plantains are golden on the bottom, 2 to 3 minutes. Turn and scatter the garlic over the plantains. Cook for another 2 to 3 minutes, or until golden on the bottom. Toss gently to coat with the garlic.

Makes 4 servings

Cook's Note: *The plantains may be easier to peel if you cut them in half through the middle crosswise.*

PER SERVING

Calories: 137
Total fat: 4.9 g
Saturated fat: 0.8 g

Cholesterol: 0 mg
Sodium: 138 mg
Dietary fiber: 2 g

Potatoes

OUR SUPER STAPLE

HEALING POWER

Can Help:

Prevent cancer

Control high blood
pressure and diabetes

Early in the history of the New World, in the Andes Mountains of Peru and Bolivia, people had a thousand names for the potato. It was that important.

In the 4,000 or so years since, the starchy tuber's reputation has peaked and dipped. The Spanish conquistadors thought the new root captivating enough to take back to the Old World. (Within a few years, potatoes became standard fare on Spanish ships because they prevented scurvy.) Once the potato arrived in Europe, though, its fortunes sagged, not because of any shortcomings of its own but because of its kinship with the deadly nightshade family, plants that had the reputation for being toxic. Potatoes were feared rather than appreciated.

Eventually, though, both botanists and diners alike learned the whole story. Potatoes aren't remotely dangerous. Plus, they're a super food staple, making them the world's number one vegetable crop.

"The potato has a little bit of almost everything," says Mark Kestin, PhD, professor of nutrition at Bastyr University and affiliate assistant professor of epidemiology at the University of Washington, both in Seattle. "You could get many of your nutritional needs met from potatoes, if you had to," he adds. Indeed. One large baked potato with the skin provides 48 percent of the Daily Value (DV) for vitamin C, about 40 percent of the DV for vitamin B_6, about 30 percent of the DV for copper, manganese, and potassium, as well as 7 grams of fiber.

Peel Power

A potato's healing abilities start in the peel, which contains an anticarcinogenic compound called chlorogenic acid, says Mary Ellen Camire, PhD, professor in the department of food science and human nutrition at the University of Maine in Orono. In laboratory studies, this particular acid has been shown to help the fiber in potatoes absorb benzo(a)pyrene, a potential carcinogen found in smoked foods such as grilled hamburgers. "The acid in the food reacts with the carcinogen by basically binding it up and making too big a molecule for the body to absorb," she explains. "In our study, it prevented the carcinogen from being absorbed almost completely."

In the Kitchen

Potatoes aren't all created equal. Some taste better baked, while others are good for soups or salads. A third type, the all-purpose potato, has been "designed" both for baking and steaming. Here's what to look for when considering potatoes:

Waxy potatoes. Known as round whites or round reds, waxy potatoes are low in starch and have a high moisture content. These potatoes keep their shape well during cooking, making them a good choice for soups, stews, and salads.

Starchy potatoes. The russet potato is a common type of starchy spud. It has a mealy, floury interior, which works well for mashing or baking.

All-purpose potatoes. Spuds like long whites are great to keep on the shelf because they can be prepared any way—baked, boiled, or steamed.

Slashing the Pressure

We don't normally think of potatoes as being high in potassium, but in fact, a baked 7-ounce spud contains more than twice the potassium of one medium-size banana. One baked potato with the skin will give you about 1,137 milligrams of potassium, almost a third of the DV for this mineral.

Potassium is important because it seems to calm the spiking effect that salt has on blood pressure. For some people, increasing potassium in their diets by eating potatoes could reduce the need for blood pressure medication, notes pharmacist Earl Mindell, RPh, PhD, professor emeritus of nutrition at Pacific Western University in Los Angeles and author of *Earl Mindell's Food as Medicine*. In one study of 54 people with high blood pressures, half added potassium-rich foods like potatoes to their diets, while the other half continued to eat their normal fare. By the end of the study, Dr. Mindell says, 81 percent of the potato eaters were able to control their blood pressures with less than half the medication they had used previously.

Recently, British scientists stumbled upon another compound inside potatoes that may help explain this veggie's extraordinary ability to help you control your blood pressure. Called kukoamines, these compounds have previously only been documented in some Chinese herbal remedies, say scientists from England's Institute of Food Research. "Potatoes have been cultivated for thousands of years, and we thought traditional crops were pretty well understood," says food scientist Fred Mellon, PhD, from the Norwich-based institute. "But this surprise finding shows that even the most familiar of foods might conceal a hoard of health-promoting chemicals."

Blood Sugar Bad Guy?

White potatoes have gotten a lot of bad press in the past few years. This veggie has been vilified by nutrition researchers who say it can send blood sugar soaring, and by nutritionists who warn that, too often, potatoes are just a vehicle for oil, butter, sour cream, and/or salt (think french fries, scalloped potatoes, and baked potatoes with the works). Women who splurged on french fries just once a week were 21 percent more likely to get diabetes than those who ate none, found a recent 20-year Harvard School of Public Health study of 84,500 women. Eating five servings per week of any white potatoes—including mashed and baked—raised the risk by 14 percent over those who ate less than half a serving per week.

But you don't have to give up spuds. Truth is, eaten in moderate quantities, with the peel on, potatoes remain a satisfying, nutritionally valuable food. In fact, the glycemic load (a measure of how much a regular serving of a food really raises your blood sugar) of a baked potato is on par with that of healthy grain foods such as barley and whole-wheat spaghetti, say blood sugar researchers from the University of Sydney, Australia. The danger? Eating potatoes every night (fried . . . or with butter) instead of choosing a variety of different veggies. (Plenty of us do just that. Potato consumption has doubled in the United States since 1970, and Americans eat more spuds than any other veggie.)

The humble spud also packs a surprising nutritional bonus—a healthy dose of vitamin C. We don't think of vitamin C as affecting our blood sugar, but there's emerging evidence that this powerful antioxidant vitamin, well-known for helping prevent heart disease, may be of help to people with diabetes. On top of this, vitamin C may also be effective in diminishing the damage to proteins caused by free radicals, dangerous oxygen molecules that damage tissues in the body.

In one study, researchers in the Netherlands found that men eating healthy diets, which were high not only in potatoes but also in fish, vegetables, and legumes, appeared to have a lower risk for diabetes. It's not yet clear what the protective mechanism is, but researchers speculate that antioxidants, including vitamin C, may play a role in keeping excess sugar out of the bloodstream.

Because potatoes are high in complex carbohydrates, they're also good for people who already have diabetes. Complex carbohydrates must be broken down into simple sugars before they're absorbed into the bloodstream. This means that the sugars enter the bloodstream in a leisurely fashion rather than pouring in all at once. This, in turn, helps keep blood sugar levels stable, which is a critical part of controlling the disease.

Further, potatoes can be key players in helping people with diabetes keep their weight down, an important benefit because being overweight makes it more difficult for the body to produce enough insulin, the hormone that helps transport sugars out of the bloodstream and into individual cells. At the same time, being overweight makes the insulin that the body does produce work less efficiently. What potatoes do is keep you full so that you're less likely to be hungry later on.

In a study of 41 hungry students at the University of Sydney in Australia, researchers found that spuds filled them up more than other foods, while at the same time delivering fewer calories. On a satiety scale that measured white bread at 100, oatmeal at 209, and fish at 225, potatoes were way ahead at 323.

GETTING THE MOST

Keep the peel. To take advantage of potatoes' cancer-fighting abilities, you really have to eat the peel, says Dr. Camire. This can be particularly important when eating grilled foods, which leave small amounts of cancer-causing substances on the food. It would be nice if you could get a fast-food burger on a potato-peel bun, says Dr. Camire. "That would help absorb the carcinogens from the grilling," she says.

A more practical solution is simply to add a baked potato or potato salad (with the peel) to your plate whenever you eat a grilled hamburger, a hot dog, or other smoky foods.

Cook them carefully. Although boiling is one of the most popular cooking methods for potatoes, it's perhaps the worst choice for preserving nutrients, since vitamin C and some B vitamins are pulled out of the potatoes and into the cooking water. In fact, boiling potatoes can result in losing about half the vitamin C, a quarter of the folate (a B vitamin), and 40 percent of the potassium, says Marilyn A. Swanson, PhD, RD, adjunct associate professor of pediatrics at Baylor College of Medicine in Houston, Texas.

If you do boil potatoes, you can recapture some of the nutrients by saving the cooking water and adding it to other foods such as soups and stews.

Baking and steaming do a good job of tenderizing potatoes, while at the same time preserving more of their nutrients. "Microwaving is your first choice," says Susan Thom, RD, a nutrition consultant in Brecksville, Ohio.

Prepare them late. Busy cooks have traditionally peeled and sliced potatoes

Doctor's Top Tip

Get a nutritional boost with Technicolor taters. Potatoes with gold, red, purple, and blue skin—and even some with gold, red, blue, orange, and purple flesh—are turning up at farmers' markets and in the produce section of supermarkets, too. They look pretty on your plate—and offer an extra dose of disease-fighting phytochemicals such as beta-carotene, lutein, and zeaxanthin, say nutrition experts from the University of California, Berkeley.

ahead of time, then submerged them in water to keep them from darkening. This may keep potatoes looking fresh, but it also strips valuable nutrients. "You lose some of the soluble vitamins in the water," says dietitian Mona Sutnick, RD, a nutrition consultant in Philadelphia.

Barbecue Oven Fries

4   medium baking potatoes
2½ tablespoons ketchup
4   teaspoons canola oil
2   teaspoons cider vinegar
2   teaspoons Worcestershire sauce
⅛   teaspoon salt

Preheat the oven to 425°F. Coat a baking sheet with cooking spray.

Scrub the potatoes and pat dry with paper towels. Cut each potato lengthwise into 5 or 6 slices, then stack the slices and cut at ¼-inch intervals to make french fries.

In a large bowl, combine the ketchup, oil, vinegar, Worcestershire sauce, and salt. Add the potatoes and toss to coat.

Spread the potatoes evenly on the baking sheet. Bake for 20 minutes, then turn and bake for 10 to 15 minutes longer, or until tender and golden. Test for doneness by inserting the tip of a sharp knife into a fry.

Makes 4 servings

PER SERVING

Calories: 185
Total fat: 4.7 g
Saturated fat: 0.3 g

Cholesterol: 0 mg
Sodium: 218 mg
Dietary fiber: 3 g

Poultry

BIRDS FOR STRONG BLOOD

HEALING POWER

Can Help:

Prevent iron-deficiency anemia

Prevent vision loss

Maintain a healthy nervous system

Prevent energy and memory problems

Keep immunity strong

Americans have long considered poultry to be a sign of prosperity. During the Depression, Franklin Delano Roosevelt promised a chicken in every pot. And every Thanksgiving we gather around a dressed turkey and show appreciation for our blessings.

A bird on the table is more than just a symbol, however. Properly prepared, poultry is an important part of a healthful diet. Without the skin, it not only is a low-fat alternative to fattier meats like beef and pork but also provides a host of disease-fighting, energy-boosting vitamins and minerals that are difficult to get from plant foods alone.

Of course, there is one caveat: That healthful piece of poultry may become a permanent part of your waistline unless you remove the skin before taking a bite. This is particularly true when buying fast food or chicken with the skin on, doused in gravy, at popular chain restaurants. For example, researchers found that a half-chicken platter at Boston Market rivaled a Big Mac, served with large fries and a chocolate milk shake, in fat, sodium, and calories.

A B-Vitamin Boost

Most of us understand the importance of getting our daily fill of the vitamin all-stars, like vitamins C and E and beta-carotene. But ask someone what the B vitamins are good for, and you'll likely get a blank stare. That's because these unsung heroes of the vitamin world don't directly prevent major health problems like heart disease and cancer—though they certainly may lend a helping hand. Mostly, they're maintenance workers; in a lot of little ways, they keep our minds and bodies working smoothly. Take away the B vitamins, and you'd find yourself fumbling through life, depressed, confused, anemic, and nervous—or worse.

Luckily, poultry is bursting with three essential B vitamins: niacin, vitamin B_6, and vitamin B_{12}.

Depending on the part of the bird you pick, chicken and turkey provide between 16 and 62 percent of the Daily Value (DV) of 20 milligrams for niacin. (Chicken

In the Kitchen

Chefs agree that the trick to making perfect poultry is to cook the bird in the skin. The melting fat from skin acts like a natural baste, keeping the meat flavorful and moist during the long cooking process.

"Poultry can be horribly dry when you cook it without the skin," says Susan Kleiner, PhD, RD, owner of High Performance Nutrition in Mercer Island, Washington. "And studies show that as long as you remove the skin when it's done cooking, the fat content of the poultry is about the same as if you had removed it beforehand."

In a hurry? Grab a rotisserie bird at the supermarket. The National Chicken Council estimates that 700 million rotisserie chickens were sold to hungry Americans in 2006 alone. True, they're higher in fat and salt than a home-cooked chicken could be, but if you remove the skin and discard the drippings, 3 ounces of white meat has just 102 calories and 2 grams of fat. And it's versatile. Dress it up by chopping the breast meat and mixing it with corn, black beans, and salsa in a microwaveable casserole dish. Top with shredded cheese and reheat for a few minutes. Or create quick curried chicken salad: Toss chunked breast meat with canola oil mayo, curry powder, sliced almonds, pineapple chunks, chopped mango, and raisins.

breast is at the high end of the scale, and turkey dark meat is at the low end.) Studies show that it may reduce cholesterol and cut the risk for heart attacks.

Poultry also contains 0.3 microgram of vitamin B_{12}, or 5 percent of the DV. Vitamin B_{12}, which is found almost solely in animal foods, is essential for healthy brain function. Get too little B_{12}, and you may find yourself feeling fatigued and experiencing memory loss and other neurological problems.

Another B vitamin, B_6, is critical for maintaining immunity. It's also necessary for making red blood cells and maintaining a healthy nervous system. Poultry provides between 0.2 and 0.5 milligram of vitamin B_6, or 10 to 25 percent of the DV.

Metal for Your Mettle

When knights went into battle, they donned suits of armor to make them stronger. Though none of us are jousting these days, we still need iron for the everyday battles of life. We just need to eat it, not wear it.

Iron is one of the most important nutrients for maximum energy and vitality. Yet many of us, especially women, fall short of the 15 milligrams needed each day, says Susan M. Kleiner, PhD, RD, owner of High Performance Nutrition in Mercer Island, Washington, and author of *The Good Mood Diet* and *Power Eating: Build Muscle, Increase Energy, Cut Fat*.

You can get between 5 and 16 percent of the iron you need each day by eating a piece of poultry. About 3 ounces of chicken leg or white-meat turkey breast provides 1.2 milligrams of iron, 8 percent of the Recommended Dietary Allowance (RDA) for women and 12 percent for men. Three ounces of roasted turkey dark meat will give you 2 milligrams, 13 percent of a woman's RDA and 20 percent of a man's.

Although iron abounds in fortified cereals, tofu, beans, and other nonmeat foods, it's not always easy for the body to absorb. By contrast, the iron in poultry (called heme iron) is easily absorbed, says Dr. Kleiner. Your body can absorb up to 15 percent more heme iron than nonheme iron, she explains. Plus, when you eat heme

---

TAKE FLIGHT ON THE WILD SIDE

Have you eaten so much chicken that you're starting to resemble Frank Purdue? Maybe it's time to leave that poultry behind and take flight with some birds of a different feather. Although they tend to be higher-priced, birds like pheasant and quail add variety to your diet while providing the same nutritional benefits as chicken or turkey.

Here's how two of the less common varieties of poultry add up. All nutritional information is based on 3-ounce servings, and the percentages of the DV or, in the case of iron, the RDA, are given.

Pheasant

Calories: 113

Fat: 3 grams

Calories from fat: 25 percent

Iron: 1 milligram (10 percent of RDA for men and 7 percent for women)

Niacin: 6 milligrams (30 percent of DV)

Vitamin B$_6$: 0.6 milligram (30 percent of DV)

Vitamin B$_{12}$: 0.7 microgram (12 percent of DV)

Zinc: 0.8 milligram (5 percent of DV)

Riboflavin: 0.1 milligram (8 percent of DV)

Vitamin C: 5 milligrams (6 percent of DV)

Quail

Calories: 123

Fat: 4 grams

Calories from fat: 31 percent

Iron: 4 milligrams (40 percent of RDA for men and 27 percent for women)

Niacin: 8 milligrams (40 percent of DV)

Vitamin B$_6$: 0.5 milligram (25 percent of DV)

Thiamin: 0.3 milligram (20 percent of DV)

Zinc: 3 milligrams (20 percent of DV)

Riboflavin: 0.3 milligram (18 percent of DV)

Vitamin C: 7 milligrams (12 percent of DV)

The New Safety Rules

Consumer Reports magazine shocked the nation in December 2006, when it announced that 83 percent of the chicken sold in supermarkets may contain bacteria that cause food-borne illness. They found bacteria in brand-name birds, store-brand birds, and organic chickens alike. "We think it's really startling," said Jean Halloran, a policy director for Consumers Union, which publishes *Consumer Reports.* "It's a very significant deterioration in food safety."

While the USDA disputed the findings as "junk science" (government studies have found that 26 to 60 percent of chickens harbor bacteria), no one disputes the fact that raw poultry is a playground for salmonella, campylobacter, and other organisms that can cause diarrhea, tummy cramps, and fever. There's no way to eliminate bacteria entirely, but these updated rules can help you keep your poultry safe and healthy:

When you buy: Choose packages that feel cool and have no tears or punctures. (Skip poultry stuffed at the store, it's too vulnerable to bacterial growth.) Put each pack in a plastic bag, so that poultry juices can't contaminate other foods. Buy poultry last; store in an ice chest if you won't be home to refrigerate it within an hour; and when you get home, unload and fridge it first.

Storage: Use or freeze poultry within 2 days. Whole birds and parts will keep, frozen, for 6 to 9 months. Ground poultry and giblets, for 3 to 4 months. (Never thaw poultry at room temperature—place it in fridge to thaw or microwave.)

Prep: Don't wash poultry—this just splashes germy juices around your kitchen (and on you). Cooking heat kills any bacteria. But do scrub tools, cutting boards, and your work area thoroughly with hot, soapy water after preparing raw chicken to prevent bacteria from multiplying. Wash your own hands frequently and dry with paper towels. Marinate birds in the fridge and toss the marinade afterward—it's a swimming pool packed with bacteria.

Cooking: Find—or buy—a food thermometer. Checking the internal temperature of poultry is the only way to ensure that it's fully cooked (going by color, texture, or juice color is unreliable, according to the USDA). Target temperatures: All poultry should be cooked to a minimum internal temperature of 165°F throughout. For whole chicken and turkey, you should check the internal temperature on the innermost part of the thigh and the thickest part of the breast.

iron, it helps your body absorb nonheme iron. That way, you get the most iron from all your food, says Dr. Kleiner.

In the Pink with Zinc

In order to stay in the pink—free from infections, colds, and other health problems that keep us home in bed watching bad daytime TV—we need strong immune systems. Getting enough zinc in the diet is critical for immunity because our infection-fighting cells require adequate stores of this trace mineral to do their job.

In addition, studies show that getting enough zinc can help slow the progression of a prevalent eye disorder called macular degeneration, which can cause irreversible vision loss, especially among the elderly.

As with iron, zinc is found in foods besides meat, like whole grains and wheat germ—but again, your body has a harder time absorbing it from plant foods than from meats, says Dr. Kleiner. "Women especially are at risk for not getting enough zinc," she says.

Eating poultry will help keep your zinc supply at the necessary levels, Dr. Kleiner says. Most poultry provides 6 to 25 percent of the 15 milligrams of zinc you need each day.

Doctor's Top Tip

Hectic day, hungry family? When the only sane meal option is the drive-thru, order grilled chicken sandwiches—not the nuggets—all around, says the American Institute for Cancer Research. "Chicken nuggets can include not just the chicken meat itself but also the skin, with several types of flour, starches, and oils," the group notes. "That makes nuggets higher in calories with about half the protein compared to an equal portion of plain cooked skinless chicken." Nuggets have four times the saturated fat and trans fats, too. (Worried that the tykes in the backseat will howl when their kids' meal doesn't come with a toy? Most chains will sell you the plastic doo-dads à la carte. Costs more, but may be worth it.)

GETTING THE MOST

Grab a drumstick. Lots of people pick around the dark meat of poultry because it's higher in fat. And that's true, concedes Dr. Kleiner, but it's also a lot higher in minerals and worth digging into occasionally.

"If you've removed the skin, you've removed the mother lode of fat anyway," she says, "and a lot of the iron and zinc are in the dark meat."

Read chicken labels carefully. Think "free-range" chicken means a friendly flock of hens pecking in the farmyard—and getting natural food, air, and sunshine that make the meat healthier? Think again. The USDA poultry labeling standards allow any bird that has outdoor access for a few minutes a day to be labeled free range. And the words "natural" and "hormone free" aren't really guarantees that a chicken was raised organically and without unnecessary medications. (The USDA already prohibits the use of hormones in the raising of chickens for home consumption.) Your best bet for finding a chemical-free bird? Look for labels that say "USDA organic," which means the chicken was raised without hormones, antibiotics, or feed grown with synthetic pesticides or fertilizers. If you'd like a happy chicken raised on grass, not a concrete-floored coop, look for labels that say "Certified Humane Raised and Handled"—a claim that's verified by a third-party group before poultry farmers can use it on the label.

Turkey Cutlets with Oregano-Lemon Sauce

1 **pound turkey breast cutlets**

3 **tablespoons all-purpose flour**

¾ **teaspoon dried oregano**

⅛ **teaspoon salt**

1 **tablespoon olive oil**

2 **cloves garlic, minced**

¼ **cup defatted reduced-sodium chicken broth**

3 **tablespoons fresh lemon juice**

Rinse the turkey and pat dry.

On a plate, combine the flour, ½ teaspoon of the oregano, and salt. Mix with a fork. Place the turkey cutlets in the flour mixture, turning to dust both sides evenly. Shake off any excess.

In a large nonstick skillet, heat the oil over medium-high heat. Add the cutlets in a single layer, and cook for 2 to 3 minutes per side, or until golden and cooked through. Check for doneness by inserting the tip of a sharp knife into a cutlet. Remove the turkey to a plate.

Add the garlic to the skillet, and cook for 10 to 12 seconds, or until fragrant. Add the broth, lemon juice, and the remaining ¼ teaspoon oregano. Cook, stirring, for 2 to 3 minutes, or until hot. Pour the sauce over the turkey.

Makes 4 servings

PER SERVING

Calories: 184	Cholesterol: 77 mg
Total fat: 4.6 g	Sodium: 124 mg
Saturated fat: 0.8 g	Dietary fiber: 0.3 g

Premenstrual Problems
FOODS FOR MONTHLY DISCOMFORT

There's probably not a woman in the country who doesn't know what "PMS" means. Yet these three letters describe a condition that's as misunderstood as it is common.

PMS, or premenstrual syndrome, is believed to affect between one-third and one-half of American women of childbearing age. There are more than 150 symptoms that may occur in women with PMS, including anxiety, breast tenderness, and food cravings. Some women get only one or two symptoms, while others are plagued by a dozen. Discomfort usually begins 10 days to 2 weeks before menstruation and eases when menstruation begins.

Doctors used to believe PMS was "all in your head." They don't think that any more. But they still aren't sure exactly what causes the dizzying array of physical and emotional problems. A variety of factors is probably involved, including swings in hormones (estrogen and progesterone), blood sugar, and the brain chemical serotonin.

Even though there's still a lot of mystery surrounding this condition, one thing is clear: What you eat can make a big difference in how you feel before your period. Here are some nutritional strategies for easing the discomfort.

Calcium's Mood-Lifting Chemistry

Researchers at the University of Massachusetts at Amherst have found evidence that a high intake of calcium and vitamin D may, in fact, not only lessen the severity of PMS symptoms but—yippee!!!—even prevent PMS from developing in the first place.

When researcher Elizabeth R. Bertone-Johnson, ScD, and her team compared women who reported developing PMS with those who had no or very mild symptoms over a 10-year period, they concluded that women who ate or drank about 1,200 milligrams of calcium and 400 IU of vitamin D daily were 30 percent less likely to develop the mood swings, bloating, pre-period cramps, and other symptoms of PMS. The calcium-plus-D group took in about four daily servings of fat-free or low-fat milk, fortified orange juice, or another low-fat dairy product such as yogurt.

While numerous other studies have linked calcium and vitamin D to a lessening of PMS symptoms, the University of Massachusetts study was one of the first to suggest that these minerals may even prevent this annoying, inconvenient, and often relationship-testing condition before it starts. And even though the researchers acknowledge that larger studies are needed, bumping up your calcium and D to these healthy levels now can't hurt—and may even help keep other health problems, such as osteoporosis and some cancers, at bay.

Calcium works to reduce PMS symptoms in a number of ways. It may help prevent the muscular contractions that cause cramping, says research psychologist James G. Penland, PhD, who has conducted calcium/PMS studies at the USDA Human Nutrition Research Center in Grand Forks, North Dakota. According to Dr. Penland, "Calcium clearly has an impact on certain brain chemicals and hormones known to affect mood."

Throughout your cycle, Dr. Penland says, it's a good idea to begin increasing your consumption of low-fat, calcium-rich foods such as fat-free or low-fat milk and low-fat yogurt. You don't need massive amounts to get the benefits—women in the studies generally took in 1,000 to about 1,340 milligrams a day, the amount in four servings of low-fat or fat-free milk, yogurt, cheese, or fortified orange juice. (Can't quite fit that much in? It's okay to take a calcium supplement.)

Magnesium for Mood Swings

Calcium isn't the only mineral that affects brain chemistry. A number of studies have found that women with PMS tend to have low levels of magnesium. Being deficient in magnesium can result in lower levels of dopamine, a brain chemical that, like serotonin, helps regulate mood, says Melvyn Werbach, MD, assistant clinical professor of psychiatry at the University of California, Los Angeles, and author of *Healing Through Nutrition* and *Nutritional Influences on Illness*. "A magnesium deficiency might also impair the metabolism of estrogen," another cause of premenstrual moodiness, he says.

In an Italian study, 28 women with PMS took 360 milligrams of magnesium a day. After 2 months, they reported having less depression, bloating, cramps, and other premenstrual symptoms. Taking 200 milligrams per day helped relieve water retention and mood swings in women in several British studies as well.

The Daily Value (DV) for magnesium is 400 to 420 milligrams for men and 310 to 320 for women (more if you're pregnant), an amount that's easy to get in food. A serving of instant oatmeal, for example, has 28 milligrams of magnesium, or 7 percent of the DV. A banana has 33 milligrams, or 8 percent of the DV, and a fillet of baked or broiled flounder has 49 milligrams, or 12 percent of the DV. Brown rice is another great source of magnesium, with a half-cup providing 42 milligrams, or 11 percent of the DV. Whole grains and dark green leafy vegetables are also high in this mineral.

Relieve Moodiness with B_6

Yet another nutrient that can help stop the emotional swings of PMS is vitamin B_6. In an English study, 32 women with PMS took 50 milligrams of vitamin B_6 a day for 3 months. They reported having less depression, irritability, and fatigue. It may be that high doses of vitamin B_6 bring premenstrual hormones into balance by lowering levels of estrogen and raising those of progesterone. And since vitamin B_6 is used by the body to manufacture serotonin, taking supplements of this vitamin may help reduce depression, Dr. Werbach says.

Numerous studies show that B_6 alleviates PMS-related depression, especially when combined with magnesium. While the DV for B_6 is 1.7 to 1.9 milligrams, it's safe to get up to 50 to 100 milligrams a day, says Dr. Werbach. If you're going with supplements, don't take more without consulting your doctor first. But you really don't need a pill to get more vitamin B_6, says Dr. Werbach. A meal consisting of 3 ounces of boneless chicken breast, a baked potato with the skin, and a banana, for example, contains nearly 2 milligrams, or 100 percent of the DV.

Calming Carbohydrates

One of the most common symptoms of PMS is the urge to binge on sugary foods, which, in turn, can lead to weight gain as well as depression and mood swings.

SMART SWAPS

There are many foods (and substances in foods) that can aggravate premenstrual pain. The problem, for many women, is how to go an entire week or more without enjoying their usual favorites. Here are some of the more-common culprits, along with some satisfying alternatives:

- Breast tenderness and increased irritability and anxiety can be caused by caffeine. Try caffeine-free colas or decaffeinated coffee, or coffee substitutes such as Postum.
- Too much salt can cause the body to retain fluids, increasing bloating and breast tenderness. Try flavoring foods with additional herbs, spices, or nonsalt seasonings, such as Mrs. Dash, and use low-salt canned and processed foods.
- Chocolate can often aggravate mood swings and breast tenderness. Use unsweetened carob instead.

It's not surprising that the sweet tooth often wakes up at a woman's time of the month. In women with PMS, that's when the body's blood sugar level is often low, explains women's health expert Susan M. Lark, MD, author of *The PMS Self-Help Book*. It's not certain why this occurs, although it appears that insulin, which moves glucose out of the bloodstream into individual cells, works more efficiently as menstruation approaches. With less glucose circulating in the bloodstream, there's less available to the brain. The brain, noting that it's low on fuel, lets the body know that it needs more, which, in body talk, loosely translates as "I need cookies!"

To quiet your body's clamor for sugar without raiding the cookie jar, it's helpful to eat complex carbohydrates. Because they're absorbed more slowly than the sugars in sweets, they help stabilize your blood sugar. And that, in turn, controls sugar cravings.

Another way in which complex carbohydrates ease premenstrual discomfort is by increasing the brain's level of serotonin, a calming chemical that regulates mood and sleep. In a small study conducted at the Massachusetts Institute of Technology in Cambridge, women with PMS reported that eating a carbohydrate-rich meal lightened their premenstrual depression, tension, and sadness and made them feel more calm and alert.

Some doctors recommend that women with premenstrual discomfort eat a small amount of whole-grain pasta, whole-grain cereal, or whole-grain bread every 3 hours, which will help keep blood sugar from falling too low. In one study, 54 percent of women who consumed a starch-based mini-meal such as bread, crackers, or cereal every 3 hours had less premenstrual discomfort.

For some women, however, it's important to avoid wheat during this time. Wheat contains gluten, a protein that tends to increase premenstrual bloating and weight gain. If this appears to be a problem for you, Dr. Lark advises that you may want to stick with rice, millet, or other nonwheat grains before your period.

There's no reason to limit yourself to bread and crackers when you're trying to get more carbohydrates. Having a bowl of whole-grain cereal, like plain granola or oatmeal, will keep you full while also keeping your sweet tooth under control. Rice cakes also make a good snack, particularly when topped with a little peanut butter or sugar-free preserves. Dried beans and other legumes are also good sources of complex carbohydrates.

In addition, fruits and vegetables are other excellent sources of complex carbohydrates. Plus, they're low in calories, so you can eat them often without worrying about your weight. Dr. Lark particularly recommends eating root vegetables, such as carrots, turnips, and parsnips, and dark green leafy vegetables like collard and mustard greens, all of which are rich in magnesium and calcium—nutrients that have been shown to ease premenstrual discomfort.

While most fruits are good for women with PMS, tropical varieties like mangoes, papayas, and pineapple are unusually high in sugar. This means they can aggravate rather than relieve food cravings. As your period approaches, you may want to stick with less-sugary fruits such as apples, oranges, or grapefruits.

The Role of Fat

Just as women often crave sweets as their periods approach, many also get a hankering for high-fat foods like doughnuts, potato chips, or ice cream. Indeed, women in the throes of PMS can get as much as 40 percent of their calories from fat, says Guy Abraham, MD, a former professor of obstetrics and gynecology at the University of California, Los Angeles, who later founded a dietary supplement company, Optimox, in Torrance, California.

More is involved than just the extra calories. The kind of fat you eat before your period—and how much of it you eat—can affect the severity of your symptoms. The worst kind of fat, not surprisingly, is the saturated kind found in red meats, whole-fat dairy foods, and many processed foods. Saturated fat causes estrogen levels to rise, which worsens virtually all PMS symptoms, says Dr. Abraham. Conversely, evidence suggests that women who eat a lot of fruits, vegetables, and whole grains but little or no meat tend to have fewer premenstrual symptoms than their carnivorous sisters.

All women, not just those with PMS, are advised to limit their consumption of fat to no more than 30 percent of total calories, with 10 percent coming from saturated fat and the rest from unsaturated fat, says Dr. Abraham.

Researchers are now looking into whether omega-3 fatty acids, fats that are found in certain types of fish, canola and olive oils, flaxseeds and flaxseed oil, and walnuts, for example, may play a role in PMS. Preliminary evidence suggests that

Doctor's Top Tip

Serious PMS? Go vegetarian. When 33 women with extreme PMS tried a strict vegan eating plan (no animal products, notably meat, fish, poultry, eggs, and dairy products) for 2 months, bloating and difficulty concentrating (two big PMS problems) decreased. And so did menstrual cramps. "For some women, the change was profound," notes lead researcher Neil Barnard, MD, president of the Washington, D.C.–based group Physicians Committee for Responsible Medicine. "Their pain was gone or dramatically reduced, something they had not experienced for years. If they needed any pain medicine at all, they needed much less than before."

Dr. Barnard suspects that the high-fiber, low-fat eating plan increases levels of sex-hormone-binding globulin—which in turn deactivates excess estrogen careening around in the bloodstream. "Our goal was to smooth out the hormonal roller coaster many of them experience each month," says Dr. Barnard.

having too few omega-3s and too much linoleic acid (an unsaturated fat) in your system can lead to an overproduction of a certain type of prostaglandin. This particular hormone-like compound can cause menstrual cramps.

Because we get so much linoleic acid from oils such as corn and safflower, some nutritionists suggest getting more omega-3s from fish such as salmon, Spanish mackerel, and chunk light tuna. You can also try using a little canola oil in cooking and using flaxseed oil in salad dressings.

In practical terms, this means using olive oil or canola oil instead of butter and substituting such things as whole-wheat bread and low-fat cream cheese for high-fat doughnuts and other snack foods. Even simple changes can help keep estrogen levels stable, thus easing the monthly woes.

Prunes

NATURE'S LAXATIVE

HEALING POWER

Can Help:

Relieve constipation

Lower cholesterol

Reduce the risk of cancer and heart disease

Would you rather have prunes . . . or dried plums? We bet you'd pick the latter. So did the California Prune Board, which officially petitioned the FDA to change the name of this sweet, chewy fruit from stodgy old "prune" to the sophisticated "dried plum" in 1999. The change drew a lot of laughs—dried plums made an appearance on *The Tonight Show* with Jay Leno and became the focus of a series of Millard Fillmore comic strips. The spiffy new moniker also boosted flagging sales by 11 percent in just 3 months, reports the renamed California Dried Plum Board.

And that's a good thing. By any name, this chewy, slightly sticky, densely sweet treat is a unique fruity package full of vitamin A, potassium, and a very special, useful fiber.

Nature's Laxative

Pharmacies stock dozens of medications for preventing and relieving constipation. But most of the time they really aren't necessary if you get in the habit of adding prunes to your daily diet. Prunes contain not just one but three different ingredients that work together to help keep your digestive system on track.

For starters, prunes are high in insoluble fiber, which is perhaps the key to preventing constipation. Since insoluble fiber isn't absorbed by your body, it stays in the digestive tract. And because it's incredibly absorbent, it soaks up large amounts of water, making stools larger and easier to pass. (Prunes also contain soluble fiber, the type that helps lower cholesterol and with it the risk of heart disease.) Just five prunes contain almost 3 grams of fiber, or about 12 percent of the Daily Value (DV).

In addition, prunes contain a natural sugar called sorbitol. Like fiber, sorbitol soaks up water wherever it can find it, says Mary Ellen Camire, PhD, professor in the department of food science and human nutrition at the University of Maine in Orono. Most fruits contain small amounts (usually less than 1 percent) of sorbitol. Prunes, however, are about 15 percent sorbitol, which explains why they're such a potent bulking agent and are often recommended for relieving constipation.

Doctor's Top Tip

Buy prune juice with added lutein. Some food makers are adding extra lutein—a phytochemical that can protect your eyes against damage wrought by sunlight—to prune juice. Even cautious nutritionists at the Center for Science in the Public Interest in Washington, D.C., say it's worth drinking.

Finally, prunes contain a compound called dihydroxyphenyl isatin, which stimulates the intestine, causing it to contract. This process is essential for having regular bowel movements.

You don't need a lot of prunes to get the benefits. One daily serving—about five prunes—is all most people need to help themselves stay regular.

All-Around Protection

As with most fruits, prunes contain generous amounts of a variety of vitamins, minerals, and other healthful compounds. In fact, they're a concentrated source of energy because they lose water during the drying process. This means that you get a lot of value in a very small package.

One of the most healthful compounds in prunes is beta-carotene. Like vitamins C and E, beta-carotene is an antioxidant, meaning that it helps neutralize harmful oxygen molecules in the body. Prunes also contain generous amounts of potassium, a mineral that's essential for keeping blood pressure down. Studies have shown that when potassium levels decline, even for short periods of time, blood pressure rises.

Prunes are a very good source of potassium, with five prunes containing 313 milligrams, which is about 9 percent of the DV. In fact, when Harvard School of Public Health researchers tracked 41,000 nurses for 4 years, they found that those who ate the most prunes, apples, oranges, and grapes had the lowest blood pressure levels.

GETTING THE MOST

For vitamins, drink the juice. Although prune juice has less fiber than the whole fruit, it's a more concentrated source of vitamins. For example, five whole prunes contain more than 1 milligram of vitamin C, while a 6-ounce glass of juice contains almost 8 milligrams. (And by the way, it's still called prune juice—not dried-plum juice.)

For regularity, eat the fruit. Since fiber is such an important part of digestive health, doctors recommend eating whole prunes, either fresh or canned, when you're trying to stay regular. While prune juice has also been used to help relieve constipation, it's somewhat less effective than the whole fruit.

Cook outside the box. Try adding whirled prunes to burgers. Texas A&M

University researchers have found that adding prune purée to hamburger meat creates a mix that's moister when cooked. Try making prune purée (use pitted prunes) in a food processor, then adding some to lean ground beef before shaping the burgers for the grill.

Baked Chicken with Prunes

1   **pound skinless, boneless chicken breast halves**

16   **pitted prunes**

¼   **cup red wine**

1   **teaspoon minced fresh rosemary**

¼   **teaspoon salt**

    Freshly ground black pepper

Preheat the oven to 350°F.

Coat a 12- × 8-inch baking dish with cooking spray. Arrange the chicken in the dish in a single layer.

In a small microwaveable bowl, combine the prunes and wine. Microwave on high power for 1 minute, or until the wine boils. Pour the mixture over the chicken. Sprinkle with the rosemary.

Bake for 30 minutes, or until the chicken is no longer pink in the center. Test for doneness by inserting the tip of a sharp knife in the center of a breast half. Sprinkle with the salt and season with pepper to taste. Remove the chicken to 4 plates. Stir the pan juices to combine the spices, and spoon over the chicken.

Makes 4 servings

PER SERVING

Calories: 215
Total fat: 2.9 g
Saturated fat: 0.8 g

Cholesterol: 63 mg
Sodium: 190 mg
Dietary fiber: 3.3 g

Psoriasis

FOODS TO STOP THE SCALES

You would think that the skin you have today is the same skin you had yesterday and the day before. But every day, millions of skin cells die, are shed, and then are replaced by healthy cells.

But in people with psoriasis, the body makes far too many skin cells, producing them about five times faster than average, which causes the skin to get thick and scaly. Doctors aren't sure what causes psoriasis, although it appears that the immune system may damage genetic material that tells skin cells how often to divide.

There's evidence that eating more produce can help control psoriasis. In a study of more than 680 people, researchers at the University of Milan in Italy found that those who ate the most carrots, tomatoes, fresh fruits, and green vegetables were much less likely to get psoriasis than folks who ate less. In fact, eating just three or more servings of carrots a week reduced the risk of psoriasis by 40 percent. Those who ate seven or more servings of tomatoes a week reduced their risk by 60 percent, and those who had two servings a day of fresh fruits reduced their risk by 50 percent. Since these foods are all sources of beta-carotene and vitamins C and E, the researchers speculate that it's the antioxidant and immune-stimulating effects of these foods that may make the difference.

Healing Strategies

For a long time, researchers have suspected that eating certain types of fish can help ease psoriasis. A British study, for example, found that people with psoriasis who ate 6 ounces of fish such as salmon, mackerel, and herring a day had a 15 percent improvement in symptoms in just 6 weeks. Experts suspect that the good omega-3 fatty acids in oily fish reduce production of inflammatory compounds.

Some doctors have noticed that psoriasis lesions improve for patients on weight-loss diets and conversely, weight gain can sometimes lead to flare-ups. Maintaining a healthy weight could help you control psoriasis.

Doctor's Top Tip

If you take the drug methotrexate for psoriasis, put even more fruit, veggies, and whole grains on your plate each day, advises the National Psoriasis Foundation. This drug can inhibit folate, an important B vitamin. Fight back by eating more chicory, asparagus, and other dark green vegetables, dried beans and peas, grapefruit and orange juice, cantaloupe, chicken livers and other organ meats, and fortified cereals.

Pumpkin

THE BETA-CAROTENE KING

HEALING POWER

Can Help:

Prevent macular
degeneration

Boost immune system

Prevent heart disease
and cancer

We have pumpkin at morning and pumpkin at noon.
If it were not for pumpkin, we should be undoon.

This is a poem that the early American colonists chanted when-ever they were overcome with appreciation for this oversize orange squash. Pumpkin was a popular food back then, and the early settlers ate a peck of it in pumpkin soup, pumpkin pie, and even pumpkin beer.

It's a different story now. We usually buy pumpkin as a Halloween decoration and then throw away the sweet, nutritious flesh. If we actually eat pumpkin at all, it's mainly in Thanksgiving and Christmas pies.

That's a darn shame, since pumpkin is more than just a giant winter squash and a carver's delight. It's also filled with powerful carotenoids like beta-carotene, which can help stop cellular damage before it leads to disease.

Good for the Eyes—and More

It's not just sheer size that earned pumpkin the title "King of Squash." A half-cup of canned pumpkin has more than 16 milligrams of beta-carotene, or 160 to 260 per-cent of the daily amount recommended by experts. Pumpkin is also a source of the eye-protecting carotenoids lutein and zeaxanthin, beta-cryptoxanthin, and alpha-carotene.

Carotenoids, which create the orange color of pumpkin, help protect the body by neutralizing harmful oxygen molecules known as free radicals. "Lutein and zea-xanthin are very potent free-radical scavengers," says Paul Lachance, PhD, professor of nutrition at Rutgers University in New Brunswick, New Jersey, and director of the university's Nutraceuticals Institute. A diet high in antioxidants can help prevent many of the diseases associated with aging, including heart disease and cancer.

Lutein and zeaxanthin aren't found only in pumpkin; they are also found in the lenses of the eyes. Studies suggest that eating foods high in these compounds may help block the formation of cataracts.

In one study, scientists at the Massachusetts Eye and Ear Infirmary in Boston compared the diets of elderly people who had advanced macular degeneration, a

In the Kitchen

Because of their size and perfect carvability, pumpkins have been destined to spend their lives on front porches rather than on dinner plates.

But pumpkins, despite their ornamental nature, are still squash, which means that they can be eaten whole, mashed, or cut into chunks for a hearty stew.

- To bake pumpkin, cut it in half (or, if it's large, into quarters), scoop out the seeds, and place the pieces, cut side down, in a baking pan. Add a little water to prevent scorching, and bake at 350°F for 45 to 60 minutes, or until easily pierced with a knife.

- To speed cooking time, pumpkin can be cut into smaller pieces and either baked in the oven, steamed, or microwaved.

- When using pumpkin for a pie, soup, or stew, you have to remove the skin. The easiest way to do this is to prepare the pumpkin for baking, then bake in a 350°F oven until the flesh is slightly soft. When the pumpkin is cool enough to handle, scoop or cut out the flesh. Discard the skin and proceed with the recipe.

condition that leads to blurred vision, to the diets of those without the disease. The researchers found that those who ate the most carotenoid-rich foods had a 43 percent lower risk of getting this condition than folks who ate the least. Among people who already had macular degeneration, those who got the most carotenoids in their diets were less likely to develop a more serious form of the disease.

The beta-carotene in pumpkin helps protect the plant itself from diseases, from getting too much sunlight, and from other naturally occurring stresses. There's strong evidence that beta-carotene can help protect people from a variety of conditions as well. Research has shown, for example, that getting more beta-carotene in the diet can help protect against a variety of cancers, including those of the stomach, esophagus, lungs, and colon. This protective effect is enhanced by phenolic acids, which are chemicals in pumpkin that bind to potential carcinogens and help prevent them from being absorbed.

The beta-carotene in pumpkin may play a role in preventing heart disease as well. Some research suggests that people with diets high in fruits and vegetables that contain beta-carotene have a lower risk of heart disease than those whose diets supplied less.

Other carotenoids have their own special powers. In a Chinese study of 63,257 women and men, those who ate the most beta-cryptoxanthin had a 27 percent reduction in lung cancer risk. Among smokers in the study, those who ate the most foods containing this carotenoid had a 3 percent lower risk for lung cancer.

The Whole Picture

In addition to its rich stores of beta-carotene and other phytonutrients, pumpkin contains generous amounts of fiber. For example, while 1 cup of cornflakes contains 1 gram of fiber, a half-cup of canned pumpkin contains more than 3 grams, or 6 percent of the Daily Value (DV).

Iron is another pumpkin mainstay. A half-cup of pumpkin provides almost 2 milligrams of iron, or about 20 percent of the Recommended Dietary Allowance (RDA) for men and 13 percent of the RDA for women. This is particularly important for women, who need to replenish their iron regularly due to menstruation.

Even richer in iron than the flesh are the pumpkin's seeds. One ounce—which consists of about 140 seeds, a huge handful—contains about 4 milligrams of iron, or about 40 percent of the RDA for men and 27 percent of the RDA for women. What's more, that ounce of seeds has as much protein—9 grams—as an ounce of meat, says Susan Thom, RD, a nutrition consultant in Brecksville, Ohio.

Pumpkin seeds are great for men's prostate issues too. Compounds found in the oil inside pumpkin seeds may help halt prostate-cell overgrowth fueled by testosterone—a condition called benign prostatic hyperplasia (BPH), which affects many men over the age of 50. Carotenoids and good fats found in pumpkin seeds may also help cut the risk for BPH. Pumpkin seeds are also a rich source of zinc, which may improve prostate function and can help protect bone density. Studies of middle-aged and older men suggest that low zinc intake may be associated with brittle, fracture-prone bones.

Of course, you don't want to eat too many pumpkin seeds, since about 73 percent of the calories (there are 148 calories in an ounce of seeds) come from fat. But when you have a taste for a crunchy, highly nutritious snack, pumpkin seeds, in moderation, are a good choice.

Doctor's Top Tip

Fresh pumpkin has a bright, sweet flavor—and it's easier to prepare than you might expect, according to the American Diabetes Association. Shop for a small pumpkin (about the size of an acorn squash) during pumpkin season, between late September and late December. Look for one that's heavy for its size, with bright color and hard skin. To prepare it, wash the outside, then cut the pumpkin into 4- to 5-inch pieces (remove the seeds, but don't remove the rind). Roast in a 350°F oven for 1 hour. Remove and cool, then scoop out the flesh. Mash with a potato masher, or purée in a blender or food processor until smooth. Use the mashed fresh pumpkin as you would canned pumpkin. A 2½-pound pumpkin provides about 2 cups of purée. It will keep in the refrigerator for up to 3 days, or it can be frozen for up to 6 months.

GETTING THE MOST

Consider it canned. Need pumpkin now? An easy, convenient alternative is to buy canned pumpkin. Nutritionally, it's almost equal to fresh.

Temper the taste. Pumpkin is among the stronger-flavored squashes, and even people who like the taste can be overwhelmed by its potent presence. To get the most pumpkin into your diet, you may want to mellow the taste. One way to do this is to add about a tablespoon of orange juice or any other citrus juice during cooking, suggests Anne Dubner, RD, a nutrition consultant in Houston.

Love your leftovers. There's no reason to force yourself to eat an entire pumpkin at one sitting—as though you could! When frozen in a freezer-proof container, pumpkin retains virtually all its goodness and nutrition.

Make your own pumpkin seed snacks. Scrape the seeds from your Halloween pumpkin, rub off the extra pumpkin flesh, and let the seeds dry overnight on a baking sheet lined with paper towels. The next day, remove the paper towel, and place the seeds on the baking sheet. Roast in a 160°F (low) oven for 15 to 20 minutes, or until the seeds are crisp and lightly browned. Season as desired.

Pumpkin Maple Pudding

1 can (16 ounces) pumpkin
1 can (12 ounces) fat-free evaporated milk
¾ cup maple syrup
1 egg
2 egg whites
1 tablespoon all-purpose flour
2 teaspoons ground cinnamon
1¼ teaspoons ground ginger
⅛ teaspoon salt
¼ cup chopped pecans

Preheat the oven to 325°F. Coat a 2½-quart baking dish or soufflé dish with cooking spray.

In a large bowl, combine the pumpkin, milk, maple syrup, egg, egg whites, flour, cinnamon, ginger, and salt. Whisk until smooth.

Pour into the prepared dish. Bake for 1 hour, or until almost set. (The pudding should still jiggle slightly in the center.)

Sprinkle with the pecans. Bake for 5 to 10 minutes longer, or until a wooden pick inserted in the center comes out clean. Remove to a wire rack to cool. Cover, and refrigerate for several hours to chill.

Makes 6 servings

Cook's Note: *For best results, serve the pudding the same day you bake it. Serve with fat-free whipped topping, if desired.*

PER SERVING

Calories: 229
Total fat: 4.4 g
Saturated fat: 0.6 g

Cholesterol: 38 mg
Sodium: 163 mg
Dietary fiber: 3.8 g

Quinoa

THE MOTHER OF ALL GRAINS

HEALING POWER

Can Help:

Fight fatigue

Prevent anemia

Regulate blood pressure

Control blood sugar

High in the Peruvian mountains centuries ago, the Incas dined on a grain so important that they named it quinoa—literally, the "mother grain."

All grains are good for health, but quinoa stands head and shoulders above the rest. It contains more protein than any other grain, and it is such a rich and balanced source of essential nutrients that food experts have called it the supergrain of the future.

Packed with Protein

Quinoa is one of the best grain sources of protein. And unlike the protein found in most grains, quinoa's protein is complete, meaning that it contains all nine amino acids that the body must get from food, says Diane Grabowski-Nepa, RD, a dietitian and nutritional counselor at the Pritikin Longevity Center in Santa Monica, California. This makes quinoa a choice grain for people who are limiting meat in their diets and who may have trouble getting enough protein.

A half-cup of cooked quinoa delivers 5 grams of protein, or 10 percent of the Daily Value (DV). "It's particularly high in the amino acid lysine," adds Grabowski-Nepa. Lysine is important for helping tissues grow and repair themselves.

A High-Energy Grain

For your blood to carry oxygen, it must have iron. When you don't get enough iron in your diet, red blood cells actually shrink, reducing the amount of oxygen they can carry. To make up the difference, the heart and lungs have to work harder. Over time, this extra exertion causes fatigue.

Quinoa can wake you up again. "Most grains have a little iron, but quinoa is a very good source," says Grabowski-Nepa. For example, a half-cup of cooked quinoa contains 4 milligrams of iron, or 40 percent of the Recommended Dietary Allowance (RDA) for men and 27 percent of the RDA for women. Compare that with a similar amount of brown rice, which has only 1 milligram of iron.

Help for Circulation

Besides providing a mineful of iron, quinoa supplies two additional nutrients, magnesium and riboflavin, which help your cardiovascular system work efficiently.

People who don't get enough magnesium in their diets have a higher risk of developing high blood pressure. In fact, doctors have found that when people deficient in magnesium start getting enough, their blood pressure improves, the blood is less likely to clot, and the heart beats more regularly. Magnesium also helps keep the linings of blood vessels supple, keeping blood pressure under control.

Quinoa can help restore your magnesium to heart-healthy standards. A half-cup of cooked quinoa contains 90 milligrams of magnesium, or 22 percent of the DV. As a fiber-rich whole grain, powerful quinoa can help keep atherosclerosis—the clogging of artery walls with fatty substances such as cholesterol—at bay and also prevent arteries from narrowing. In the Estrogen Replacement and Atherosclerosis Trial study of 200 postmenopausal women, Tufts University researchers found that those who ate at least six servings of whole grains each week enjoyed these benefits.

A bonus: Getting sufficient magnesium as well as riboflavin, another vitamin found in quinoa, can also reduce the frequency of migraine headaches.

A Gluten-Free Good Guy

The American and Canadian dietetic societies recently released a recommendation that people with gluten intolerance could safely include quinoa in their diets. The grain had long been the subject of controversy among people with gluten intolerance.

In the Kitchen

While wheat, rice, and other grains are all prepared in similar ways, quinoa is smaller and more delicate and must be treated a little bit differently. Here's what chefs advise:

Wash it well. As quinoa grows, it develops a natural, protective coating called saponin, which sometimes has a bitter taste. To wash away the residue, rinse quinoa before you start cooking.

Watch the time. Quinoa cooks more quickly than other grains, and because of its delicate texture, it can get twice as mushy when you overcook it. To get the proper consistency, bring 2 cups of water to a boil, add 1 cup of quinoa, reduce the heat to low, and cook, covered, for 10 to 15 minutes, or until the grains are tender but still slightly crunchy and all the liquid has been absorbed.

Use a little, get a lot. Some folks balk at the price of quinoa, which is quite a bit more expensive than other grains. But because it plumps up a lot during cooking—up to four times its original volume—a little goes a long way.

Doctor's Top Tip

Add quinoa to your arsenal of blood-sugar-lowering foods. Instead of bread with dinner, prepare a quick-cooking pot of quinoa. This fast grain's fiber and protein give it a low glycemic load, according to researchers at the University of Sydney, Australia. That's good news: Carbohydrates with a low glycemic load help keep blood sugar low and steady, reducing between-meal cravings and cutting the risk for diabetes and heart disease.

While the protein in quinoa itself doesn't contain gluten, experts had warned that quinoa could be packaged in plants that also produce wheat products, raising the risk for gluten contamination. The team of dietitians who studied quinoa concluded that contamination is not likely.

GETTING THE MOST

Explore the possibilities. People often use grains only for side dishes because they're not sure what else to do with them. But quinoa is soft and somewhat bland, meaning that you can include it in almost any recipe. Adding quinoa to soups, pasta dishes, or stuffings, for example, makes it easy to get more of its nutritional power in your diet every day, says Grabowski-Nepa.

Keep it cold. While most grains are good keepers, quinoa spoils quickly. To preserve the nutrients and the good taste, it's best to buy quinoa only in small amounts and store it in an airtight container in the refrigerator or another cool, dark place.

Southwestern Quinoa and Chickpea Salad

1 cup quinoa

1¾ cups water

4 teaspoons olive oil

1 cup canned chickpeas, rinsed and drained

1 medium tomato, seeded and chopped

3 tablespoons fresh lime juice

2 tablespoons minced fresh cilantro

½ teaspoon ground cumin

1 clove garlic, minced

⅛ teaspoon salt

Place the quinoa in a fine strainer, and rinse well with cold water. Drain and transfer to a medium saucepan.

Add the water, and bring to a boil over medium heat. Cover, reduce the heat to low, and simmer for 15 minutes, or until the quinoa is tender but still slightly crunchy. If all the water has not been absorbed, drain it through a fine strainer.

Transfer the quinoa to a medium bowl. Drizzle with the oil, and toss to coat. Add the chickpeas, tomato, lime juice, cilantro, cumin, garlic, and salt. Toss well.

Makes 4 servings

PER SERVING

Calories: 271
Total fat: 8.4 g
Saturated fat: 0.9 g

Cholesterol: 0 mg
Sodium: 219 mg
Dietary fiber: 6.4 g

Raisins

TURN DOWN HIGH BLOOD PRESSURE

HEALING POWER

Can Help:

Cut cancer risk

Keep cardiovascular
system healthy

Improve digestion

Lower blood pressure

Protect teeth

Raisins may not be much to look at, but they do have an illustrious history. Prehistoric cave dwellers attributed religious powers to raisins. They made raisin necklaces and decorations and drew pictures of raisins on cave walls. As early as 1000 BC, the Israelites used them to pay taxes to King David. Just try that with the IRS!

Raisins occupy a much humbler place in society today. But they're just as useful as ever. Backpackers and hikers appreciate raisins for being a high-energy, low-fat, very convenient snack.

Raisins fit easily in a lunch box, and they don't get as mushy as bananas if you accidentally leave them in your desk drawer. And they almost never go bad, even when they're in the pantry for months at a time.

Raisins offer more than just convenience. Studies suggest that they can help lower blood pressure and cholesterol and even play a role in keeping digestion and blood healthy.

Sweet Treat for Your Ticker . . . and Your Arteries

How can a tiny box of raisins protect your entire cardiovascular system—from the tiniest artery to your heart itself? Credit the mix of fiber, minerals, and phytochemicals inside each wrinkly little fruit.

In one study, researchers at Johns Hopkins Medical Institutions in Baltimore gave 87 African American men either potassium supplements or blank pills. Those who were given the potassium saw their systolic pressure (the higher number) drop almost seven points, while their diastolic pressure (the lower number) went down almost three points. While the amount of potassium given in the study was quite high—you would have to eat about 3 cups of raisins to get the same amount—smaller amounts are also beneficial. Just ¼ cup of raisins contains 272 milligrams of potassium, or almost 8 percent of the Daily Value (DV).

"All Americans, but particularly those who are over the age of 40, ought to be consuming a fair number of foods that contain high levels of potassium, such as

In the Kitchen

There's very little nutritional difference between black and golden raisins. (The black variety has more thiamin, while the golden seedless type has a bit more vitamin B_6.) The main difference between them is the way they are dried.

- **Black, or sun-dried, raisins** are actually dried in the sun. This is what gives them their dark, shriveled look. They're used for both baking and snacking.
- **Golden seedless raisins** are dried by exposing them to the fumes of burning sulfur in a closed chamber, which gives them their golden hue. They're usually used for baking—in fruit cakes, for example—because of their attractive appearance.

Both types of raisins are extremely durable. As long as they are kept tightly wrapped, they will keep in the pantry for several months and for a year or more when stored in the refrigerator or freezer. You'll know they've gone bad if you spot white sugar crystals collecting on the surface.

It's common for raisins to dry out a bit during storage. Don't throw them out. Steaming them for about 5 minutes will restore much of the missing moisture and make them plumper. Or if you're going to use them for baking, let them sit in hot water or fruit juice for about 5 minutes, then add them to the recipe.

---

raisins," recommends Donald V. Schlimme, PhD, professor emeritus of nutrition and food science at the University of Maryland in College Park.

Like other dried fruits, raisins are a good source of dietary fiber, with nearly 2 grams of fiber in ¼ cup, or about 8 percent of the DV. Great at easing everyday digestive complaints like constipation and hemorrhoids, fiber can also tackle one of the biggest health threats Americans face: heart disease.

In one study done at the Health Research and Studies Center in Los Altos, California, researchers asked people with high cholesterol levels to eat 3 ounces of raisins (a little more than a half-cup) a day as part of a high-fiber, low-fat diet. After a month, the participants' total cholesterol dropped an average of more than 8 percent, while their harmful low-density lipoprotein (LDL) cholesterol levels dropped 15 percent.

The soluble fiber in raisins seems uniquely able to mingle with bile acids in the intestines—lowering cholesterol by whisking this cholesterol-infused digestive juice out of the body. (Your body then pulls more cholesterol out of circulation to build new bile acids.) In a test tube study conducted at the University of Maine, researchers found that the fiber binds effectively with bile acids.

FOOD ALERT

A Color for Caution

The process that gives golden raisins their pleasant hue may cause serious problems for some people.

During processing, golden raisins are exposed to sulfites, the same compounds that are sometimes used to keep salad bar produce from turning brown. It wasn't until the mid-1980s that researchers discovered that some people are sensitive to these compounds, which can cause asthma attacks or other allergic-type reactions.

"Anyone who is sulfite-sensitive should stay clear of golden seedless raisins," says Mark McLellan, PhD, dean of research for the University of Florida's Institute of Food and Agricultural Sciences and director of the Florida Agricultural Experiment Station in Gainesville, Florida.

A New Cancer Fighter

Catechins of the sort found in raisins (and in other fruits and vegetables) reduced intestinal tumors by at least 70 percent in a Weill Medical College of Cornell University lab study that fed this powerful antioxidant to lab mice. Experts have plenty of reason to believe catechins protect people, too: When researchers compared the diets of 2,000 cancer patients with 2,000 people without cancer, they found that people with the highest consumption of foods from plants (fruits, vegetables, grains, and legumes) had the lowest risk of colon cancer. Meanwhile, researchers from London's National Research Centre have found that low intake of fruit, including dried fruits such as raisins, was associated with increased cancer risk in women.

Other studies suggest that the fiber and tartaric acid in sun-dried raisins play an important role in colon health. When 16 healthy men and women ate two servings of raisins per day, levels of bile acids in the colon decreased while food and waste sped through more quickly. That's good news, because bile acids are thought to enhance the growth of cancer cells. "We found a significant, positive correlation between consuming sun-dried raisins and a change in some colon cancer risk factors," said Gene Spiller, PhD, lead study author and a researcher at the Health Research and Studies Center in Los Altos, California. "Eating as little as two servings—or 1 cup—of raisins resulted in beneficial changes in colon function that may help combat the estimated 130,000 new cases of colorectal cancer expected to be diagnosed this year."

Iron and More

When we think of iron-rich foods, things such as red meat and liver usually come to mind. But raisins may be a better source of iron, particularly for people who eat little or no meat. "If someone were to ask me what food other than red meat I would recommend for high iron, I would say raisins," says Dr. Schlimme.

Iron is essential for the creation of hemoglobin in red blood cells, which the body uses to transport oxygen. Although iron is readily available in food, women who are menstruating or pregnant often need extra amounts of the mineral.

A quarter-cup of raisins has 0.8 milligram of iron, which is more than 8 percent of the Recommended Dietary Allowance (RDA) for men and 5 percent of the RDA for women.

GETTING THE MOST

Have a raisin combo. Raisins contain a type of iron called nonheme iron, which is harder for the body to absorb than the heme iron found in meats. Eating raisins along with foods high in vitamin C, however, helps improve the absorption of nonheme iron.

Shop for convenience. To get the most raisins in your diet, nutritionists often recommend buying the snack-size packs. Due to their small size and the fact that raisins almost never go bad, they're perfect for tossing in your purse, glove compartment, or desk drawer, and eating whenever you are in the mood for a quick snack.

Doctor's Top Tip

Eat raisins for healthier teeth. If you've avoided raisins as a between-meal snack due to worries that their sticky sweetness would promote cavities, now hear this: New research from the University of Illinois at Chicago suggests that phytochemicals in raisins, including oleanolic acid and betulinic acid, actually fight bacteria responsible for cavities and gum disease, by preventing them from adhering to teeth. "Moreover, raisins contain primarily fructose and glucose, not sucrose, the main culprit in oral disease," notes lead study author Christine Wu, PhD, professor at the university's College of Dentistry. Now go toss a couple of boxes of raisins into your briefcase or backpack!

Raisin Coffeecake Ring

COFFEECAKE

- 1½ cups raisins
- ½ cup fresh orange juice
- 2 teaspoons vanilla extract
- ¼ teaspoon ground cinnamon
- 2 teaspoons unsalted butter
- 1 pound frozen whole-wheat or white bread dough, thawed

GLAZE

- 2 tablespoons fresh orange juice
- 3 tablespoons confectioners' sugar
- 1 teaspoon unsalted butter

To make the coffeecake: In a medium saucepan, combine the raisins, orange juice, vanilla extract, and cinnamon. Cook over medium heat, stirring frequently, until the raisins have absorbed all the liquid, 5 to 7 minutes. Remove from the heat, and stir in the butter. Cover, and set aside.

Coat a baking sheet with cooking spray. On a work surface, pat and stretch the dough into a 12- × 6-inch rectangle.

Spread evenly with the raisin mixture, leaving about ½ inch uncovered along 1 long side. Starting with the other long side, roll the dough tightly. Pinch the edges together to seal them.

Transfer the dough to the baking sheet, forming it into a ring. Pinch the ends together. Use a sharp knife to cut into the ring at 12 intervals about 1½ inches apart (cut almost but not all the way through the dough). Spread the cuts out slightly so the filling is visible.

Cover the dough loosely with plastic wrap, and set aside in a warm spot for 2 to 4 hours, or until doubled in bulk.

Preheat the oven to 350°F. Remove the plastic wrap, and bake the dough for 20 to 25 minutes, or until golden. Leave on the baking sheet until you make the glaze.

To make the glaze: In a small microwaveable bowl, combine the orange juice, sugar, and butter. Microwave on high for about 30 seconds, or until the butter melts. Whisk until smooth. Brush over the warm coffeecake. Transfer the coffeecake to a wire rack to cool.

Makes 12 slices

PER SLICE

Calories: 172	Cholesterol: 3 mg
Total fat: 2.6 g	Sodium: 168 mg
Saturated fat: 0.6 g	Dietary fiber: 3 g

Rhubarb

RELIEF FROM CONSTIPATION

Now let us all praise the Rhubarb . . .
Its roseate stalks are a treat
Especially when stewed or otherwise brewed
In concoctions delectably sweet.

"In Praise of Rhubarb"—Cynthia Francisco

HEALING POWER

Can Help:

Lower cholesterol

Prevent cancer

Boost immunity

Ease digestive problems

Cool hot flashes

Granted, not many of us get sufficiently excited enough about this tart, acidic plant to praise all of its virtues in verse. If you're suffering from constipation, however, rhubarb just might be able to give you something to sing about after all.

And you might not be the only one singing. Research shows that people with high cholesterol and low immunity may want to join the rhubarb chorus. Also, although more research is needed, evidence suggests that rhubarb may help fight certain cancers.

Before going any further, though, take heed of this critical caution: You should eat only the rhubarb stalks. Rhubarb leaves contain extraordinarily high levels of oxalates as well as another, as-yet-unidentified toxin. The oxalates can cause stomach irritation and kidney problems. When used properly, however, rhubarb is a wonderfully healthy food that you'll certainly want to try.

Garden-Variety Laxative

It's folklore, but most experts agree: Eating rhubarb works against constipation because this member of the buckwheat family is a good source of fiber.

"People have historically used rhubarb for constipation by eating it stewed or in pies, but they didn't know why it worked," says Tapan K. Basu, PhD, professor of nutrition at the University of Alberta in Edmonton, Canada. "Today, we know it's a good source of fiber."

The fibrous rhubarb stalks contain large amounts of insoluble fiber—more than 2 grams in a half-cup serving—which add the bulk necessary to keep your bowels moving on a regular basis.

Ronald L. Hoffman, MD, director of the Hoffman Center for Holistic Medicine in New York City and author of *Seven Weeks to a Settled Stomach*, offers this rhubarb recipe for when you're waiting for nature's call: Chop 3 stalks fresh raw rhubarb (removing and discarding the toxic leaves), and mix with 1 cup apple juice, ¼ peeled lemon, and 1 teaspoon honey. Put all the ingredients in a blender and purée until smooth. (Because raw rhubarb is very tart, you may want to add other juices to the recipe to soften the flavor.) Drink as necessary.

Flushing Out Cholesterol

Rhubarb, along with other fiber-rich foods such as oat bran and beans, can sop up cholesterol and flush it from your body before it gets a chance to stick to your artery walls, clogging them and contributing to heart disease.

In one study, researchers at the University of Alberta found that rhubarb fiber significantly reduces cholesterol, especially the harmful low-density lipoprotein (LDL) cholesterol, and also lowers triglycerides, which are potentially dangerous fats in the bloodstream. People who participated in the study consumed 27 grams of fiber-dense powdered rhubarb stalks a day for 30 days.

"How much rhubarb you need to eat to get the same effect, we don't know yet," says Dr. Basu, who was the study's lead researcher. "But we can say that rhubarb

In the Kitchen

In an effort to keep its tartness under control, most people pour mountains of sugar on rhubarb before the first spoonful reaches their mouths, adding a lot of empty calories to an otherwise healthy food.

To enjoy rhubarb while keeping the pre-sweetening to reasonable levels, here's what chefs advise:

Give it some juice. Many cooks stew rhubarb in orange or pineapple juice, which subdues the tartness and gives a pleasant hint of sweetness.

To stew rhubarb, chop the stalks into bite-size pieces. Put the pieces in a large saucepan, adding about a half-cup of water or apple or orange juice for every 3 to 4 cups of rhubarb.

Cook for about 15 minutes, or until the rhubarb is tender.

Add some spice. Adding spices is a sugar-free way to tame rhubarb's bite. Good choices include orange zest, rosewater, ginger, and cinnamon.

Pair rhubarb with other fruits. To sweeten rhubarb without using a ton of sugar, combine it with sweeter fruits such as strawberries, suggests the University of Alaska Cooperative Extension Service. If cooking with green rhubarb, adding a few cranberries will produce a brilliant pink hue. And keep some frozen rhubarb on hand—you can add chopped rhubarb to other fruits if you don't have enough berries for a pie or cobbler.

contains an effective kind of fiber, so eating it certainly can't hurt."

Tumor-Squelching Potential

Although the evidence is still preliminary, research indicates that rhubarb may contain compounds that can help prevent cancer.

In the only published study on rhubarb's effectiveness against cancer, researchers at the University of Mainz in Germany tested raw rhubarb juice, along with the juices of various other vegetables and fruits, against cancer-causing agents. They found that rhubarb ranked close to the top in preventing cell mutations that commonly lead to cancer.

Although this early research is promising, researchers still aren't sure if drinking rhubarb juice—or eating the whole stalk—will produce the same beneficial effects as those seen in test tubes.

A Tart Burst of Protection

Rhubarb contains vitamin C, an antioxidant vitamin that attacks and immobilizes free radicals, oxygen molecules that are the damaging force behind heart disease, some cancers, and certain "symptoms" of aging, like wrinkles or macular degeneration.

In addition, vitamin C has been shown to help keep the bad LDL cholesterol in your body from oxidizing—the process that allows it to stick to artery walls. It also plays an important role in the formation of collagen, a protein that makes up skin and connective tissue and helps keep skin smooth. Plus, vitamin C is a known immunity booster, helping your body stave off colds and infections.

A half-cup of cooked rhubarb delivers almost 4 milligrams of vitamin C, or nearly 7 percent of the Daily Value (DV).

GETTING THE MOST

Bet on red. Because of its tartness, most people would have a tough time downing more than a few bites of rhubarb. Here's a shopping tip that may help. Generally,

> ## Doctor's Top Tip
>
> An extract of rhubarb long used by German women to douse hot flashes is showing promise in scientific studies. Researchers from Health Research Services Ltd. in St. Leon-Rot, gave 109 perimenopausal women with frequent hot flashes either a rhubarb-extract tablet or a dummy pill for 12 weeks. After just 4 weeks, the rhubarb group reported 5½ fewer flashes per day. How does it work? No one's quite sure, but scientists at the University of Pittsburgh Medical Center say that rhubarb contains a plant estrogen called lindleyin that may help balance out the big hormone swings that happen during menopause. While it's too early to recommend a supplement, it's another reason to enjoy this sweet-tart treat when it's in season in early summer.

FOOD ALERT

Stop the Stones

If you're prone to kidney stones, you might want to pass on the rhubarb pie. Rhubarb contains high levels of oxalates, mineral salts that aren't processed in the body but instead are passed in the urine. For people who are sensitive to oxalates, eating too much rhubarb or other high-oxalate foods can cause the minerals to accumulate, possibly leading to oxalate-containing kidney stones.

the redder the stalk, the sweeter the taste, and the more you can eat with the least "pucker effect." Skip stalks with yellowish spots or green areas for best taste. And if the stalks seem tough, remove the outer fibers with a vegetable peeler, suggests the Pennsylvania State Agricultural Extension Service.

Store unwashed. Rhubarb stalks will keep in the fridge for up to 2 weeks. If you've got an abundance in your home garden, or happen to have picked up a bushel at an early-spring farmers' market, try this "individual quick-freezing method" for the surplus: Spread a single layer of cut rhubarb on trays, freeze until firm, then pack the cut pieces loosely in airtight bags or containers. You can take out just what you need when it's time to cook. Rhubarb keeps for about 9 months in the freezer.

Protect the flavor. Cook rhubarb in glass, enamel, or stainless steel. Pans made of aluminum or other metal cookware may impart a metallic taste to your final dish. (Anodized aluminum, however, is good to use—the surface doesn't react to the acids in rhubarb.) Store in glass containers.

Rice

A GOOD GRAIN FOR YOUR HEART

If there were just one food in every cook's pantry, it would probably be rice. This grain is the main ingredient in cuisines around the globe, with an estimated 40,000 varieties available worldwide. In the United States, you can buy white and brown basmati rice from India and Pakistan (not to mention Texmati from Texas), Arborio rice from Italy, Valencia rice from Spain, and "sticky" rice from Japan to name just a few.

HEALING POWER

Can Help:

Reduce cholesterol

Lower the risk of colon and breast cancer

Keep digestion regular

The most nutritious kind of rice is brown rice, which contains abundant amounts of fiber, complex carbohydrates, and essential B vitamins, says Maren Hegsted, PhD, professor emeritus of human nutrition and food at Louisiana State University in Baton Rouge.

And that's not all. Whole grains such as brown rice retain all four parts of their original grain kernel—the germ, the bran, a protective layer called the aleurone, and the starchy endosperm—intact. White rice only has the high-carb, nearly zero-fiber endosperm. What's missing? Not just fiber, but also hundreds of health-protective phytochemicals, vitamins, and minerals. According to the American Institute for Cancer Research, whole grains can have 10 times the amount of vitamin E; four times the potassium, magnesium, and zinc; three times the vitamin B_6, and twice the selenium of refined grains. No wonder eating at least three servings a day cuts your risk for heart disease, diabetes, cancer, and overweight.

Strike at the Source

We often forget that the body actually needs small amounts of cholesterol for functions such as making cell walls, for example, and for manufacturing essential hormones. To supply the necessary amounts, the liver produces cholesterol every day. But when we eat a high-fat diet, the body churns out more cholesterol than it can use. And that is when the risk of heart disease goes up.

Getting more brown rice, Dr. Hegsted says, can help keep this from happening. A compound in the bran layer of rice, called oryzanol, has been shown to reduce the body's production of cholesterol. In fact, this compound is chemically similar to cholesterol-lowering medications.

Doctor's Top Tip

Make your own instant brown rice, the easy way. Brown rice takes nearly three times longer to cook than white rice (45 minutes versus about 15), putting it out of reach for time-pressed weeknight cooks. One option: Use instant or quick-cooking brown rice, which delivers the same 2 grams of fiber per half-cup serving, and cooks in just 10 to 15 minutes. (Look for a brand with no added trans fats.)

But to get all the nutrition that real, minimally processed brown rice has to offer, even when your time is short, plan ahead. University of Nebraska, Lincoln, extension agent Alice Henneman, MS, RD, suggests cooking extra rice when you have time, then freezing the surplus in small containers. Reheat it in a microwave oven. "To do so, add 2 tablespoons of liquid per cup of cooked rice," she advises. "Cook frozen rice for 2 minutes on high power for each cup, then fluff with a fork." You're getting all of the nutrients brown rice has to offer this way. It's just not clear whether the processing required to create fast-cooking varieties disturbs the grain's nutrient-packed layers.

In a study at Louisiana State University, people ate 100 grams (about 3½ ounces) of rice bran a day for 3 weeks. At the end of the study, levels of harmful low-density lipoprotein (LDL) cholesterol went down 10 percent, while levels of beneficial high-density lipoprotein (HDL) cholesterol stayed relatively high. That translates into a 30 percent reduction in heart risk. "In combination with a low-fat diet, brown rice is one of the best foods you can eat for lowering cholesterol," says Dr. Hegsted.

A Digestive Sponge

Brown rice is darker and more chewy than its light-colored cousin because it's wrapped in a nutritious outer skin—the part of the grain that's highest in fiber. A half-cup of brown rice contains about 2 grams of fiber, Dr. Hegsted says.

Fiber offers powerful protection against type 2 diabetes. Studies show that eating at least three daily servings of brown rice and other whole grains cuts the risk for this condition 21 to 30 percent. Why? Fiber slows digestion and keeps blood sugar low and steady. In contrast, carbohydrates from refined grains send blood sugar soaring after a meal, triggering the release of more insulin to force the sugar into cells. Over time, higher blood sugar and insulin levels put you in the danger zone for diabetes—and also for high blood pressure and even some forms of cancer.

The fiber in brown rice is the insoluble kind that acts like a sponge in the intestine, soaking up large amounts of water, says Dr. Hegsted. This causes stools to get larger and wetter, so they pass more easily. In addition, larger stools move more quickly through the colon. This means that any harmful substances that they contain have less time to damage cells in the colon wall, which may reduce the risk of cancer. Some researchers estimate that if people would increase the amount of fiber in their diets to 39 grams a day, the risk for colon cancer could drop 31 percent.

Manufacturers often promise that their rice will cook up perfect every time, which suggests that some rice, at least, is coming to the table sticky and wet, or, worse, dry and hard. Here's a strategy for making perfect rice every time, no matter what kind you buy:

Leave it alone. It's almost impossible for cooks not to stir or investigate a pot of rice while it cooks. The problem is, stirring rice frequently before it's done damages the grains and can make the finished product soft and gummy. (Arborio rice, however, is meant to be stirred during cooking.)

Choose your liquid. While rice is customarily cooked in plain water, many chefs prefer to use flavored liquids, which add depth and complexity to the finished dish. Chicken and beef broths are ideal cooking liquids. Or you can simply add a squeeze of lemon, a splash of flavored vinegar, or a sprinkling of herbs to the water.

Avoid overcooking. To prevent rice from overcooking, it's a good idea to check it just before you think it's done. If the rice still looks a little wet, it needs an extra minute or two (or more) to absorb excess water.

Other research has refuted the high-fiber, less colon cancer connection. But that doesn't mean you should switch to white rice. When researchers studied 61,000 Swedish women for 15 years, they found that those who consumed more than $4\frac{1}{2}$ servings of whole grains daily had a 35 percent lower risk of colon cancer. Why? It could be the combination of high fiber as well as lignans and phenolic compounds in whole grains, which may discourage the growth of cancer cells.

What's good for the colon is also good for the breasts. Since the fiber in brown rice binds with estrogen in the digestive tract, there's less of the hormone circulating in the bloodstream. This is important because high levels of estrogen have been shown to trigger changes in cells that can lead to breast cancer. A study by Australian and Canadian researchers found that women who ate 28 grams of fiber a day had a 38 percent lower risk of developing breast cancer than those getting half that amount.

GETTING THE MOST

Keep it cool. Since brown rice is filled with oils, it quickly turns rancid when stored at normal room temperature, Dr. Hegsted says. To preserve the healing compounds, be sure to store brown rice in an airtight container in the refrigerator, where it will stay fresh for up to a year.

Save the water. Many of the important nutrients in brown and white rice leach into the water during cooking. To get these nutrients on your plate instead of pouring them down the drain, let rice cook until all the water is absorbed.

Use it "dry." Since the niacin and thiamin in fortified white rice are found on the outer layer of the grain, rinsing rice before cooking will wash these nutrients away. It's best to go straight from the bag into the cooking water. The exception is when you're using imported rice, which may contain more impurities than the domestic kinds.

Chinese-Style Ginger Rice with Chicken

½ cup instant brown rice

2 cups plus 2 tablespoons water

¼ teaspoon salt

1¼ pounds boneless, skinless chicken breast halves, cut into 1-inch pieces

3 tablespoons reduced-sodium soy sauce

Freshly ground black pepper

1 bag (16 ounces) frozen stir-fry vegetables

½ teaspoon ground ginger

In a medium saucepan combine the rice, 2 cups of the water, and the salt. Bring to a boil over high heat. Reduce the heat to low, cover, and simmer until the liquid has been absorbed, about 10 minutes. Remove from the heat, and let stand for 5 minutes, covered.

Meanwhile, in a large microwaveable bowl, toss the chicken with 1 tablespoon of the soy sauce, and season to taste with pepper. Cover with a lid or vented plastic wrap, and microwave on high power, stirring twice, until no longer pink, 3 to 5 minutes.

Add the frozen vegetables, ginger, remaining 2 tablespoons water, and remaining 2 tablespoons soy sauce. Cover, and microwave on high power, stirring 2 or 3 times, until the vegetables are heated through, about 5 minutes.

Fluff the rice with a fork. Serve the chicken and vegetables over the rice.

Makes 4 servings

PER SERVING

Calories: 241
Total fat: 2 g
Saturated fat: 0.5 g

Cholesterol: 82 mg
Sodium: 549 mg
Dietary fiber: 2 g

Sea Vegetables
PROTECTION FROM THE DEEP

HEALING POWER
Can Help:
Inhibit tumor growth
Boost immunity
Prevent macular degeneration

When the Beatles were crooning "Octopus's Garden" back in 1969, they almost certainly weren't extolling the virtues of seaweed, or sea vegetables, as they're called by those who harvest and consume them today. But given what we've learned about these valuable plants, they probably should have been.

Eaten regularly, sea vegetables can be a valuable source of essential vitamins and minerals. In addition, they contain a variety of protective compounds that may help ward off some serious health threats, such as cancer.

A Traditional Cancer Fighter

For perhaps thousands of years, sea vegetables have been used in Asian cultures to prevent and treat cancer. As is often the case, research now indicates that there is more than a little scientific evidence supporting these ancient healing methods. "We need more clinical studies, but so far, there have been some interesting population and animal studies showing that sea vegetables can prevent tumors," says Alfred A. Bushway, PhD, professor of food science at the University of Maine in Orono, who believes that sea vegetables may be partially responsible for the lower cancer rates in countries like Japan, where sea vegetables are as ubiquitous as our potato.

Japanese researchers studied the effects of extracts from eight different kinds of sea vegetables on cells that had been treated with potent cancer-causing agents. The results showed that sea vegetables may have tumor-squelching power.

Two types of leafy sea veggies—kelp and dulse—have been reported to reduce the risk of intestinal or mammary cancer in animal studies. When nutrition researchers at Ryerson University in Toronto studied the effects of extracts of these sea plants on human cervical cancer cells, the results were intriguing. After 72 hours, dulse extracts inhibited cervical cancer cell growth by up to 78 percent while kelp slowed cell growth and division by up to 69 percent. What's at work? In another study, lead researcher Yvonne Yuan, PhD, associate professor of nutrition at Ryerson University in Toronto, Canada, reported that red dulse contains powerful antioxidants that may work in the body to combat cell-damaging free radicals.

FOOD ALERT

Danger from the Deep

Although sea vegetables contain an array of healing nutrients, they also contain iodine and sodium, which, in large amounts, aren't so helpful.

You need small amounts of iodine for processing protein and carbohydrates. In addition, the thyroid gland requires iodine to regulate growth and development. But a little goes a long way: You only need about 150 micrograms a day.

Sea vegetables, however, may contain many times that amount. People who eat a lot of sea vegetables may find themselves getting too much iodine—1,000 micrograms a day is considered the upper limit—which can make the thyroid work less efficiently, says Alfred A. Bushway, PhD, of the University of Maine in Orono.

Another mineral that sea vegetables carry by the boatload is sodium. Too much sodium can cause high blood pressure in people who are sensitive to it.

If you're sensitive to sodium, says Dr. Bushway, rinsing sea vegetables prior to cooking will reduce the sodium content by about 10 to 20 percent. Soaking them in water will reduce the levels of sodium even more, by about 50 to 70 percent, depending on the variety you're using.

Kelp for Your Blood and Heart

If you want your blood to have the strength of the sea itself, a dose of vegetables from its waters can help.

One ounce of kelp, a thin, tender sea vegetable often used in soups and stir-fries, provides 51 micrograms of folate, or 13 percent of the Daily Value (DV) for this B vitamin, which helps break down protein in the body and aids in the regeneration of red blood cells. An ounce of nori, the sea vegetable frequently used in sushi, provides 42 micrograms of folate, or 11 percent of the DV of this vital nutrient.

Kelp also contains magnesium, a mineral that has been found to keep high blood pressure in check, especially among people who are sensitive to sodium. One ounce of kelp has more than 34 milligrams, or almost 9 percent of the DV for this heart-healthy nutrient.

A Sea of Immunity

You don't see too many whales swimming around with the sniffles. Maybe that's because of all the sea vegetables they're skimming off the ocean's swells.

Certain varieties of sea vegetables are packed with important vitamins that boost immunity and help fend off a host of diseases.

Topping this list is the nutritious nori. One ounce of raw nori contains 11 milligrams of infection-fighting vitamin C, or more than 18 percent of the DV. Vitamin C is an antioxidant nutrient widely known for its ability to sweep up harmful, tissue-damaging oxygen molecules called free radicals.

An ounce of nori also delivers nearly 1,500 IU of vitamin A, or 30 percent of the DV. Studies show that vitamin A not only builds immunity but also can safeguard against night blindness and vision problems associated with aging, such as macular

In the Kitchen

The first time you pull a flat, green sheet of dried nori from its wrapper, your reaction almost certainly will be, "How the heck am I supposed to eat this?"

Although seaweed, which is sold in health food stores and Asian markets, does look strange, it's surprisingly easy to work with. It's important, however, to know which kind you're getting, since each is handled somewhat differently.

Alaria. Also known as wakame, this is the seaweed traditionally used in miso soup. When using it for salads or pasta dishes, simply soften it in water for 2 to 3 minutes and cut it into slivers. Alaria can be quite chewy, but cutting away the stiff midrib will help make it tender.

Dulse. Dried dulse has deep red wrinkled leaves, which can be eaten straight from the package. (It can be quite salty, however, so you may want to rinse it first.) Like nori, dulse is typically snipped and added to soups, stews, and pasta dishes. It is also available in ready-to-use flakes.

Hijiki. One of the stronger tasting sea-weeds, hijiki (also spelled "hiziki") resembles black angel hair pasta in its packaged form. To tame its wild briny flavor, soak it for 10 to 15 minutes, then drain; it will quadruple in size when hydrated. Chefs recommend simmering hijiki for about 30 minutes or until tender, then adding it to salads, vegetables, or bean dishes. It can also be drizzled with sesame oil and eaten as a side dish.

Kelp. Sold in wide, dried, dark green strips, kelp (similar to the Japanese kombu) is often added to soups and stews as a replacement for salt. To add seasoning to bean and grain dishes, chefs will sometimes add strips of kelp. Also, roasted kelp chips make a great garnish.

Nori. Also known as laver, nori is sold in paper-thin, green, dried sheets. It has a mildly briny flavor and is generally used to wrap around sushi, float in soups, or accentuate the flavor of salads and pasta. When adding nori to a dish, use scissors to cut it into strips. You can also tear it with your hands. Sprinkle it into the food, stirring to keep it from clumping.

Doctor's Top Tip

Sprinkle ready-to-eat sea vegetables on rice, salads, or soups. Look for cans of furikake in your local Asian grocery store. Often mistaken by Westerners for goldfish food, furikake is a dry Japanese condiment, made of chopped seaweed, sesame seeds, and other ingredients, which is meant to be sprinkled on top of rice. It doesn't take a lot of sea vegetables to get the benefits. "Nutritional studies indicate that as little as ¼ ounce of dried sea vegetables can make a significant nutritional contribution to your diet," says Alfred A. Bushway, PhD, of the University of Maine in Orono.

degeneration. In addition, vitamin A can protect against several kinds of cancer.

A word of caution: Ignore infomercials and health food store claims that sea vegetables can "regenerate" your body, normalize thyroid function, or cut food cravings. According to the American Cancer Society, these claims simply aren't true. Promises that sea plants can cure tuberculosis, fibromyalgia, cancer, asthma, or diabetes could lead you into dangerous waters. Enjoying sea vegetables as you would veggies grown on land makes nutritional sense. Regarding them as medicine doesn't.

Good News for Vegans

If you're among the strictest of vegetarians, meaning that you don't eat meat, meat products, dairy products, or eggs, you may want to add some sea vegetables to your palette of land vegetables. It's a helpful way to ensure that you're getting adequate amounts of vitamin B_{12}, a nutrient most commonly found in meat.

Although there is some controversy about how much vitamin B_{12} sea vegetables provide, experts agree that those who regularly dine on these vegetables have higher levels of vitamin B_{12} in their blood than those who do not.

In one study of 21 strict vegetarians, researchers found that those who ate sea vegetables regularly had blood levels of vitamin B_{12} twice as high as those who didn't eat the vegetables.

Without adequate amounts of vitamin B_{12}, you can experience fatigue, memory loss, and nerve damage resulting in tingling in the feet and hands. Although few people are at risk for vitamin B_{12} deficiency, it can be a concern for strict vegetarians and for some elderly people who have trouble absorbing this vital nutrient.

GETTING THE MOST

Rinse lightly. Dried sea vegetables also provide trace minerals, including potassium. But they're on the surface, so experts recommend using a light touch when rinsing them prior to cooking. "Some people soak and rinse the life out of their sea vegetables," says Dr. Bushway. "We just recommend light rinsing. Otherwise, you'll lose a lot of the surface minerals, like potassium."

Invest in stock. The best way to retain the maximum amount of nutrients is to make soup out of your sea vegetables, says Dr. Bushway. "When sea vegetables are used in soups, some of the minerals are released into the broth," he says. "The remainder provide valuable fiber and unique phytochemicals, such as the alginate found in kelp."

The best way to include more sea vegetables in your diet is to experiment. "Add small, bite-size pieces to salads, soups, stews, grain dishes, stir-fries, and sandwiches," says Carl Karush of Maine Coast Sea Vegetables in Franklin.

Kelp and Potato Chowder

1 tablespoon canola oil

1 large onion, finely chopped

7 cups water

4 medium boiling potatoes, peeled and finely chopped

1 cup finely crumbled dried kelp (about ¾ ounce)

⅛ teaspoon salt

Freshly ground black pepper

In a Dutch oven, heat the oil over medium-high heat. Add the onion, and cook, stirring frequently, until golden, 8 to 10 minutes.

Add the water, potatoes, kelp, and salt. Bring to a boil. Partially cover, reduce the heat to low, and simmer until the potatoes are tender, 30 to 35 minutes. Season to taste with pepper.

Makes 6 servings

PER SERVING

Calories: 116
Total fat: 2.5 g
Saturated fat: 0.2 g

Cholesterol: 0 mg
Sodium: 208 mg
Dietary fiber: 2.7 g

Shellfish

HEALTH ON THE HALF SHELL

HEALING POWER

Can Help:

Prevent anemia

Boost immunity

Prevent heart disease

For most folks, shellfish like lobster, shrimp, scallops, and oysters are luxuries—foods to be reserved for special occasions. For one thing, shellfish are expensive, often costing twice as much (or more) as other fish. Shellfish also have a reputation for containing boatloads of cholesterol and a sea of sodium, both of which health-conscious diners usually try to avoid.

While it's true that shellfish are high in cholesterol and sodium, these aren't the health threats that scientists once thought they were, says Robert M. Grodner, PhD, professor emeritus in the department of food science at Louisiana State University in Baton Rouge. In addition, shellfish contain good amounts of vitamins, minerals, and other healthful compounds that more than offset their slight nutritional downside.

Good for the Heart

People who eat a lot of seafood fare even better than vegetarians when it comes to heart health. In one study, seafood eaters with high concentrations of omega-3s in their blood had significantly lower blood pressure and lower levels of cholesterol and triglycerides—blood fats that in large amounts can increase the risk of heart disease—than vegetarians who didn't eat shellfish. Although many of the studies on omega-3s have focused on fish like salmon and mackerel, all fish, including shellfish, contain some omega-3s. In fact, eating six medium oysters five to seven times a month will provide all the omega-3s your heart needs.

Omega-3s love your heart and blood vessels. These fatty acids improve the electrical stability of the heart, guarding against deadly out-of-rhythm heart beats, notes researcher Dariush Mozaffarian, MD, DrPH, a cardiologist at Harvard Medical School and the author of a recent study finding that people who eat just two fish meals per week cut their risk of heart disease death by a respectable 36 percent. Omega-3s also make the linings of blood vessels function better and may improve the way cells respond to insulin, the hormone that tells cells to absorb blood sugar. Insulin problems raise the risk for diabetes and heart disease.

Scallops, as well as other shellfish, give your cardiovascular system a boost of

In the Kitchen

Shellfish are extremely perishable. Even when properly stored, they stay fresh for only a day or two. In addition, they cook very quickly. The difference between "just right" and "yuck" is often measured in minutes—or less. Here are a few tips for having the freshest catch every time:

Buy them live. Since shellfish go bad so quickly, it's best to buy them live and cook them the same day. To keep them fresh after bringing them home from the store, be sure to store them in the refrigerator until you're ready to start cooking.

Check for doneness. Few foods are less appetizing than undercooked shellfish. Lobsters and crabs turn bright red when they're done, usually in about 15 to 20 minutes. Clams, mussels, and oysters are nearly done when the shells open. Letting them cook for another 5 minutes will finish the job.

---

vitamin B_{12}—one serving of scallops packs a third of your daily needs. In its heart-protecting role, vitamin B_{12} helps your body deactivate the amino acid homocysteine before it can harm the thin inner lining of artery walls and set the stage for a buildup of artery-clogging plaque.

What about cholesterol? Shrimp's quirky cholesterol count—about 200 milligrams in 12 large ones, which is about the same as the cholesterol in one large egg—could make you pass up this low-cal delicacy. But for most of us, shrimp should get the green light: In a definitive Rockefeller University study, shrimp raised bad low-density lipoprotein (LDL) cholesterol by 7 percent, but also boosted good high-density lipoprotein (HDL) cholesterol even higher and decreased heart-threatening blood fats called triglycerides by 13 percent. Researchers concluded that when they took all of shrimp's effects on blood fats into consideration, the bottom line is that shrimp's a heart-smart treat. In contrast, eating two eggs raised LDL levels 10 percent but didn't have the same positive effects on other blood fats.

And don't be deterred by the sodium in shellfish, either. As you would expect of creatures from the sea, shellfish contain quite a bit—about 150 to 900 milligrams in a 3-ounce serving, depending on the type. But unless your doctor has suggested that you reduce the sodium in your diet, shellfish shouldn't be a problem. One serving of shellfish is well within the Daily Value (DV) of 2,400 milligrams of sodium.

Multivitamins in a Shell

Aside from their role in protecting the heart, shellfish are incredibly rich sources of a variety of essential (and hard-to-find) vitamins and minerals. The large amounts of vitamin B_{12} in shellfish are important to your health for other reasons. The body uses this nutrient to keep nerves healthy and make red blood cells. When levels of vitamin B_{12} slip, the body (and mind) can literally short-circuit, causing memory loss, confusion, slow reflexes, and fatigue. In fact, what's thought to be senility in older people is sometimes nothing more than a lack of vitamin B_{12}.

Three ounces of crab contains 10 micrograms of vitamin B_{12}, or 167 percent of the DV. Clams are even better, with 3 ounces—about nine small steamed clams—providing 1,400 percent of the DV.

With the exception of shrimp, shellfish also contain a lot of zinc, which is essential for keeping the immune system strong. Oysters are the best source, with six oysters containing about 27 milligrams, or almost 181 percent of the DV.

It's sometimes hard to get enough iron from foods, which is why about 20 percent of Americans are low in this important mineral. But if you can muster up enough muscle to lift a mussel to your mouth, you'll get much of the iron you need to help prevent iron-deficiency anemia. Three ounces of mussels provides about 6 milligrams of iron, or 60 percent of the Recommended Dietary Allowance (RDA) for men and 40 percent of the RDA for women.

Finally, many shellfish are good sources of magnesium, potassium, and vitamin C. The vitamin C is a great bonus because it helps the body absorb more of the iron found in these foods.

FOOD ALERT

Hazards on the Half-Shell

Shellfish are nutritious and delicious. But unless they're prepared with care, they can also be dangerous.

In order to eat and breathe, shellfish such as clams and oysters filter 15 to 20 gallons of water a day through their shells. When the water contains bacteria, like the potentially harmful *Vibrio vulnificus*, the shellfish become contaminated and have the ability to make you sick.

This doesn't mean that you can't eat shellfish safely. Since the bacteria are readily killed by heat, cooking your catch will prevent potential problems. While this is bad news for lovers of oysters on the half-shell, there may be an alternative, at least in the future. Laboratory studies suggest that dousing raw oysters with hot sauce will kill the bacteria. Until further research is done, however, it's best to be safe and eat your shellfish cooked.

Brain Food That's Fun to Eat

Your brain's got one of the highest concentrations of omega-3 fatty acids in your entire body. These long chains of fat molecules are woven into the membranes of brain cells, helping to send and receive the electrical and hormonal signals that translate into thoughts and feelings. "Researchers who look at problems like postpartum depression, schizophrenia, and depression are finding associations between lower levels of seafood intake and a greater likelihood of problems," notes researcher Susan E. Carlson, PhD, professor of dietetics and nutrition at the University of Kansas Medical Center in Kansas City. "And lab studies are showing that when you change the composition of brain cell membranes, so that there's less good fat in the mix, the membranes don't send and receive signals as well."

GETTING THE MOST

Eat them with vitamin C. Since your body is better able to absorb the iron in foods when you eat them with vitamin C, include vitamin C–rich foods such as broccoli or peppers on the shellfish menu.

Mix and match. Because shellfish are usually considered a luxury item, most people eat only a handful or two at a time. An easy way to include more of them in your diet is to toss them together in one big, briny stew, says Dr. Grodner. "It can be a mighty healthful meal," he says.

Doctor's Top Tip

For low-pollution, eco-friendly shellfish, go for these varieties: farmed scallops, blue or New Zealand green mussels, butter or Pacific littleneck clams, Northern shrimp, and spotted prawns. Eat with confidence! These shellfish are low in contaminants and raised with environmentally friendly methods that don't pollute surrounding waters or endanger other sea creatures, advises Bill Chameides, PhD, chief scientist for the Environmental Defense Fund. Dungeness and stone crabs are also recommended. But do exercise a little caution with lobster—mercury content means you should limit your children's meals of lobster to two or three per month.

Seafood Stew

2 tablespoons olive oil

1½ cups chopped onions

1 tablespoon minced garlic

1 can (28 ounces) plum tomatoes with basil (with juice)

2½ cups water

1 cup reduced-sodium vegetable juice

¼ cup no-salt-added tomato paste

1 teaspoon dried oregano

8 ounces Dungeness or blue crabmeat

9 ounces medium shrimp, peeled and deveined

8 ounces chopped clams (with juice)

1 tablespoon chopped parsley

In a Dutch oven, heat the oil over medium heat. Add the onions and garlic. Cook, stirring frequently, until the onions soften, about 5 minutes. Add the tomatoes (with juice), breaking up the tomatoes with the back of a spoon.

Add the water, vegetable juice, tomato paste, and oregano. Stir to mix. Bring to a boil, then reduce the heat to low. Cover and cook for 30 minutes.

Meanwhile, pick over the crabmeat, and discard any bits of shell. Place the crabmeat in a fine strainer. Rinse with cold water and drain.

Add the crabmeat, shrimp, and clams to the pot. Increase the heat to medium-high. As soon as the stew returns to a boil, remove it from the heat. Set aside, covered, until the shrimp are opaque in the center, about 5 minutes. Test by cutting a shrimp in half.

Sprinkle with the parsley.

Makes 6 servings

Cook's Note: *Serve the stew with plenty of whole-grain bread for dipping in the sauce.*

PER SERVING ————————————

Calories: 227	Cholesterol: 108 mg
Total fat: 6.6 g	Sodium: 481 mg
Saturated fat: 0.9 g	Dietary fiber: 2.7 g

Smoking

OUTSMARTING THE EVIL WEED

Apparently there aren't a lot of smokers thumping melons or scrutinizing tomatoes at the local supermarket. Experts aren't sure why, but smokers don't eat as many fruits and vegetables as nonsmokers do. But the more fruits and vegetables you eat, studies show, the better your odds of escaping the ravages of the smoker's "big three"—heart disease, stroke, and cancer.

You don't have to eat boatloads of bananas or bushels of Brussels sprouts to get the benefits. Eating just one fruit or a serving of vegetables a day may slightly cut your risk of lung cancer, and having nine or more servings a day can have a significant impact.

There are two reasons that fruits and vegetables should get top billing on a smoker's plate. First, they're packed with antioxidants, powerful nutrients that protect against smoking-related diseases like heart disease and cancer. Plus, produce is loaded with phytonutrients, compounds found in plants that show promise for preventing or even treating these diseases. Just how powerful are the antioxidants in produce? In a Chinese study of 63,257 women and men, those who ate the most fruits and vegetables loaded with the antioxidant beta-cryptoxanthin had a 27 percent reduction in lung cancer risk. But smokers in the study who ate the most foods containing this carotenoid cut their risk by 37 percent.

Understanding the Danger

Bananas turn brown. Cooking oils turn rancid. Our bodies eventually decay. Yech—it's not a pretty image. In all these cases, the damage is caused by the same thing: highly reactive, dangerous molecules called free radicals.

Although free radicals occur naturally, their numbers are greatly increased by such things as pollution and exposure to cigarette smoke—either as a smoker or as someone who breathes in secondhand smoke on a regular basis. The result? Damage caused by free radicals contributes to a host of age-related maladies like heart disease, cancer, and a type of vision loss called age-related macular degeneration.

The danger's not just for smokers. It's for anyone exposed to cigarette smoke. Secondhand smoke—which includes both the smoke exhaled by smokers and "sidestream smoke" from the end of a lit cigarette, pipe, or cigar—contains over 4,000

THE BEST PROTECTION

The USDA recommends that we eat at least five servings of fruits and vegetables a day. But because tobacco smoke depletes valuable nutrients from the body, smokers "ought to eat at least twice that amount," says James Scala, PhD, a nutritionist and author of *If You Can't/Won't Stop Smoking*.

While it's always best to eat a wide variety of fruits and vegetables, some foods have been found to be especially protective.

Citrus fruit. Smoking one cigarette destroys between 25 and 100 milligrams of vitamin C, says pharmacist Earl Mindell, RPh, PhD, professor emeritus of nutrition at Pacific Western University in Los Angeles and author of *Earl Mindell's Food as Medicine*. "It would be a good idea to eat a fruit or vegetable that's rich in vitamin C for every cigarette you smoke," he says.

Cruciferous vegetables. Broccoli, cauliflower, watercress, and other members of this vegetable family contain compounds called indoles and isothiocyanates, which in laboratory studies have been shown to slow the growth of cancers.

Soy foods. Tofu, tempeh, and other soy foods contain a number of cancer-fighting substances, including genistein and protease inhibitors. In Japan (where people eat large amounts of soy), more than 60 percent of men over age 20 smoke, yet the incidence of lung cancer is much lower than it is here, says Dr. Mindell.

Strawberries, grapes, and cherries. These fruits are rich in ellagic acid, a phytochemical that has been shown to destroy hydrocarbons, potentially cancer-causing chemicals in cigarette smoke.

Tomatoes. Inside tomatoes is a substance called lycopene, which has powerful antioxidant abilities. In fact, tomatoes appear to provide more cancer protection than other fruits or green vegetables.

---

chemical compounds, including 60 known or suspected to cause cancer. Breathing this stuff in causes an estimated 46,000 deaths from heart disease in nonsmokers who live with smokers and about 3,400 lung cancer deaths in nonsmoking adults.

It would seem logical that taking an antioxidant supplement would offer all the protection you'd need. But a famous and tragic study of 29,133 male smokers from Finland proves dramatically that getting your antioxidants from food is the way to go. The men took high-dose supplements of beta-carotene, alpha-tocopherol, both, or nothing for several years. Men taking the supplements had an 18 percent increased risk for lung cancer. Another beta-carotene supplementation study for smokers was cut short when researchers found an increased risk of lung cancer for smokers. Experts can't fully explain why, but they suspect that antioxidants like beta-carotene work when they're in their original, natural package—and come with hundreds of other phytonutrients. In other words, a carrot is better for you than a capsule. Since these two earlier studies were done, more recent studies of smaller doses of vitamins A, C, and E have found no advantage to taking them as separate supplements and, in some cases, found increased risk of death, though researchers could not pinpoint the cause.

"People who eat more fruits and vegetables get half the lung cancer per given amount of smoking compared with the people who eat less. So there's clearly some big interaction. Plus smoking depletes all your antioxidants. It's well known that it's an oxidative stress," notes Bruce Ames, PhD, professor of biochemistry and molecular biology and director of the National Institute of Environmental Health Sciences Center at the University of California, Berkeley.

The Main Players

While supplements may not be a smart way to get extra antioxidants, plenty of research shows that a diet rich in fruits, vegetables, whole grains, and nuts—all top sources of a wide range of antioxidant compounds—certainly is. If you smoke, you need these foods even more than a nonsmoker does. The body pulls antioxidants out of the blood and into the lungs in a valiant attempt to neutralize free-radical damage, says Gary E. Hatch, PhD, a research pharmacologist and branch chief of the pulmonary toxicology branch of the Environmental Protection Agency. "The cells in the lungs of a smoker are loaded with a lot more antioxidants than those of a nonsmoker," he explains. "The antioxidants are trying to protect the airways from the onslaught of these noxious chemicals."

Those antioxidants that have been linked with lower cancer rates include beta-carotene (which the body converts to vitamin A), vitamins C and E, and the mineral selenium.

Beta-carotene. Abundant in orange and yellow fruits and vegetables such as apricots, cantaloupes, carrots, pumpkins, and squash, beta-carotene from foods seems to protect against "smokers' cancers"—those of the colon, kidneys, skin, and lungs, says James Scala, PhD, a nutritionist and author of *If You Can't/Won't Stop Smoking*. Study after study shows that low levels of beta-carotene are associated with a greater cancer risk, including the risk of lung cancer.

Vitamin C. Found in strawberries, papaya, citrus fruits, and many other foods, vitamin C has been found to protect against a variety of cancers as well as heart disease and stroke, says pharmacist Earl Mindell, RPh, PhD, professor emeritus of nutrition at Pacific Western University in Los Angeles and author of *Earl Mindell's Food as Medicine*.

Doctor's Top Tip

Protect your heart with a mixed vegetable salad or coleslaw every day. In a study of 22 smokers and nonsmokers, those who ate more carrots, pear tomatoes, cabbage, green beans, and spinach protected bad low-density lipoprotein (LDL) cholesterol against oxidation—the damage that leads to clogged arteries—14 percent longer, says lead study author Anne-Marie Roussel, PhD, a nutrition researcher at the Université Joseph Fourier in Grenoble, France.

Vitamin E. Concentrated in wheat germ and wheat germ oil, vitamin E helps keep cell walls intact so it's harder for marauding free radicals to push their way in. More important, it also neutralizes free radicals, says Dr. Scala.

Selenium. Found in most fruits and vegetables, especially garlic, onions, and other bulb vegetables, selenium works with vitamin E to neutralize free radicals.

The Case for Produce

The evidence is strong (and getting stronger) that people who eat lots of fresh fruits and vegetables have a lower risk of developing lung and other cancers than people who eat less produce.

In a Japanese study, for example, researchers found that men who ate raw vegetables every day slashed their lung cancer risk by about 36 percent. Those who ate fruit every day reduced their risk of lung cancer by 55 percent.

Even the men who were smokers benefited. Smokers who ate fruit, raw vegetables, and green vegetables every day reduced their lung cancer risk by 59 percent, 44 percent, and 52 percent, respectively.

The benefits of produce aren't only in relation to lung cancer either. A high intake of fruits and vegetables has been linked to lower risks of just about every type of cancer.

Secondhand Protection

It's not only smokers who need extra dietary protection. Research has shown that secondhand smoke can be dangerous for people who live or work with those who light up. According to a study led by Susan Taylor Mayne, PhD, professor of chronic disease epidemiology at the Yale School of Public Health, eating 1½ additional servings of raw fresh fruits or vegetables a day may slash the risk of lung cancer from secondhand smoke by as much as 60 percent.

"Eating fruits and vegetables is associated with a decrease in risk, regardless of the amount of passive smoke that nonsmokers are exposed to," says Dr. Mayne. Particularly good choices are cantaloupes, carrots, and broccoli, which are loaded with beta-carotene.

Soy Foods

HELP FOR WEIGHT LOSS

HEALING POWER

Can Help:

Control weight

Lower heart disease risk

"Soy to the World" sang out headlines in the 1990s, when study after study suggested that this venerable Asian food might have near-magical powers to protect against heart disease, cancer, hot flashes, and brittle bones. But flash forward to 2006, where one dour headline—"Soyanara"—tells the sad tale. Has this promising superfood become a has-bean?

Maybe not.

Soy's no miracle cure. A growing stack of research studies shows that soy doesn't significantly reduce cholesterol, can't guard against breast cancer or protect you from prostate cancer, and probably does little to build bones or cool hot flashes. But there are still plenty of good reasons to enjoy soy. This amazingly versatile food is packed with nutritional good guys like fiber, omega-3 fatty acids, low-fat protein, and a slew of important vitamins and minerals. And, it's low in saturated fat, cholesterol, and calories. Choose soy, and you get many of the health benefits usually found only in fruits and vegetables: Soy can help cut your risk for heart disease, and since it is lower in fat and calories than meat, it can also help you control your weight (if you eat tofu instead of a cheeseburger, for example). That's good news, because soy seems to be here to stay. Once hidden in Asian supermarkets and health food stores, soy is decidedly mainstream. Sales of soy foods in the United States have skyrocketed—from $300 million in 1992 to $3.9 billion by 2004. Just check out the soy yogurts, soy baby formula, and soy milk crowding the shelves of your local grocery store.

The new bottom line on soy? Choose it if you're looking for new alternatives to high-fat mainstream proteins like meats and cheeses. Skip it—guilt-free—if you never loved the taste or the texture. And if you're at risk for breast cancer or prostate cancer, exercise a little caution (the jury's still out on whether plant hormones in soy might stimulate tumor cells). Here's what you need to know.

The Party's Over

Soy foods faced big setbacks in 2005, when a US government panel said there wasn't clear evidence that soy could guard against heart disease, ease menopause, or protect

In the Kitchen

You've seen tofu in the produce section of your supermarket. But how do you eat this pale, spongy stuff?

Almost any way you want. The advantage of tofu is that while it has little taste of its own, it takes on the flavor of whatever it's cooked with. You can use it with meats and in soups, vegetable dishes, and even desserts.

There are two main types of tofu, firm and soft. Which one you buy depends on how you're going to use it.

- **Firm tofu** has had much of the water removed, giving it a solid consistency. It's usually used when you want the tofu to keep its shape, as in recipes for stir-fries, casseroles, or mock meatballs.
- **Soft (also called silken) tofu** contains more water than the firm variety, giving it a soft, creamy texture. It's usually used for making dips, salad dressings, and desserts.

Both types of tofu should be rinsed with cold water before using. If you're not planning to use the tofu immediately after opening the container, or if you buy it fresh from an open container at an Asian market, rinse it daily and keep it submerged in fresh water. You can also keep it frozen.

After rinsing, press out excess water with your hands or by placing the tofu between several layers of paper towels and pressing with your palm. Removing the excess water will help the tofu maintain its shape during preparation.

---

bones from osteoporosis. In response, the National Institutes of Health said it would stop paying for new soy studies. That fall, soy producers withdrew a petition that asked the FDA to permit food labels to claim that soy protein helps prevent cancer. Behind these changes were new studies that put soy in perspective.

Modest cholesterol benefits. An American Heart Association review of soy research concludes that a daily dose of soy might cut cholesterol by just 3 percent. The panel said the slight drop was probably due to soy's fiber and low fat, not to estrogen-like isoflavones in the bean.

No significant help for hot flashes. "Out of eight randomized controlled trials of soy foods, only one found a significant reduction in the frequency of hot flashes," says a report from Oregon State University's Linus Pauling Institute. While three out of five studies of soy isoflavone extracts found that isoflavones did help, they only cooled hot flashes by about 10 to 20 percent. And soy didn't improve vaginal dryness at all.

Questionable for cancer protection. While eating soy foods in childhood may help protect against breast cancer in adulthood, studies have found that eating

THE JOY OF SOY

Don't know tofu from tempeh? Here are some of the most common soy foods, along with a few suggestions for using them.

Edamame and soy nuts. Edamame are tender, young green soybeans—you can buy them frozen or sometimes find them, still in the shell, at farmers' markets. They're delicious when lightly steamed as a snack or side dish. Soy nuts are simply soy beans that have been soaked, then baked until brown and crunchy. They're a nice change of pace if you like crunchy snack foods.

Meat substitutes. If you want to cut back on meat while getting more soy, look for "mock" meats, like cold cuts, bacon, sausage, franks, and burgers. These are mainly made from soy, and in some cases, they are virtually indistinguishable from the real thing.

Soy flour. Made from roasted, ground soybeans, soy flour can replace some of the wheat flour used for baking. Nutritionists advise buying defatted soy flour, which contains less fat and more protein than the full-fat variety.

Soy milk. A creamy, milk-like drink made from ground, soaked soybeans and water, it's sold plain and in a variety of flavors. Some people prefer "lite" soy milk. It's lower in fat than the regular kind.

Tempeh. These chunky, tender cakes are made from fermented soybeans that have been laced with mold, giving them their distinctively smoky, nutty flavor. You can grill tempeh or add it to spaghetti sauce, chili, or casseroles.

Texturized soy protein. Made from soy flour, this meat substitute can replace part or all of the meat in meat loaf, burgers, and chili.

Tofu. A creamy white, cheeselike food made from curdled soy milk, tofu comes in firm and soft varieties and can be used in virtually anything from soups to desserts.

You will find soft and firm varieties of tofu at most supermarkets in the produce section. Other soy foods are available at specialty and health food stores.

soy as an adult didn't seem to help at all, say Linus Pauling Institute experts. Researchers had thought the plant estrogens—called isoflavones—in soy could protect against breast cancers triggered by more potent human estrogens, but studies showed that it doesn't seem to help. When researchers at the Kimmel Cancer Center at Johns Hopkins University in Baltimore reviewed 18 studies on soy and breast cancer, they found that women who ate large quantities of soy may have lowered their risk by 15 percent. But the researchers say women in different studies ate different amounts of soy, so they can't draw any conclusions.

Doctor's Top Tip

Have soy in place of foods high in animal fats. "Soy products such as fresh or frozen soybeans (edamame), tofu, soy butter, soy nuts, and some soy burgers could be beneficial to heart health when they displace foods such as hamburgers, cheese, and other sources of saturated fat from the diet," says Alice Lichtenstein, ScD, head of the American Heart Association's nutrition committee and director of the Cardiovascular Nutrition Laboratory at the Jean Mayer USDA Human Nutrition Research Center on Aging at Tufts. "Heart disease is a major problem—using soy protein instead of animal protein is still a win."

The idea had been that soy isoflavones would lock onto estrogen receptors on cells, blocking more powerful human estrogens and stopping the growth of estrogen-sensitive breast cancers. It was also thought that isoflavones could dock at testosterone receptors, blocking hormone-stimulated prostate cancer changes. But research hasn't shown this to be true.

Soy Safety

Experts urge some caution with soy products—especially for women who've had breast cancer or are at risk. The reason? The isoflavones, which researchers worry could have an impact on estrogen-fueled breast cancers. Soy experts from the National Cancer Institute say there's not yet enough evidence to say whether soy foods or supplements increase risk for developing breast cancer, or having a recurrence. Prostate cancer survivors should be cautious, too, say Tufts University cancer experts.

But what if you don't have cancer risk and like soy? Nutritionists with the Center for Science in the Public Interest say that even if you like soy, don't have more than 50 to 70 milligrams of isoflavones a day. That's the equivalent of 1 to 2 (8-ounce) cups of soy milk or 6 to 9 ounces of tofu.

Good Reasons to Try Soy

For most of us, soy foods like tofu, tempeh, and other meat replacements made with soy can be a healthy change from higher-fat meats and cheeses. "There are lots of reasons to add soy to your diet just from a basic nutritional perspective," says prominent soy researcher Mark Messina, PhD, of Loma Linda University in California.

For example, a half-cup of tofu provides about 20 grams of protein, or 40 percent of the Daily Value (DV). The same half-cup supplies about 258 milligrams of calcium, or more than 25 percent of the DV, and 13 milligrams of iron, or 87 percent of the Recommended Dietary Allowance (RDA) for women and 130 percent of the RDA for men.

While soy foods are moderately high in fat, most of the fat is polyunsaturated. Soy foods contain little of the artery-clogging saturated fat found in meat and many dairy foods, says Dr. Messina.

GETTING THE MOST

Add it last. When cooking with tofu or other soy products, always add them late in the cooking process. Researchers speculate that cooking at high heats for extended periods of time may reduce or eliminate many of the nutritional benefits.

Shop for power. While it's best to eat soy foods in their unadulterated form, there are times that you may have a taste for a ready-made vegetable burger or breakfast sausage. When buying processed soy foods, make sure that they contain "soy protein," "hydrolyzed vegetable protein," or "textured vegetable protein," which are all acceptable sources of phytoestrogens. By contrast, don't expect too much from products containing soy protein concentrates.

Soy Fruit Smoothie

2 cups vanilla-flavored soy beverage, well chilled

1 cup frozen sliced peaches

1 medium banana, cut into chunks

8 medium strawberries

¼ teaspoon ground cinnamon

Ice cubes (optional)

In a blender, combine the soy beverage, peaches, banana, strawberries, and cinnamon. Blend until smooth and creamy. Add a few ice cubes, if desired, and blend again.

Makes 2 servings

Cook's Notes: *If you are concerned about calories, use a "lite" soy beverage. This recipe can easily be doubled and prepared in batches for more people.*

PER SERVING

Calories: 248
Total fat: 3.3 g
Saturated fat: 0.6 g

Cholesterol: 0 mg
Sodium: 122 mg
Dietary fiber: 4.8 g

Mocha Tofu Pudding

2 packages (10½ ounces each) silken tofu

⅔ cup packed light brown sugar

5 tablespoons unsweetened cocoa powder

1¼ teaspoons vanilla extract

⅛ teaspoon ground cinnamon

2 teaspoons instant coffee powder

2 teaspoons boiling water

Rinse and drain the tofu and pat dry with paper towels. Place the tofu in a food processor. Add the brown sugar, cocoa, vanilla extract, and cinnamon. In a cup, mix the coffee powder and water, stirring to dissolve. Add to the food processor. Process until smooth, stopping occasionally to scrape down the sides of the container.

Spoon into small dessert dishes. Cover and refrigerate for at least 30 minutes, or until the pudding firms up.

Makes 6 servings

PER SERVING

Calories: 133

Total fat: 3.6 g

Saturated fat: 0.4 g

Cholesterol: 0 mg

Sodium: 43 mg

Dietary fiber: 1.6 g

Spices

PROTECTIVE FLAVORINGS

In biblical times, mustard seeds were thought to cure everything from toothaches to epilepsy. (Some people even sniffed ground mustard seeds because sneezing was thought to purge the brain.) Saffron, black pepper, fenugreek, and many other spices were also prized for their healing powers.

As it turns out, the ancients had an uncanny sense of which spices were most likely to be effective. "Researchers have identified many substances in spices that offer health benefits," says Melanie Polk, RD, director of nutrition education at the American Institute for Cancer Research. In fact, researchers are studying the healing potential of many kitchen spices, including black pepper, cumin, cloves, cinnamon, nutmeg, fenugreek, and turmeric.

The National Institute of Nutrition in India, for example, has found that turmeric contains compounds that may help prevent cancer. The research is so promising, in fact, that India's National Cancer Institute has proposed a public education campaign to promote greater use of this aromatic spice. (Read more on turmeric below.)

Unlike herbs, which come from the leaves of plants, spices are made from the buds, bark, fruits, roots, or seeds. The drying process doesn't appear to diminish their healing powers. When properly stored, spices can retain their active ingredients for months or even years.

Research into the world of spices is very new, Polk says, so scientists are only beginning to understand their healing potential. But what has been discovered so far is impressive.

Defense against Cancer

Spices contain an abundance of compounds called phytochemicals, or phytonutrients, many of which may help prevent normal, healthy cells from turning into cancer. And the ways in which these compounds work are as varied as the spices themselves.

Many spices, for example, contain antioxidants, substances that block the effects of free radicals in the body. Free radicals are harmful oxygen molecules that punch holes in healthy cells, sometimes causing genetic damage that can lead to cancer.

> **HEALING POWER**
> **Can Help:**
>
> Protect against cataracts
>
> Prevent cancer
>
> Lower cholesterol and triglycerides
>
> Prevent excessive blood clotting

Turmeric is a very rich source of antioxidants, including a compound called curcumin. In animal studies, curcumin has been shown to reduce the risk of colon cancer by 58 percent. Other research suggests that it may work against skin cancer as well.

What's more, some spices have the ability to help neutralize harmful substances in the body, taking away their cancer-causing potential. Nutmeg, ginger, cumin, black pepper, and coriander, for example, have been shown to help block the effects of aflatoxin, a mold that can cause liver cancer.

Finally, some spices appear to be capable of killing cancer cells outright. In laboratory studies, for example, compounds from saffron were placed on human cancer cells, including cells that cause leukemia. Not only did the dangerous cells stop growing, but the compounds appeared to have no effect on normal, healthy cells.

Since the research is still very new, researchers can't predict which spices or how much of different spices you might need to reduce your risk of getting cancer. "The best advice for now," Polk says, "is to use a variety of spices, especially for replacing salt and fat in your food."

Keeping Arteries Clear

There is good evidence that getting more spices in your diet can help cut your risk for heart disease. Some of the same compounds in spices that prevent free radicals from damaging healthy cells also prevent them from damaging cholesterol. This is important, because when cholesterol is damaged, it's much more likely to stick to artery walls.

In the Kitchen

Despite their robust appearance, spices don't last forever. And even when they're fresh, they're often reluctant to give up their full range of flavors. Here are a few ways to get the best tastes every time:

Stock up often. If you haven't bought spices since the last time you moved, it's probably time to throw out the old ones and start fresh. Ground spices lose their flavor quickly, usually in about 6 months. Whole spices, however, will keep their flavors for a year or two. Fresher is better, of course, but spices retain their health-promoting properties for several months or longer.

Store them carefully. Exposure to light, moisture, and air will quickly rob your spices of their delicious flavors. To keep them fresh, store them in airtight containers in a cool, dry place, preferably kept away from direct light.

Boost the flavor. To make a spice's natural flavors stand out even more, toast it briefly in a dry skillet until it's slightly brown and aromatic.

Cloves, for example, contain the powerful antioxidants kaempferol and rhamnetin. The curcumin in turmeric can also protect the arteries. Turmeric, incidentally, may provide double protection because it not only blocks free radicals but also has been shown to lower levels of triglycerides—dangerous blood fats that, in large amounts, appear to raise the risk of heart disease.

Yet another way in which certain spices keep cholesterol levels down is by trapping cholesterol-containing substances in the intestine. Fenugreek, for example, contains compounds called saponins, which bind to cholesterol and cause it to be excreted from the body. In one study, for example, scientists found that animals given fenugreek had drops in cholesterol of at least 18 percent.

It's not only high cholesterol that can raise the risk for heart disease. Another potential problem is platelets—small, cell-like components in blood that aid in clotting. While platelets are essential for stopping bleeding, sometimes they get too active and begin forming excessive clots in the bloodstream. If a clot gets large enough to block an artery, the result can be a heart attack or even a stroke.

At least five spices—turmeric, fenugreek, cloves, red chile peppers, and ginger—have been shown to help prevent platelets from clumping. In fact, a compound in ginger called gingerol has a chemical structure somewhat similar to aspirin's, which is a proven clot-busting drug.

Cutting Diabetes Risk

Cinnamon improves your body's ability to obey insulin and take up glucose (blood sugar), report researchers at the USDA's Beltsville Human Nutrition Research Center in Maryland. It also cuts heart-threatening triglycerides and bad low-density lipoprotein (LDL) cholesterol. At work is a compound in this spice called methylhydroxy chalcone polymer, which makes cells absorb glucose faster and convert it more easily into energy. When 30 women and 30 men with type 2 diabetes received either cinnamon or a placebo capsule (dummy pill) every day for 40 days, researchers found that the cinnamon group's blood sugar levels had fallen by 18 to 29 percent, their LDL cholesterol dropped 7 to 17 percent, their triglycerides fell 23 to 30 percent, and their good high-density lipoprotein (HDL) cholesterol rose slightly.

A Promising Future

Since spices contain a large number of compounds, researchers have just begun mapping their healing powers. But research from around the globe indicates that the list of benefits will only keep growing.

Researchers at the National Cancer Institute, for example, have found that the curcumin in turmeric can help prevent HIV, the virus that causes AIDS, from

Sprinkle cinnamon on your morning coffee . . . or toast . . . or oatmeal. A half-teaspoon of cinnamon each day could cut your triglycerides and total cholesterol by 12 to 30 percent while it boosts your body's ability to store blood sugar, reports researcher Richard A. Anderson, PhD, a research chemist with the USDA Human Nutrition Research Center in Beltsville, Maryland. You could also double the amount you use in baked goods' recipes, sprinkle it on baked sweet potatoes, add it to chilis and curries for authentic flavor, or create a zero-carb, low-calorie cinnamon sugar mix by blending together a sugar substitute like Splenda with equal parts ground cinnamon.

multiplying. Research has shown, in fact, that when people with AIDS were given curcumin, the illness progressed at a slower rate.

Curcumin has also been shown to protect the eyes from free radicals, which are one of the leading causes of cataracts. In fact, a laboratory study found that curcumin was able to reduce free-radical damage to the eyes by 52 percent. Other studies have found that curcumin supplements could ease the pain and inflammation of rheumatoid arthritis.

There's growing evidence that ginger, too, could help quell the inflammation associated with some forms of arthritis. In several studies, women and men with osteoarthritis and rheumatoid arthritis who took ginger extracts experienced a significant reduction in pain and as a result, needed less of their pain medications and anti-inflammatory drugs. (A reality check: They still rated ibuprofen as a better pain reliever than ginger!) Lab studies confirm that compounds in ginger inhibit inflammation, suggesting it could help cut risk for health problems like heart disease, cancer, and Alzheimer's disease, as well as arthritis.

The gingerol in ginger relaxes blood vessels. This spice has a long history of use easing stomach upsets. Now, researchers at the University of Michigan are studying whether ginger can help ease nausea for cancer patients undergoing chemotherapy. "Ginger has been shown to be effective in a number of clinical trials against nausea and vomiting associated with motion sickness, pregnancy, and postoperative recovery," says lead investigator Suzanna Zick, ND, MPH. "With this trial, we hope to determine its efficacy and safety for chemotherapy-induced nausea and vomiting. "We hope ginger will be effective for patients who continue to experience delayed nausea and vomiting despite treatment with other antinausea drugs," Dr. Zick adds.

On another front, spicy, red-hot paprika shows promise for cutting cancer risk, due to the anti-inflammatory and antioxidant properties of the compound capsaicin.

And a powerful, inflammation-fighting, numbing compound in cloves called eugenol has made it a top choice in products used by dentists during root canal surgery. It may even help cut risk for digestive system cancers.

Finally, researchers at the University of Wales College of Medicine discovered that a strain of black pepper called West African black pepper appears to produce changes in the brains of mice that can reduce the severity of seizures.

"We only have information on a few spices so far," Polk says. "But no doubt, we'll be uncovering similarly exciting information about many others in the future."

Indian-Style Spice Mix

8 **teaspoons dry mustard**

4 **teaspoons ground fenugreek**

4 **teaspoons ground cumin**

2 **teaspoons ground cloves**

2 **teaspoons ground coriander**

2 **teaspoons ground ginger**

2 **teaspoons ground turmeric**

½ **teaspoon ground cinnamon**

In a small bowl, combine the mustard, fenugreek, cumin, cloves, coriander, ginger, turmeric, and cinnamon. Mix well to blend. Store in a small, airtight jar in a cool, dark cupboard or the refrigerator.

Makes ½ cup

Cook's Notes: *Ground fenugreek is available in Indian groceries, some specialty food shops, and health food stores.*

You could easily double this recipe. The spice mixture is delicious enough—and versatile enough—to keep on hand in the kitchen. It's excellent as a rub for broiled or pan-cooked meats, fish, and poultry (rub the mixture over the food generously before cooking). Or use it as a flavoring for steamed cauliflower, carrots, and other vegetables. To bring out the flavor, toast the spice mix briefly in a dry skillet just before using.

Spiced Potato Cakes

3   large baking potatoes

2   teaspoons canola oil

1   cup chopped onions

4   teaspoons Indian-Style Spice Mix (page 589)

¾   cup fat-free plain yogurt

¼   cup fat-free egg substitute

2   teaspoons unsalted butter

¼   teaspoon salt

Scrub the potatoes and pat dry with paper towels. With a fork, pierce each potato in 3 or 4 places. Arrange the potatoes, spoke fashion, in a microwave oven on top of a paper towel. Microwave on high power for 10 minutes. Turn the potatoes, and rotate from the front to the back of the microwave. Microwave for 8 to 10 minutes, or until the potatoes are tender. Test for doneness by inserting the tip of a small, sharp knife into a potato. Let the potatoes stand for 5 minutes.

Halve the potatoes lengthwise. Use a large spoon to scrape all the flesh into a medium bowl; discard the skins. Mash with a fork and set aside.

In a large nonstick skillet, heat the oil over medium-high heat. Add the onions and cook, stirring frequently, until they start to turn golden, about 5 minutes. Add the spice mix, and cook for 30 seconds, or until fragrant.

Remove from the heat and transfer to a large bowl. Add the yogurt, egg substitute, butter, and salt. Stir to combine. Add the potatoes. Mix well.

Wipe the skillet with a paper towel, and coat with cooking spray. Heat over medium-high heat. Drop the potato mixture into the skillet in 4 mounds, patting the mixture with a spatula to make thick cakes. Cook until golden on the bottom, about 5 minutes. Turn and cook until golden on the second side, about 3 minutes.

Makes 4 servings

PER SERVING ──────────────

Calories: 243	Cholesterol: 5 mg
Total fat: 4.9 g	Sodium: 171 mg
Saturated fat: 1.4 g	Dietary fiber: 3.9 g

Squash

PACKED WITH BETA-CAROTENE— AND MORE

HEALING POWER

Can Help:

Prevent lung problems

Reduce the risk of
endometrial cancer

Judging from ancient remains found in Mexican caves, folks have been eating squash for at least 7,000 years. Squash was one of the nourishing "three sisters" in early Native American diets. (The other two were corn and beans.) And the vegetable was considered so important that squash were often buried with the dead in order to provide them with nourishment on their final journey.

In the mid-1700s, George Washington and Thomas Jefferson both grew squash on their estates, and in the 1800s, merchant seamen carried home exotic new varieties from their travels throughout the Americas—introducing a wide range of squash shapes, colors, and sizes to America's kitchen gardens and dinner tables.

It has taken science a few thousand years to prove what early Americans knew from experience: Squash is almost overloaded with nourishing compounds. In fact, squash contains such a rich array of vitamins, minerals, and other compounds that scientists have just begun to map its healing potential. "I don't think anybody really knows all the good substances there are in squash," says Dexter L. Morris, MD, PhD, associate professor in the department of emergency medicine at the University of North Carolina School of Medicine at Chapel Hill.

When researchers talk about the healing powers of squash, what they're usually referring to is winter squash, such as Hubbard, acorn, and butternut, which are distinguished by their deep yellow and orange flesh colors. Pale summer squash, by contrast, while low in calories and a decent source of fiber, is generally regarded as a nutritional lightweight, at least until future research proves otherwise.

"Not long ago, I was saying that apples and onions didn't have much in them," admits Mark Kestin, PhD, professor of nutrition at Bastyr University, and an affiliate associate professor of epidemiology and public health at the University of Washington, both in Seattle. Then researchers discovered a variety of heart-saving flavonoids, and the produce suddenly looked rich. "Summer squash may have some incredible substance we haven't discovered yet," he says.

In the Kitchen

A winter squash may be full of beta-carotene, vitamin C, and other healing compounds, but it doesn't readily give them up. The squash is encased in a tough, leathery skin, which requires a sharp knife and a strong hand to cut all the way through. And if your hand should slip—look out!

Here's how to make cutting it a little easier: Rather than trying to cut the raw, tough skin, partly bake the squash first. When the skin softens—usually after about 20 minutes at 375°F—cut the squash open and clean it out. Then put it back in the oven until it's tender.

Microwave winter squash. No time to cook squash for 45 minutes? No problem. Cut an acorn squash in half, remove the seeds and fiber, then turn it upside down on a microwaveable pan with a small amount of water in the bottom. Cook on high power for 3 to 5 minutes, then test for doneness by pricking through the skin with a fork (if it's soft, it's ready to eat). Still tough? Cook for another 3 to 5 minutes. Serve with a little olive oil and brown sugar, or purée the squash in a blender with chicken stock and spices, then heat for a creamy squash soup.

Create healthier "pasta." Instead of high-calorie, high-carb noodles, serve your favorite tomato sauce over the luscious, low-calorie, high-fiber strands of spaghetti squash. For 6 cups of strands, wash, then bake a 3¼-pound whole squash at 375°F for 1½ hours or until it is tender. Cool, slice in half lengthwise, and scoop out the seeds. Then scrape the inside of the squash with a fork to remove the yummy strands.

Color Them Healthy

Two of the most popular winter squashes, the bumpy-skinned Hubbard squash and the deeply tanned butternut squash, are both rich in vitamin C and beta-carotene, antioxidants that can help prevent cancer, heart disease, and certain age-related conditions, such as macular degeneration. Eating a half-cup of baked butternut squash will provide more than a quarter of the Daily Value (DV) for vitamin C and 40 to 66 percent of the beta-carotene recommended by experts.

For people with asthma, squash and other foods rich in vitamin C can be powerful breath savers. "People who have more C in their diets over time have fewer lung ailments. The vitamin gets transported to the lining of the lung and serves as an antioxidant there," explains Gary E. Hatch, PhD, a research pharmacologist and branch chief of pulmonary toxicology at the Environmental Protection Agency.

Dr. Hatch recommends that everyone get at least 200 milligrams daily of dietary vitamin C, which is about the amount in 1½ cups of baked butternut squash.

On the beta-carotene front, "there are tons of studies showing that eating vegetables rich in beta-carotene" is good for you, says Dr. Morris. Doctors in Italy and Switzerland studied the diets of more than 1,000 of their countrywomen. Preliminary research suggests that women who got the most beta-carotene—5.5 milligrams a day, which is about the amount in 1 cup of baked winter squash—had half the risk of endometrial cancer as those who ate the least. Beta-carotene can also cool off inflammation and may help ease inflammatory conditions, including not only asthma but osteoarthritis and rheumatoid arthritis as well.

Comfort Food with a Protective Punch

New research reveals that compounds tucked into the colorful flesh of winter squash—and to a lesser extent in the skin of summer squashes such as zucchini—may help battle a wide variety of medical conditions. Squash extracts lessen urinary and sexual problems associated with enlarged prostate in men. And a carotenoid called beta-cryptoxanthin, found in brilliant orange foods such as winter squash, cut the risk of lung cancer by 27 to 37 percent in a massive study of 63,247 Chinese women and men.

Furthermore, rich stores of vitamin A in winter squash may help guard against emphysema in smokers by replenishing supplies depleted by compounds in tobacco

---

DELICIOUS CHOICES

When shopping for squash, most of us think of the old standbys, like acorn or spaghetti squash. But supermarkets these days often have many varieties to choose from. Here are some squashes you may want to try:

- **Buttercup squash** look like little drums wearing pale beanies, which match the stripes running down their green skin. About 3 pounds on the average, buttercup squash is mild and sweet, but sometimes dry.
- **Calabaza squash**, a giant type from the West Indies, wind up in markets cut into huge hunks that show off their neon-orange flesh. This is a sweet squash that is best puréed or cooked with other foods.
- **Delicata squash's** skin is the color of heavy cream, but it's daubed and striped with green and sometimes orange, and the flesh is yellow and sweet.
- **Golden nugget** looks like Cinderella's carriage at midnight—a big pumpkin turned small. It's mildly sweet and only has enough flesh for one serving.
- **Sweet dumpling squash**, barely bigger than a good-size apple, are cream-colored and scalloped with mottled green. They're often baked and served whole.

Doctor's Top Tip

Cook several varieties and colors of summer squash together, suggests the Centers for Disease Control and Prevention. The look is colorful and appealing, and you're covering more nutritional bases, since each color has a slightly different ratio of the healthful phytochemicals called carotenoids.

smoke, say Kansas State University researchers. Low levels of vitamin A have been associated with higher emphysema risk; eating A-rich foods may explain why some smokers never develop this debilitating lung ailment.

Think of squash as a giant, naturally balanced vitamin-and-mineral supplement. For one thing, it's got blood-pressure-lowering potassium. For another, squash contains the B vitamin folate, which helps cut risk for birth defects in babies. Folate may also help deactivate a compound called homocysteine that's been linked with higher rates of heart attack and stroke. Homocysteine can damage the delicate inner lining of blood vessels, setting the stage for artery-clogging atherosclerosis. In addition, the fiber in winter squash can help keep cholesterol in check and improve gastrointestinal woes such as diarrhea and constipation.

GETTING THE MOST

Eat the peel. While zucchini and other kinds of summer squash don't have the rich nutrient stores of winter squash, they do contain a lot of fiber, but only if you eat the peel. A half-cup of unpeeled, uncooked summer squash contains more than 1 gram of fiber.

Think outside the pan. Marinate and grill summer squash, or grate it in a food processor and add it to summer salads or to muffins. Experiment with adding a variety of spices, such as dill, lemon pepper, chili powder, or basil and garlic to your squash dishes. Or simply slice summer squash and serve it on a tray of crudités with dip.

Shop for color. There's a huge variability in the amount of beta-carotene found in squash. It can range anywhere from about 0.5 milligram to about 5 milligrams, even in the same kind of squash.

As a rule, experts say, the darker the squash, the more beta-carotene it contains. The shell of an acorn squash, for example, should be an intensely deep dark green. Butternut squash should be a butterscotch tan, and Hubbards should be almost glow-in-the-dark orange.

Buy it ahead of time. The hard skin that makes winter squash such a challenge to cut also helps protect the flesh inside. This means that you can store winter squash for a month or more in a cool, well-ventilated place before the nutrients start to diminish. In fact, storing squash actually causes the amount of beta-carotene to increase, according to nutrition expert Densie Webb, RD, PhD, coauthor of *Foods for Better Health* and *The Dish on Eating Healthy and Being Fabulous*.

Zucchini with Garlic and Oregano

1½ pounds zucchini

1½ teaspoons olive oil

  4 cloves garlic, minced

  1 large tomato, seeded and diced

  ¾ teaspoon dried oregano

  ¼ teaspoon salt

     Pinch of freshly ground black pepper

Trim the zucchini and cut it into ¼-inch-thick slices.

In a large skillet, heat the oil over medium heat. Add the garlic, and cook for 30 seconds, or just until fragrant. Add the zucchini, and toss to mix. Add the tomato and oregano, and toss well. Reduce the heat to medium-low, cover, and cook until the zucchini softens, about 5 minutes. Add the salt and pepper to taste, and stir gently.

Makes 4 servings

Cook's Note: *If desired, sprinkle the zucchini with grated Parmesan cheese before serving.*

PER SERVING

Calories: 48
Total fat: 1.9 g
Saturated fat: 0.3 g

Cholesterol: 0 mg
Sodium: 141 mg
Dietary fiber: 2.2 g

Acorn Squash with Bread Stuffing

2 large acorn squash (about 1½ pounds each)

4 teaspoons olive oil

1 cup minced onions

5 slices stale bread, cut into ½-inch cubes

¾ teaspoon ground savory

¼ teaspoon freshly ground black pepper

Preheat the oven to 375°F.

Cut each squash in half lengthwise. Scoop out and discard the seeds. Place the squash halves, cut side down, in a large baking dish. Add ½ inch of water to the pan. Bake for 25 to 30 minutes, or until the squash halves can be pierced with the tip of a sharp knife but are still fairly firm.

Meanwhile, in a large nonstick skillet, heat the oil over medium heat. Add the onions, and cook until softened, about 5 minutes. Stir in the bread, savory, and pepper. Cook until the bread starts to brown slightly. Stir in ¾ cup water, then add up to ¼ cup more water to make the bread moist but not wet.

Remove the squash from the oven. Turn the halves over, and spoon the bread mixture into the cavities. Pour enough hot tap water into the pan to return the level to about ½ inch.

Continue to bake the squash for 20 to 30 minutes, or until it is tender and the filling is golden. Test for doneness by inserting the tip of a sharp knife into the squash.

Makes 4 servings

Cook's Note: *Use stale wheatberry or multi-grain bread for a really flavorful, nutritious stuffing.*

PER SERVING

Calories: 256
Total fat: 6.2 g
Saturated fat: 1 g

Cholesterol: 0 mg
Sodium: 182 mg
Dietary fiber: 12 g

Stomach Upset
CALMING THE QUEASIES

One of life's ironies is that many of the foods we like best, like creamy chocolate éclairs or a feast of roast turkey, stuffing, and gravy, are the same ones that our stomachs like least, at least when we overindulge. And overindulge we do—with family, friends, and co-workers—more than a few times a year. This is why our festive feasts sometimes end not with a glass of wine but with a spoonful of Pepto-Bismol or a glass of bubbly Alka-Seltzer (instead of champagne!).

Getting too much food in your system at one time is a common cause of stomach upset because your body has trouble handling the sudden increase in volume, says William Ruderman, MD, a gastroenterologist in private practice in Orlando, Florida. Eating too much fat at once can also be a problem because it may trip the nausea sensor in your brain, which sends those miserable, queasy sensations down to your stomach.

High-fat foods are bad in yet another way. They temporarily weaken a small muscle at the base of the esophagus, the tube leading from the mouth to the stomach. This allows digestive juices, which normally stay in the stomach, to surge upstream, causing heartburn or nausea, says Marie Borum, MD, professor of medicine and director of the division of gastroenterology at George Washington University Medical Center in Washington, D.C. The combination of heartburn and that too-full feeling can take the cheerful bloom off any social evening.

Two of the best ways to keep your stomach calm are to eat a little bit less at meals and to cut back on your intake of fatty foods, especially fried meats, says Dr. Borum. But if your stomach's already upset, what you really need is something that will take the queasiness away fast. As it turns out, foods, especially bland foods, can do that, too.

"I recommend starting with water, then moving on to toast, broth, bland soup, or soft-boiled eggs," says Dr. Borum. "Naturally, you also want to avoid the hard-to-digest foods like ice cream or fried chicken."

When even bland foods are hard to get down, don't even try to eat, Dr. Borum adds. There's nothing wrong with going without food for 4 to 6 hours. Many people are reluctant to skip meals, but a temporary fast can actually be very soothing. In fact, that may be just the right thing to help your stomach recover.

MERRY, MERRY, QUITE CONTRARY

Good food, good drink, and good company—who doesn't like a good party? But making too many trips to the punch bowl can leave your stomach wishing you'd spent the night playing solitaire.

While there's no real cure for "morning-after stomach," there are a few foods that will help ease the discomfort of a hangover. Here are some examples that you can try in a pinch.

Keep it plain. Having a slice of plain bread—without butter, peanut butter, or cream cheese—will help buffer acids in the stomach that can lead to nausea, according to Marie Borum, MD, professor of medicine and director of the division of gastroenterology at George Washington University Medical Center in Washington, D.C. In addition, bland foods like bread and pasta are very easy to digest, which can help keep an upset stomach calm.

Drink like a fish. Getting more water into your system can help relieve the nausea and dehydration that may be caused by excessive drinking. If you've been drinking alcohol, in fact, it's a good idea to have plenty of water before going to bed at night because it can help prevent some of the discomfort you might experience the next morning.

One of the most popular remedies for an upset stomach is also one of the oldest. Studies show that ginger can sometimes work better than over-the-counter drugs to settle a somersaulting stomach. "Ginger is the one herbal treatment that's pretty widely accepted as effective," says Marvin Schuster, MD, founder of the Marvin M. Schuster Digestive and Motility Disorders Center at Johns Hopkins Bayview Medical Center in Baltimore.

While fresh ginger is effective, it's really too spicy to use to get the amounts that are necessary for healing. An easier strategy, says Dr. Schuster, is to brew a cup of ginger tea. Grate 2 teaspoons of fresh ginger, and let it steep in hot water for 10 minutes. Strain the tea, then drink it until you feel better. For many people, just 1 cup is enough to do the trick.

Another beverage that may help settle your stomach is Coca-Cola. The ingredients in Coke are top secret, so no one really knows why so many people reach for the "real thing" when their stomachs are flip-flopping. Still, drinking Coke does seem to be helpful, says Dr. Borum. "Coke is also high in sugar, which is important if you've already been sick and need hydration," she adds.

One problem with having an upset stomach is that it's often difficult even to drink water without feeling sicker. To keep yourself from getting dehydrated, try keeping a small piece of ice in your mouth, Dr. Borum suggests. This will allow some water to enter your system, but not so much that it will upset your stomach even more. Sometimes sipping extremely cold liquids may do the trick. Or take small, frequent sips every 15 to 30 minutes (this is easier on an upset tummy and promotes absorption).

Dieting and have stomach upset? Don't soothe your tummy with "sugar-free" foods. These sweets and drinks are often made with sugar alcohols like sorbitol, xylitol, mannitol, and maltitol, which can cause gas and bloating—and even act as a laxative.

And if your stomach is queasy, be sure to skip nonsteroidal anti-inflammatory drugs (NSAIDs). Ibuprofen (including Advil and Motrin) and aspirin can further upset your tummy. Use acetaminophen if you need a pain reliever.

Doctor's Top Tip

If you're not just nauseous, but also vomiting, make an effort to stay hydrated. Drink small, steady amounts of clear liquids, suggests the National Institutes of Health. If you've been sick for several hours, switch to diluted fruit juice, a sports drink like Gatorade, or broth. Your body may be depleted of fluids and also short on electrolytes like potassium and sodium, which help cells function and communicate. You can create your own rehydration drink by mixing together ¾ teaspoon of table salt, 1 teaspoon of baking powder, 4 tablespoons of white sugar, 1 cup of orange juice, and 1 quart of water. Take small, frequent sips.

Stress

GETTING EASE WITH Bs

Late for work—grab a doughnut. The report's due—pour another cup of coffee. The children are yelling—take an ice cream break. Stress is all around us, and food often provides a welcome, if momentary, break. Unfortunately, the foods we often turn to in times of stress, like coffee and sweets, have a way of making us feel even more frazzled later on.

It doesn't have to be this way. Research has shown that eating more of some foods and less of others can cause stress hormones in the body to decline. Making slight changes in your diet will produce physical changes in the brain that can make the world's problems just a little bit easier to handle.

Calming Carbohydrates

Mashed potatoes. Fresh-baked bread. A steaming plate of pasta. These are just a few of the "comfort foods" that many of us instinctively turn to in times of stress. As it turns out, our instincts are dead-on. Researchers have found that foods high in carbohydrates produce changes in the brain that can take the edge off stress.

During emotionally trying times, the brain quickly uses up its supply of serotonin, a chemical that imparts feelings of well-being. When serotonin levels fall, negative feelings tend to rise, says Joe Tecce, PhD, a neuropsychologist and associate professor of psychology at Boston College in Chestnut Hill, Massachusetts.

Eating foods that are high in carbohydrates, like pasta, bagels, or baked potatoes, can quickly raise low serotonin levels, making you feel less stressed and more relaxed, says Dr. Tecce. And here's a little carbohydrate bonus: As serotonin levels rise, appetite usually decreases, which means that you're less likely to eat your way through hard times.

A Zoo Story

Next time you visit the monkey house, take a moment to admire our swinging cousins. They turn somersaults, hang from trees, and generally appear to be having a great time. They don't have to deal with carpools or bills, which could explain their lack of stress. Then again, maybe it's all the bananas they've been eating.

Research suggests that foods high in vitamin B_6, such as bananas, potatoes, and prunes, can relieve irritability and stress, making people (and maybe monkeys) feel just a little bit better. In one study, Dr. Tecce and his colleagues at the Jean Mayer USDA Human Nutrition Research Center on Aging at Tufts University in Boston lowered vitamin B_6 levels in a group of volunteers. The people became increasingly irritable and tense.

Vitamin B_6 improves mood by raising levels of dopamine, a chemical in the brain that is related to feeling good. When you don't get enough vitamin B_6 in your diet, dopamine levels fall, and you can experience negative feelings. In addition, people who don't get enough vitamin B_6 may produce too little serotonin, which will make them feel even worse.

It's not yet clear how much vitamin B_6 you might need to help keep stress levels down, says Dr. Tecce. It seems likely, however, that the Daily Value (DV) of 2 milligrams is probably enough. It's very easy to get this much vitamin B_6 in your diet. One banana, for example, has 0.7 milligram, or 35 percent of the DV; a half-cup of chickpeas has 0.6 milligram, or 30 percent of the DV; and a baked potato has 0.4 milligram, or 20 percent of the DV.

The Caffeine Crash

Just about anywhere there are people hard at work, there will also be a coffeepot. And the more stress these people feel, the more likely they are to hit the joe. In a study of almost 300 people, for example, researchers at the University of Minnesota in Morris found that half of them drank more coffee or caffeine-containing soft drinks during high-pressure times.

Caffeine produces a quick zing that can momentarily make you feel more relaxed and confident. Fairly quickly, however, it stimulates the production of cortisol, a stress hormone that raises blood pressure and heart rate. This can make you feel more stressed than you did before, says William Lovallo, PhD, professor of psychiatry and behavioral sciences at the University of Oklahoma Health Sciences Center in Oklahoma City.

It doesn't take potfuls of coffee to rev up your stress levels, Dr. Lovallo adds. In a study of 48 men, Dr. Lovallo and his colleagues found that those drinking just 2 to 3 cups had a significant increase in blood pressure.

This doesn't mean that you have to give up your favorite drinks, Dr. Lovallo adds. But when the pressure's on, switching to drinks without caffeine will help keep you calmer and more in control.

And while you're filling your cup, put the lid back on the sugar. Within minutes after eating sweets, blood sugar levels start to fall. "When your blood sugar is going up and down, you are more susceptible to moodiness and irritability," says Peter

Doctor's Top Tip

You can get off the carb/stress/ carb roller-coaster by eating high-fiber, low-sugar foods at meals and snacks. When adult volunteers in a diet study at Children's Hospital Boston ate low-glycemic foods (high-fiber, low-sugar foods that keep blood sugar low and steady), they not only lost weight faster, but their moods and energy levels stayed higher, reports lead study author David Ludwig, MD. If this strategy can help you get through the physical stress of losing weight, it may also help you withstand the fattening cookie urges of daily stresses, too.

Miller, PhD, professor of psychiatry and behavioral sciences at the Medical University of South Carolina in Charleston and former executive director of the Hilton Head Health Institute in Hilton Head Island, South Carolina.

The Stress-Cookie Connection

There's a good reason we head for the cookies, chocolate, or (fill in your favorite stress-busting food) when we are under pressure. Eating sugar- and fat-rich foods helps blunt the effects of our physiological response to chronic stress.

During chronic stress, levels of glucocorticoid hormones increase. Researchers at the University of California, San Francisco, found that rats with elevated glucocorticoid levels engage in pleasure-seeking activities such as eating fat and sugar. When they do so, they gain abdominal fat.

Eating comfort foods puts the brakes on a key element of chronic stress. In the short term, it may be worth gaining a couple of pounds to calm down. In the long term, however, fixing the source of the stress or finding alternatives such as yoga or meditation are healthier.

The other problem with the stress/carb connection: roller-coaster cravings. First, blood sugar soars (and you feel great). Then your pancreas pumps out a big dose of insulin, which pushes all that sugar into your cells, and blood sugar plummets. You feel cranky again . . . so you reach for more cookies. The result? More crankiness . . . and finally difficulty fitting into your favorite jeans.

Stroke

A HEALTHY-BRAIN DIET

The most frightening thing about stroke is how suddenly it can strike. People who have had a stroke say there's often no discernible warning, no sign—just a split-second sense that something has suddenly gone wrong.

But even though the stroke itself comes out of the blue, the problems that cause it can be years in the making. Stroke occurs when blood, and the oxygen and nutrients it contains, stop reaching parts of the brain—thanks usually to a blood clot blocking a tiny artery in your brain or, less often, when an artery ruptures and blood is lost.

High blood pressure, high cholesterol, diabetes, and a dangerous prediabetic condition called metabolic syndrome all raise your risk—and they're all factors that can be reduced significantly by choosing the right foods. "Your diet plays a critical role in preventing stroke," says Thomas A. Pearson, MD, PhD, professor of epidemiology and chairman of the department of community and preventive medicine at the University of Rochester in New York.

In a study of more than 87,000 nurses, for example, researchers at the Harvard School of Public Health found that women who ate the most fruits and vegetables were 40 percent less likely to have a stroke than those who ate the least. In another study, this one conducted at the University of California, San Diego, researchers discovered that people who ate a single serving of potassium-rich fruits or vegetables a day were also able to cut their risk of stroke by 40 percent.

These six eating strategies offer powerful protection:

Calm high blood pressure with dairy and potassium. High blood pressure (135/85 or higher) doubles your risk for a stroke. Here's why. Pummeled by high-speed bloodflow, arteries in the brain thicken and can ultimately squeeze shut. Under pressure, small arteries may rupture. High blood pressure also ups the risk for developing clot-producing plaque in artery walls. If everyone with high blood pressure in the United States brought it under control, more than 300,000 strokes annually could be prevented.

Your food plan? Include low-fat dairy products and plenty of potassium-rich foods in your diet. Not only does potassium fight high blood pressure (something 50 million of us suffer from), it also appears to make blood less likely to clot, which can reduce the risk of stroke even more. Not sure what foods are good sources of potassium? Fat-free and 1% milk, low-fat yogurt, vegetable juice cocktail, baby limas, kidney beans, and lentils are all rich in potassium. So are baked potatoes, prune juice, dried peaches, and Swiss chard.

Milk is another beverage that appears to play a role in reducing the risk of stroke. In one large study, researchers from the Honolulu Heart Program found that men who did not drink milk were twice as likely to have a stroke as those who drank at least 16 ounces daily. When reaching for the carton, however, be sure that it contains low-fat or fat-free milk, since the saturated fat in whole milk may offset its benefits.

Reverse metabolic syndrome with smart meal combos. Metabolic syndrome is a combination of prediabetic conditions including insulin resistance—which occurs when your cells stop responding quickly to insulin's command to absorb blood sugar—plus slightly high blood pressure, blood sugar, and triglycerides, plus low levels of good high-density lipoprotein (HDL) cholesterol. Nearly everyone with this condition—and there are at least 40 million Americans at risk for metabolic syndrome—is overweight. Having metabolic syndrome doubles stroke risk.

What fights it? Eating high-fiber, low-sugar foods, lean protein, good fats such as nuts, oily cold-water fish (or fish oil capsules), and flaxseed. Eating fruits, vegetables, and grain products low on the glycemic index (a ranking system based on how foods affect your blood sugar levels) also keeps blood sugar and insulin levels lower. This can cut cravings and help you lose weight and can almost instantly make cells throughout your body more sensitive to insulin's signals. Foods to avoid: doughnuts, sugary soft drinks, and white bread, which send sugar levels soaring, fast. Foods to embrace: most whole grains, beans, fruits, and vegetables, which digest more slowly and so release sugar into the bloodstream at a leisurely rate. You can also slow the rise in blood sugar after a meal by combining a high-fiber or high-protein food with a refined carbohydrate—for example, have some navy beans with instant rice.

Lose weight. Not only what you eat but how much you eat can play a role in controlling stroke. Overweight raises a woman's stroke risk by 75 percent. Obesity raises it by 100 percent. The stroke connection: When Harvard University researchers compared body weight and stroke risk in 116,759 nurses, they found that overweight women were two to four times more likely to have high blood pressure, diabetes, and high cholesterol.

Furthermore, being overweight is perhaps the leading cause of high blood pressure, which vastly increases stroke risk. In fact, people with high blood pressure are five times more likely to have a stroke than those whose blood pressures are normal. In addition, being overweight makes you more likely to develop diabetes, which also increases the risk of stroke.

Get serious about treating diabetes with slow carbs. Having diabetes makes a woman's risk for stroke two to four times higher than normal. An even more potent threat for women than men, diabetes seems to up women's stroke odds by raising their blood pressure and boosting their odds for brain-threatening blood clots.

What's the best food strategy? Keep diabetes under control by choosing "good," "slow," complex carbohydrates like fruits, vegetables, and whole grains. These keep blood sugar lower and steadier and also help control levels of insulin in your body. Experts suspect that surges of insulin after a meal heavy in refined carbs contribute to biochemical changes in the body that promote high blood pressure and blood clot formation—two big stroke risks.

Rebalance your cholesterol profile with better fats. High levels of bad low-density lipoprotein (LDL) cholesterol and low levels of good HDL cholesterol both raise stroke risk. A lack of good HDL leaves your body unable to haul away the bad-guy LDL, giving it free rein to lodge inside the lining of artery walls and start the process that leads to clogged arteries.

For lower LDL and higher HDL levels, eat less saturated fat and more good fats. Choosing olive and canola oil over other fats for cooking, and snacking on a small handful of walnuts can help maintain healthy HDL levels. (Add exercise to really give 'em a boost.)

At the same time, skip full-fat milk, cheese, sour cream, and ice cream . . . and turn down that fat-marbled prime rib. What you don't eat can be just as important as what you do, adds Dr. Pearson. Research has shown, for example, that people getting the most fat in their diets—especially the saturated fat in meats and other animal foods—are much more likely to have a stroke than those eating more healthful foods. This is because a diet that's high in saturated fat raises cholesterol levels. Cholesterol, which is notorious for clogging arteries in the heart, can also block blood vessels in and leading to the brain.

"Reducing saturated fat intake is the most powerful dietary maneuver you can make to lower cholesterol levels," says John R. Crouse, MD, professor of medicine and public health sciences and currently associate director of the Wake Forest University School of Medicine General Clinical Research Center.

For most people, limiting meat servings to 3 or 4 ounces a day, using little (or no) butter, switching to low-fat dairy foods, and avoiding high-fat snacks is all it takes to keep cholesterol at healthy levels.

And choose lots of produce, too. When researchers from the well-known Framingham Heart Study group scrutinized the diets of more than 830 men, they found that for every three servings of fruits and vegetables people ate every day, their risk of stroke declined 22 percent.

Doctor's Top Tip

Dropping just a few pounds can cut stroke risk. You don't have to be model-thin to stay healthy, says Thomas A. Pearson, MD, PhD, of the University of Rochester. Losing 10 to 20 pounds is often enough to lower blood pressure and with it, the risk of having a stroke.

There are several reasons that fruits and vegetables are so beneficial for preventing stroke. For one thing, they're high in fiber, which has been shown to lower cholesterol. And according to epidemiologist Michael Hertog, PhD, of the National Institute of Public Health and Environmental Protection in the Netherlands, these foods also contain powerful antioxidants, which help prevent the harmful LDL cholesterol from sticking to artery walls and blocking bloodflow to the brain. Foods especially high in antioxidants include garlic, onions, kale, carrots, Brussels sprouts, broccoli, blueberries, plums, cherries, oranges, and red grapes.

It doesn't take a lot of antioxidant-rich foods to get the benefits. In the Nurses' Health Study, for example, Harvard researchers found that women who got as little as 15 milligrams of beta-carotene daily, about the amount in one large carrot, reduced their risk of stroke.

Along with fruits and vegetables, tea (both the green and black varieties) is an excellent source of flavonoids. When Dr. Hertog studied more than 550 men ages 50 to 69, he found that those who got most of their flavonoids from tea were able to reduce their risk of stroke by 73 percent, compared with those who got the least of these healthful compounds. He found that those who drink at least 5 cups of tea daily can reduce their stroke risk by more than two-thirds, compared with those who drink less than 3 cups a day.

Sweet Peppers

PICK A PECK FOR HEALTH

HEALING POWER
Can Help:
Prevent cataracts
Reduce the risk of heart disease

Due to the growing interest in ethnic cuisines, sweet peppers, which range in color from dark green to fire engine red, depending on how long they're left on the vine, aren't found only in salad bars anymore. They're also being used in soups, sauces, stir-fries, purées, and pasta dishes. Peppers do more than add a sweet high note to recipes. They're also filled with nutrients that have been shown in studies to battle cataracts and heart disease. And unlike their fiery-tempered siblings, the chile peppers, sweet peppers are mild enough to eat in large amounts, so you can easily reap their health benefits.

Stuffed with Antioxidants

Even though sweet peppers such as bell peppers, pimientos, and frying peppers don't get as much attention as broccoli, cauliflower, and other powerhouse foods, they're among the most nutrient-dense vegetables you can buy, especially when it comes to vitamin C and beta-carotene. (As a rule, the redder the pepper, the more healthful beta-carotene it contains.)

Bite for bite, few vegetables contain as much beta-carotene (which is converted to vitamin A in the body) as the sweet red pepper. This is important because beta-carotene plays a key role in keeping the immune system healthy. It's also a potent antioxidant, meaning that it fights tissue-damaging oxygen molecules known as free radicals, which scientists believe contribute to major health foes like heart disease and cataracts.

Sweet red peppers are such a good source of beta-carotene, in fact, that a group of German researchers has classified them as a "must-eat" food for people trying to get more of this antioxidant. One pepper has 4 milligrams of beta-carotene, or 40 to 66 percent of the recommended daily amount of 6 to 10 milligrams.

Both sweet red and green peppers also contain generous amounts of vitamin C, another powerful antioxidant. A half-cup of chopped green pepper (about half a pepper) contains 45 milligrams of vitamin C, or 74 percent of the Daily Value (DV). Sweet red peppers are even better, with the same-size serving providing 142 milli-

In the Kitchen

Some like it hot—and some don't. If you prefer peppers that are sweet to those that make you sweat, here are a few varieties you may want to try:

- **Bell peppers**, which are now available in almost every color of the rainbow, can be eaten raw, grilled, baked, or stir-fried.
- **Frying peppers** have a mild, sweet taste, and their thin walls make them perfect for sautéing and using as a topping for toasted Italian bread.
- **Hungarian yellow wax (banana) peppers**, which resemble the fruit both in color and shape, have a mild, sweet taste, and are often used in salads and sandwiches.
- **Paprika peppers**, which are dried to make the spice, can also be fried, stuffed, or eaten raw.
- **Pimientos** are squat, heart-shaped peppers that aficionados claim are the best-tasting peppers you can buy. While they're often used commercially for stuffing olives, you can buy them fresh in some specialty produce markets from late summer to fall.

grams of vitamin C, or 236 percent of the DV. That's more than twice the amount that you'd get from a medium-size orange.

The combination of vitamin C and beta-carotene can provide potent protection. These two compounds work together in your body to disarm free radicals. In a study of more than 900 people, Italian researchers found that those who ate sweet peppers and other foods rich in beta-carotene regularly were significantly less likely to have cataracts than those who did not.

Some limited studies appear to indicate that eating a diet high in antioxidants may also reduce the risk of developing age-related macular degeneration, a leading cause of blindness in the United States. More research is needed, but it's not too soon to eat more fruits and vegetables high in the eye-protecting antioxidants lutein and zeaxanthin, including red, green, and yellow/orange bell peppers.

Another antioxidant found in abundance in red peppers is beta-cryptoxanthin, an orange-red carotenoid that can significantly cut risk for lung cancer.

GETTING THE MOST

Cook them lightly. Since vitamin C is fragile, it's readily destroyed during cooking. Eating peppers raw will provide the most of this nutrient. Beta-carotene, on the other hand, needs a little heat to release it from the pepper's fiber cells. To get the most of both nutrients, it's a good idea to steam, sauté, or microwave peppers until they're softened but still have a little crunch.

Add some fat. In order for beta-carotene to be absorbed into the bloodstream, it needs to be accompanied by a little fat. Drizzling peppers with a touch of olive oil, before or after cooking, will help you get the most of this important compound. If you're eating raw peppers, dunking them in a bit of dip will also help the beta-carotene be absorbed.

Mix 'em up. Even though peppers are one of the healthiest vegetables going, few people eat enough of them to get the full benefit. The easiest way to get more peppers in your diet is to use them as an ingredient in various recipes. You can use peppers to add a sweet punch to pasta dishes and meat loaf, for example.

Layer in a salad or a main dish. Eating a broad range of fruits and vegetables and whole grains packed with a wide variety of cancer-fighting antioxidants is a smart health strategy promoted by the American Institute for Cancer Research. Creating layered salads and entrées that include peppers is a smart way to put this plan on your plate. For example, create triple-tiered salads with a bed of mixed greens, topped with your favorite beans, topped with thinly sliced red bell peppers. Make a casserole that includes a layer of sautéed mixed peppers with onions.

Raise a glassful. Another way to get more peppers in your diet is to make them into juice. The juice from two green bell peppers contains 132 milligrams of vitamin C, three times the amount you'd get from the usual half-cup serving of chopped green pepper. Although pepper juice isn't very appetizing on its own, it adds a sweet zip to other juices, such as carrot juice. Try mixing four or five carrots with two green bell peppers in a juicer for a supercharged antioxidant cocktail.

Doctor's Top Tip

Roasting red bell peppers gives them a rich, full, extra-sweet, and slightly smoky flavor. Mayo Clinic dietitians suggest creating this culinary treat at home by placing washed, seeded bell peppers on a baking sheet lined with aluminum foil. Broil in the oven, turning frequently with tongs, until the skin blackens all over, about 10 minutes. Transfer the peppers to a bowl, cover, and let steam until the skin loosens, about 10 minutes. Peel and refrigerate, covered, until needed.

Sautéed Bell Peppers

1 green bell pepper

1 red bell pepper

1 yellow bell pepper

2 teaspoons olive oil

1 tablespoon balsamic vinegar

⅛ teaspoon salt

Freshly ground black pepper

Cut the green, red, and yellow peppers in half lengthwise. Remove and discard the ribs and seeds. Cut the peppers lengthwise into ¼-inch-wide strips.

In a large skillet, heat the oil over medium-high heat. Add the peppers, and cook until they just begin to soften, 2 to 3 minutes. Remove from the heat, and sprinkle with the vinegar and salt. Season to taste with pepper. Toss and serve warm.

Makes 4 servings

PER SERVING ─────────────────────────

Calories: 44

Total fat: 2.4 g

Saturated fat: 0.3 g

Cholesterol: 0 mg

Sodium: 77 mg

Dietary fiber: 1.5 g

Sweet Potatoes

PACKED WITH ANTIOXIDANTS

HEALING POWER

Can Help:

Preserve memory

Control diabetes

Reduce the risk of heart disease and cancer

Have you ever wondered how Scarlett O'Hara maintained her 19-inch waist? One secret may have been sweet potatoes. Before Scarlett went to a barbecue, her nanny dished up sweet potatoes to keep her from filling up on fattening party fare. We can almost hear Scarlett's gentle protest—"Why, I can't eat a thing!"—as she pushed away temptation, filled up as she was by those sweetly nutritious, oddly shaped little tubers.

Sweet potatoes are more than just a filling food, of course. A member of the morning glory family (except in name, they're not related to white potatoes), they contain a trio of powerful antioxidants: beta-carotene and vitamins C and E. This means that they can play a role in preventing cancer and heart disease. And because sweet potatoes are rich in complex carbohydrates and low in calories—there are 117 calories in a 4-ounce serving—experts recommend them for controlling weight and weight-related conditions like diabetes.

A Package of Protection

Experts often recommend sweet potatoes for their high amounts of beta-carotene. A 4-ounce serving will provide more than 14 milligrams of beta-carotene. They are an easy way to get the heart-health and cancer-fighting benefits into your diet, says Pamela Savage-Marr, RD, a health education specialist at Oakwood Health Care System in Dearborn, Michigan.

As do vitamins C and E and other antioxidants, beta-carotene helps protect the body from harmful oxygen molecules known as free radicals, says Dexter L. Morris, MD, PhD, associate professor in the department of emergency medicine at the University of North Carolina School of Medicine at Chapel Hill. Eating sweet potatoes and other foods that are rich in beta-carotene helps neutralize these molecules before they damage various parts of the body, such as the blood vessels or certain parts of the eye.

In a study of almost 1,900 men, Dr. Morris and his colleagues found that men who had the most carotenoids in their blood—not just beta-carotene but also such phytonutrients as lutein and zeaxanthin—had 72 percent fewer heart attacks than

In the Kitchen

Is that thing really a sweet potato? Sweet potatoes come in all shapes and sizes, so don't be surprised if the veggie touted by that name at your supermarket looks a little different from month to month. Sweet potatoes can have skin that's white, yellow, orange, red, or even purple. Inside, the flesh may be yellow or deep orange. But don't call it a yam—true yams are grown in South America, the Caribbean, and Africa. They have brown or black outer skin and flesh that's off-white, purple, or red and tastes sweeter than that of a sweet potato. Most "yams" sold in US supermarkets are really sweet potatoes.

Because they are cured (meaning that they are kept in high humidity and temperatures for about a week and a half) by growers before they are shipped to market, sweet potatoes are excellent keepers and will stay fresh for about a month after you bring them home from the store. It's important, however, to store them carefully to prevent them from going bad.

Keep them cool. Sweet potatoes should be stored in cellars, pantries, or basements, where temperatures stay around 45° to 55°F.

(Don't put them in the refrigerator, since this shortens their shelf life.) When sweet potatoes are stored at room temperature, they'll keep for about a week.

Store them dry. Sweet potatoes will spoil once they get wet. That's why it's best to store them dry, then wash them only when you're ready to start cooking.

Treat them gently. Sweet potatoes spoil quickly when they get cut or bruised, so don't buy them if they look damaged. At home, treating them gently will help ensure their longevity.

Bake a big batch. Baked sweet potatoes will keep in the refrigerator for 7 to 10 days. To bake, scrub the potatoes, dry them, and pierce the skins in several places. Place them on a baking sheet covered with aluminum foil (to catch dripping juices) and bake at 350°F for about 1 hour. Any leftovers can be reheated in a microwave oven or mashed with trans-fat-free margarine (buy a brand that's low in saturated fat, too) and a dab of brown sugar for a quick side dish later in the week.

---

those with the lowest levels. Even smokers, who need all the protection they can get, showed the benefits: Those who got the most of these protective compounds had 25 percent fewer heart attacks than those who got the least.

Sweet potatoes are also a rich source of vitamin C, with a 4-ounce serving providing 28 milligrams, or nearly half the Daily Value (DV). In addition, the same-size serving provides 6 IU of vitamin E, or 20 percent of the DV. "That's a very difficult nutrient to get from natural sources," says Paul Lachance, PhD, executive director of the Nutraceuticals Institute at Rutgers University in New Brunswick, New Jersey.

Controlling Blood Sugar

Since sweet potatoes are a good source of fiber, they're a very healthful food for people with diabetes. The fiber indirectly helps lower blood sugar levels by slowing the rate at which food is converted into glucose and absorbed into the bloodstream. And because sweet potatoes are high in complex carbohydrates, they can help people control their weight, which also helps keep diabetes under control.

The connection between weight and blood sugar levels is not a casual one. About 85 percent of people with type 2 (non-insulin-dependent) diabetes are overweight. Since sweet potatoes are so satisfying, you're less likely to reach for other, fattier foods.

The resulting weight loss can cause a dramatic improvement. In fact, losing even 5 to 10 pounds will help some people maintain normal blood sugar levels, says internist Stanley Mirsky, MD, associate clinical professor of metabolic diseases at Mount Sinai School of Medicine in New York City and author of *Controlling Diabetes the Easy Way*.

> ### Doctor's Top Tip
>
> Choose sweet potatoes over white potatoes. Harvard School of Public Health nutritionists say it's always smart to choose a more colorful vegetable over a less colorful one. That alone would make sweet a better choice than white when it comes to potatoes. The sweet potato's orange flesh is a richer source of beta-carotene and vitamins. But there's a new reason: Sweet potatoes are better for your blood sugar. Despite their name, and a flavor so divine it makes a good dessert, sweet potatoes don't raise your blood sugar as high, or as fast, as white potatoes do.

Good for the Mind

In addition to fiber and antioxidant vitamins, sweet potatoes also contain the B vitamins folate and B_6. These are the vitamins that may give the brain a boost in performing some of its functions, which can diminish as we age.

In a study at the Jean Mayer USDA Human Nutrition Research Center on Aging at Tufts University in Boston, researchers looked at the levels of folate and vitamins B_6 and B_{12} in the blood of 70 men ages 54 to 81. Men with low levels of folate and B_{12} had higher levels of an amino acid called homocysteine. High levels of homocysteine were linked to poorer performances on spatial tests such as copying a cube or a circle or identifying patterns.

GETTING THE MOST

Shop for color. When buying sweet potatoes, always choose those with the most intense, lush orange color. The richer the color, the greater the jolt of beta-carotene, says Mark Kestin, PhD, professor of nutrition at Bastyr University and affiliate assistant professor of epidemiology at the University of Washington, both in Seattle.

Have a little fat. While some vitamins dissolve in water, beta-carotene requires the presence of fat to get through the intestinal wall, says John Erdman, PhD, a beta-carotene expert and professor of food science and human nutrition at the University of Illinois in Urbana-Champaign. In most cases, you'll get the necessary amount of fat, usually 5 to 7 grams, in other foods you'll be having with your meal, he explains.

Sesame Sweet Potatoes

2 **pounds sweet potatoes**

2 **teaspoons sesame seeds**

1 **bunch scallions, chopped**

1 **tablespoon olive oil**

2 **cloves garlic, minced**

1 **tablespoon reduced-sodium soy sauce**

1 **tablespoon packed light brown sugar**

1 **teaspoon dark sesame oil**

Scrub the sweet potatoes and pat dry with paper towels. With a fork, pierce each potato in 3 or 4 places. Place the potatoes, in spoke fashion and with the thinner ends pointing toward the center, on a paper towel in a microwave oven. Microwave on high power for 5 minutes. Turn the potatoes.

Microwave for 5 to 8 minutes more, or until the potatoes can easily be pierced with the tip of a sharp knife but are still firm. Set aside until cool enough to handle. Peel, then cut into thick slices.

Place the sesame seeds in a large nonstick skillet. Stir over medium heat for 30 seconds, or until golden. Stir in the scallions, olive oil, and garlic. Cook for 30 seconds longer, or until fragrant. Add the soy sauce, brown sugar, and sesame oil. Cook until the sugar melts, about 10 seconds. Add the sweet potatoes to the pan, and toss to coat. Cook for 1 minute to heat through.

Makes 6 servings

PER SERVING

Calories: 208	Cholesterol: 0 mg
Total fat: 5.6 g	Sodium: 275 mg
Saturated fat: 0.8 g	Dietary fiber: 4.7 g

Tangerines
PEEL A LITTLE PROTECTION

HEALING POWER
Can Help:
Prevent heart disease
Reduce the risk of cancer

At one time or another you've probably used canned mandarin oranges—tiny, doll-like sections of orange fruit that look precious and perfect. You can imagine them coming all the way from China, where most citrus fruits actually got their start.

Mandarin oranges are really small tangerines, or to be more precise, tangerines are really mandarin oranges, since tangerine isn't a formal botanical term. So mandarin oranges—we'll still call them tangerines—are actually no more exotic than a lunchbox fruit.

But their benefits are anything but commonplace. Tangerines contain an abundance of impressive healing compounds. Like oranges, they are rich in vitamin C. One tangerine has 26 milligrams, or 43 percent of the Daily Value (DV). Tangerines also contain a compound called beta-cryptoxanthin, which turns into vitamin A in the body. Eight ounces of tangerine juice can provide up to 1,037 IU of vitamin A, or more than 20 percent of the DV.

This combination of nutrients has antioxidant powers—that is, it can help stop harmful oxygen molecules called free radicals from causing cell damage in the body, which can lead to everything from wrinkles and heart disease to cancer, says Bill Widmer, PhD, a research scientist with the Florida Department of Citrus Research Center in Lake Alfred.

Protection against Cancer

What makes tangerines really exciting to researchers are two compounds, tangeretin and nobiletin, which appear to be extremely potent against certain types of breast cancer.

In Japan, researchers at the Tokyo College of Pharmacy found that tangeretin could inhibit the growth of leukemia cells, essentially by causing them to program their own deaths. Better yet, the compound wasn't toxic to healthy cells, which is an important goal for any cancer treatment.

Doctor's Top Tip

Put two tangerines in your briefcase, purse, or backpack. And keep a dozen more in a bowl on the counter. Keeping fruit within easy reach ups the odds that you'll eat more of it every day, according to the Mayo Clinic.

In the Kitchen

We often think of tangerines as being little more than small oranges, but they have a world of tastes and textures all their own. Here are some varieties that you may want to give a try:

- **Fairchilds** are the first tangerines of the season, available from mid-October through December. They're wonderfully easy to peel.
- **Dancy tangerines** have a sweet flavor and a discomfiting number of seeds. They, too, are easy to peel.
- **Honey tangerines** are sweet enough to make you forget butterscotch. They're very juicy and can have an abundance of seeds.
- **Mandarins** have a light orange color and a deliciously complex, sweet flavor. The Satsuma and the Royal are the two varieties.
- **Tangelos** are a cross between a tangerine and a grapefruit. They often have a knob at one end like a little topknot. As you would expect, given their parentage, they're both tart and sweet, and very juicy. Orlandos and Minneolas are popular Tangelo types.

GETTING THE MOST

Save the peel. While the flesh of tangerines contains a goodly share of healing compounds, most of the tangeretin and nobiletin are concentrated in the peel. To add more of these nutrients to your diet, use a microplane zester to finely grate the colored part of the peel (the zest), then stir the zest into a glass of juice, mix it into rice and pasta dishes, or sprinkle it on salads. You'll get extra-zingy flavor along with the extra nutritional benefits.

Try something new. Tiny tangerines—no bigger than a grape—are just beginning to arrive in Western supermarkets, though they've long been an upper-class delicacy in China.

Buy a box of a tangerine relative, the clementine. Not quite a tangerine, the sweet juicy clementine is a cross between a sweet orange and a Chinese mandarin. Grown in Spain, Morocco, and other parts of North Africa, clementines seem like a splurge—they almost always come in small, decorative crates and cost anywhere from $5 to $8 per box. Why they're worth it: Easy to peel, seedless, and a pleasure to eat, the clementine is an easy way to boost your daily fruit intake. Kids love 'em, too.

Drink up. Although tangerines are in season only from October to May, you may want to enjoy tangerine juice during the off-season. When you go to the supermarket, look for ready-made juices or frozen concentrates that have had tangerine juice added to them.

Glazed Tangerines with Almonds

4 **large tangerines**

2 **tablespoons chopped almonds**

1 **tablespoon packed light brown sugar**

1 **teaspoon grated fresh ginger**

Preheat the broiler. Coat a broiler pan with cooking spray.

Grate the zest from 2 of the tangerines, and place it in a small bowl. Add the almonds, brown sugar, and ginger. Stir to mix.

Peel the tangerines, and discard the peel. Separate the fruit into sections. Arrange close together on the broiler pan, and sprinkle evenly with the almond mixture.

Broil 6 inches from the heat until the topping bubbles and is lightly browned, about 1 to 2 minutes. Serve warm.

Makes 4 servings

PER SERVING

Calories: 70
Total fat: 2.3 g
Saturated fat: 0.2 g

Cholesterol: 0 mg
Sodium: 2 mg
Dietary fiber: 1.7 g

Tea

A CUP OF GOOD HEALTH

HEALING POWER

Can Help:

Control cholesterol

Prevent stroke and heart disease

Reduce tooth decay

Prevent intestinal cancer

What would you think if a man in a string tie and a long, black coat came up to you and said, "Psss-ss-st. Wanna buy a drink that stops cancer of the skin, lung, stomach, colon, liver, breast, esophagus, and pancreas? And cancer of the small intestine? And heart disease and stroke? And cavities—did I say cavities?"

"Snake oil salesman": That's what you'd think.

Well, Mister Snake Oil would be more right than wrong. Laboratory studies have shown that tea has indeed stopped tumors from forming. The risk of stroke and heart disease tumbles when you drink tea. And tea does have clout against cavities.

Tea contains hundreds of compounds called polyphenols. These compounds act like antioxidants—that is, they help neutralize harmful oxygen molecules in the body known as free radicals, which have been linked to cancer, heart disease, and a number of less serious problems, such as wrinkles.

"In general, polyphenols are very, very good antioxidants. But the best polyphenols are in tea, which has a lot of them," says Joe A. Vinson, PhD, professor of analytical chemistry at the University of Scranton in Pennsylvania. "They make up nearly 30 percent of tea's dry weight."

This may help explain why tea is the most popular beverage in the world.

Arterial Protection

Blocked arteries (and the heart attacks, high blood pressure, and strokes they can lead to) don't happen all at once. They're typically preceded by years of steadily increasing damage, in which the body's dangerous low-density lipoprotein (LDL) cholesterol oxidizes and gradually makes arteries stiff and narrow.

That's where tea can help. In studies, Dr. Vinson found that the polyphenols in tea were extremely effective in preventing cholesterol from oxidizing and fouling blood vessels. In fact, one of the polyphenols in tea, epigallocatechin gallate (EGCG), was able to neutralize five times as much LDL cholesterol as vitamin C, the strongest of the antioxidant vitamins.

One reason that tea's polyphenols are so effective is that they can work in two places at once, blocking the harmful effects of oxidized LDL cholesterol both in the bloodstream and at the artery walls, "where LDL really produces atherosclerosis," says Dr. Vinson.

In a Dutch study of 800 men, researchers found that those who ate the most flavonoids, a large phytochemical family that includes tea's polyphenols, had a 58 percent lower risk of dying from heart disease than those who ate the least. When the results were further analyzed, it was revealed that the healthiest men were those getting more than half their flavonoids from black tea, with onions and apples contributing most of the rest.

You don't need to drink rivers of tea to get the benefits. In the Dutch study, the healthiest men drank about 4 cups of tea a day.

Just as tea helps protect arteries leading from the heart, it has a similar effect on those in or leading to the brain, says Dr. Vinson.

In another large study, Dutch researchers looked at the diets of 550 men ages 50 to 69. As in the heart study, the men who had the highest flavonoid levels—those who drank almost 5 cups of black tea a day or more—were 69 percent less likely to have a stroke than the men who drank less than 3 cups of black tea a day. This finding is backed up by a new Japanese study finding that people who drank at least 5 cups of green tea daily had a whopping 62 percent lower risk of dying from clot-caused strokes. Experts think that the antioxidants in green tea help keep platelets—sticky cells that clump together to form clots—sliding safely past each other. No clots, no stroke.

Help against Cancer

Every time you grill a hamburger, compounds called heterocyclic amines form on the surface of the food. In the body, these chemicals turn into more dangerous forms, which can cause cancer, says John H. Weisburger, MD, PhD, vice president for research and director of the Naylor Dana Institute for Disease Prevention at the American Health Foundation in Valhalla, New York.

Enter the tea polyphenols. Inside the body, these compounds help prevent the formation of potential carcinogens, Dr. Weisburger says. In other words, they help stop cancer before it starts.

Cancer researcher Hasan Mukhtar, PhD, of the department of dermatology at the University of Wisconsin in Madison, has seen tea stop cancer at each stage of its life cycle, arresting both its growth and spread. And where cancerous tumors have already formed, he has seen tea shrink them.

Studying the effects of green tea on sunburned skin in laboratory animals, Dr.

THE COLOR OF TEA

Green tea. Black tea. Vanilla maple tea. French vanilla tea. Raspberry tea. Black currant tea. Apricot tea. Which tea has the most healing polyphenols?

It doesn't matter. As long as it's real tea and not herbal tea, which doesn't contain leaves from *Camellia sinensis*, the tea plant, there's very little difference among them, says tea researcher Joe A. Vinson, PhD, of the University of Scranton in Pennsylvania. After all, they all contain leaves from the same plant.

They're not identical, however. The lightest leaves, green and white, are minimally processed and, in general, retain more disease-protective polyphenols and other antioxidants. But darker teas contain healthy theaflavins, which form when their polyphenols ferment and turn orange-red. Here's a brief look at the various "real" teas:

Black. The color refers to the leaves; the beverage is deep amber. Black tea varieties include Darjeeling and Earl Grey; flavors range from spicy to flowery. Black tea may lower the risk of heart disease and colon cancer; it can also inhibit bacteria that cause cavities and bad breath.

Green. If you find the flavor too "grassy," try jewel green matcha or Japanese sencha. Green tea has been shown in numerous studies to help prevent many kinds of cancer, lower cholesterol, and boost immunity.

Oolong. Midway between green and black tea in color, flavor, and antioxidant action, oolong has a fresh floral or fruity aroma. Drinking 3 cups a day may help relieve itchy skin rashes.

Pu-ehr (poo-air). This dark red tea has an earthy flavor reminiscent of coffee and tobacco. It's considered a delicacy in China (you can purchase it online), where its processing is a highly guarded secret. The most oxidized of teas, pu-ehr is said to mellow and improve with age, like wine. It may help reduce cholesterol.

White. Rare and somewhat expensive, this least-processed tea has an extremely subtle flavor. But it does contain more antioxidants than other teas. Test tube studies show that it can block DNA mutations (which trigger tumor formation). A study on rats discovered it prevented precancerous colon tumors.

Mukhtar found that the animals given tea developed one-tenth as many tumors as those given water. (Even when the tea-treated animals developed tumors, they were often benign, not cancerous.) What's more, tea was equally effective whether given as a drink or applied to the skin. Some cosmetics companies have started adding green tea to skin products for its potential protective benefits.

Good for the Teeth

Having a toothache generally isn't a big deal, unless it's *your* toothache. Tea can help prevent the pain, since it contains numerous compounds, polyphenols as well as tannin, that act as antibiotics. In other words, tea is great for mopping up the bacteria that promote tooth decay.

Tea also contains fluoride, which provides further dental protection. When researchers at Forsyth Dental Center in Boston tested a variety of foods for their antibacterial qualities, they found that tea was far and away the most protective.

Japanese researchers at Kyushu University in Fukuoka, Japan, have identified four components in tea—tannin, catechin, caffeine, and tocopherol (a vitamin E–like substance)—that help increase the acid resistance of tooth enamel. This quartet of compounds was made even more effective with the addition of extra fluoride. The extra oomph made tooth enamel 98 percent impervious to the action of acids on the teeth.

GETTING THE MOST

Steep three and see. When you brew tea, it takes 3 minutes for it to release the health-promoting compounds. That's also the amount of time researchers use in their studies on tea. Although longer steeping causes more compounds to be released, "those compounds are bitter. And a bigger dose doesn't necessarily put twice as much of them in the body," says Dr. Vinson.

Bag it. Tea aficionados always use loose tea. No easy tea bags for them. But the pulverized contents of tea bags actually release more polyphenols than the larger loose leaves. That's because the tiny particles in the bag yield more surface area for polyphenols to dissolve into hot water.

Pick your flavors. Although green tea has been more thoroughly researched than the black variety (mainly because the first studies were done in China and Japan, where green tea is the preferred brew), both kinds show equally salutary effects, says Dr. Vinson.

If you prefer decaffeinated tea, by all means drink up. The removal of caffeine has little effect on tea's polyphenol content, so little is lost in the translation, Dr. Vinson says.

The same goes for bottled teas, iced tea, and teas made from mixes, Dr. Vinson adds. In fact, some soft drink and juice companies have been so impressed with tea's benefits that they've begun fortifying their beverages with green tea. Check out your health food store for new products.

Doctor's Top Tip

If you're a sneezer, drink more green tea. In laboratory tests, Japanese researchers have found that the abundant and active antioxidant compound in green tea, epigallocatechin gallate (EGCG), blocks the biochemical process involved in producing an allergic response. "If you have allergies, consider drinking it," says Hirofumi Tachibana, PhD, associate professor of chemistry at Kyushu University in Fukuoka, Japan. Dr. Tachibana suspects that green tea may be useful against a wide range of sneeze-starting allergens, including pollen, pet dander, and dust. Go for two to three mugs a day.

Hold the milk—at least for now. One preliminary study in Italy found that adding milk to tea, as the British do at tea time, blocked tea's antioxidant benefits. "There is some evidence that milk protein binds to some of the tea compounds and blocks their absorption. But those compounds could get unbound in the stomach. So we're not so sure milk is bad," says Dr. Vinson.

Keep it fresh. If you make your own iced tea, drink it within a few days, suggests Dr. Vinson. "And make sure you cover it to keep it fresh when you refrigerate it," he advises. "My experience tells me not to keep iced tea for more than a week because the concentration of compounds falls off. You get to the point where about 10 percent has been lost or changed."

Have tea with meat. Since tea's polyphenol compounds help to block the formation of cancer-causing chemicals, it's a good idea to enjoy a tea party after eating fried or charred meat.

Drink it iced, too. Many bottled and powdered iced teas retain spectacular antioxidant levels. In one *Prevention* magazine analysis of antioxidants in various commercial iced teas, even the lowest-scoring convenience iced teas contained at least as many antioxidants as fruits and vegetables, such as strawberries and spinach! But highest honors went to home-made iced tea—cold-brewed refrigerator tea and classic hot-brewed tea that was then chilled came in almost dead even with each other for antioxidant levels. (One tip: Shake cold-brewed tea before removing tea bags, it seems to knock more antioxidants into the liquid.)

Tea-Poached Figs

20 dried Calimyrna figs

¾ cup water

½ cup apple cider

1 strip orange zest (1 × ½ inch)

1 cinnamon stick (2 inches long)

4 orange pekoe tea bags

Cut off and discard the stems of the figs. Pierce each fig in 1 or 2 places with the tip of a sharp knife.

In a medium saucepan, combine the water, cider, orange zest, and cinnamon stick. Bring to a boil over medium heat. Remove from the heat, and add the tea bags. Let stand, stirring occasionally, until the mixture looks like brewed tea, about 5 minutes. Press the tea bags with a spoon to extract the liquid. Discard the tea bags.

Add the figs to the tea. Cook over medium heat until the liquid comes to a simmer, 1 to 2 minutes. Reduce the heat to low, and cook, stirring occasionally, until the figs are plump and moist, about 5 minutes.

Transfer the figs and liquid to a heatproof bowl. Discard the orange zest and cinnamon stick. Let cool. Serve the figs with the liquid.

Makes 4 servings

PER SERVING

Calories: 253	Cholesterol: 0 mg
Total fat: 1.1 g	Sodium: 13 mg
Saturated fat: 0.2 g	Dietary fiber: 8.7 g

Thyroid Disease
FOODS FOR HORMONAL HEALTH

Goiter. Bulging eyes. Overweight. Say "thyroid," and one of these words probably pops into your brain. Yet few of us know what this gland actually does until something goes wrong with it.

The thyroid is a butterfly-shaped gland that wraps around the windpipe and sits just below the Adam's apple. It produces hormones that help control the body's metabolism—how you burn calories and use energy. This means that the thyroid gland has a direct effect on your weight, energy levels, and your ability to absorb nutrients from food. When the thyroid produces the right amount of hormones, all is well. But when it produces either too much hormone or too little, it can interfere with all these bodily processes.

Thyroid disease is almost always treated with medications that regulate the amount of hormones the gland produces. But it can take several months for the medication to start working. During this time, your body may not be able to adequately metabolize certain nutrients, such as iodine, calcium, fat, and protein. So your doctor may recommend adjusting your diet in the meantime. Once the medication has corrected the problem, however, you can follow a normal, healthy diet.

A Delicate Balance

As we've seen, the thyroid's main job is to regulate metabolism. When there's enough thyroid hormone in your blood, the thyroid "shuts off," just as an air conditioner turns off when a room reaches the right temperature. When your body needs more thyroid hormone, the gland kicks in again.

In people with thyroid disease, this internal switch doesn't work properly. If you have a condition called hypothyroidism, the gland doesn't produce enough thyroid hormone. The body stages a slowdown. You may feel cold or tired, your hair and skin may become dry, and you may gain weight. For reasons that aren't clear, women are 10 times more likely than men to develop this condition.

By contrast, people with a condition called *hyper*thyroidism produce too much thyroid hormone, causing the body to speed up. Common symptoms include weight loss, a pounding heart, and skin that's hot and sweaty. Again, women are far more likely than men to develop this condition.

Obviously, the different types of thyroid disease require different nutritional strategies while the medication is taking effect.

The Iodine Tightrope

The thyroid gland depends on iodine, which is found in food, to manufacture thyroid hormone. It doesn't take much. The iodine in your body makes up less than 0.00001 percent of your body weight. But your thyroid can't do its job without even this tiny amount of this trace mineral.

So hungry is the thyroid gland for iodine that when it doesn't get enough, it gradually grows larger as it tries to suck up as much iodine as it can. Eventually, it gets large enough to be seen from the outside. This swelling is called a goiter.

In developing countries, where iodine in the diet is in short supply, goiters are common. But in the United States, where there's plenty of iodine in food—not only in iodized salt but also in bread and milk—this type of goiter is rare.

But iodine still causes problems in this country. In fact, the average American consumes too much. This isn't a problem when the thyroid is working normally. But for those with thyroid disease, it can cause the gland to churn out too little (or not enough) of its essential hormones.

When you've recently started taking thyroid medication, your doctor may recommend that you avoid iodine-rich foods, like shellfish and spinach. Once the medication has fully taken effect, however, you can resume your normal diet.

Another food that you may want to avoid is kelp. While some alternative practitioners suggest eating kelp to treat thyroid problems, mainstream physicians generally advise against it. Kelp (a kind of seaweed) has large amounts of iodine, which could make things worse.

Stay Regular with Fiber

For people with an underactive thyroid, the entire body—including the digestion—slows down. This, in turn, can result in constipation, a common symptom in those with this condition.

To help keep digestion regular, it's wise to eat plenty of fiber-rich foods. The fiber in fruits, vegetables, and whole grains helps keep food moving through the system. But some experts advise people with underactive thyroids to avoid certain vegetables before treatment and early in their treatment, because they may depress thyroid function. According to University of Maryland experts, these include broccoli, cabbage, Brussels sprouts, cauliflower, kale, spinach, turnips, beans, and mustard greens.

Thyroid experts recommend 20 to 35 grams of fiber a day. You don't have to

Doctor's Top Tip

Be sure to take hypothyroid drugs on an empty stomach. Some foods and supplements can interfere with your body's ability to absorb synthetic thyroid hormone. These include iron supplements, calcium supplements, soybean flour, as well as some antacids, ulcer drugs, and cholesterol-lowering medicines, say Mayo Clinic thyroid experts. Your best strategy for avoiding interactions: Take thyroid meds several hours before or after having any of these.

make a science out of it. Eating three to five servings of vegetables (preferably raw), two to four servings of fresh fruits, and six to 11 servings of whole-grain bread, cereal, grains, or legumes every day should provide an adequate amount of fiber.

Bone Up with Calcium

We've been talking about people with underactive thyroids. Those with overactive glands have different concerns. One of the most significant is the risk of developing bone-thinning osteoporosis, says Deah Baird, ND, a naturopathic doctor in private practice in Portland, Oregon.

When the thyroid gland is overactive, calcium is removed from the blood and excreted in the urine, explains Dr. Baird. This is serious because the body compensates by removing calcium from the bones to make up the difference.

To prevent bone problems, it's important to eat a diet high in calcium, says Dr. Baird. Low-fat and fat-free dairy foods, including milk, cheese, and yogurt, are all good sources, as are dark green leafy vegetables, such as collard greens and spinach. Having 1 cup fat-free yogurt and 1 cup cooked greens, accompanied by a glass of fat-free milk, will provide you with the Daily Value (DV) of 1,000 milligrams of calcium. Since people with an overactive thyroid frequently lose weight, it's important to eat a well-balanced diet with enough calories to maintain a healthy weight. For those who are allergic to dairy, it's a good idea to take a calcium supplement or add nondairy sources of calcium to the diet, she adds.

Bone loss can also be a concern for people who take synthetic thyroid hormone for hypothyroidism. Even just a little excess hormone can lead to bone loss if it's not caught for several years. So be sure to get the regular checkups and tests your doctor recommends to ensure your dose is exactly right.

Untreated hypothyroidism can lead to a condition called carotenemia, in which beta-carotene from the fruits and vegetables you eat isn't metabolized into vitamin A and instead builds up, discoloring the skin (especially the palms and soles). According to the Thyroid Foundation, this doesn't really pose a health risk. Once hypothyroidism is corrected with thyroid hormone, carotenemia stops.

Feeding a Faulty Thyroid

If it weren't so dangerous, having an overactive thyroid gland might be considered the world's greatest weight-loss aid. Most people with overactive thyroids need to eat 15 to 20 percent more calories than a person with a healthy gland, at least until the medication takes effect. Those with serious problems may need to eat twice as much as they once did—sometimes more than 3,000 calories a day—just to maintain the energy and weight they had before.

Some thyroid doctors advise patients just beginning treatment for hyperthyroidism to eat foods high in fat and protein to prevent their overactive metabolisms from burning away needed fat and muscle. Meat, fish, poultry, whole milk, cheese, butter, nuts, and seeds are good sources of both fat and protein.

Of course, this no-holds-barred eating strategy is only for the short term. Once the medication becomes fully active and the thyroid hormone levels are back to normal, you'll need to eat fewer calories, or you'll gain weight. Sometimes, though, this can be tough. Appetite may be one of the last things to settle back to normal levels after treatment begins. So you may keep on eating extra calories but not burn them off . . . and gain unwanted pounds. Talk with your doctor about your calorie needs and how to stick with a sensible eating plan. One idea: Gradually cut back on fat and refined carbohydrates as your thyroid function normalizes, keep on eating fruits, vegetables, and moderate portions of whole grains so you feel full and satisfied after meals.

By contrast, people with an underactive gland may need only half the calories of other adults. They'll also want to limit their consumption of fatty foods. People with underactive thyroids tend to have higher levels of cholesterol and triglycerides, which can increase their risk of cardiovascular disease. Eat plenty of complex carbohydrates, such as whole-grain breads, cereals, fruits, and vegetables as well as fat-free milk and low-fat or fat-free cheese and yogurt.

Again, this special diet is only for the short term. With the proper medication, thyroid levels will return to normal, and you'll be able to eat as many calories as you did before your thyroid malfunctioned.

The Benefits of Produce

We saw earlier how the fiber in fruits and vegetables can help relieve symptoms caused by an underactive thyroid gland. As it turns out, there are additional substances in vegetables, particularly cabbage, that may aid an overactive gland as well. Research suggests that these compounds may help the gland slow down naturally, says Dr. Baird.

Members of the brassica family of vegetables, including broccoli, cabbage, Brussels sprouts, cauliflower, kale, mustard greens, and turnips, as well as soybeans, peanuts, millet, and spinach, contain goitrogens—chemicals that block the thyroid's ability to use iodine. With less iodine, the gland naturally produces less thyroid hormone, Dr. Baird explains.

Since cooking may deactivate the goitrogens in vegetables, it's a good idea, when you're eating for thyroid disease, to have your vegetables raw. An alternative to eating raw vegetables is to drink them, since juices contain large amounts of the healing compounds. It's not clear how much you'd need to drink to have a positive effect on the thyroid. A good starting place would be to have an 8-ounce glass of vegetable juice every day.

Vegetable juices are very easy to make. Wash the vegetables well, cut them into pieces to fit the opening in the juicer, and drop them in. You can make a single-ingredient juice, or mix and match vegetables to create your own flavors. Many people include carrots and celery in their juices because these are considered "universal mixers."

Tomatoes

PROTECTION FOR THE PROSTATE

HEALING POWER

Can Help:

Reduce the risk of cancer and heart disease

Prevent cataracts

Keep older people active

If it weren't for Colonel Robert Gibbon Johnson, America might never have tasted the tomato.

For centuries, tomatoes, which are members of the deadly nightshade family, were thought to be toxic, capable of causing appendicitis, cancer, and "brain fever." But Colonel Johnson, an admittedly eccentric gentleman, thought otherwise. After a trip overseas in the early 1800s, he returned to Salem, New Jersey, with tomatoes and a plan to liberate this lush, red fruit from its fearsome reputation.

Never one to miss a dramatic opportunity, Johnson announced to the townsfolk that on September 26, 1820, he would eat not just one but an entire basket of tomatoes. Public excitement was high, and some 2,000 spectators arrived to watch Johnson commit what they were certain would be suicide.

He lived, of course, and tomatoes went on to become our favorite fruit. Better yet, tomatoes contain compounds that may help prevent a number of serious conditions, from heart disease and cancer to cataracts.

Cellular Protection

Tomatoes contain a red pigment called lycopene. This compound appears to act as an antioxidant—that is, it helps neutralize cell-damaging oxygen molecules called free radicals before they cause damage. Almost no one reaps more benefits from tomatoes than Italians, who eat them in one form or another virtually every day. While cooked tomatoes with a touch of oil have the highest levels of lycopene, even raw tomatoes offer powerful protection. Researchers in Italy found that people who ate seven or more servings of fresh, uncooked tomatoes a week had a 60 percent lower chance of developing stomach, colon, or rectal cancers than folks who ate two servings or less.

In one large US study of nearly 48,000 men, Harvard researchers found that men who ate at least 10 servings a week of tomatoes, whether raw, cooked, or in sauce, were able to cut their risk of developing prostate cancer by 45 percent. Ten servings sounds like a lot, but when they're spread out over an entire week, it's probably not

FOOD ALERT

Trouble on the Vine

As nutritious as tomatoes are, for some people they're simply too hard to handle.

They're a common cause of allergies, causing symptoms such as hives, asthma, and headaches, says Richard Podell, MD, clinical professor in the department of family medicine at Robert Wood Johnson Medical School in New Providence, New Jersey. For some people, the problem with tomatoes is simply their acidity; eating them may make their stomachs upset or cause mouth irritation.

It's particularly important to avoid tomatoes if you're allergic to aspirin—at least until you get your doctor's okay. This is because tomatoes contain chemicals called salicylates, which are the active ingredients in aspirin. While most aspirin-sensitive people do not react to the salicylates in foods, you could be the exception, and allergic reactions can be quite serious, or even fatal, says Dr. Podell.

much more than you're getting now. A single serving, after all, is only a half-cup of tomato sauce, which is about the amount of sauce on a slice of pizza.

"Lycopene is a very strong antioxidant," says Meir Stampfer, MD, coauthor of the study and professor of epidemiology and nutrition at the Harvard School of Public Health. "For some reason, lycopene concentrates in the prostate. Men with high levels of lycopene in their blood are at lower risk for prostate cancer."

Lycopene may help cut risk by inhibiting the growth and replication of cancer cells. New lab research from the University of Illinois at Urbana-Champaign suggests lycopene may also shift the balance of male hormones that can fuel prostate cancer. It may also stop cancer before it starts by protecting genes from damage caused by free radicals. But recent studies don't agree on how protective lycopene really is. One landmark National Cancer Institute study that tracked the health and diets of 29,361 men for 4 years found only a 17 percent reduction in prostate cancer risk for those who ate pizza once a week compared with those who ate pizza less than twice a month. Of note: Among the men with a family history of prostate cancer, risk dropped if they ate more tomato products that come with a smidge of fat, such as spaghetti sauce or foods containing tomato sauce such as lasagna or pizza.

Reality check: Lycopene, tomatoes, and sauce aren't magic bullets. Recently, the FDA allowed food manufacturers to print only watered-down health claims on tomato products—claims so mild that experts expect they may never show up on the label of your favorite brand of spaghetti sauce. According to a 2-year-long government analysis, there's only limited evidence that eating a half-cup to a full cup of tomatoes or sauce a week cuts prostate risk. The FDA also concluded that it's highly unlikely or uncertain that tomatoes and sauce could prevent gastric, ovarian, or pancreatic cancer.

The bottom line? No single nutrient or food is so powerful that it can single-handedly stop big health threats. But don't give up on salads and order another cheeseburger. A new line of research suggests there's actually strength in numbers: Serious health benefits come when you eat a rainbow-hued diet rich in a variety of fruits, vegetables, and whole grains. In an intriguing new lab study from the Netherlands, lycopene plus vitamin E—a combination you'd get from tomato sauce and whole-wheat pasta—inhibited the growth of prostate cancer cells.

Research also suggests that getting more lycopene in the diet may help older people stay active longer. In a study of 88 nuns ages 77 to 98, researchers found that those who got the most lycopene were the ones least likely to need help with daily activities such as getting dressed and walking.

In the Kitchen

Come February, the juiciest, vine-ripe tomatoes are but a wistful summer memory. Cheer up. Even when fresh tomatoes are out of season, sun-dried tomatoes are a great way to get the delicious taste all year and are a nice change of pace from the Roma, grape, and cherry tomatoes you can find just about year-round in the supermarket.

Unfortunately, sun-dried tomatoes can be expensive. To enjoy their rich taste without paying an exorbitant price at the supermarket, you may want to take advantage of the abundance of vine-ripened tomatoes available in summer, at a low price, and dry some yourself. Here's how:

1. Choose ripe, unbruised tomatoes. Wash thoroughly and cut off the stems and butt ends.

2. Place each tomato on its side, and cut into ¼-inch slices.

3. Put the slices on a baking sheet, and place in a 120° to 140°F oven for about 24 hours. The tomatoes are done when they're leathery, yet still pliable.

4. Pack the dried tomatoes into small jars, plastic freezer bags, or plastic containers, and refrigerate or freeze until you're ready to use them. If you're using glass jars, make sure they're at room temperature before putting them in the freezer to prevent them from breaking.

Be sure to discard any tomatoes that develop black, yellow, or white spots, which could be mold that sometimes develops during the drying process.

Doctor's Top Tip

Order your pizza with "double the sauce, please." When epidemiologist Mahyar Etminan, PharmD, of Royal Victoria Hospital in Montreal, analyzed 22 major studies of tomatoes, lycopene, and prostate cancer risk, he concluded that cooked tomatoes—as sauce, soup, stewed tomatoes, or in a sauté for example—were more protective than raw. The lycopene in tomatoes is located in the cell walls. Cooking tomatoes in a little bit of oil causes the cell walls to burst, releasing more of the healing lycopene.

New Discoveries

In the not-too-distant future, doctors may be recommending tomatoes as a way of preventing lung cancer. Tomatoes contain two powerful compounds, coumaric acid and chlorogenic acid, that may help block the effects of nitrosamines, which are cancer-causing compounds that form naturally in the body and "are the most potent carcinogen in tobacco smoke," says Joseph Hotchkiss, PhD, professor of food chemistry and toxicology at Cornell University in Ithaca, New York.

Until recently, scientists believed that it was the vitamin C in fruits and vegetables that helped neutralize these dangerous compounds. But a study conducted by Dr. Hotchkiss and his colleagues revealed that tomatoes blocked the formation of nitrosamines even after the vitamin C was removed from the fruit.

The protective coumaric and chlorogenic acids found in tomatoes are also found in other fruits and vegetables, like carrots, green peppers, pineapples, and strawberries. Dr. Hotchkiss speculates that these compounds may be one of the reasons that people who eat more fruits and vegetables have a lower risk of developing cancer.

Additional Protection

Lemons and limes are not the only fruits that are high in vitamin C. Tomatoes also contain loads of this powerful vitamin, which has been shown to help relieve conditions ranging from cataracts and cancer to heart disease. One medium-size tomato provides almost 24 milligrams, or 40 percent of the Daily Value (DV) for this vitamin.

Tomatoes are also a good source of vitamin A, which has been shown to boost immunity and help prevent cancer. One medium tomato provides 766 IU of vitamin A, or 15 percent of the DV.

In addition, a tomato provides 273 milligrams of potassium, or 8 percent of the DV for this mineral. Each tomato also contains about 1 gram of iron, or 7 percent of the Recommended Dietary Allowance (RDA) for women and 10 percent of the RDA for men. While the amount of iron is relatively small, your body is able to absorb it very efficiently when it's taken with the abundant vitamin C that's also in the tomatoes.

GETTING THE MOST

Shop for color. When buying fresh tomatoes, look for a brilliant shade of red. Ripe red tomatoes can have four times more beta-carotene than green, immature ones.

Shop for convenience. You don't have to buy fresh tomatoes—or those pale impostors that hit the supermarket come February—to get the healing benefits. Lycopene can withstand the high heats used in processing, so canned tomatoes and tomato sauce both contain their full complement of this helpful compound.

Get four-season fresh tomatoes (that taste good). Check out the cherry, grape, and Roma tomatoes that are for sale 12 months of the year in the produce section of your supermarket. They taste great, are juicy, and make great snacks. They taste like summer, even when vine-ripened local tomatoes are months away.

Have a little fat. "If you eat a tomato with a little bit of fat, like olive oil, you'll absorb the lycopene better," says Dr. Stampfer.

Classic Tomato Sauce

- 2 teaspoons olive oil
- 1 cup chopped onions
- 2 cloves garlic, minced
- 1 can (28 ounces) crushed tomatoes in purée
- 2 tablespoons no-salt-added tomato paste
- 1½ teaspoons dried basil
- ½ teaspoon dried thyme

In a Dutch oven, heat the oil over medium-low heat. Add the onions and garlic. Cook, stirring occasionally, until the onions soften, about 8 minutes. Add the tomatoes, tomato paste, basil, and thyme. Partially cover, and cook over medium heat until the tomatoes are softened, about 30 minutes.

Makes about 4 cups

Cook's Note: *This sauce is perfect served over whole-wheat pasta, couscous, quinoa, brown rice, or baked potatoes.*

PER CUP

Calories: 111	Cholesterol: 0 mg
Total fat: 2.4 g	Sodium: 495 mg
Saturated fat: 0.3 g	Dietary fiber: 4.4 g

Tropical Fruits
EXOTIC HEALING

HEALING POWER

Can Help:

Aid in digestion

Prevent heart disease
and cancer

The next time you're pushing your shopping cart past the pineapples, pause for a moment to check out their tropical neighbors. From October to January, you'll find perfect pomegranates. Guavas, masquerading as oversized lemons and limes, make their appearance in summer and again in winter. And all year long, you'll find papayas, which look like pears on steroids, as well as mangoes in hues ranging from a rather unripe green to a ripe, rosy orange. Despite their unfamiliar appearance, tropical fruits offer many of the same benefits as their homegrown kin—and then some. Not only are they high in fiber, but they also contain an array of powerful compounds that can help fight heart disease and even cancer.

While dozens of tropical fruits are grown worldwide, the ones you're most likely to find in this country are mangoes, papayas, guavas, and pomegranates.

Mango Magic

You don't really chew a mango—you slurp it up. But even though this exceedingly juicy fruit, which tastes like peach and pineapple mixed together, only sweeter, is messy to eat, it's well worth the effort.

Mangoes, like many fruits, contain large amounts of vitamin C. What makes them really special is that they also contain a lot of beta-carotene. Both vitamin C and beta-carotene are antioxidants—meaning they can block the effects of harmful oxygen molecules called free radicals. This is important because free radicals can damage healthy tissues throughout the body. What's more, they also damage the body's low-density lipoprotein (LDL) cholesterol, making it more likely to stick to the lining of artery walls and increase the risk of heart disease.

One mango contains almost 5 milligrams of beta-carotene, or 50 to 83 percent of the recommended amount of 6 to 10 milligrams, and 57 milligrams of vitamin C, or 95 percent of the Daily Value (DV). It's a very healthful mix. In an Australian study, people were given juice containing both beta-carotene and vitamin C every day for 3 weeks. Researchers found that the LDL cholesterol in the juice drinkers suffered less damage than before they started drinking up.

In a recent University of Florida study, mango extracts inhibited the growth of cancer cells in test tubes. "We can't say these compounds from mangoes are going to prevent cancer in humans because those studies haven't been done," says Susan Percival, PhD, a University of Florida nutrition and immunity specialist. "But what we can say about the mango is that it contains potent antioxidants, and it would be a good part of a healthy diet."

It's not only antioxidants that make mangoes good for the heart. They're also high in fiber, with one mango supplying almost 6 grams of fiber—more than you'd get in 1 cup of cooked oat bran. What's more, nearly half of the fiber in mangoes is the soluble kind. Study after study has shown that getting more soluble fiber in the diet can help lower cholesterol and reduce the risk of heart disease, high blood pressure, and stroke. The insoluble fiber in mangoes is also important, because it causes stools—and any harmful substances they contain—to move through the body more quickly. This means that eating more mangoes can play a role in reducing the risk of colon cancer.

The Power of Papayas

On the outside, they look like yellow or orange avocados. On the inside, you'll find beautiful yellow-orange flesh that hints at the healing power within.

In the Kitchen

The one problem with tropical fruits, at least for American shoppers, is knowing how to pick the best ones. Here's how to get the best taste every time:

Take a sniff. Tropical fruits should smell sweet and fragrant, even before they're cut. So put your nose to work before putting them in your cart. If the smell is weak, the taste will be disappointing, too.

Keep them cool, not cold. When tropical fruits need a little time to ripen, it's best to store them in a cool, dry place. But don't put them in the refrigerator, since cold literally kills the flavor.

Find the right combination. Fruit salads, yes; gelatin salads, no. It's not a good idea to combine raw papaya or pineapple with gelatin. The enzymes in the raw fruit will break down the protein in the gelatin and keep it from setting.

Avoid pomegranate stains. Rather than wrestle with the fruit itself, keep the mess to a minimum by slicing off the crown of the fruit, then cutting the remaining pomegranate into sections, says the California-based Pomegranate Council. Put the sections into a bowl of water. Roll the juice-filled arils out of the submerged sections with your fingers. Discard the fibers and skin, drain off the water, and enjoy this ancient treat.

Papayas are packed with carotenoids, natural plant pigments that give many fruits and vegetables their beautiful hues. But carotenoids do much more than pretty up a plate. They can, quite literally, save your life.

The carotenoids in papayas are extremely powerful antioxidants. Studies have shown that people who eat the most carotenoid-rich foods like papayas have a significantly lower risk of dying from heart disease and cancer.

Many fruits and vegetables contain carotenoids, but papayas are way ahead of the pack. In one study, German researchers rated 39 foods according to their carotenoid content. Papayas came out on top, with half a fruit providing almost 3.8 milligrams of carotenoids. By contrast, grapefruits (which came in second) have 3.6 milligrams, and apricots have 2.6 milligrams.

Papaya also contains a number of protease enzymes, such as papain, which are very similar to enzymes produced naturally in the stomach. Eating raw papaya during or after a meal makes it easier for the body to digest proteins, which can help ease an upset stomach. Papaya may play a role in preventing ulcers as well. In a laboratory study, animals given high doses of stomach-churning drugs were less likely to get ulcers when they were fed papaya for several days beforehand. While similar research hasn't been done in people, it seems likely that having a little papaya each day could help counteract the irritating effects of aspirin and other anti-inflammatory drugs.

In another new study, Russian researchers have found that papaya extracts speed wound healing. They speculate that papaya's antioxidant action may protect tissue from ongoing damage during the healing process.

Great Guavas

It's not always easy to find guavas in the supermarket, but these pink or yellow, lemon-size fruits, which are often available in gourmet, Hispanic, or Indian markets, are definitely worth the search.

What makes guavas so special is a carotenoid called lycopene. For a long time, lycopene took a backseat to a related compound called beta-carotene. But studies now suggest that lycopene may be even more powerful than its more-famous kin. In fact, lycopene is one of the strongest antioxidants, says Paul Lachance, PhD, professor of nutrition and executive director of the Nutraceuticals Institute at Rutgers University in New Brunswick, New Jersey.

In laboratory studies, Israeli scientists found that lycopene was able to quickly block the growth of lung and breast cancer cells. And in a large study of almost 48,000 men, Harvard researchers found that men who got the most lycopene in their diets had a 45 percent lower risk of developing prostate cancer than those getting the least. While tomatoes have long been admired for their high lycopene content, and studies on its effects often produce conflicting results, guavas are a far better source, with at least 50 percent more lycopene in a single fruit. When researchers at the USDA's Citrus and Subtropical Products Laboratory in Winter Haven, Florida, compared the antioxidant content of 14 South Florida tropical fruits, red guava came out on top.

Finally, when it comes to dietary fiber, guava is truly a superstar, containing about 9 grams per cup. That's more fiber than you'd get in an apple, apricot, banana, and nectarine combined. This has drawn the attention of heart researchers, since getting more fiber in the diet is one of the best ways to lower cholesterol.

In a study of 120 men, Indian researchers found that those who ate five to nine guavas a day for 3 months had a drop in total cholesterol of almost 10 percent. Better yet, their levels of healthful, high-density lipoprotein cholesterol actually rose 8 percent.

Doctor's Top Tip

Prostate cancer survivors and men at risk for this cancer should try to sip 8 ounces of 100 percent pomegranate juice a day. "This is not a cure, but we may be able to change the way prostate cancer grows," says said Allan Pantuck, MD, associate professor of urology at UCLA's Jonsson Cancer Center, and lead author of a study finding that pomegranate juice slowed the rise in prostate cancer biomarkers.

Popular Pomegranates

Exotic and a tad mysterious (how do you eat one without making a huge mess?), pomegranates originated in tropical Asia and have been grown for thousands of years throughout the Mediterranean and the Middle East. Popular at Thanksgiving and Christmas, fresh pomegranates have a leathery exterior; inside are hundreds of magenta "arils"—sacs full of this fruit's distinctive sweet-tart-earthy juice. Bottled, the juice is available year-round.

Rich in antioxidants, pomegranate phytochemicals may help guard against heart-threatening atherosclerosis. When researchers at Rambam Medical Center in Haifa, Israel, tested compounds from pomegranates in lab studies, they found that these flavonoids protected particles of bad LDL cholesterol against oxidation—the first step in the development of gunky plaque that builds up in artery walls.

Moreover, a daily glass of pomegranate juice slowed the rise of cancer markers called prostate-specific antigens (PSAs) to one-quarter their usual rate in a 3-year University of California, Los Angeles, study of 50 men who had undergone surgery or radiation for prostate cancer. When prostate cancer is present, PSA levels normally double every 15 months; for juice drinkers, it took 54 months. Researchers announced they had also seen a slowdown in PSA–doubling rates for men with early-stage prostate cancer who had chosen a "watchful waiting" strategy rather than surgery, radiation, or hormone treatment. Antioxidants in the juice may protect healthy cells while isoflavones may trigger the death of cancerous cells, experts suspect.

GETTING THE MOST

Add a little fat. The lycopene in guavas is absorbed more efficiently when it's eaten with a little fat. Spooning yogurt on sliced guava, for example, will help you get the most lycopene, while adding a hint of richness to this tangy fruit.

Keep the heat down. Tropical fruits are often used as ingredients in recipes such as sauces for meat dishes. Unfortunately, the heat used in cooking destroys some of the vitamin C, says Donald V. Schlimme, PhD, professor emeritus of nutrition and food science at the University of Maryland in College Park. To get the most vitamins, he recommends eating tropical fruits raw—the way nature intended.

Store them carefully. Tropical fruits that are exposed to air and sunlight will quickly give up their vitamin C. Keeping the fruits in a cool, dark place will help keep them fresh while preserving this vital nutrient.

Ulcers

EATING FOR RELIEF

Gone are the days when doctors treated ulcers by putting people on a bland diet consisting of milk, cream, and eggs. The idea was that this bland fare would somehow neutralize excess stomach acid, which was caused, it was thought, by stress or frequent meals of three-alarm chili, and allow the ulcers to heal.

As it turns out, most ulcers are caused by a nasty bacterium called *Helicobacter pylori*—a tummy-damaging foe that can't be vanquished with a bland diet. Still, if you have an ulcer, what you eat and drink does affect how you feel, says Isadore Rosenfeld, MD, clinical professor of medicine at New York Hospital–Cornell Medical Center in New York City, and author of *Doctor, What Should I Eat?* Some foods, like coffee (including decaf), stimulate the secretion of stomach acid, which can delay healing and make the pain of ulcers worse. On the other hand, a number of foods may help protect the stomach's protective lining from attack. And choosing the right foods during ulcer treatment can make you more comfortable and even help ulcers heal faster.

The Head Healer

Cabbage is one of the oldest folk remedies for ulcers, dating back to Roman times. In 1949, a group of researchers at Stanford University School of Medicine decided to put this virtuous vegetable to the test. In the study, 13 people with ulcers drank 1 liter (about a quart) of raw cabbage juice every day. They healed six times faster than people whose only treatment was the standard bland diet.

Cabbage contains glutamine, an amino acid that increases bloodflow to the stomach and helps strengthen its protective lining.

It's an extremely effective ulcer treatment, says Michael T. Murray, ND, a naturopathic doctor, professor at Bastyr University in Seattle, and author of *Natural Alternatives to Over-the-Counter and Prescription Drugs*. The healing usually takes place in less than 1 week, he adds.

During an ulcer flare-up, Dr. Murray says, you should drink the juice from half a head (about 2 cups) of cabbage each day. If you prefer to chew your medicine, eating the same amount of raw cabbage is equally effective. Don't cook the cabbage, however, since heat destroys its anti-ulcer abilities.

Produce Protection

Your body produces extremely powerful acids to digest the food you eat. While the lining of your stomach and duodenum—the top of your small intestine—can usually protect itself from these acids, *H. pylori* can weaken it so that acids reach and erode the stomach or intestinal wall. Two-thirds of all ulcers that develop in the stomach and upper intestinal tract are caused by *H. pylori*. Most of the others are the results of overuse of over-the-counter or prescription nonsteroidal anti-inflammatory drugs—NSAIDs—such as ibuprofen or aspirin.

Many people have *H. pylori* infections. But not everyone who has an infection will develop an ulcer. Fiber may tip the ulcer odds in your favor. When Harvard School of Public Health researchers tracked 47,806 men ages 40 to 75 for 6 years, they discovered that eating fruits and vegetables helped protect against the development of duodenal ulcers—ulcers in the delicate lining of the upper part of the small intestine.

How much? Men who ate seven servings of produce a day had a 33 percent lower risk for ulcers than guys who had less than three daily helpings of fruit and vegetables. Men who ate the most had a 45 percent lower risk compared to those whose diets were more focused on meat, fat, and refined carbohydrates. And those who ate the most soluble fiber—the kind that becomes gel-like in your gastrointestinal system—cut risk by 60 percent. And getting plenty of vitamin A—from fruits and vegetables, as well as supplements—slashed risk by 57 percent. Why would fiber protect the stomach lining? Even experts at the Institute of Medicine in Washington, D.C.—a medical group that advises the federal government—aren't quite sure, but they suspect it has something to do with fiber's ability to slow down the process of digestion. This may prevent stomach acids from rushing into your small intestine and damaging it.

A Sweet Solution

When ulcer pain hits, most people are more likely to reach for a bottle of antacid than a spoonful of honey. But a dose of honey goes down a lot easier than that chalky white stuff, and it may do more than a bit of good.

Honey has been used in folk medicine for all kinds of stomach troubles. Researchers at King Saudi University College of Medicine in Saudi Arabia found that raw, unprocessed honey strengthens the lining of the stomach. And a laboratory study at the University of Waikato in New Zealand found that a mild solution of honey made from the nectar of the manuka flower, native to New Zealand, was able to completely stop the growth of ulcer-causing bacteria. Some experts recommend using only raw, unpasteurized honey for easing an ulcer, since heat-processed honey doesn't contain any of the beneficial substances. Try taking 1 tablespoon of raw, unprocessed honey at bedtime on an empty stomach. You can do this every day to help the ulcer heal. Continue this sweet treatment indefinitely to help prevent ulcers from coming back, he adds.

Healing Cultures

Yogurt is one of the great healing foods. It has been used successfully for treating yeast infections, easing lactose intolerance, and boosting immunity. There's reason to believe that it may play a role in preventing ulcers as well.

Yogurt's healing ability stems from the living stowaways it contains—live, healthful bacteria in every creamy cupful. These are friendly bacteria that will compete with the bacteria that cause ulcers. The helpful bacteria in yogurt, such as *Lactobacillus bulgaricus* and *L. acidophilus*, hustle for elbow room inside the stomach. Get enough of these beneficial bacteria in your system, and the ulcer-causing bacteria will find themselves outnumbered and unwelcome.

In addition, a natural sugar in yogurt called lactose breaks down into lactic acid during digestion. This helps restore a healthful acidic environment in the intestines.

When you have an ulcer, try eating 1 cup of yogurt three or four times a day for a couple of weeks, recommends Dr. Rosenfeld. When you combine yogurt therapy with any medical treatment you may be using, you can expect to shorten the course of your ulcer by about a third.

Incidentally, when buying yogurt, look for brands labeled "live and active cultures," which contain the beneficial live bacteria.

A Whole-Diet Plan

Even though you can help heal an ulcer by eating specific, healing foods, there's really no substitute for an overall healthful diet—even when you're clearing up your ulcer with antibiotics that fight *H. pylori* or by switching your pain reliever to something that won't damage your gastrointestinal system.

For starters, help yourself to a plantain. This cousin to the banana contains an enzyme that stimulates mucus production in the stomach lining, strengthening its natural defenses. When buying plantains, look for those that are green and slightly unripe, because these are thought to contain more of the healing enzymes.

It's also a good idea to take advantage of fiber. Getting lots of fruits, whole

> ### Doctor's Top Tip
>
> You can cut duodenal ulcer risk by eating more beans, carrots, and oranges.
>
> These foods are high in soluble fiber, which in some way protects the upper part of your small intestine from damage, notes nutrition researcher Walid Aldoori, ScD, medical director at Wyeth Consumer Healthcare in Mississauga, Ontario, Canada.

grains, legumes, and vegetables in your diet can help prevent or even heal ulcers. This is because these foods contain generous amounts of dietary fiber, which encourages the growth of the stomach's protective mucous layer. Dr. Rosenfeld recommends getting at least 35 grams of fiber every day, although the Daily Value (DV) for fiber is 25 grams.

Even though doctors once recommended milk as the cornerstone of anti-ulcer diets, it was bad advice. Milk not only increases stomach acid production, but some people are allergic to it, and food allergies may cause ulcers, according to Dr. Murray.

While you're making basic changes in your diet, don't forget to look at some of the obvious problem areas. Even though the caffeine in coffee doesn't cause ulcers, it can make you more susceptible to getting them. Along with cigarettes and alcohol, it can also make existing ulcers worse, says Dr. Rosenfeld.

Urinary Tract Infections

FLUSHING OUT THE PLUMBING

For a long time, doctors dismissed food cures for urinary tract infections (UTIs) as being nothing but folklore. But there's increasing evidence that what you drink can play a role in preventing and even treating these painful conditions.

UTIs occur when bacteria take up residence in the bladder or urethra (the tube through which urine flows), causing painful or frequent urination. More common in women than men, UTIs are usually treated with antibiotics, which can clear up the problem in a few days.

Research suggests, however, that drinking cranberry juice will not only help prevent UTIs but also speed recovery if you're already sick. In one study, researchers in Boston gave 153 women either 10 ounces of cranberry juice or 10 ounces of a look-alike fluid every day for 6 months. They found that women drinking the cranberry juice were 58 percent less likely to develop UTIs than those drinking the phony fluid.

Researchers believe that women who are prone to UTIs may have "stickier" cells in the urethra, making it easier for bacteria to hold on. It appears that cranberries contain a substance, which hasn't yet been identified, that acts like a nonstick coating for these cells, making the bacteria more likely to slip away. The inner lining of the bladder simply becomes more slippery.

Incidentally, it's not only cranberry juice that works against UTIs. Scientists believe that blueberry juice and lingonberry juice may have similar effects.

While you might get some benefit from eating whole berries, juices are a more convenient way to get more of the protective compounds. That's why doctors recommend that women who frequently get UTIs

Doctor's Top Tip

Have a cup of unsweetened cranberry juice a day and a carton of plain yogurt or a serving of aged cheese three times a week. Researchers in Finland found that women who followed this dietary pattern were 34 to 80 percent less likely to develop a bladder infection.

Which type of cranberry juice is best? Skip those labeled "cocktail"—they contain loads of high-fructose corn syrup. Go for a tart 8-ounce glass of unsweetened cranberry juice. "It doesn't cure an infection once it's established, but it can possibly prevent one," notes Michael L. Guralnick, MD, assistant professor of urology at the Medical College of Wisconsin in Milwaukee.

THE ACID TEST

When scientists first started investigating cranberry juice as a cure for urinary tract infections (UTIs), they suspected that its high acid content was probably responsible. Acidic urine, they reasoned, would provide a less hospitable environment for bacteria.

Soon people were trying to ease infections with other high-acid substances, such as vitamin C or large amounts of oranges and tomatoes.

As it turns out, acid may not be the answer. In fact, some doctors believe that creating a high-acid environment just irritates an already-inflamed bladder. In fact, the National Institutes of Health recommends that if you have a UTI or are prone to UTIs, you should avoid fluids that irritate the bladder, such as alcohol, citrus juices, and drinks containing caffeine.

It still isn't certain whether women with UTIs should eat, avoid, or simply not worry about having acidic foods. But doctors do recommend listening to your body. If you have an infection and find that certain foods, like citrus fruits, tomatoes, aged cheese, spicy foods, and coffee, make it more painful to urinate, you're better off leaving them alone until the infection has gone away.

should drink 10 ounces of cranberry juice—or, if you can find it, blueberry juice—every day.

Wash Away Infection

Even if you don't have juice in the refrigerator, there's another liquid strategy for preventing UTIs. Drinking eight 8-ounce glasses of water a day will help your body wash away bacteria before they cause infection.

Drinking water is particularly important when it's time for your annual pelvic exam. Many women get UTIs after the exam, possibly because the instruments can irritate the vagina and push bacteria nearer to the urethral opening, where they're more likely to cause infection. Having two big glasses of water—one before the exam and one after—and then using the bathroom will help keep the urinary tract free of bacteria.

Vegetarian Diets
EATING FOR A LONG LIFE

When people first started experimenting with meatless cooking in the 1960s, meals were often colorless, tasteless, or both. After all, there's only so much you can do with brown rice-and-lentil loaf or tofu on a bed of alfalfa sprouts.

HEALING POWER
Can Help:
Lower cholesterol levels
Prevent vision loss
Reduce the risk of cancer and heart disease

But the "nuts-and-berries" approach of the early years has pretty much gone the way of the Volkswagen minibus. With over a quarter-century's experience to learn from, cooks today are combining fruits, vegetables, grains, and legumes in exciting new ways. The tastes are so good, in fact, that even large restaurant chains are now offering meatless meals.

The result? Over 30 million Americans—including one in three teens—say they've tried vegetarian eating, according to the American Dietetic Association. What is it that they like? The health benefits—and how good the food tastes.

Although vegetarian menus have changed, one thing has stayed the same. A plant-based diet—which is low in saturated fat and high in fiber, antioxidant vitamins, and a powerful array of protective chemicals—is the ultimate prescription for a longer, healthier life, says Virginia Messina, MPH, RD, a dietitian in Port Townsend, Washington, and coauthor of *The Vegetarian Way*.

Research studies show that vegetarians have lower rates of cancer, heart disease, high blood pressure, type 2 diabetes, and obesity than meat eaters. British researchers say vegetarians have a 20 percent lower risk of fatal heart disease and a 40 percent lower risk of cancer.

Other studies have found even more protection. Nearly 40 years ago, a large study of 27,530 Seventh-Day Adventists, whose religion advocates a meatless diet, provided the first scientific link between vegetarian diets and better health. Researchers were amazed to discover that among the vegetarian Adventists, death rates from cancer were 50 to 70 percent lower than among other Americans.

Since then, study after study has confirmed the benefits of vegetarian eating.

In China, for example, where people eat little or no meat, diseases such as heart disease, breast cancer, and diabetes are far less common than in this country. "If we had diets similar to this in America, they could prevent 80 to 90 percent of the chronic, degenerative diseases that people get before age 65," says T. Colin Campbell, PhD, professor emeritus of nutritional biochemistry at Cornell University in Ithaca, New York, and director of the landmark 20-year China-Oxford-Cornell Diet and Health Project, which has helped uncover the benefits of a low-meat or no-meat diet. The study's bottom line? "People who ate the most animal-based foods got the most chronic disease," Dr. Campbell notes. "People who ate the most plant-based foods were the healthiest and tended to avoid chronic disease. These results could not be ignored."

Naturally Lean

One thing that makes vegetarian meals so healthful is what they *don't* have—all the saturated fat and cholesterol that come from meat. In fact, while most Americans get about 36 percent of their total calories from fat, vegetarians get less, usually between 30 and 34 percent. And most of the fat they do get is the healthier polyunsaturated and monounsaturated kind—and not the dangerous saturated fat that comes from animal foods.

In one study, researchers put 500 people on a vegetarian diet. After 12 days, cholesterol levels had dropped an average of 11 percent.

In the Kitchen

Meat, for all its drawbacks, has one thing going for it: It's very high in flavor. When you take meat off the menu, you have to put the taste back in. To make meatless meals with "big" flavors, chefs recommend using an abundance of herbs, spices, spice mixtures, and flavorful liquids, like balsamic vinegar. Here are a few taste enhancers you may want to try:

- Adding a teaspoon of curry paste to beans and grains will impart a deep, aromatic flavor.
- A splash of vinegar—balsamic and tarragon vinegars are popular choices— adds a tart sparkle to steamed vegetables, like broccoli or Brussels sprouts.

- Mustards aren't just for hot dogs and burgers. Adding a tablespoon of gourmet mustard to beans, grains, or even salad dressings lends a bit of "bite" and a hint of tartness. Flavored mustards will pump up the tastes even more.
- Fresh herbs provide an intensity of flavor that you just can't get with dried. You can buy fresh parsley, dill, thyme, oregano, and cilantro at most supermarkets. Health food stores will usually have a wider selection.
- There are literally dozens of hot sauces with names like "Prairie Fire" or "Raging Passion." If you like your food hot, these work well with almost anything, from soups and stews to casseroles.

It's not just the lack of saturated fat that makes vegetarian meals so healthful. It's also the "good" fats that are used to replace it. Studies have shown, for example, that both polyunsaturated and monounsaturated fats, which are found in olive oil, canola oil, nuts, seeds, and many other plant foods, can lower levels of cholesterol when they're used to replace saturated fat in the diet. And the omega-3 fatty acids found in some plant foods, such as walnuts and flaxseed, can further protect against heart disease by helping to keep artery walls flexible and supporting the electrical "system" within the heart that regulates a healthy heartbeat.

The Powers of Plants

For years, doctors have been pleading with Americans to eat more fruits, vegetables, whole grains, and legumes, the same foods that vegetarian meals include in abundance. Most plant foods are loaded with antioxidants, such as beta-carotene and vitamins C and E, which are essential for protecting the body from disease. In addition, many plant foods contain an abundance of phytonutrients, natural plant compounds that appear to lower the risk for cataracts, heart disease, and many other serious problems.

In one study, for example, researchers found that people who got the most carotenoids, the plant pigments that are found in dark green and deep orange, yellow, and red fruits and vegetables, had half the risk of developing macular degeneration (the leading cause of irreversible vision loss in older adults) as people getting less.

Vegetarian diets cut the risk of breast, colon, ovarian, and prostate cancer in a number of studies. The magic ingredients include a slew of cancer-fighting phytochemicals. The naturally lower levels of saturated fat in most vegetarian diets (except those that rely heavily on cheese) sidestep a problem inherent in meat-rich diets: High-saturated-fat diets seem to promote production of a form of estrogen called estradiol, which is linked to breast cancer. In one study, women who ate the most animal fats had a one-third higher risk of breast cancer than those who ate the least. And another study found that vegetarians have higher levels of "natural killer cells"—special white blood cells that attack cancer cells—in their bloodstreams.

But even if you took all the nutrients out of plant foods, the vegetarian diet would still have an edge because of all the dietary fiber it contains. The average American gets only 12 to 15 grams of fiber a day, while vegetarians get as much as three times that amount, Messina says.

It's almost impossible to exaggerate the importance of getting enough dietary fiber. Because it isn't absorbed by the body, fiber passes through the digestive tract, adding bulk to stools and helping them move more swiftly. This does more than prevent constipation. The more quickly stools and any harmful substances they

Doctor's Top Tip

Vegans—vegetarians who shun all animal foods including dairy and eggs—are at high risk for deficiencies of B$_{12}$, a vitamin crucial for a healthy nervous system. Some studies show that the body's stores of B$_{12}$ drop by one-third within just 2 months of adopting a vegan diet. That's because plant foods don't contain this important nutrient, which binds to animal proteins, warns Lindsay Allen, PhD, director of the USDA Western Human Nutrition Research Center at the University of California, Davis. Depleting your body's supply can lead to neurological problems. If you're a vegan, or eat very little meat and dairy on a regular basis, take a B$_{12}$ supplement every day, or be sure to eat a breakfast cereal fortified with it. The Daily Value for B$_{12}$ is 6 micrograms.

contain move through the colon, the less likely they are to do cellular damage that could lead to cancer.

In addition, one type of fiber, called soluble fiber, forms a gel in the intestine that helps prevent fat and cholesterol from passing through the intestinal wall and into the bloodstream. In a study of more than 43,000 men, for example, researchers found that those who added just 10 grams of fiber a day to their diets—about 25 percent of the amount vegetarians get each day—decreased their risk of heart disease by almost 30 percent.

Vegetarian diets seem to guard against other health issues, too, including kidney stones, gallstones, and asthma. How? High-protein diets packed with meat prompt your body to excrete more calcium, oxalate, and uric acid—the main building blocks of kidney stones. Meat-rich diets seem to double the odds for gallstones in women, too, and may actually threaten bone density by prompting the excretion of calcium. And vegetable-based meals cut the frequency and severity of asthma attacks in a Swedish study of 24 women and men with this breathing problem.

Staying in Balance

A vegetarian diet can provide all the nutrients your body needs, including protein. This is even true for strict vegetarians, who may avoid eggs, milk, or other animal foods entirely. The proteins in meats are complete, meaning that they contain all the amino acids you need. The proteins in legumes and grains, however, may be low in one or more of the amino acids. But because legumes and grains contain some amino acids, eating a variety of these foods throughout the day will provide the proper balance.

Apart from protein, there is one nutrient that people following a strict vegetarian diet have to be aware of. Vitamin B$_{12}$, which the body uses to make red blood cells, is found only in animal foods. People who don't get enough vitamin B$_{12}$ get tired and weak, a condition doctors call pernicious anemia.

But you can get plenty of vitamin B$_{12}$ by eating foods fortified with this nutrient, such as fortified cereals, fortified soy milk, or B$_{12}$-enriched nutritional yeast.

Braised Vegetable Medley

4 teaspoons olive oil

4 medium potatoes, cut into large chunks

6 ounces small button mushrooms

16 baby carrots

1 package (9 ounces) frozen artichoke hearts

4 cloves garlic, sliced

1½ cups vegetable broth

¼ teaspoon salt

¼ cup water

1½ tablespoons minced fresh dill

Freshly ground black pepper

In a Dutch oven, heat the oil over medium heat. Add the potatoes, mushrooms, and carrots. Cook until the vegetables begin to lightly brown, about 5 minutes.

Add the artichokes, garlic, broth, and salt. Cover and reduce the heat to low. Cook until the potatoes and carrots are very tender, 30 to 35 minutes. Add up to ¼ cup water if the vegetables begin to dry out.

Add the dill, and season to taste with pepper. Stir gently to mix.

Makes 4 servings

Cook's Note: *For a heartier meal, serve the vegetables over cooked couscous.*

PER SERVING

Calories: 181
Total fat: 5.3 g
Saturated fat: 0.8 g

Cholesterol: 0 mg
Sodium: 187 mg
Dietary fiber: 7.1 g

Spiced Tofu with Spinach and Tomatoes

16 ounces firm regular tofu

2 teaspoons canola oil

1¾ cups chopped onions

1½ tablespoons grated fresh ginger

1 tablespoon minced garlic

1½ teaspoons ground cumin

2 medium tomatoes, cut into 8 wedges each

⅓ cup water

1 bag (6 ounces) washed and trimmed spinach, torn into bite-size pieces

¼ teaspoon salt

Rinse and drain the tofu, and cut it into 1-inch cubes. Place the tofu on several layers of paper towels, then cover with several more paper towels. Press down lightly to remove some of the liquid. Set aside.

In a large nonstick skillet, heat the oil over medium heat. Add the onions, and cook, stirring frequently, until golden, about 6 to 8 minutes.

Increase the heat to medium-high. Add the tofu, ginger, garlic, and cumin. Cook for 3 to 4 minutes, or until the tofu starts to brown. Add the tomatoes, and stir. Cook for 1 minute longer. Add the water.

Add the spinach, a handful at a time; add more spinach as the first batch starts to cook down. Cook just until the spinach is wilted. Sprinkle with the salt.

Makes 4 servings

Cook's Note: *Serve with cooked rice or toasted pita bread.*

PER SERVING

Calories: 163
Total fat: 8.3 g
Saturated fat: 1 g

Cholesterol: 0 mg
Sodium: 174 mg
Dietary fiber: 4 g

Water

WASH AWAY KIDNEY STONES

Run your car without water in the radiator, and it will come to a steaming halt. Yet people who wouldn't dream of letting their cars run dry often walk around without enough water in their own radiators. And because every cell in the body requires fluids to dissolve and transport vitamins, minerals, sugar, and other chemicals, not drinking enough water can leave you feeling like a run-down Ford.

HEALING POWER

Can Help:

Cut heart disease risk

Reduce the risk of kidney stones

Restore energy

Prevent constipation

The average person loses about 2 percent of his body weight (about 1½ quarts of water) in urine, perspiration, and other body fluids every day. To replace these fluids, doctors advise drinking at least eight glasses of water, milk, or juice a day—more if you're a large person, over age 55, sick with a cold, or simply active.

To make sure you drink enough, the brain has special sensors in a part of the brain called the thalamus, which monitor blood levels of sodium. When concentrations of sodium rise, it means that water levels are low. The brain then sends a signal, in the form of thirst, that says it's time to head to the water cooler.

This system usually works well. As we age, however, the thirst sensor gets less sensitive, so we don't always drink enough, says Lucia Kaiser, PhD, RD, a cooperative extension specialist at the University of California, Davis. Plus, sometimes we get so busy, we don't take time to drink. That can cause serious problems, ranging from kidney stones and constipation to fatigue. Let's take a look at a few of the ways in which water can keep us healthy.

Prevent Heart-Threatening Clots

"Not drinking enough water can be as harmful to your heart as smoking," warns Jacqueline Chan, DrPH, professor at Loma Linda University in California, who found a surprising connection between quaffing H_2O and reduced risk for heart disease. In an analysis of the thirst-quenching habits and health histories of 20,000 Seventh-Day Adventists from California, Dr. Chan found that men who drank three or four glasses of water per day had a 40 percent reduction in risk of coronary heart disease, while women who drank the same number had a 43 percent risk reduction.

For men, more was better: Getting five or more glasses of water a day cut risk 62 percent, but only reduced women's risk 39 percent.

The risk reduction was greater than that found for other famous heart-protecting steps such as quitting smoking, reducing cholesterol, exercising, or maintaining a healthy weight, the researchers say. And it surpasses the benefits of taking a daily low-dose aspirin or having a glass of wine. (Of course, the best way to get water's benefits is in addition to other healthy habits, not in place of them!)

Other fluids, including coffee, soda, milk, and caffeinated sodas didn't cut heart risk; Dr. Chan thinks that while water thins the blood and therefore cuts clotting risk, other beverages actually draw water from the blood because they cannot be digested until their concentration is reduced. "People need to be made aware that there is a difference, at least for heart health, whether they get their fluids from plain water or from sodas," she says.

The researchers speculate that if a water habit improved heart health for already-healthy Adventists, who generally follow a vegetarian eating plan and don't smoke, then it may be even more helpful for other Americans.

Stopping Stones

Men say it's the worst pain they've ever known. Women say they'd rather have the pain of childbirth. Both men and women agree that once you've had a kidney stone, you never want to get another one.

Getting enough water, doctors say, will help ensure you never do. Normally, many of the wastes in the body are dissolved in fluids and carried out in the urine. But when you don't drink enough water, the wastes may become concentrated, forming crystals that can bond together and form kidney stones.

"I tell people to think of the insides of their bodies as they would their kitchens," says Bernell Baldwin, PhD, an instructor in applied physiology at Wildwood Lifestyle Center and Hospital in Georgia and science editor of *Journal of Health and Healing*. "You can't expect your body to be able to clean up its dishes without giving it enough water."

Here's an easy test to tell if you're getting enough water. Look at your urine. Except in the morning, when you haven't had fluids all night, it should be pale yellow or even clear. If it's dark, that means wastes are too concentrated, and you should be drinking more water.

Fluid Movements

Another way in which water helps remove wastes from the body is by keeping the stools soft, which helps prevent constipation, says Dr. Baldwin. When you don't drink enough, stools become hard and dry, and it takes longer for them to move through your system.

Constipation isn't merely uncomfortable, Dr. Baldwin adds. Studies have shown that constipation may lead to other problems, such as hemorrhoids, diverticular disease, or even colon cancer.

"You should drink two glasses of water about a half-hour before eating breakfast," Dr. Baldwin advises. "This not only hydrates your body but also primes your system, flushing out wastes and getting it ready for food."

Wash Away Fatigue

We think of fatigue as being caused by not getting enough sleep or working too hard. But in many cases, the problem is even more basic: not getting enough water.

Here's what happens. When you don't drink enough, cells throughout your body start getting a little dry. To quench their thirst, they draw water from the most convenient place—the bloodstream. This leaves the blood thick, sludgy, and harder to pump. The extra work involved in pumping the blood can cause energy levels to decline, Dr. Baldwin says.

You don't have to run completely dry to feel the effects. In a small study of cyclists, researchers found that their performance levels dropped when they lost as little as 2 percent of their body weight in fluids—the equivalent of about six glasses of water.

Wash Away Weight

One of the nicest benefits of drinking more water is that it can help you lose weight. For one thing, many of us think it's time to eat when, in fact, we're merely thirsty. Drinking water is a great way to quell hunger pangs. In addition, when you drink with meals, you're more likely to take in fewer calories, says Dr. Kaiser.

Water can help in yet another way. When you drink cold water (40°F or cooler) you actually burn calories, because the body has to raise the temperature of the water to 98.6°F. In the process, it burns slightly less than 1 calorie per ounce of water. So if

Doctor's Top Tip

Drink more when the temperature soars or if you've been exercising. Exercising outside in hot and humid conditions can be hard on your heart, because when your body sweats in order to cool itself, it draws fluid from your blood. In response, your heart must work harder to pump a smaller volume of blood. Drink 8 ounces of water before, during, and again after you exercise, suggests the American Heart Association.

One caveat, though: There is a dangerous condition called dilutional hyponutremia, which occurs when some exercisers drink too much water without replacing the electrolytes that they sweat or urinate out. If you run marathons or bike for long distances in hot weather, or do other intense sports, discuss proper water intake with your doctor or trainer.

you toss back eight glasses of cold water a day, you'll burn about 62 calories. That adds up to 434 calories a week, according to Ellington Darden, PhD, author of *A Flat Stomach ASAP.*

GETTING THE MOST

Eat for drink. Drinking isn't the only way to get more water in your diet. Many foods are also very high in moisture. Having soups or stews, for example, can be a big help toward getting your daily water allowance, says Dr. Kaiser. "For even more fluid, add some crunchy vegetables like celery and peppers to these dishes," she says.

Pick some fruit. Juicy fruits like watermelons, cantaloupes, oranges, and grapefruits are mostly water, so they're an excellent (and convenient) way to get more water in your diet, Dr. Kaiser says.

Choose your drinks carefully. Recent guidelines from the National Academy of Sciences say that you can count caffeinated drinks and alcoholic beverages toward your daily water total, along with juices and decaffeinated coffee and tea. But caffeine and alcohol are diuretics, meaning they pull more water out of your body than they put in. So to net 2 cups of water by drinking coffee, you'd have to drink 3 cups of coffee. Better to drink a glass of water for every caffeine- or alcohol-containing drink.

Watercress

A BOUQUET OF PROTECTION

Looking for something special to make for Valentine's Day? Give your sweetie a special treat by saying "sayonara" to chocolates, "arrivederci" to lobster, and "hello" to a fresh bouquet of watercress.

This delicate green, with dime-size leaves and a pungent, peppery flavor, is more than just a celebration salad. First, it's a cruciferous vegetable (meaning that its flowers have four petals, resembling a cross). The crucifers, including broccoli and cauliflower, are well-known for their cancer-fighting potential. Watercress is also a dark green leafy vegetable, meaning that it's packed with beta-carotene, a nutrient that helps ward off heart disease and diseases associated with aging, such as cataracts.

Watercress has a long pedigree as a healthy superfood. Anglo-Saxons munched it to prevent baldness. Roman emperors ate it to help them make bold decisions. In Crete, watercress has an ancient reputation as an aphrodisiac. Irish monks called it "pure food for sages." And the Victorians prized it as a cure for headaches and hiccups.

Snuffing Out Cancer

This spicy green is a traditional filling for dainty sandwiches served at a proper English high tea. If you ever find yourself faced with the choice of watercress or cucumber sandwiches at a fancy tea, go for the watercress—and say yes to second helpings. Population studies show that people who eat plenty of cruciferous vegetables, like watercress, have lower rates of cancer. Watercress researchers will tell you that this crucifer is particularly potent against lung cancer caused by smoking or breathing secondhand smoke. Scientists have found that when they included phenethyl isothiocyanate (PEITC), a natural compound found in watercress that gives this food its peppery flavor, in the daily diets of laboratory animals and exposed them to cancer-causing chemicals found in tobacco smoke, the animals were 50 percent less likely to develop lung cancer tumors than animals given their regular diet, without PEITC.

HEALING POWER

Can Help:

Reduce the risk of lung cancer

Prevent heart disease

Decrease the risk of cataracts

Prevent wrinkles

Encouraged by the results, the scientists recruited 11 smokers to see if watercress would have similar effects in people as it did in the laboratory.

It did. "We got results with humans that were consistent with what we saw in laboratory animals," says Stephen Hecht, PhD, professor of cancer prevention at the University of Minnesota Cancer Center in Minneapolis.

Watercress is the richest food source of PEITC. More than 50 research studies have shown that it seems to prevent cancer-causing agents—including some of those found in tobacco smoke—from being metabolized by the body to become carcinogens. It also seems to trigger enzymes that disarm carcinogens. But watercress seems to have other anticancer compounds hiding in its tiny green leaves as well. British researchers have discovered that it contains methylsulphinylalkyl glucosinolate—which also turns off the development of cancer and seems to make this salad green twice as potent a cancer fighter.

The catch, of course, is that you have to eat a lot of watercress for it to be effective. And watercress won't necessarily protect you from other cancer-causing chemicals in tobacco smoke, adds Dr. Hecht.

"The volunteers in our study ate 2 ounces of watercress at each meal, three meals a day. That's a pretty hefty sandwich or a large salad—more than you would normally eat at one sitting. And you would have to do it several times a day," says Dr. Hecht.

Of course, no one is telling you that eating watercress is going to wash away smoke's toxic effects. No food on the planet can. But adding watercress to your daily diet may be a step in the right direction while you work on clearing the smoke from your life.

In the Kitchen

With its tiny, delicate leaves and thick stems, watercress looks quite a bit different from other salad greens. But with a little care, you can use this lively member of the mustard family the same way you would any leafy green.

To keep watercress fresh, refrigerate it in a plastic bag. Or refrigerate it stems-down in a glass of water, and cover it with a plastic bag. It will keep for up to 5 days.

When using watercress, unless you're adding it to soup stock, use only the leaves and the thinner stems. Otherwise, the pungent, peppery flavor may be overpowering.

Incidentally, this is one green you don't want to skimp on. Watercress shrinks substantially during cooking, and what may look like a big pile on the counter may almost disappear on the plate. Plan on cooking one bunch per person.

Other Benefits

Along with keeping cancer cells at bay, watercress also helps fight another major public health enemy—heart disease.

Like other dark green leafy vegetables, watercress is packed with beta-carotene, an antioxidant nutrient that has been linked to lower rates of heart disease. In fact, watercress has more beta-carotene than broccoli or tomatoes. It's also packed with the vision-guarding phytochemicals lutein and zeaxanthin. As a bonus, a 1-cup serving of watercress also provides 24 percent of the Daily Value (DV) for vitamin C, another valuable disease-fighting antioxidant vitamin.

The antioxidants, which include beta-carotene and vitamins C and E, help sweep up cell-damaging oxygen molecules from your body. Keeping lots of beta-carotene in your bloodstream seems to be the ticket to lowering your risk of heart attack, certain cancers, and ailments associated with aging, such as cataracts and wrinkles.

> ### Doctor's Top Tip
>
> Pair watercress with delicately flavored foods to accent its fresh, peppery bite. The Mayo Clinic suggests sprinkling it over sliced fresh or grilled pears, or chopping watercress and adding it to mushroom soup.

GETTING THE MOST

Eat it raw. Watercress is best eaten in its natural state, fresh and crisp. When cooked, it loses its ability to release PEITC. "Fortunately, most people don't cook it," says Dr. Hecht. "Your dose of that active ingredient is less in a cooked vegetable than a raw one."

Use it often. Chances are that you'll never eat the 6 ounces of watercress a day that you need to extract the maximum healing benefit, says Dr. Hecht. But you can put a hefty amount in your diet simply by using it more often. For example, it makes a tasty replacement for lettuce in sandwiches and salads.

Wheat

THE E GRAIN

HEALING POWER

Can Help:

Improve digestion

Reduce the risk of heart disease and cancer

Forget corn, oats, rice, or rye. For Americans, wheat is by far the number one grain. The average American, in fact, eats 148 pounds of wheat, in the form of pasta, bread, bagels, and cereals, a year.

One reason that we eat so much wheat is that it's a remarkably versatile grain. Even if you don't care for bread, there are literally dozens, if not hundreds, of common recipes that call for wheat. It has a light flavor that works well in all kinds of foods, from the flakiest biscuits to the heartiest polentas.

It's our good fortune that wheat is nutritious as well as delicious. In fact, it's one of the most healthful foods you can buy. Like all grains, wheat is rich in vitamins, minerals, and complex carbohydrates.

But what makes wheat truly special is that it contains one thing that many foods do not: vitamin E. This is important because vitamin E is mainly found in cooking oils such as safflower and canola oils. As a result, getting the Daily Value (DV) of 30 IU of vitamin E can be tricky unless you choose your foods carefully, says Susan Finn, PhD, chairperson of the American Council for Fitness and Nutrition.

Eating more wheat makes it just a little bit easier. It's worth doing, Dr. Finn adds, because vitamin E may play a direct role both in lowering cholesterol and in preventing it from sticking to the lining of artery walls, which can help reduce the risk of heart disease.

A Vitamin for the Heart

Every day, the body produces an enormous number of free radicals, which are harmful oxygen molecules that have lost an electron. As a result, these molecules go zipping through the body, grabbing extra electrons wherever they can find them. In the process, they damage cholesterol in the bloodstream, making it sticky and more likely to cling to artery walls—the first step in causing heart disease.

Research has shown that eating more wheat can help stop this process from getting started. In a study of 31,000 people, for example, researchers found that those who ate the most whole-wheat bread had a much lower risk of heart disease than those who ate white bread.

Doctors speculate that the vitamin E in wheat causes the liver to produce less cholesterol, says Michael H. Davidson, MD, executive medical director of Radiant Research in Chicago. In one study, for example, people with high cholesterol were given 20 grams (about a quarter-cup) of wheat germ a day for 4 weeks. (Most of the vitamin E in wheat is concentrated in the germ layer.) Then, for 14 weeks after that, they upped the amount to 30 grams. At the end of the study, researchers found that their cholesterol levels had dropped an average of 7 percent.

Wheat germ is a very concentrated source of vitamin E, with a little less than 2 tablespoons providing 5 IU, or about 16 percent of the DV. Oat bran and whole-wheat breads and cereals also contain vitamin E, although in smaller amounts than the germ.

Body-Wide Benefits

If you remember the oat bran frenzy of a few years ago, you already know that this grain is prized for its high fiber content. But oats aren't the only way to get a lot of

In the Kitchen

Much of the wheat in our diets comes from bread and breakfast cereals, but there are many other kinds of wheat as well. To get the most of this nutritious, delicious grain, here are a few variations you may want to try:

- **Bulgur** is made from whole-wheat kernels that have been parboiled and dried. Used either whole or cracked, it makes a great side dish and is often used as a substitute for rice.
- **Cracked wheat**, like bulgur, is made from the entire grain. However, it's milled more thoroughly and is broken into small pieces, which allows it to cook more quickly. Cracked wheat is often

used as a hot cereal. It can also be used to add a nutty crunch to other cereals or to casseroles.

- **Wheat germ** is the embryo, or the sprouting part, of the grain. It's a super source of both vitamin E and fiber. You can add wheat germ when baking breads or casseroles. Some people even use it as a topping for yogurt or ice cream. Because wheat germ contains a lot of oils, however, it spoils rapidly unless it's kept in the refrigerator.
- **Rolled wheat** is made by rolling the whole grains into flat little flakes. Rolled wheat is often used for making hot cereal or as an ingredient in baked goods.

fiber in your diet. Wheat bran, in fact, contains more than 1½ times the fiber of oat bran, and that's good news for your health.

The type of fiber that is in wheat, called insoluble fiber, absorbs lots of water as it passes through the intestine, causing stools to get larger and heavier. The larger stools pass through the body more quickly—which means that any harmful substances they contain have less time to damage cells in the colon, says Beth Kunkel, PhD, RD, professor of food and nutrition at Clemson University in South Carolina.

When researchers analyzed more than 13 international studies involving more than 15,000 people, they found that those who got the most fiber had a substantially lower risk of developing colon cancer. The researchers estimated that if people would increase the amount of fiber in their diets to 39 grams a day, their risk of colon cancer might drop as much as 31 percent.

One serving of a whole-grain cereal (look for the words "whole wheat" or "whole oats" as the first ingredient on the ingredients list) can have 4 to 7 grams of fiber per serving and also gives you a range of nutrients found only in whole grains: a dose of niacin, thiamin, riboflavin, magnesium, phosphorus, iron, and zinc, as well as protein and some good fat. Wheat germ is also a good fiber source, with a little less than 2 tablespoons providing more than 1 gram. Bulgur, whole-wheat pasta, and cracked wheat (which is used to make tabbouleh) are other good fiber finds, says Dr. Finn.

In other studies, whole grains such as whole wheat cut risk for type 2 diabetes. Just three servings a day reduced risk by 21 to 30 percent. Grains reduce insulin resistance—a prediabetic condition in which cells resist insulin's signals to absorb blood sugar. Eating more whole grains can improve your insulin sensitivity in just 6 weeks.

Whole wheat can help guard against cancer, too. Eating more whole grains can cut the risk of gastrointestinal tract cancers, including cancers of the mouth, throat, stomach, colon, and rectum. But by how much? One review of 40 studies has found that diets rich in whole grains slashed cancer risk 34 percent. Moms who eat more whole wheat during pregnancy may help their children resist cancer, too, suggests a Georgetown University lab study. When pregnant rats were fed more whole wheat, anticancer genes in their offspring were more active. When the young rats were exposed to carcinogens, they were less likely to develop breast cancer than those whose mothers hadn't been fed diets packed with whole wheat.

On a day-to-day basis, more whole wheat (and other whole grains) can make life more comfortable—preventing constipation by softening and bulking up stools. Diets rich in whole grains and fiber may also cut risk for diverticulosis—a condition in which small pouches form in the colon.

Whole Wheat Versus White

If you haven't given up the white bread habit yet, we've got even more reasons why you should make the switch. According to data collected by the USDA, whole wheat's got nearly five times more fiber, twice the calcium, seven times more magnesium, and about 10 percent more niacin than enriched bleached all-purpose white flour.

GETTING THE MOST

Buy it whole. To get the most vitamin E and fiber from wheat, it's important to buy foods containing wheat germ or whole wheat, which contain the outer, more-nutritious parts of the grain. Once wheat has been processed—when making white bread or "light" cereals, for example—most of the protective ingredients are lost, says Dr. Finn.

Find it in new places. Choose whole-wheat pasta, and bake with whole-wheat flour instead of white flour (or go half-and-half). Choose whole-wheat snack crackers, tortillas, and dinner rolls. And look for breakfast cereals like shredded wheat and wheat flakes, too.

Doctor's Top Tip

Food manufacturers sometimes make it difficult to tell if you've really got a whole-wheat product, or a look-alike, warn Harvard School of Public Health nutrition experts. Your whole-wheat bread, pasta, or cereal's the real thing if it meets one of these criteria: Whole wheat is the first ingredient; there are at least 3 grams of fiber per serving; the label's got this claim: "Diets rich in whole-grain foods and other plant foods and low in total fat, saturated fat, and cholesterol may reduce the risk for heart disease and certain cancers," which means it is at least 51 percent whole grain by weight.

Whole-Wheat Pancakes

1¼ cups whole-wheat flour

¼ cup toasted wheat germ

1½ teaspoons baking powder

½ teaspoon ground cinnamon

⅛ teaspoon salt

1½ cups fat-free milk

¼ cup fat-free egg substitute

1 tablespoon unsalted butter, melted

In a large bowl, combine the flour, wheat germ, baking powder, cinnamon, and salt. Mix well. Add the milk, egg substitute, and butter. Mix just until the ingredients are blended. Do not overmix.

Coat a large nonstick skillet with cooking spray. Heat over medium-high heat until a drop of water dropped into the skillet sizzles. Using a ¼-cup measuring cup as a ladle, scoop out slightly less than ¼ cup of batter for each pancake. Drop the batter into the pan, being careful not to crowd the pancakes.

Cook for 2 minutes, or until the edges begin to look dry. Flip and cook for 1 minute, or until browned on the bottom. Remove from the pan.

Take the skillet off the heat, and coat it with more cooking spray. Continue until all the batter is used.

Makes 4 servings (3 pancakes each)

Cook's Note: *Place the pancakes on a baking sheet in a 175°F oven to keep them warm until all are cooked. Serve with maple syrup or honey, if desired.*

PER SERVING ————————————————

Calories: 221	Cholesterol: 10 mg
Total fat: 4.5 g	Sodium: 325 mg
Saturated fat: 2.1 g	Dietary fiber: 5.5 g

Wine

THE SECRET TO A HEALTHY HEART

HEALING POWER

Can Help:

Prevent heart disease and stroke

Control intestinal bacteria

Ever since man discovered the fruits of fermentation, wine has been a welcome guest, not just at the dinner table but also at weddings, religious rituals, and even doctors' offices.

Only recently, however, have scientists begun to investigate the actual health benefits of sipping Chianti with your ziti. And the findings they've uncorked are enough to make any wine lover raise his glass and say, "Salut!"

Used in moderation, wine, particularly the red varieties, can help lower cholesterol and fight hardening of the arteries and heart disease. In addition, studies suggest that it can kill the bacteria that cause food poisoning and traveler's diarrhea. Obviously, experts don't recommend that people start guzzling wine rather than sipping it or that people who don't drink should suddenly start. Rather, what the evidence suggests is that moderate drinking can be a helpful addition to a healthy diet.

Fruit of the Vein

For years, researchers looked with amazement across the Atlantic as their French allies indulged in cigarettes, buttery croissants, and fat-laden pâtés—and were still 2½ times less likely to develop heart disease than their supposedly healthier American counterparts.

Researchers are still investigating the so-called French paradox, but it appears likely that the French have healthier hearts at least partly because of their penchant for red wines. These wines are rich in compounds that help lower cholesterol and prevent harmful low-density lipoprotein (LDL) cholesterol from sticking to the lining of artery walls—the process that leads to heart disease. Red wines also help keep blood platelets from sticking together and forming dangerous clots.

Dual-Action Heart Protection

The ways in which red wine keeps your pump primed are complex. There is more than one chemical compound at work, and some of these compounds have more than one benefit, say researchers.

For starters, the alcohol in red wine may be beneficial. For example, people who drink small amounts of alcohol seem to have increased protection from heart disease, studies show.

The reason, say researchers, is that ethanol, or alcohol, in spirited drinks raises levels of good, heart-protecting high-density lipoprotein (HDL) cholesterol.

But if raising HDL cholesterol were the only benefit, drinking red wine wouldn't be any more effective than, say, quaffing a shot of scotch or a mug of beer. And while beer and other alcoholic drinks have some benefits, wine's the only one with health-promoting polyphenols.

The reason wine seems to offer superior protection is that it contains powerful flavonoids such as quercetin. Along with other potentially protective compounds like resveratrol, it apparently helps prevent the body's dangerous LDL cholesterol from oxidizing. This, in turn, makes bad LDL cholesterol less likely to stick to artery walls.

In lab studies, resveratrol has been shown to slow aging in mice, protect against weight gain, and boost endurance. How? Resveratrol seems to improve the functioning of mitochondria—tiny power plants inside every cell in your body.

"Flavonoids in red wine are more powerful than vitamin E, which everyone knows is an important antioxidant," says John D. Folts, PhD, professor of medicine and director of the coronary thrombosis laboratory at the University of Wisconsin Medical School in Madison.

Keeping LDL cholesterol in check is a good start against heart disease, but that's not all the quercetin in wine does, says Dr. Folts. It also helps prevent platelets in blood from sticking together. Indeed, a study led by Dr. Folts and his colleagues found that when red wine was given to laboratory animals, it eliminated potentially dangerous clots, which can cause heart attacks and stroke.

"Red wine performs double duty, giving you two major benefits in one place," says Dr. Folts.

Color Counts

When researchers talk about the healing benefits of wine, they're usually referring to red wine. When it comes to heart health, researchers say, light wines pale in comparison to their robust red brethren.

In a laboratory study at the University of California, Davis, for example, researchers found that red wines could prevent anywhere from 46 to 100 percent of LDL cholesterol from oxidizing, while white wines were not as protective. Similarly, laboratory studies suggest that white wine lacks the clot-blocking ability of red, says Dr. Folts.

THE BENEFITS WITHOUT THE BOOZE

For every connoisseur of fine bouquets and vintages, there's someone who would just as soon skip the sherry and sip something sans alcohol.

If nonalcoholic wine is your toast of choice, you're in luck. Except for the alcohol, which is extracted during processing, these beverages contain the same active ingredients as "real" wines, including quercetin and resveratrol, two compounds that show healing potential.

When drinking for health, experts say, pick nonalcoholic wines the same way you do their spirited counterparts, by the darkness of their hue. Many of the protective compounds are also the ones that give the beverage its crimson color.

Why is red wine so much superior to its paler counterpart? It's all in the making, say experts.

When vintners make wine, they throw everything in the vat—not just grapes but also the skins, seeds, and stems. They're all mashed up to create a chunky mixture called must, which is where the healthy flavonoids reside.

"The longer the must ferments in the alcohol, the more of these compounds release into the wine, says Dr. Folts. With white wine, the must is taken out early so that the wine never darkens. With red wine, the must is kept in a long time, and the wine picks up a lot of flavonoids."

UC Davis researchers have found that some red wines are also rich in saponins, which lower heart disease risk by binding to cholesterol and preventing their absorption. Saponins may also cool bodywide inflammation, which could also lower heart disease and cancer risk.

Researcher Andrew Waterhouse, PhD, professor of enology (wine chemistry) at UC Davis found that red wines contain 3 to 10 times more saponins than whites. The richest source was red Zinfandel, followed by Syrah, Pinot Noir, and Cabernet Sauvignon. The two white varieties in the study, Sauvignon Blanc and Chardonnay, contained less.

The saponins may come from the waxy grape skins and seem to dissolve into the wine during fermentation. Wines with the highest alcohol content also had the most saponins.

In moderation, wine may help you maintain a healthy weight. When researchers at the Mayo Clinic tracked drinking behavior and weight in 8,200 women and men, they found that those who enjoyed one to two alcoholic beverages a day were 54 percent less likely to be obese than teetotalers. Nondrinkers and ex-drinkers were twice as likely to be obese. "People who have a glass of wine or beer each day often have it with the evening meal, and it could be that a drink replaces a later, high-calorie evening snack," speculates study coauthor Jim Rohrer, PhD.

But more didn't translate into extra-slim physiques: Those who swallowed four or more drinks per day were about 50 percent more likely to be obese than non-drinkers.

Wine against Infection

When you were a kid, you probably ran into your share of bacteria that resulted in nasty bouts of the runs. At the same time, you probably spent a lot of time running away from your mother as she chased you with drippy pink spoonfuls of bismuth subsalicylate, better known as Pepto-Bismol.

Even today, experts advise taking a shot of the pink stuff while traveling to help prevent bacterial infections that can cause traveler's diarrhea. If only it didn't taste so bad! Wouldn't it be nice if you could exchange that chalky, neon liquid for something a bit more palatable—like a nice glass of Chardonnay?

You might be able to, say scientists from Tripler Army Medical Center in Honolulu. Intrigued by the use of wine as a digestive aid throughout history, the researchers tested red wine, white wine, and bismuth subsalicylate against some of the meanest intestinal germs, including shigella, salmonella, and *Escherichia coli*. They found that both red and white wine were more effective than the drug for wiping out harmful bacteria.

FOOD ALERT
The Grapes of Wrath

Everyone knows that having a glass too many of red wine can leave you wishing your head were attached to someone else's body.

But for some people with a tendency toward migraine headaches, even a little wine can cause a lot of headache. Red wine contains substances called amines, which cause blood vessels in the brain to constrict and then expand. In sensitive people, this can result in eye-popping headaches.

Although white wine contains fewer headache-producing amines than the red varieties, it doesn't contain as many healing compounds either. So if headaches are a problem for you, you may want to ask your doctor if a nonalcoholic wine will allow you to enjoy the great tastes without the pain.

More research is needed, but it appears likely that sipping a little wine with your vacation meals could help bolster your intestinal health so that you aren't slowed down by a case of the runs.

GETTING THE MOST

Know when to say when. The most important tip for getting the maximum health benefits from your wine cellar is knowing when to put your glass down, say the experts. The daily limit is one 5-ounce glass a day for women and two 5-ounce glasses a day for men. Experts agree, however, that if you're at risk for over-indulging—or if you have a personal or family history of alcoholism—you're better off skipping alcohol entirely.

Go for the gusto. When you're scanning the shelves for the wine with the highest levels of heart-healthy compounds, go for the full-bodied, robust varieties, advises Dr. Waterhouse.

"There is a close relationship between the level of tannin, the substance that makes wine dry, and the level of healing compounds in red wines," says Dr. Waterhouse. Three of the most heart-healthy wines are Cabernet Sauvignon, Petite Sirah, and Merlot.

Doctor's Top Tip

Nibble a wine drinker's favorite foods. When researchers from Denmark's National Institute of Public Health analyzed 3.5 million sales at 98 Danish supermarkets, they discovered another reason why wine drinkers are healthier: The Danish wine drinkers bought more healthy foods such as olives, fruits, vegetables, poultry, veal, beef, milk, and low-fat cheese. In contrast, beer drinkers bought more prepared foods, cold cuts, sausages, pork, lamb, chips, sugar, butter, margarine, and soft drinks, says Morten Groenbaek, MD, PhD, deputy director of research at the institute.

Wound Healing
REPAIRING THE DAMAGE

No one makes it through the bumper-car ride of life without getting cuts and scrapes along the way. In fact, doctors estimate that Americans get more than 12 million cuts and other wounds every year.

If you happen to be among the walking wounded, you can count yourself fortunate that the skin is usually able to heal itself in deft displays of regeneration. But for healing to occur, you have to eat the right foods. Nutrients such as protein, vitamin C, and zinc are the building blocks for new skin. If you don't get enough of them in your diet, it takes longer for wounds to heal, says Judith Petry, MD, medical director of the Vermont Healing Tools Project in Brattleboro.

A Strong Foundation

Protein is essential for healing cuts and wounds, but it isn't always available where you need it most. Only about 10 percent of the body's protein is found in the skin, while the rest is used elsewhere in the body.

"Protein gets used for energy before it goes to healing," says Michele Gottschlich, PhD, RD, director of nutrition services for the Shriners Burns Institute in Cincinnati.

When your body goes into healing mode, the need for protein can double. Suppose, for example, that you normally get 50 grams of protein a day. After burning yourself, you may need to increase that amount to 100 grams in order to heal properly, Dr. Gottschlich says. This means increasing your daily intake of protein-rich foods to 8 to 10 servings instead of the usual 4 to 6 servings that nutritionists recommend for general well-being. The amount of protein your body needs for healing depends largely on the severity of the wound. If you're recovering from massive burns, for example, you may want to increase your protein intake by stirring nonfat dry milk into milk, cereal, soups, and gravies, having desserts made with eggs, such as pudding or custard, and adding shredded cheese to vegetable dishes.

Meats are among the best sources of protein. A 3-ounce serving of flank steak, for example, has 23 grams of protein, or about 46 percent of the Daily Value (DV). If you don't want to eat meat, you can also get protein from fish, beans, nuts, and grains.

"Tofu is also an impressive source of protein," adds Dr. Gottschlich. A 4-ounce serving has more than 9 grams, about the same amount you'd get from 1¼ ounces of ground beef.

Seize the Vitamin C

Orange juice is a favorite home remedy for colds because the vitamin C it contains helps strengthen immunity. What works for sniffles will work for wounds as well. If you aren't getting enough vitamin C in your diet, your susceptibility to infection quickly increases.

In addition, vitamin C is essential for strengthening collagen, the tissue that holds skin cells together. When you don't get enough vitamin C in your diet, collagen gets weaker, and wounds heal more slowly. "Tissue integrity, the actual strength of the skin, relies on vitamin C," says Vincent Falanga, MD, professor of dermatology at Boston University School of Medicine.

In a study at the Burn Center of Cook County Hospital in Chicago, researchers found that laboratory animals that got extra vitamin C in their diets had better blood circulation and less wound swelling than those getting less.

Whether you have a cut, a burn, or any other kind of wound, it's a good idea to get at least 500 milligrams of vitamin C a day, or about eight times the DV of 60 milligrams, says Dr. Falanga. In fact, it doesn't hurt to get even more—up to 1,000 milligrams a day, he says. This is particularly true for older folks and those who smoke, since these people are often low in vitamin C.

It's easy to get a lot of vitamin C from foods. Good sources include orange juice, strawberries, broccoli, cantaloupe, tomatoes, bell peppers, and potatoes. A half-cup serving of red bell peppers, for example, has 95 milligrams of vitamin C, or 158 percent of the DV, while an orange has nearly 70 milligrams, or 116 percent of the DV. For a superb vitamin C kick, grab a guava. One guava contains 165 milligrams of vitamin C, or 275 percent of the DV.

Think Zinc

Many Americans don't get enough zinc, a mineral that helps tissues grow and repair themselves. In fact, slow wound healing is often a telltale sign that you're not getting enough of this important mineral.

The DV for zinc is 15 milligrams. This doesn't sound like a lot, but getting enough zinc can be tricky, since only about 20 percent of the zinc in foods is absorbed during digestion, says Ananda Prasad, MD, PhD, professor of medicine at Wayne State University School of Medicine in Detroit. However, eating zinc-rich foods along with protein from animal foods will help the absorption of zinc, he says.

Doctor's Top Tip

Heal faster with a broccoli and beef stir-fry. "Protein helps speed burn healing by rebuilding collagen, a building block of skin tissue," notes Michele Gottschlich, PhD, RD, director of nutrition services for the Shriners Burns Institute in Cincinnati. Vitamin C (found in good amounts in broccoli) also helps rebuild collagen, she says.

An excellent source of zinc is oysters, with ½ cup providing 8 milligrams, or 54 percent of the DV. Wheat germ is also good, with 1⅔ tablespoons containing about 2 milligrams, or 13 percent of the DV.

Call in the Skin Helpers

Sip more H_2O. Water keeps skin hydrated, important while helping to heal burns, Dr. Gottschlich notes. Sip eight 8-ounce glasses a day.

Focus on omega-3 fatty acids. Fats help your body build new cells—and they become part of every cell membrane. Go for oily fish, walnuts, and flaxseed.

Get a full range of vitamins and minerals. If your diet's not always up to par (and nobody's is perfect!), consider taking a multivitamin as an insurance policy against a shortfall of important vitamins and minerals, Dr. Gottschlich suggests. These include B vitamins, which help your body use energy from carbohydrates to rebuild tissue; vitamin K, which helps blood clot; and vitamin A, which helps collagen form supportive nets and skin cells reproduce.

Yeast Infections

HEALING CULTURES

For a long time, women have been telling each other how effective yogurt is for clearing up yeast infections. Doctors have always been skeptical, but that's about to change. In a small study at Long Island Jewish Medical Center in New York, women who got frequent yeast infections were given 1 cup of yogurt every day for 6 months. At the end of the study, researchers found that the rate of yeast infections had dropped by 75 percent.

The yogurt used in the study contained live cultures of bacteria called *Lactobacillus acidophilus,* which are "friendly" bacteria that help control the growth of yeast in the intestines and vagina, explains Paul Reilly, ND, a naturopathic doctor and adjunct instructor at Bastyr University in Seattle. Eating yogurt helps restore the vagina's natural environment, so yeast infections are much less likely to recur.

For most women, the amount of yogurt used in the study—1 cup a day—is plenty, Dr. Reilly adds. The one challenge may be finding yogurt that contains *L. acidophilus* bacteria, since most national yogurt brands contain other types of organisms. In fact, even when you do find a supermarket yogurt that contains *L. acidophilus,* the concentration may be too low for it to be effective. Your best bet, says Dr. Reilly, is to buy the yogurt at health food stores, which usually have a good selection to choose from.

Nature's Penicillin

Through the ages, garlic has been used for disinfecting wounds, stopping dysentery, and even treating tuberculosis. Here's another feather in its cap. Research suggests that garlic can help cure yeast infections as well as prevent them from coming back.

Garlic contains dozens of chemical compounds, among them ajoene, allicin-alliin, and diallyl sulphide, which have proven power against fungal infections. In a laboratory study at Loma Linda University in California, animals with yeast infections were given either a placebo (inactive) saline solution or a solution made with aged garlic extract. Two days later, animals in the saline group were still infected. Those in the garlic group, however, were completely free of the fungus.

Garlic has been shown to kill the yeast fungus on contact. In addition, garlic appears to stimulate the activity of neutrophils and macrophages, immune system cells that battle infection.

Doctor's Top Tip

If you're fighting boomerang yeast infections, choose plain or artificially sweetened yogurt. In a surprising study, researcher Betsy Foxman, PhD, of the University of Michigan's School of Public Health, found that women who ate acidophilus-rich products had a higher risk for another yeast infection. She suspects that the sugars in sweetened yogurt may provide food for the yeast you're trying to discourage—and may overpower the "good" yeast-fighting acidophilus bacteria.

Even though the animals in the study were given aged garlic extract, fresh garlic is also effective, says Dr. Reilly. For treating and preventing yeast infections, he recommends eating several cloves to a bulb of garlic a day. You don't have to eat it raw to get the benefits, he adds. Garlic retains some of its strength when it's baked, microwaved, or sautéed. To be most effective, however, the cloves should be crushed or chopped, since this releases more of the active compounds.

Boosting Your Defenses

The research is still preliminary, but evidence suggests that eating more foods containing beta-carotene and vitamins C and E can help prevent yeast infections. Researchers at Albert Einstein College of Medicine in the Bronx found that women with yeast infections had significantly less beta-carotene in their vaginal cells than women without the infections. The researchers speculate that women with higher levels of beta-carotene may be more resistant to the fungus. And according to Dr. Reilly: "Vitamins C and E stimulate the immune system to activate specialized cells, which are a primary defense against things like yeast," he says.

You can get plenty of beta-carotene and vitamin C simply by eating a variety of fruits and vegetables. Vitamin E, however, is found mainly in vegetable oils. To get more vitamin E in your diet without all the fat, Dr. Reilly recommends having several servings a day of nuts and seeds. An even better source is wheat germ.

A Sweet Problem

For women who frequently get yeast infections, sugary foods can be a real problem because yeast, it appears, likes sweets just as much as we do, Dr. Reilly says.

Research has shown that women who eat a lot of honey, sugar, or molasses get more yeast infections than women who eat less. It makes sense because eating sugar raises the amount of sugar in the bloodstream, which provides a perfect medium for yeast to thrive. For some women, even the natural sugars in fruit and milk can be a problem, says Carolyn DeMarco, MD, a physician in Toronto and author of *Take Charge of Your Body: Women's Health Advisor.* "I tell women who are susceptible to yeast infections to think about cutting back on their intake of fruits and to avoid fruit juices completely," Dr. DeMarco says.

Yogurt

THE BENEFITS OF BACTERIA

HEALING POWER

Can Help:

Prevent yeast infections

Boost immunity

Heal and prevent ulcers

If someone suggested that you swallow a spoonful of live bugs, you wouldn't do it on a bet. But what if they told you that every spoonful would provide dramatic improvements in your health?

Millions of Americans willingly eat millions of live organisms every day when they open containers of yogurt. Yogurt is positively brimming with bacteria—the live and active cultures that you read about on the label. Research has shown that these "friendly" bacteria can strengthen the immune system and help ulcers heal more quickly. Scientists have also found it may promote a longer life: A 5-year-long study of 162 elderly people found that those who ate yogurt and drank milk four or more times a week were 38 percent less likely to die during the study period.

And all that good bacteria may keep us more comfortable, day in, day out, as well. The bacteria also may help prevent recurrent yeast infections, says Eileen Hilton, MD, an infectious disease specialist and president of the Biomedical Research Alliance of New York. And even if you took the bacteria out of yogurt, it would still be a super source of calcium—better, in fact, than a serving of low-fat milk.

Stopping the Yeast Beast

If you've ever had a yeast infection, you know that you never want to get another one. Eating more yogurt, Dr. Hilton says, may help prevent them from occurring (provided it's sugar-free or plain!).

Yeast infections occur when a fungus that normally lives in the vagina suddenly multiplies, causing itching, burning, and other uncomfortable symptoms. A study at Long Island Jewish Medical Center suggests that eating live-culture yogurt, especially yogurt containing bacteria called *Lactobacillus acidophilus*, may help keep the fungus under control.

In the study, women who frequently had yeast infections were asked to eat 8 ounces of yogurt a day for 6 months. At the end of the study, the rate of yeast infections had dropped significantly. The women were so satisfied, in fact, that when researchers asked them to stop eating yogurt, many of them refused to give it up.

The Long Island researchers speculate that eating yogurt helps keep the vagina's natural bacterial environment in balance, making it harder for the yeast fungus to thrive. Additional studies need to be done, Dr. Hilton adds, but in the meantime, women who are trying to prevent yeast infections may want to try eating 1 cup of yogurt a day—the same amount that was used in the study.

It's important, however, to eat yogurt that contains live cultures, Dr. Hilton adds. Yogurt that has been heat-treated doesn't contain bacteria and probably won't be effective. Read the label to find out if your brand has been heat-treated.

Help for Immunity

You probably remember the television commercials for yogurt that featured hearty, 100-year-old Russians hiking up rocky peaks with energy to spare. The ads were an exaggeration, of course, but yogurt's healthful reputation is not.

The same bacteria in yogurt that help prevent yeast infections can also strengthen the immune system. In one study, for example, researchers at the University of California, Davis, found that people who ate 2 cups of yogurt a day for 4 months had about four times more gamma interferon, a protein that helps the immune system's white blood cells fight disease, than people who did not eat yogurt. "Gamma interferon is the best mechanism the body has to defend itself against viruses," says Georges Halpern, MD, PhD, professor emeritus in the department of internal medicine at the University of California, who was author of the study.

In a more recent study of 33 women in their twenties who ate yogurt every day for 4 weeks, the number of infection-fighting T lymphocytes in their blood increased 30 percent, report researchers from the University of Vienna, Austria. Their immune cells were also able to fight infection with more force—a benefit that persisted for 2 weeks after the women stopped eating the yogurt.

There's more evidence that yogurt may work against bacterial infections. In a laboratory study conducted by researchers at the Netherlands Institute for Dairy Research, animals given yogurt had much lower levels of salmonella bacteria, a common cause of food poisoning, than animals given milk. What's more, the bacteria that did survive had little impact on the animals given yogurt, while those given milk got much sicker.

It's not entirely clear why yogurt helped protect the animals from disease. Apart from its immunity-boosting effects, researchers speculate that yogurt's high calcium content may create an unfavorable environment in which the bacteria can't thrive.

Ulcer Relief

Since most ulcers are caused by bacteria, the usual treatment is to give large doses of antibiotics. But there's good evidence that eating plenty of live-culture yogurt can keep ulcer-causing bacteria under control.

When you eat yogurt, the beneficial bacteria take up residence inside the digestive tract. Once in place, they begin competing with the harmful bacteria that cause ulcers. This makes it more difficult for the ulcer-causing germs to thrive.

In addition, yogurt contains a natural sugar called lactose, which breaks down into lactic acid during digestion. The lactic acid helps restore a healthful environment in the intestine.

Even if you already have an ulcer and are taking medication, eating yogurt will make the treatment more effective. The organisms that are in many yogurts tend to act like antibiotics in the stomach, lactobacillus experts suspect.

If you have an ulcer, try eating between 1 and 4 cups of yogurt a day, recommends Isadore Rosenfeld, MD, clinical professor of medicine at New York Hospital–Cornell Medical Center in New York City and author of *Doctor, What Should I Eat?* Just be sure to buy yogurt that says "live and active cultures" on the label.

> ### Doctor's Top Tip
>
> Treat the kids to (low-fat) yogurt. Researchers at the University of Tennessee who tracked the weight and eating habits of 52 children for 8 years found that those who ate the most calcium-rich foods had the healthiest body weights. Getting just two dairy servings a day could cut a kid's risk for being overweight by up to 70 percent, says lead study author Jean Skinner, PhD, a researcher in the university's nutrition department.

Smart for Your Heart

In a study of the eating habits and health of 5,996 women and men by researchers at Rush University Medical Center in Chicago, levels of homocysteine—a compound in the blood that's been linked with heart attacks—were 6.4 times lower for people who ate yogurt more than 15 times a month than for people who avoided yogurt.

Yogurt packed with live cultures may also rebalance your cholesterol. A small study of 17 women from the University of Austria in Vienna found that eating 36 ounces of yogurt a day for 4 weeks raised good high-density lipoprotein (HDL) cholesterol significantly while lowering bad low-density lipoprotein (LDL) cholesterol at the same time.

Calcium without Pain

Even though the large amounts of calcium in low-fat milk make it one of the most healthful foods you can find, many people simply can't drink a lot of it. In fact, doctors estimate that more than 30 million Americans don't have enough of the enzyme (lactase) needed to digest the sugar (lactose) in milk.

Yogurt, however, is an easy-to-digest alternative. Even though yogurt does contain lactose, the live bacteria help the body break it down, so it's less likely to cause discomfort, says Barbara Dixon, RD, a nutritionist in Baton Rouge, Louisiana, and author of *Good Health for African Americans*. And when it comes to calcium, yogurt is a super source, with 1 cup of plain low-fat yogurt providing 414 milligrams, or more than 40 percent of the Daily Value (DV). Compare that with low-fat milk, with just 300 milligrams per serving.

As it turns out, yogurt contains a special protein called lactoferrin that helps the body build and maintain bone. It promotes the growth of cells inside bone called osteoblasts and also keeps them alive 50 to 70 percent longer, studies suggest.

GETTING THE MOST

Eat it soon. When buying yogurt, check the "sell by" date, and select the latest dated one you can find. Store the yogurt unopened in the refrigerator. Yogurt with live cultures should keep for about 10 days past the "sell by" date.

Eat it cold. Since the bacteria in yogurt can't withstand high heat, it's best to eat your yogurt cold. When you do use yogurt for cooking—when making a sauce, for example—add it when the dish is finished cooking and has been removed from the heat.

Herbed Yogurt Cheese Dip

2 cups fat-free plain yogurt

2 ounces reduced-fat cream cheese

1½ tablespoons minced fresh chives

1 tablespoon minced fresh basil

¼ teaspoon coarsely ground black pepper

Line a strainer with 2 layers of cheesecloth, and set it over a large bowl. Spoon the yogurt into the strainer. Cover, and refrigerate for at least 12 hours, or until the yogurt is the consistency of cream cheese. You should have about 1 cup of yogurt cheese and 1 cup of drained liquid. (Discard the liquid or use as directed in the Cook's Notes.)

Place the yogurt cheese, cream cheese, chives, basil, and pepper in a food processor. Process until well blended. Spoon into a small bowl. Cover, and refrigerate for at least 1 hour to allow the flavors to blend.

Makes 1 cup

Cook's Notes: *Use yogurt that does not contain gums as thickeners; they will prevent it from draining.*

The liquid drained from the yogurt (called whey) can be used in place of milk in pancake, muffin, and quick-bread batters.

Serve the dip with raw vegetables, or use it as a spread on low-fat crackers.

PER 2 TABLESPOONS ———————————

Calories: 42	Cholesterol: 6 mg
Total fat: 1.6 g	Sodium: 54 mg
Saturated fat: 1 g	Dietary fiber: 0 g

Yucca

THE BLOOD BUILDER

HEALING POWER

Can Help:

Prevent heart disease

Reduce the risk of cancer

Prevent cataracts

Keep skin smooth

Everyone knows about tapioca, but you may not have heard of manioc, cassava, or yucca. Don't let the strange names confuse you. They're all the same food, although the name is different in different parts of the world.

In the United States, what we call yucca is a long, brown, tropical vegetable (a tuber, actually) with rough skin. It's not much in the looks department, but inside is a mild, crisp, white flesh that resembles a potato's. The tapioca we make into pudding is made from dried, ground yucca. Yucca can also be boiled and mashed just like a potato.

Yucca is the world's number two vegetable crop, after potatoes. It's prepared and enjoyed dozens of different ways: boiled, fried, or fermented into a soup called *foufou* in Africa; used as a roasted flour called *farinha de mandioca* in parts of Brazil; baked then sliced into crunchy chips in India; and made into noodles and pastries in Thailand. This starchy vegetable has been sustaining humankind for thousands of years; recently, archeologists found evidence of manioc on stone tools at a 4,500-year-old settlement in coastal Ecuador.

In the United States, yucca is still little-known outside ethnic supermarkets. But it's starting to attract a following. For one thing, this tuber is as tough as nails—it's uniquely full of iron, plus the vitamin C that helps your body absorb it. It's also a very good source of magnesium, which is needed to protect your bones, heart, arteries, and blood pressure.

Help for Iron Maidens

Iron is an essential mineral that helps your cells get enough oxygen. Men rarely have a problem getting enough iron in their diets. But women of childbearing age lose a lot of iron due to menstruation. In fact, 20 percent of women in this country (as well as 50 percent of pregnant women and 3 percent of men) may have low iron stores, says Sally S. Harris, MD, a clinical faculty member at Stanford Medical School. Low iron levels make you feel run-down. Over time, it can lead to iron-deficiency anemia.

In the Kitchen

With its unfamiliar looks, yucca can be a daunting presence when you're cooking it for the first time. Don't be intimidated; it's no more complicated than cooking a potato.

- To peel yucca, first cut it into 2- or 3-inch sections. Using a paring knife, slit the skin (both the upper and lower layer), then work the blade underneath to loosen it. Grab the loose skin with your fingers, and peel it off.
- Slice each piece in half lengthwise, and remove the tough fiber that runs down the middle.

- Put the pieces in a deep pot and cover with cold water. Bring the water to a boil, then reduce the heat to maintain a steady simmer.
- After 20 minutes, test for doneness using a thin, sharp knife. When it penetrates the flesh easily, the piece is done. (Not all pieces will cook at the same rate, so you may want to check them individually.)
- Drain and serve as you would potatoes: in pieces, mashed, or with your favorite toppings.

Although iron is easy to get from meat, most of us are trying to eat less meat these days. There's simply not a lot of iron in vegetables, and the type of iron they do contain (called nonheme iron) isn't readily absorbed by the body unless it's also accompanied by vitamin C.

Yucca, however, is a veritable iron mine. A half-cup of cooked yucca contains more than 2 milligrams of iron, or 13 percent of the Recommended Dietary Allowance (RDA) for women and 20 percent of the RDA for men. And because it also contains large amounts of vitamin C—almost 21 milligrams, or 35 percent of the Daily Value (DV)—the iron is much easier to absorb.

Natural Cholesterol Control

When researchers from the government-affiliated Food and Nutrition Research Unit in the Philippines tested the cholesterol-lowering potential of five popular Philippine root vegetables—sweet potato, cassava, taro, purple yam, and spiny yam—and six different types of legumes—kidney bean, peanut, mung bean, green pea, chickpea, and pigeon pea—in 20 people with high cholesterol, cassava (yucca) was the clear winner. "Among the root crops," the researchers reported, "only cassava showed a significant decrease in LDL-cholesterol [low-density lipoprotein] levels." Levels fell an average of 15 points for people who ate cassava daily for 2 weeks.

Doctor's Top Tip

If you'd like to try cooking with raw yucca, ask if it's a sweet variety—this type can be peeled and then baked, boiled, fried, or roasted, say experts at the University of Florida–based Florida Extension Service. While other varieties of yucca must be processed first to remove a poisonous substance called cyanogenic glucoside, sweet varieties are safe.

Additional Benefits

The vitamin C in yucca does more than help contribute to your iron stores. It's also a powerhouse vitamin that has been shown to help prevent heart disease, cancer, and age-related conditions such as cataracts. Vitamin C plays a role in forming collagen, the fibrous protein that keeps skin supple. It has also been shown to reduce the duration and severity of colds and other viral infections.

Yucca appears to have additional healing powers apart from its vitamin content. In parts of the Amazon, yucca is made into a poultice and used to relieve chills and fever. It has also been used in the Amazon to soothe sore muscles, and when mixed in a bath, to treat sterility in women.

Index

Underscored references indicate boxed text.

A

Acerola
  health benefits of, 1–2
  preparing and eating, 2, 2
Acesulfame potassium, 48
Acetaminophen, 598
Acetyl-L-carnitine, 10
Acid reflux, insomnia and, 358
Advanced glycation endproducts
    (AGEs), 7, 8
Aging
  advanced glycation endproducts
    and, 7, 8
  longevity, 3, 6–8
  nutritional deficiencies in, 5–6
  positively affected by
    antioxidants, 3–5
    calorie restriction, 6–8
    green tea, 263
    nutrient-dense foods, 6
Alaria, 567
Alcohol. *See also* Beer; Wine, red
  and heart health, 108, 328–29
  may cause
    birth defects, 100
    deficiency diseases, 209
    dehydration, 654
    gout, 298
    hemorrhoids, 330
    infertility, 353
    insomnia, 358
    memory problems, 419
    ulcers, 642
    urinary tract infections, 644
  moderation in, 329
  positively affects
    diabetes, 219
  wine vs. beer drinkers, 667
Allergies, airborne. *See* Hay fever
Allergies, food
  about, 268–69
  breastfeeding and, 269

  common, 195, 268, 630
  eating in restaurants and,
    270–71
  food labels and, 270
  may cause
    earaches, 269
    rheumatoid arthritis, 40–41
  positively affected by
    green tea, 622
    probiotics, 270
Almonds
  for
    cholesterol, 179, 182
    heart health, 446
  Glazed Tangerines with Almonds,
    617
  Spiced Almond Cereal Snack Mix,
    448
Alpha-carotene, 144, 364
Alpha-linolenic acid, 391, 404
Alpha-tocopherol. *See* Vitamin E
Aluminum, 11
Alzheimer's disease
  aluminum and, 11
  free radicals and, 278
  incidence of, 9
  positively affected by
    acetyl-L-carnitine, 10
    antioxidants, 9, 18, 365–66
    B-complex vitamins, 9–10
    curcumin, 511
    currants, 203
    folate, 58
    fruits and vegetables, 418
    Mediterranean diet, 10–11
    vitamin C, 366
    vitamin E, 366
Anaphylaxis, 269
Anchovies, 258
Anemia
  foods to prevent, 13, 394–96
  headaches and, 320
  incidence of, 13

  iron for, 13, 14, 15
  pernicious, 16, 397, 648
  signs of, 13
Anorexia, pellagra and, 209
Antioxidants
  for
    Alzheimer's disease, 9, 365–66
    asthma, 62–63
    heart health, 327–28
    LDL cholesterol, 365
    memory problems, 418
  aging and, 3–5, 18
  foods high in
    artichokes, 43–44
    basil, 77
    beans, 84
    beets, 89
    blueberries, 606
    broccoli, 280, 606
    Brussels sprouts, 606
    carrots, 280, 606
    cherries, 606
    gogi berries, 278
    grapes, 606
    guavas, 636–37
    kale, 606
    leafy vegetables, 280
    olive oil, 461
    onions, 606
    oranges, 606
    peppers, 280
    plums, 606
    pomegranates, 637
    red wine, 133
    spinach, 280
    sweet potatoes, 280
    tangerines, 615
    tomatoes, 629–31
    wheat germ, 280
  free radicals and, 18–19
  smoking and, 575–77
  supplements, 273–74, 275
Appendicitis, 25–26

Curcumin *(cont.)*
  being studied for
    Alzheimer's disease, 511
    arthritis, 511
Currants
  Apple-Currant Chutney, 206
  health benefits of, 203–5
  preparing and using, 204,
    205
Cyclamate, 49

D

Daily Values (DVs), 272–73
Dairy. *See also* Milk; Yogurt
  for
    Alzheimer's disease prevention,
      419
    blood pressure, 603–4
    dental health, 211–12
    diabetes prevention, 221
    gout, 298
    osteoporosis, 473–76, 626
  may cause
    constipation, 193
    diarrhea, 225
    gas, 289
    infertility, 353
    irritable bowel syndrome,
      360
Dandelion greens, 311, 348
DASH diet, 70, 104, 106–7
Decongestants
  black tea, 189
  chicken soup, 167–69, 189
  chile peppers, 172–73, 189
Dental health
  foods for
    black tea, 213
    cheese, 213
    dairy, 211
    garlic, 286
    raisins, 212, 555
    tea, 621
  nutrition for, 211–12
  sweet foods and, 212–13
Depression
  possible causes of
    excessive caffeine, 216,
      235
    sugar, 216, 235
    premenstrual, 535

preventing, with
  carbohydrates, 215
  fish, 214–15
  shellfish, 573
Desserts
  Apple Crumble with Toasted-Oat
    Topping, 33
  Chocolate Mint Pudding Cake,
    390
  Double-Berry Sundaes, 97
  Double-Ginger Gingerbread, 295
  Figs Stuffed with Orange Anise
    Cream, 253
  Flax Banana Bread, 267
  Frozen Chocolate-Banana Pops, 72
  Mocha Tofu Pudding, 584
  Oatmeal-Apricot Cookies, 454
  Pineapple with Almond Cream
    Topping, 516
  Pumpkin Maple Pudding, 547
  Raisin Coffeecake Ring, 556
  Strawberry Tart with Oat-
    Cinnamon Crust, 98
DHA, 273
Diabetes
  adversely affected by
    juice fasting, 367
    saturated fats, 382
  artificial sweeteners and, 49
  belly fat and, 379
  chromium and, 222–23
  controlling, with
    avocados, 65–66
    beans, 82–83
    buckwheat, 120–21
    bulgur, 124
    carbohydrates, 218–19, 223, 223
    fiber, 219–20
    oranges, 471
    sweet potatoes, 613
  diet for, 217, 605
  glycemic index and, 218–19
  high triglycerides and, 65
  magnesium for, 223
  pregnancy and, 101
  preventing, with
    beer, 219
    brown rice, 562
    coffee, 183
    dairy, 221
    fiber, 562
    pectin, 498
    potatoes, 524–25

whole grains, 660
    wine, 219
  stroke and, 605
  vitamins for, 208, 220–22
Diarrhea
  causes of, 224–27
  fluids at first sign of, 224
  preventing, with
    squash, 594
    wine, 666–67
  tips for travelers, 226
  treating, with
    apples, 224
    bland foods, 224
    honey, 342–43
    wine, 225
Diets
  Asian diet, 51–55
  gluten-free, 156–58
  low-carb, 377–80
  low-fat, 382–88
  Mediterranean diet, 403–7
  vegan, 40–41, 568, 648
  vegetarian, 645–48
Digestion. *See also* Constipation; Gas
  positively affected by
    basil, 78
    bulgur, 125
    currants, 205
    fiber, 74, 125
    papayas, 636
    pineapple, 514–15
    plantains, 518–19
    raisins, 553
Dips
  Herbed Yogurt Cheese Dip, 677
Diseases, deficiency, 207–10
Diverticulitis, 228, 230
Diverticulosis
  causes of, 229–30
  incidence of, 228
  popcorn and seeds and, 229
  preventing, with
    apples, 31
    fiber, 31, 229–30
    fruits and vegetables, 229, 230
    whole grains, 660
Docosahexaenoic acid (DHA), 273
Dopamine, 214, 231, 601
Dopar, 484
Dramamine, 292–93
D-tagatose, 227
Dulse, 565, 567

E

Earaches, food allergies and, <u>269</u>
Echinacea, for colds, 334
Edamame. *See also* Soy
  cooking tips, <u>581</u>
  Edamame and Escarole Salad, 87
Eggs, 339
Eicosapentaenoic acid (EPA), 273
Elderberries, <u>94</u>, 95
Ellagic acid, 93, 198, 204, 447, 510,
  <u>576</u>
Emphysema, 593–94
Endive, 263
Endometrial cancer, preventing with
  Brussels sprouts, 115
  flaxseed, 265–66
  squash, 593
Enova cooking oil, <u>238</u>
EPA, 273
Equal artificial sweetener, 48
Erections, vitamin E and, 21–22
Erythritol, 227
Esophageal cancer, preventing with
  onions, 465
  pumpkin, 544
  vitamin C, 375
  walnuts, 447
Estrogen. *See also* Phytoestrogens
  isoflavones and, 502
  during menopause, 421–22
Eugenol, 78
Exercise
  anemia and, 395
  as antioxidant booster, <u>279</u>
  for carpal tunnel syndrome, 142
  Gatorade and, <u>438</u>
  in Mediterranean countries, 404–5
  water during, <u>653</u>, 654
Expectorants. *See* Chile peppers
Eye health. *See also* Cataracts;
    Macular degeneration
  foods for
    apricots, 36
    asparagus, 59
    cantaloupe, 135
    carrots, 144–45
    fish, 256
    greens, 310–11
    nori, 567–68
  free radicals and, 278
  low-fat diet for, 386

vitamin A for, 36, 59–60, 567–68
vitamin C for, 148

F

Fasting
  to remove toxins, 367
  for upset stomach, 597
Fat, dietary. *See also* Foods, high-fat,
    may cause; Omega-3 fatty
    acids
  fat substitutes, 236–39
  gallstones and, 281
  in low-fat diet, 382–88
  monounsaturated
    in avocados, 65–66
    benefits of, 325
    for heart health, 388, 404
    to lower LDL, <u>181</u>
    for lupus, 393
  polyunsaturated
    benefits of, 325
    for heart health, 388
  saturated
    arthritis and, 39–40
    foods high in, 387
    health problems due to, 382
    heart disease and, 383, 387
    high cholesterol and, <u>181</u>
    lupus and, 392–93
    macular degeneration and, 386
    memory problems and, 417–18
    obesity and, 382
  trans fats
    disease and, <u>281</u>
    gallstones and, <u>281</u>
    heart disease and, 325, 387–88
    mental functioning and, 420
  triglycerides and, 236
Fatigue
  brain chemicals and, 231–32
  causes of, 234–35
  in premenopausal women, 232
  preventing, with
    fruits and vegetables, 232
    iron, 232
    small, frequent meals, 233
    vitamin C, 232
    water intake, 653
Fava beans, 483–84
Fenugreek, 587
Ferulic acid, 123, 450

Feverfew, 334
Fiber, dietary, 240–47
  for
    appendicitis, 25–26
    blood pressure, 44, 107–8, 241
    blood sugar, 44, 219–20, 471,
     487
    cancer prevention, 44, 134, 471
    cholesterol, 44, 179, 251, 471
    colon cancer prevention, 44, 134
    constipation, 190–91, 471,
     539–40
    diabetes, 219–20, 487
    diarrhea, 471
    digestion, 74
    diverticulosis, 229–30
    fibrocystic breasts, 249
    heart health, 44, 179, 251
    hypothyroidism, 625–26
    intestinal polyps, 125
    irritable bowel syndrome,
     361–62, <u>362</u>
    kidney stone prevention, 370–71
    Parkinson's disease, 483
    ulcers, 640, 641–42
  adding gradually, 191, 229–30,
    <u>246</u>, 290
  in Asian diet, 53
  foods high in
    apples, 31, 247, 328
    apricots, 36
    artichokes, 44–45
    bananas, 72
    barley, 74
    beans, 81, 83, 85, 134, 220, 247,
     328
    berries, 95, 247, 328
    broccoli, 111
    brown rice, 562–63
    Brussels sprouts, 134, 220, 247
    bulgur, 124–25
    chart, <u>244</u>–<u>45</u>
    currants, 205
    figs, 251, 328
    guavas, 637
    mangoes, 635
    melons, 412–13
    nuts, 447
    oats, 451
    okra, 134, 457
    oranges, 471
    peaches, 328
    plantains, 519

O

Pineapple *(cont.)*
  bromelain extract, 513
  culinary tips for, 514, 515
  Pineapple with Almond Cream
    Topping, 516
Pistachios, 178, 447
Pizza
  Broccoli Pesto Pizzas, 113
Plantains
  for
    blood pressure, 517–18
    heart health, 517
    immune system health, 519–20
    stroke prevention, 517
    ulcers, 518–19, 641
  allergies to, 519
  culinary tips for, 518, 520
  Plantains with Garlic and Thyme,
    521
PMS. *See* Premenstrual syndrome
Polyps, intestinal
  bulgur for, 125
  folate for, 412
  melons for, 412–13
Pomegranates
  avoiding stains from, 635
  health benefits of, 637–38
  juice of, for
    memory problems, 419
    prostate cancer, 505, 637,
      637–38
  Steak and Spinach Salad with
    Pomegranate Dressing, 313
Popcorn, diverticulosis and, 229
Pork
  as beef alternative, 400
  for herpes, 339
  recipes
    Dijon Pork Chops with
      Cabbage, 12
    Horseradish-Spiked Pork and
      Apples, 401
Potassium
  for
    blood pressure, 106, 603
    muscle cramps, 438
    stroke prevention, 603–4
  foods high in
    apricots, 106
    avocados, 67, 106
    bananas, 106, 438
    beans, 84, 106, 604
    buckwheat, 120
    figs, 252

lentils, 604
melons, 413
milk, 430, 604
plantains, 517
potatoes, 106, 438, 604
prunes, 540, 604
raisins, 552–53
shellfish, 106, 572
squash, 594
Swiss chard, 604
tomatoes, 632
yogurt, 604
Potatoes
  for
    blood pressure, 523
    cancer prevention, 511, 522
    immune system health, 669
    kidney stone prevention, 369
    muscle cramps, 438
    stress, 600
  blood sugar and, 524
  colored, 525
  culinary tips for, 525–26
  grilled foods and, 522, 525
  hay fever caution, 315
  in low-carb diet, 378
  peels of, 525
  recipes
    Barbecue Oven Fries, 526
    Creamy Potato Soup, 431
    Kelp and Potato Chowder, 569
    Spiced Potato Cakes, 590
Poultry. *See also* Chicken; Turkey
  bacteria and food safety, 530
  culinary tips for, 528
  dark meat of, 531
  for iron deficiency, 528–29
Prebiotics, 348
Pregnancy
  alcohol use during, 100
  diabetes and, 101
  fish caution, 256
  fish for, 256, 257–58
  folate for, 45, 57, 99, 410–11
Premenstrual syndrome (PMS)
  adversely affected by
    high-fat foods, 537
    linoleic acid, 538
    wheat, 536
  positively affected by
    calcium with vitamin D, 533–34
    carbohydrates, 216, 535–37
    magnesium, 432–33
    millet, 432–33

omega-3s, 537–38
parsley, 485
vitamin B$_6$, 535
symptoms of, 533
Probiotics
  for allergies, 270
  foods high in, 348
  for immune system health, 348
Prostate cancer
  lycopene and, 23, 35
  preventing, with
    beer, 133
    broccoli, 109–10
    cabbage, 128
    cauliflower, 150
    chile peppers, 172
    cranberries, 198
    greens, 309
    guavas, 636
    onions, 465
    pink grapefruit, 131
    pomegranate juice, 505, 637,
      637–38
    red wine, 133
    saponin-rich foods, 511
    tea, 54
    tomatoes, 629, 631
    vegetables, 115
    vegetarian diet, 647
    walnuts and pecans, 447
    watermelon, 131
  soy, pros and cons of, 506, 579
Protein
  for
    fatigue, 231–33
    weight loss, 480, 481
    wound healing, 668
  at breakfast, 234
  foods high in
    nuts, 447
    oats, 453
    pumpkin seeds, 545
    quinoa, 548
Prunes
  for
    constipation, 192–93, 539–40
    stress, 600
  Baked Chicken with Prunes, 541
  culinary tips for, 540–41
Psoriasis
  fish for, 542
  fruits and vegetables for, 542
  weight control and, 542
Psyllium seeds, 361

for protection against effects of
smoking, <u>576</u>
as source of lycopene, 131–32, 629
Toppings
Bing Cherry Topping, 166
Citrus Honey, 344
Garlicky Sour Cream Topping,
288
Walnut and Red Pepper Pasta
Topping, 448
Total cereal, 416
Trailblazer fat substitute, 237
Traveler's diarrhea, <u>226</u>
Triglycerides
dietary fat and, 236
HDL levels and, 182
lowering, with
avocados, 65–66
beans, 82
cinnamon, 587, <u>588</u>
corn bran, 195
fish, 182, 255
garlic, 284, 334, 509
grape juice, 305
omega-3 fatty acids, 182, 255,
326
onions, 509
peas, 494–95
rhubarb, 558
turmeric, 587
Tryptophan
foods high in, 356
insomnia and, 356
mood and, 215
Tuna
albacore, caution about, 258
Mediterranean Tuna Wrap, 260
for omega-3s, 182, 214–15
as source of niacin, 358
Turkey
for insomnia, 356
recipes
Mustard Greens with Smoked
Turkey, 314
Pear and Smoked Turkey Salad,
493
Turkey Cutlets with Oregano-
Lemon Sauce, 532
turkey sausage, <u>400</u>
Turmeric
for
cancer prevention, 510, 586
eye health, 588
heart health, 587

HIV, 587–88
prostate cancer prevention, 150
rheumatoid arthritis, 588
in cooking, <u>511</u>
Zyflamend, <u>511</u>
Turnip greens, 311, <u>503</u>
Turnips
for cancer prevention, <u>505</u>
for hyperthyroidism, 628
Tyramine, headaches and, <u>321</u>

U

Ulcers
causes of, 639, 642
preventing, with
basil, 78
chile peppers, 174
papayas, 636
plantains, 641
treating, with
cabbage, 639
fiber, 640, 641–42
honey, 342, 640–41
plantains, 518–19
yogurt, 641, 674–75
Ultraviolet light, 278
Uric acid
role in gout, 296–97
vitamin C and, 298–99
Urinary tract infections (UTIs)
preventing and treating, with
blueberry juice, 643–44
cranberry juice, 95–96,
200–201, <u>643</u>, 643–44
lingonberry juice, 643
parsley, 485
water intake, 644
Urine odor, after eating asparagus, <u>58</u>
USDA Food Guide Pyramid, 377
UTIs. *See* Urinary tract infections

V

Vegan diet
for rheumatoid arthritis, 40–41
sea vegetables in, 568
vitamin B$_{12}$ and, <u>648</u>
Vegetable dishes. *See* Side dishes
Vegetarian diet
culinary tips for, <u>646</u>
health benefits of, 645–48

pernicious anemia and, 16, 397,
648
for rheumatoid arthritis, 40–41, <u>41</u>
vitamin B$_{12}$ and, 648
Venison, 400
Vitamin A
for
dental health, 212
eye health, 36, 144–45, 519–20
immune system health, 59–60,
345
infections, 350
skin health, 59
ulcers, 640
foods high in
apricots, 36
asparagus, 59
carrots, 350
kale, 350
mustard greens, 350
nori, 567
plantains, 519
spinach, 350
squash, 350, 593–94
tangerines, 615
Vitamin B$_2$. *See* Riboflavin
Vitamin B$_6$
for
Alzheimer's disease, 10
immune system health, 345, 528
memory problems, 416–17
migraines, 319
nervous system, 528
stress, 600–601
in aging, 5
foods high in
baked potatoes, 417, 535
bananas, 10, 319, 417, 535, 600
buckwheat, 121
chicken, 535
chickpeas, 5, 10, 417, 601
figs, 252–53
plantains, 519
potatoes, 5, 10, 319, 600
poultry, 10, 417, 528
prunes, 600
sweet potatoes, 613
swordfish, 319
mood and, 601
Vitamin B$_{12}$
for
Alzheimer's disease, 10
immune system health, 345
memory problems, 416–17, 528